KU-733-561

Psychological Approaches to Rehabilitation after Traumatic Brain Injury

Psychological Approaches to Rehabilitation after Traumatic Brain Injury

Edited by Andy Tyerman and Nigel S. King

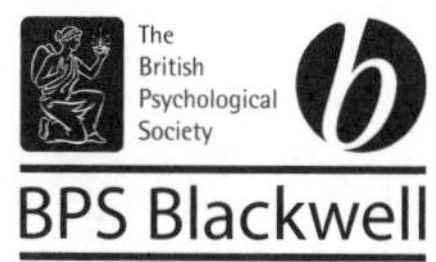

A BPS Blackwell book

BLACKWELL PUBLISHING
350 Main Street, Malden, MA 02148-5020, USA
9600 Garsington Road, Oxford OX4 2DQ, UK
550 Swanston Street, Carlton, Victoria 3053, Australia

First published 2008 by The British Psychological Society and Blackwell Publishing Ltd

1 2008

Library of Congress Cataloging-in-Publication Data

Psychological approaches to rehabilitation after traumatic brain injury / edited by Andy Tyerman and Nigel S. King.
p. ; cm.
Includes bibliographical references and index.
ISBN 978-1-4051-1167-6 (hardback : alk. paper) 1. Brain–Wounds and injuries–Patients–Rehabilitation–Great Britain. 2. Brain–Wounds and injuries–Patients–Mental health services–Great Britain. 3. Brain–Wounds and injuries–Complications–Great Britain. I. Tyerman, Andy. II. King S., Nigel, 1966- III. British Psychological Society.
[DNLM: 1. Brain Injuries–rehabilitation–Great Britain. 2. Brain Injuries–complications–Great Britain. 3. Brain Injuries–psychology–Great Britain. 4. Mental Health Services–Great Britain. WL 354 P974 2007]

RC387.5.P76 2007
617.4′810443–dc22

2007030475

A catalogue record for this title is available from the British Library.

Set in 10 on 12 pt Sabon
by SNP Best-set Typesetter Ltd., Hong Kong
Printed and bound in Singapore
by Markono Print Media Pte Ltd

The publisher's policy is to use permanent paper from mills that operate a sustainable forestry policy, and which has been manufactured from pulp processed using acid-free and elementary chlorine-free practices. Furthermore, the publisher ensures that the text paper and cover board used have met acceptable environmental accreditation standards.

For further information on
BPS Blackwell, visit our website:
www.bpsblackwell.com

Contents

List of Contributors

Mrs Sandra Barton
Clinical Nurse Specialist/Family Specialist
Community Head Injury Service
Buckinghamshire Primary Care Trust
The Camborne Centre
Jansel Square
Aylesbury
Bucks HP21 7ET

Mr David Carew
Chief Psychologist
Department of Work & Pensions
6th Floor, The Adelphi
1–11 John Adam Street
London WC2N 6HT

Mrs Katherine N. Carpenter
Consultant Clinical Neuropsychologist
Russell Cairns Unit
Level 3, West Wing
John Radcliffe Hospital
Headley Way
Headington
Oxford OX3 9DU

Rev'd Dr Joanna Collicutt McGrath
Heythrop College
University of London
Kensington Square
London W8 5HQ

Ms Sylvia Collumb
Employment Co-ordinator
Mental Health Partnership
NHS Greater Glasgow & Clyde
Dalian House
350 St Vincent Street
Glasgow G3 8YZ

Dr Audrey Daisley
Consultant Clinical Neuropsychologist
Dept of Clinical Neuropsychology
Oxford Centre for Enablement
Nuffield Orthopaedic Centre
Windmill Road
Oxford OX3 7LD

Professor Jonathan J. Evans
Professor of Applied Neuropsychology
Section of Psychological Medicine
Academic Centre
Gartnavel Royal Hospital
1055 Great Western Road
Glasgow G12 0XH

Dr Camilla Herbert
Consultant in Neuropsychology and Rehabilitation
Brain Injury Rehabilitation Trust
Kerwin Court
Five Oaks Road
Slinfold
West Sussex RH13 0TP

Dr Roger Johnson
Clinical Neuropsychologist
Coldbeck Farmhouse
Ravenstonedale
Kirkby Stephen
Cumbria CA17 4LW

Dr Nigel S. King
Consultant Clinical Neuropsychologist & Clinical Tutor
Community Head Injury Service
Buckinghamshire Primary Care Trust
The Camborne Centre
Jansel Square
Aylesbury
Bucks HP21 7ET

Dr Pat McKenna
Consultant Clinical Neuropsychologist
Rookwood Hospital
Fairwater Road
Llandaff
Cardiff CF5 2YN

Mr Robert Merriman
Senior Quality Assurance Manager
Disabilities Trust
2 Bennell Court
West Street
Comberton
Cambridgeshire CB3 7DS

Professor Michael Oddy
Director of Clinical Services & Consultant in Neuropsychology and Rehabilitation
Brain Injury Rehabilitation Trust
Kerwin Court
Five Oaks Road
Slinford
West Sussex RH13 0TP

Professor M. Jane Riddoch
Behavioural Brain Sciences Centre
School of Psychology
University of Birmingham
Edgbaston
Birmingham B15 2TT

Mrs Sue Stoten
Occupational Therapist & Brain Injury Case Manager
Anglia Case Management
4–5 Ticehurst Yard
Beyton Road, Tostock
Bury St Edmonds
Suffolk IP30 9PH

Dr Andy Tyerman
Consultant Clinical Neuropsychologist & Head of Service
Community Head Injury Service
Buckinghamshire Primary Care Trust
The Camborne Centre
Jansel Square
Aylesbury
Bucks HP21 7ET

Mrs Ruth Tyerman
Programme Manager, Working Out
Community Head Injury Service
Buckinghamshire Primary Care Trust
The Camborne Centre
Jansel Square
Aylesbury
Bucks HP21 7ET

Mr Peter Viney
Former Placement Consultant
Community Head Injury Service
Buckinghamshire Primary Care Trust
The Camborne Centre
Jansel Square
Aylesbury
Bucks HP21 7ET

Dr Guinevere Webster
Clinical Psychologist
National Spinal Injuries Centre
Stoke Mandeville Hospital
Aylesbury
Bucks HP21 8AL

Dr W. Huw Williams
Senior Lecturer
School of Psychology
University of Exeter
Washington Singer Laboratories
Perry Road
Exeter EX4 4QG

Professor Barbara A. Wilson
Senior Scientist
MRC Cognition & Brain Sciences Unit
Box 58
Addenbrook's Hospital
Hills Road
Cambridge CB2 2QQ

Dr Claire Willson
Clinical Neuropsychologist
Community Brain Injury Team
Rookwood Hospital
Fairwater Road
Llandaff
Cardiff CF5 2YN

Professor Rodger Ll. Wood
Department of Psychology
University of Wales, Swansea
Singleton Park
Swansea SA2 8PP

Dr Andrew D. Worthington
Consultant in Neuropsychology & Rehabilitation
Brain Injury Rehabilitation Trust
West Heath House
54 Ivyhouse Road
West Heath
Birmingham B38 8JW

Acknowledgements

We wish to express our deep appreciation to all the people with traumatic brain injury and their relatives who have shared their experiences with us over the years, especially those who have agreed to be reported as illustrative examples, which so enrich the book.

We also wish to express our gratitude to the following: the British Psychological Society for commissioning the original project; the chapter authors for their excellent contributions and for their patience; the reviewers for their valuable comments; and the Vale of Aylesbury Primary Care Trust, Oxford Doctoral Course in Clinical Psychology and BPS Blackwell for their support.

1

Introduction to Traumatic Brain Injury

Nigel S. King and Andy Tyerman

Introduction

Traumatic brain injury (TBI) is a major area of health and social care need. In the UK it is estimated that around a million people each year attend accident and emergency departments with an injury to the head. The annual incidence of hospital admissions after head injury is estimated to be 229 per 100,000 in England. This includes 356 per 100,000 for children (aged 0–15), 178 per 100,000 for adults (aged 16–75), and 384 per 100,000 for older adults (aged 75 and over) (Tennett, 2005). Whilst 75–85 per cent of such injuries are mild in nature (Kraus & Nourjah, 1988; Miller & Jones, 1985), the incidence of moderate or severe TBI is estimated to be 25 per 100,000 (RCP/BSRM, 2003). Outcome ranges from complete recovery to persistent coma or death. Prevalence of disability from TBI is estimated to affect 100–150 per 100,000 (British Society of Rehabilitation Medicine, 1998), affecting one family in 300 (Lancet, 1983).

TBI often results in complex impairments that interact across a number of domains – physical, sensory, cognitive, behavioural and emotional. However, in the long term it is the psychological rather than the physical difficulties that cause most restrictions. These typically involve difficulties in: (1) maintaining positive relationships with family and friends; (2) maintaining occupational activities; and (3) making long-term adjustment to impairments and disabilities and their wide-ranging personal, family and social effects. The critical importance of the psychological effects of TBI and the need for psychological services to assist their management has long been recognised (e.g. British Psychological Society, 1989; British Society of Rehabilitation Medicine, 1998; Medical Disability Society, 1988; Royal College of Physicians, 1986; RCP/BSRM, 2003). It is imperative that professionals from all rehabilitation disciplines are familiar with them.

The publication of the *National Service Framework for Long-term Conditions* (Department of Health, 2005) provides a strategic framework for developing services for adults with TBI and other neurological conditions over the next decade within the National Health Service (NHS) in the UK. This links with recent clinical guidelines covering early assessment and management (NICE, 2003), rehabilitation (RCP/BSRM, 2003) and vocational assessment/rehabilitation (RCP/JCP/BSRM, 2004). As such, it is timely to address the ways in which psychological approaches to rehabilitation after TBI can be implemented. This book attempts to achieve this across five broad areas: (1) service provision; (2) cognitive rehabilitation; (3) behavioural and emotional interventions; (4) vocational rehabilitation; and (5) family interventions. By focusing on practical applications it is hoped that the book will be useful not only to clinical psychologists but to all professionals involved in rehabilitation for people with TBI and their families.

In this chapter we shall outline briefly the nature of TBI, its psychological effects and current service provision for adults in the UK (with a focus on psychological approaches to rehabilitation), and then introduce the other 18 chapters in this book.

The Nature of Traumatic Brain Injury

Traumatic brain injury has been defined as 'brain injury caused by trauma to the head including the effects of direct complications of trauma notably hypoxaemia, hypotension, intracranial haemorrhage and raised intracranial pressure' (British Society of Rehabilitation Medicine, 1998). Head injury has been defined as 'trauma that carries some risk of damage to the brain' (Field, 1976).

There are two main types of head injury – open and closed: open head injury occurs when the skull and protective linings of the brain are damaged and the brain is exposed; closed head injury occurs when the skull and protective linings of the brain are not penetrated. In the UK, TBI is predominantly of a closed, blunt-impact nature arising from sudden changes in velocity (e.g. acceleration/deceleration injuries from road traffic accidents), assaults or falls. Open, penetrating injuries (e.g. arising from gunshot wounds or bomb blasts) are uncommon in the UK but frequently occur in war zones.

Severe TBI often involves some skull fracture. This may be simple, compound (open), comminuted (involving a shattering of the bone into a number of pieces) or depressed (when a skull fragment has been pushed through the linings of the brain into the brain substance). The latter injuries are likely to occur when the head makes contact with a sharp rather than flat surface (e.g. kerb) or when the head is hit with an object (e.g. hammer), which concentrates the force on a small area of the skull. The damage to the underlying brain may be primary (i.e. occurring at the time of injury) or secondary (i.e. due to subsequent complications).

Primary brain damage

There are two main types of primary brain damage: haemorrhagic contusions (areas of bruising) and diffuse axonal injury (widespread damage to axons). Contusions are more common after falls and direct blows while axonal injury is more common after acceleration/deceleration injuries such as road traffic accidents.

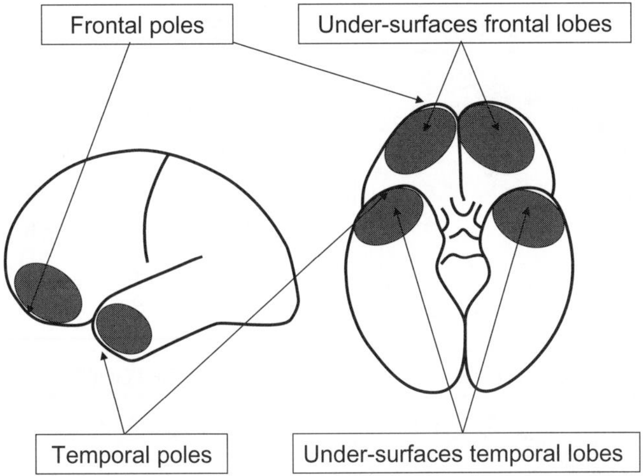

Figure 1.1 Common sites of contusion

Haemorrhagic contusions on the crests of the gyri of the cortex can occur under the point of impact (especially after depressed skull fractures) or directly opposite it ('contrecoup' injury), but are seen most often on the under-surfaces of the frontal lobes and around the pole of the temporal lobes, where the brain impacts on the sharpest and most confined parts of skull (see Figure 1.1). Haemorrhage occurs when the blood vessels supplying oxygen are ruptured.

Diffuse axonal injury refers to widespread tearing or shearing of axons in the white matter due to violent movement of the largely unrestrained brain, causing stretching and compressing of axons (i.e. the part of the neuron which conveys impulses from the cell body to the next neuron in the chain). Diffuse axonal injury is considered to be the more important mechanism of primary brain damage.

Secondary brain damage

There are two main types of secondary brain damage: extracranial (i.e. outside the skull) and intracranial (i.e. inside the skull).

Extracranial causes of secondary brain damage include respiratory failure, hypoxia (insufficient oxygen) or hypotension (loss of blood flow). Even a short period of loss of blood flow to part of the brain will set up a chain reaction leading to death of neural tissue (ischaemia). As such, protecting the airway, maintaining breathing and controlling bleeding are the first priorities in accident and emergency departments.

Intracranial causes of secondary damage include haemorrhage (bleeding); haematomas (collections of blood following haemorrhage); cerebral oedema (brain swelling); infection (after open wounds); and hydrocephalus (build up of cerebrospinal fluid). Haemorrhage in particular can quickly transform a seemingly mild TBI into a life-threatening event. Haemorrhage and resultant haematoma can occur

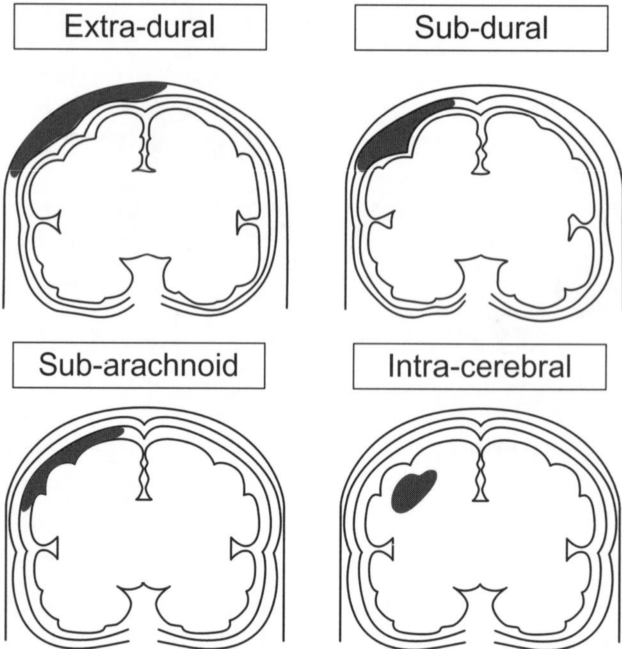

Figure 1.2 Types of haemorrhage

both above and below the two outer coverings of the brain (the dura mater and arachnoid mater), as well as within the brain itself (see Figure 1.2):

- an extra-dural haematoma is a collection of blood inside the skull but outside the dura mater (the outer covering of the brain);
- a sub-dural haematoma lies underneath the dura mater but outside the arachnoid mater (the middle covering of the brain);
- a sub-arachnoid haemorrhage is bleeding under the arachnoid mater into the sub-arachnoid space where cerebrospinal fluid flows; and
- an intra-cerebral haemorrhage is bleeding within the brain itself.

Raised intracranial pressure, resulting from swelling of the brain within the confines of the skull, may lead to a reduction in cerebral blood flow or brain compression which, if unchecked, may lead to death. Hydrocephalus (resulting from disruption to the flow or absorption of cerebrospinal fluid) can arise acutely in the early days or weeks of recovery or develop gradually in the months or years post-injury. A further neurological complication is that of post-traumatic epilepsy, which is experienced by an estimated 5 per cent of people admitted to hospital after TBI. Identified risk factors for post-traumatic epilepsy include early seizure, cerebral haematoma and depressed skull fracture. For a summary of the nature of TBI see, for example, McGlashan (2002), Ponsford (1995) or Povlishock and Katz (2005). For an overview of early management of TBI, see Smith (1996).

Severity of traumatic brain injury

The severity of TBI is usually measured by: (i) depth of unconsciousness – usually measured immediately after resuscitation on the Glasgow Coma Scale (GCS); (ii) length of unconsciousness (i.e. GCS <9); (iii) presence of neurological signs (e.g. paresis or damage revealed by neuro-imaging techniques); and/or (iv) length of post traumatic amnesia (PTA) (i.e. the period of time between injury and regaining continuous day-to-day memory for events). The classification of GCS and PTA is detailed in Table 1.1.

After a mild or moderate TBI about 50 per cent will experience one or more of a range of 'post concussional symptoms'. These may include headaches, fatigue, dizziness, irritability, nausea, sensitivity to light and/or noise, blurred/double vision, poor memory, poor concentration, slowed thinking, sleep disturbance, tinnitus, anxiety, depression or frustration. These symptoms may be caused by organic and/or psychological factors. Whilst, for most, full recovery occurs within a few days to three months, 5–10 per cent will have persisting symptoms after a year, which may lead to vocational and other long-term consequences. Post-traumatic stress symptoms may also occur, e.g. phobic avoidance of situations associated with the injury. A vicious circle can easily develop where anxiety, depression, irritability or frustration exacerbates the symptoms, leading to increased distress and reduced coping, which in turn causes further exacerbation of symptoms (King & Tyerman, 2003).

The disabilities associated with severe TBI are extremely varied, and encompass both physical (i.e. motor and sensory deficits) and psychological changes (e.g. cognitive impairment, loss of behavioural control and altered emotional response). For some these will be quite subtle and only evident: (i) under stress; (ii) in busy work environments; and/or (iii) when skills or emotional/behavioural control is under pressure (e.g. on formal testing or in demanding situations). Improvement typically takes place gradually over a period of months and years. The most rapid recovery is usually seen within the first 6–12 months with more patchy improvement thereafter. Some degree of permanent impairment is likely after more severe injuries. The majority of recovery occurs within the first two years such that significant difficulties at two years rarely resolve naturally thereafter, although limited improvement can sometimes be experienced up to and beyond five years post-injury. However, positive adjustments leading to improved function can be facilitated many years post-injury, as people with TBI are helped to develop greater understanding and management of long-term difficulties. This is especially

Table 1.1 Severity of head injury

Severity	Glasgow Coma Scale	Post-traumatic amnesia
Mild	13–15	<1 hour
Moderate	9–12	1–24 hours
Severe	3–8	1–7 days
Very severe	N/A	1–4 weeks
Extremely severe	N/A	>4 weeks

so when people have received only limited early rehabilitation, either in scope or duration.

Psychological Effects of TBI

The effects of TBI have similarities with other neurological conditions but also distinct features in terms of onset, symptom profile and course (Tyerman & King, 2004). Physical disability ranges from general paralysis (affecting all four limbs, speech, swallowing, etc.), through to more specific changes (e.g. paralysis down one side of the body) or subtle reductions in strength, coordination and balance. Sensory disturbances (such as double vision, visual field deficits and reduced sensation, taste and smell) are quite common. Whilst less common, hearing deficits also occur. Many people with TBI are troubled by headaches and fatigue, and some by other specific changes (e.g. sleep disturbance, altered sexual response, etc.). For a summary of physical effects of TBI, see Mathers *et al.*, 2002. It is the psychological changes however that predominate, reflecting a combination of primary neuropsychological and secondary psychological effects. These include complex interactions between cognitive, behavioural and emotional changes.

Cognitive impairment

After TBI the most common cognitive difficulties are in the areas of attention and concentration, new learning/memory, speed of information processing and executive functioning (i.e. reasoning, planning, problem solving, self-awareness and self-monitoring). Subtle difficulties with language skills (e.g. comprehension, verbal fluency, word finding) are also quite common. More marked impairment of language skills (e.g. receptive or expressive dysphasia, acquired dyslexia, etc.) and other specific impairment (e.g. visuo-perceptual, spatial and constructional difficulties) are less common but can occur as a result of focal injury or after severe generalised damage. Becoming aware of confusing changes in cognitive skills can be a highly disturbing experience. Difficulties with communication, memory, visuo-perceptual/spatial-motor function and executive/attentional skills are addressed in detail in chapters 6–9.

The characteristic reduction in awareness after TBI, which often reflects a complex and dynamic interaction of neurological and psychological factors, poses a particular challenge and necessitates 'unique and specialized neuropsychological interventions' (Trexler *et al.*, 2000). Loss of awareness may prevent the person from recognising impairments, from accepting the observations of family and friends or from accepting the results of formal assessments, thereby reducing engagement in rehabilitation and the use of coping strategies. The application of coping strategies will also be affected by the interaction of cognitive impairment, behavioural/emotional volatility and difficulties in psychological adjustment. Even with awareness, people with executive difficulties commonly struggle to adapt strategies to new situations, make appropriate decisions or problem solve about difficult situations. As such, disruption to executive function is of particular importance, not only in its direct effects on independence and control, but also in the limitations imposed on insight, understanding, use of compensatory strategies and long-term adjustment (Tyerman & King, 2004).

Behavioural/emotional changes

A wide range of behavioural and emotional changes may be experienced after TBI, reflecting an interaction of primary neurological damage and secondary psychological effects. Common primary changes include irritability and intolerance, aggressive outbursts, disinhibition, impulsivity, emotional lability and mood swings. In contrast, others may experience passivity, lack of initiation and/or a flattening of emotional response. Equally, a wide range of emotional reactions may be experienced, such as frustration and anger, fear and anxiety, depression, loss of confidence/self-esteem. Some people, most commonly those with mild or moderate TBI, also experience post-traumatic stress disorder (PTSD). There can also be subtle and confusing changes in the experience and expression of emotion. Behavioural difficulties, common emotional difficulties, PTSD and difficulties with psychological adjustment are reviewed in chapters 10–13.

Early on some people experience the emotional impact of the consequences of TBI in terms of their loss of skills, roles and control over one's life, the slow pace of progress and the uncertain extent of future recovery. Others in early rehabilitation however may appear unconcerned about their predicament owing to limited insight into the extent of cognitive and behavioural/emotional difficulties, unrealistic expectations of a full recovery and/or psychological denial. As such, anxiety, depression and loss of confidence may surface only later when the person has developed greater insight and/or attempted and struggled to resume former family, work and social roles.

Social and family effects

Whilst recovery and adjustment to TBI may continue over several years, the complex array of physical, cognitive, behavioural and emotional difficulties are such that people with TBI often face major restrictions in independence, occupation, leisure and social life. This is often mirrored by substantial impact upon the family.

Some people with TBI lose the capacity for independent living, contribute less to family life in terms of practical, social, parental and marital roles and experience a much reduced leisure and social life. Return to education, training or work represents a major challenge. Reduced cognitive and motor speed, limited concentration, unreliable memory, headaches and/or fatigue renders many uncompetitive in their previous work or training, whilst specific effects (e.g. visual field deficits, communication difficulties, executive difficulties, loss of behavioural or emotional control) may preclude a return to specific occupations. Those returning to work may have difficulty in sustaining work over time and/or have difficulty in securing and coping with alternative employment. Those unable to return to paid employment may struggle to find alternative occupation appropriate to their interests and needs. Return to previous occupation is discussed in chapter 14 and return to alternative occupation in chapters 15 and 16.

Primary carers of people with TBI often experience high levels of stress and distress, often amidst marked changes in family relationships, roles and functioning. As family life changes in response to the difficulties and needs of the person with TBI, the occupational, leisure and social lives of other family members may falter. Family relationships often become strained as a result of the changes in the person with TBI. These often include the need for supervision, reduced communication and social skills, behavioural difficulties, emotional vulnerability and resultant disruption to household routines and family activities. Changes in arousal may disrupt sexual relations and partners may find the behaviour of the person with TBI incompatible with that of a sexual partner. Partners often struggle to cope with the competing needs of the person with TBI, children, home and work, with some feeling trapped in a relationship they no longer find rewarding. Some couples adjust positively, others remain close but with less fun and intimacy. However, for some the extent of change is such that the person and/or partner are unable to adjust and the relationship breaks down. Changes in the person and impact on the family may also have a major impact on siblings and children. The impact of TBI on the family and related services are discussed in chapters 17 and 18 and for child relatives specifically in chapter 19.

Traumatic Brain Injury Services

People with the most severe head injuries are likely to be transferred to regional neuroscience services for neurosurgical intervention and care before returning to their local general hospital. However, the majority of people with TBI are treated in the general hospital. Whilst some general hospitals have arrangements for follow-up of clients with TBI, many have no such provision. Some of the more severely injured will receive a period of specialist post-acute neurological in-patient rehabilitation. Once discharged back into the community, specialist rehabilitation services in the UK are very patchy. Some people will be seen for rehabilitation in hospital out-patient departments or through hospital outreach teams, some will be referred to a specialist brain injury team or case manager and others will be seen by specialist neurorehabilitation or local generic rehabilitation services.

Rehabilitation is a process of active change through which a person who has become disabled acquires the knowledge and skills needed for optimal physical, psychological and social function. Rehabilitation services use all means to minimise the impact of disabling conditions and to assist disabled people to achieve their desired level of autonomy and participation in society (British Society of Rehabilitation Medicine, 1998). Rehabilitation after TBI requires input from an interdisciplinary team (including medicine, clinical neuropsychology, nursing, occupational therapy, physiotherapy, speech and language therapy), in liaison with acute services, the primary care team, Social Services and a range of community services. Core brain injury rehabilitation typically focuses initially on promoting optimal independence through provision of assistive devices and interventions to address the following areas of difficulty:

- symptom management;
- mobility and motor skills;
- sensory function;
- personal and domestic independence;
- communication and social skills;

- cognitive function;
- behavioural control; and
- emotional well-being.

Some TBI services also provide ongoing rehabilitation to promote optimal community reintegration through interventions and support. These might: assist a return to work, education, driving, leisure or social life; help with family and sexual relationships; or facilitate psychological adjustment. Provision of specialist education, counselling and support for relatives is sometimes provided. Community rehabilitation however is underdeveloped in the UK, with provision focusing on physical disability and few services specialising in interventions addressing cognitive and behavioural difficulties (McMillan & Ledder, 2001). As such, many people with TBI currently do not receive the required community rehabilitation and long-term support. The *National Service Framework for Long-term Conditions* (Department of Health, 2005) however gives a clear outline of how TBI services in the NHS need to be developed over the next decade and means that there is now an excellent opportunity for TBI services to be more consistent and coordinated across the UK.

Neuropsychological assessment and interventions are vital components of brain injury rehabilitation. Drawing on a combination of specialist neuropsychological knowledge and core training, clinical neuropsychology provides the following key functions (British Psychological Society, 1989):

a. to carry out detailed assessments of cognition, emotion, behaviour and social competence;
b. to devise and implement training programmes to address these difficulties;
c. to liaise with educational agencies and employers; and
d. to provide and advise about long-term care and facilitate long-term personal, family and social adjustment.

An updated report (British Psychological Society, 2005), outlines a proposed acquired brain injury service network (see Figure 1.3). Key recommendations include the need for: a brain injury service network/care pathways; early assessment and treatment by specialist staff; specialist facilities for people with high physical dependence, severe challenging behaviour and for those who are minimally responsive; post-acute community rehabilitation service; and integration of brain injury and vocational rehabilitation services.

In the UK clinical neuropsychologists work with people with TBI in a range of settings across the care pathway – in regional neuroscience centres, in-patient neurological rehabilitation centres, community neurorehabilitation or specialist community brain injury teams and in specialist services focusing specifically on cognitive, behavioural and/or vocational needs after acquired brain injury (Carpenter & Tyerman, 2006). For an outline of the role of the clinical neuropsychologist, see British Psychological Society, 2004. In developing rehabilitation interventions, clinical neuropsychologists have drawn on a wide range of theoretical approaches (e.g. neuropsychological, cognitive–behavioural, behaviour modification and humanistic psychotherapy). For a review of the principles and theoretical approaches to neuropsychological rehabilitation, see Prigatano (1999) and Wilson (2002, 2004).

Understanding and managing the psychological effects of TBI is important not only for those directly involved in psychological interventions but for other members

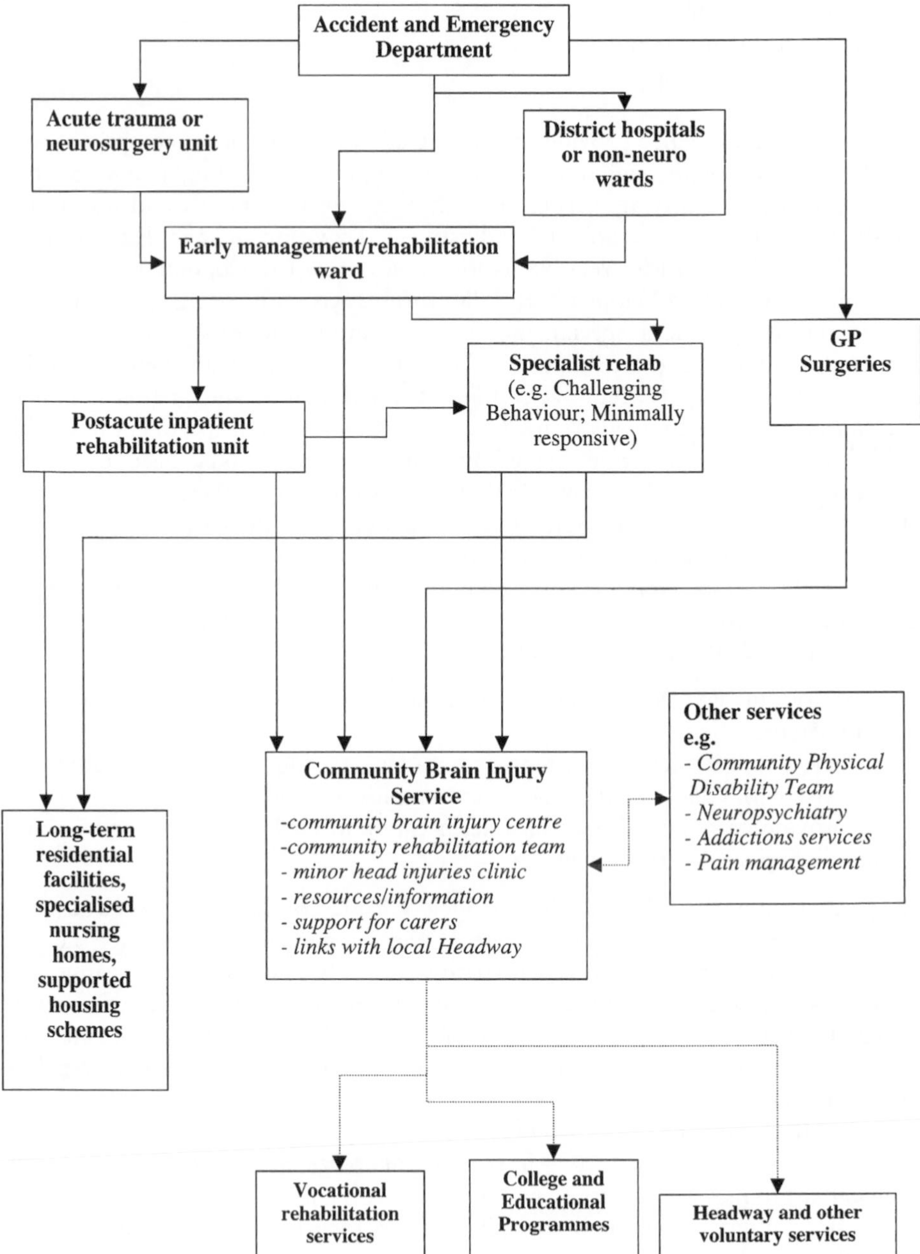

Figure 1.3 The ABI Service Network (reproduced with permission from the British Psychological Society, 2005)

of the rehabilitation team and other agencies. This is reflected in an expanding literature addressing the integration of psychological approaches with other therapies within the rehabilitation team. An excellent example is provided by Campbell (2000) who describes the impact of cognitive and behavioural difficulties on the provision of physical therapy, with illustrative examples and management suggestions. The nature and management of cognitive, behavioural and emotional difficulties should therefore be key elements of staff training in brain injury rehabilitation across all disciplines (see Jackson & Manchester, 2001).

Psychological Approaches to Rehabilitation after TBI

In summary, TBI commonly results in a complex and highly disabling array of impairments that have a dramatic impact on the person and those close to them. Many people with TBI and their families therefore require treatment and support across a range of contexts – acute hospital, in-patient rehabilitation, residential, out-patient and community settings. The aims of rehabilitation services are to promote optimal recovery, independence and participation and to facilitate long-term personal, family and social adjustment. Very significant psychological challenges are faced by the person with TBI and those close to them. This book describes psychological approaches to rehabilitation to assist people with TBI and their relatives in meeting these challenges.

The book covers five broad areas. Part I, 'Service Provision', has chapters on the role of psychological approaches in acute, in-patient rehabilitation, community rehabilitation and residential settings. Part II, 'Cognitive Rehabilitation', has chapters on communication disorders, memory, visuo-perceptual and spatial-motor disorders, and executive/attentional difficulties. Part III, 'Behavioural and Emotional Interventions', has chapters on behavioural difficulties; fear, anxiety and depression; TBI and post-traumatic stress disorder; and facilitating psychological adjustment. Part IV, 'Vocational Rehabilitation', has chapters on return to previous employment, vocational rehabilitation and supported employment/job coaching. Part V, 'Family Interventions', has chapters on TBI and the family; working with families – a community service example; and familial brain injury – impact on and interventions with children. The chapters have been written by recognised experts in their respective fields in the UK and reviewed by both a clinical neuropsychologist and a member of a relevant professional group.

The practical emphasis of the book means that it concentrates on providing ideas and references for applying psychological approaches in these domains and on signposting clinicians to pragmatic resources to aid their work. The extensive use of case study material illustrates how these approaches have been used in day-to-day practice. As such, the outcome literature is attended to only when it enhances the practical emphasis of the book. Fuller accounts of the effectiveness of cognitive and psychological rehabilitation methods, both generally and for traumatic brain injury in particular, have been well described elsewhere (e.g. Carney & Coudray, 2005; Halligan & Wade, 2005; Trexler, 2000; Williams & Evans, 2003).

It is hoped that the book will stimulate the development and provision of interventions by clinical neuropsychologists and others which address the psychological effects of TBI and thereby improve the quality of life of people with TBI and their relatives. In developing and providing such services it is vital that we contribute, whenever possible, to our collective knowledge about the effectiveness of such interventions through systematic feedback, case studies, service evaluation and outcomes studies.

Recommended Reading

Christensen, A-L. & Uzzell, B.P. (2000). *International handbook of neuropsychological rehabilitation.* New York: Kluwer Academic/Plenum Publishers.
Edited book including chapters on acute management/recovery, neuropsychological assessment, neuropsychological rehabilitation – four general chapters and nine chapters outlining specific programmes in the USA, South America and Europe.

Goldstein, L.H. & McNeil, J.E. (2004). *Clinical neuropsychology: A practical guide to assessment and management for clinicians.* Chichester: Wiley.
Edited book outlining current practice in clinical neuropsychology in the UK. Chapters on neuroscience; neuropsychological assessment; areas of cognitive function; working with children, adults and the law; and rehabilitation (four chapters).

Johnstone, B. & Stonington, H.H. (2001). *Rehabilitation of neuropsychological disorders. A practical guide for rehabilitation professionals.* Philadelphia: Psychology Press.
Edited book by US authors on assessment/rehabilitation including practical management strategies for areas of cognitive impairment – includes chapters on attention, memory, executive, visuospatial and language disorders.

Ponsford, J., Sloan, S. & Snow, P. (1995). *Traumatic brain injury: Rehabilitation for everyday adaptive living.* Hove: Lawrence Erlbaum Associates.
Practical account with case examples – chapters on TBI mechanisms and sequelae, impaired consciousness, cognitive difficulties, communication/interpersonal skills, behavioural problems, return to the community, psychological adjustment, working with families and TBI in children.

Wilson, B.A. (Ed.) (2003). *Neuropsychological rehabilitation: theory and practice.* Hove: Psychology Press.
Edited book (UK/international authors). Includes chapters on attention, executive deficits, memory, language, emotional disorders, social rehabilitation, behaviour disorders, dementia, TBI in children, reduced awareness states, and service delivery.

Wood, R.Ll. & McMillan, T.M. (2001). *Neurobehavioural disability and social handicap following traumatic brain injury.* Hove: Psychology Press.
Edited book (predominantly UK authors) outlining the nature, assessment and management of neurobehavioural disability and social handicap after TBI. Includes specific chapters on challenging behaviour and dysexecutive syndrome.

Useful Resources

www.dh.gov.uk/longtermnsf
The section of the Department of Health website on the National Service Framework (NSF) for Long-term (Neurological) Conditions includes access to the NSF (and its 11 quality

requirements), a list of regional and local PCT Leads for the NSF and a good practice guide including examples of good practice for each quality requirement.

www.hdipub.com
The HDI publishers' website provides access to a selection of TBI publications including the HDI Professional series (25 booklets on specific aspects of TBI and their management) and the HDI Coping Series (5 booklets for TBI clients/families).

www.headway.org.uk
Headway, the brain injury association (UK), website provides information on the nature of TBI, local Headway groups and branches, the range of Headway publications and a list of personal injury solicitors in the UK.

www.ukabif.org.uk
UK Acquired Brain Injury Forum website provides a directory of rehabilitation services in the UK plus information on membership, the ABI All Party Parliamentary Group, forthcoming conferences/events and links to other organisations.

References

British Psychological Society (1989). *Working party report on services for young adult patients with acquired brain damage.* Leicester: British Psychological Society.

British Psychological Society (2004). *Commissioning clinical neuropsychological services.* Leicester: British Psychological Society – Division of Neuropsychology.

British Psychological Society (2005). *Clinical neuropsychology and rehabilitation services for adults with acquired brain injury.* Leicester: British Psychological Society – Division of Neuropsychology .

British Society of Rehabilitation Medicine (1998). *Rehabilitation after traumatic brain injury.* A working party report. London: British Society of Rehabilitation Medicine.

Campbell, M. (2000). *Rehabilitation for traumatic brain injury. Physical therapy practice in context.* London: Churchill Livingstone.

Carney, N. & Coudray, H. (2005). Cognitive rehabilitation outcomes for traumatic brain injury. In P.W. Halligan & D.T. Wade (Eds.) *Effectiveness of rehabilitation for cognitive deficits* (pp.295–317). Oxford: Oxford University Press.

Carpenter, K. & Tyerman, A. (2006). Working in clinical neuropsychology. In J. Hall & S. Llewellyn (Eds.) *What is clinical psychology?* (4th edn, pp.273–295). Oxford: Oxford University Press.

Department of Health (2005). *The national service framework for long-term conditions.* London. Department of Health. www.dh.gov.uk/longtermnsf.

Field, J.H. (1976). *Epidemiology of head injuries in England and Wales with particular reference to rehabilitation.* London: HMSO.

Halligan, P.W. & Wade, D.T. (Eds.) (2005). *Effectiveness of rehabilitation for cognitive deficits.* Oxford: Oxford University Press.

Jackson, H. & Manchester, D. (2001). Towards the development of brain injury specialists. *NeuroRehabilitation, 16*, 27–40.

King, N.S. & Tyerman, A. (2003). The neuropsychological presentation and treatment of head injury and traumatic brain injury. In P.W. Halligan, J. Marshall & U. Kischka (Eds.) *Oxford handbook of clinical neuropsychology* (pp.487–505). Oxford: Oxford University Press.

Kraus, J.F. & Nourjah, P. (1988). The epidemiology of mild uncomplicated brain injury. *Trauma, 28*, 1637–1643.

Lancet (1983). Caring for the disabled after head injury. *The Lancet, II*, 948–949.

Mathers, T., McGlashan, K., Vick, K. & Gravell, R. (2002). Physical issues following head injury. In R. Gravell & R. Johnson (Eds.) *Head injury rehabilitation: A community team perspective* (pp.70–111). London: Whurr Publishers.

McGlashan, K. (2002). Setting the scene. In R. Gravell & R. Johnson (Eds.) *Head injury rehabilitation: A community team perspective* (pp.37–69). London: Whurr Publishers.

McMillan, T.E. & Ledder, H. (2001). A survey of services provided by neurorehabilitation teams in South East England. *Clinical Rehabilitation*, *15*, 582–588.

Medical Disability Society (1988). *A working party report on the management of traumatic brain injury*. London: The Royal College of Physicians.

Miller, J.D. & Jones, P.A. (1985). The work of a Regional Head Injury Service. *The Lancet*, 18 May, 1141–1141.

NICE (2003). *Head injury. Triage, assessment, and early management of head injury in infants, children and adults*. London: National Institute of Clinical Excellence.

Ponsford, J. (1995). Mechanisms, recovery, and sequelae of traumatic brain injury: A foundation for the REAL approach. In J. Ponsford, S. Sloan & P. Snow (Eds.) *Traumatic brain injury: Rehabilitation for everyday adaptive living* (pp.1–31). Hove: Lawrence Erlbaum.

Povlishock, J.T. & Katz, D.I. (2005). Update of neuropathology and neurological recovery after traumatic brain injury. *Journal of Head Trauma Rehabilitation*, *20*, 76–94.

Prigatano, G.P. (1999). *Principles of neuropsychological rehabilitation*. New York: Oxford University Press.

RCP/BSRM (2003). *Rehabilitation following acquired brain injury: National clinical guidelines* (L. Turner-Stokes, Ed.). London: Royal College of Physicians/British Society of Rehabilitation Medicine.

RCP/JCP/BSRM (2004). *Vocational assessment and rehabilitation after acquired brain injury. Inter-agency guidelines*. Report of an inter-agency advisory group on vocational rehabilitation after brain injury (A. Tyerman & M. Meehan, Eds.). London: Royal College of Physicians, Jobcentre Plus and British Society of Rehabilitation Medicine.

Royal College of Physicians (1986). *Physical disability in 1986 and beyond*. London: The Royal College of Physicians.

Smith, M. (1996). Acute care. In F.D. Rose & D.A. Johnson (Eds.) *Brain injury and after: Towards improved outcome* (pp.21–48). Chichester: Wiley.

Tennett, A. (2005). Admission to hospital following head injury in England: Incidence and socio-economic determinants. *BioMedCentral Public Health* (March 2005), *5*, 21.

Trexler, L.E. (2000). Empirical support for neuropsychological rehabilitation. In A-L. Christensen & B.P. Uzell (Eds.) *International handbook of neuropsychological rehabilitation* (pp.137–150). New York: Kluwer Academic.

Trexler, L.E., Eberle, R. & Zappala, G. (2000). Models and programs of the Center for Neuropsychological Rehabilitation: Fifteen years experience. In A-L. Christensen & B.P. Uzzell (Eds.) *International handbook of neuropsychological rehabilitation* (pp.215–229). New York: Kluwer Academic/Plenum Publishers.

Tyerman, A. & King, N.S. (2004). Psychological interventions for neurologically impaired individuals. In L.H. Goldstein & J. McNeil (Eds.) *Clinical neuropsychology; A practical guide to assessment and management for clinicians* (pp.385–404). Chichester: Wiley.

Williams, W.H. & Evans, J.J. (Eds.) (2003). Biopsychosocial approaches in neurorehabilitation: Assessment and management of neuropsychiatric, mood and behavioural disorders. *Neuropsychological Rehabilitation*, *13*, Special Issue 1–2.

Wilson, B.A. (2002). Towards a comprehensive model of cognitive rehabilitation. *Neuropsychological Rehabilitation*, *12*, 97–210.

Wilson, B.A. (2004). Theoretical approaches to cognitive rehabilitation. In L.H. Goldstein & J. McNeil (Eds.) *Clinical neuropsychology: A practical guide to assessment & management for clinicians* (pp.345–366). Chichester: Wiley.

Part I

Service Provision

2

Acute Neuropsychological Rehabilitation Services

Katherine N. Carpenter

Introduction

Traumatic brain injury poses unique problems both for those that survive the experience and for the families, carers and clinicians faced with the task of helping with their rehabilitation. Recent data on admission to hospital following head injury in England give an incidence rate of 229 per 100,000 (Tennant 2005). This rate varied by a factor of 4.6 across Strategic Health Authorities (SHAs) and Primary Care Trusts (PCTs) and there is a strong argument for the planning of head-injury-related services to be based on local rather than national incidence figures. Reliable data on admission rates to regional neuroscience centres versus District General Hospitals (DGHs) are lacking. The majority of admissions will be for mild head injury but these may nevertheless have significant sequelae to warrant rehabilitation.

A blow to the head with a blunt object, or blunt impact of the head against an object in association with acceleration/deceleration forces, can result in *primary* brain injury which occurs on impact and is irreversible, and *secondary* brain injury which occurs as a result of potentially treatable systemic complications. Primary brain injury therefore includes skull fracture, cerebral contusion and diffuse axonal injury. Secondary brain injury encompasses intracranial haematoma, brain swelling, raised intracranial pressure, infection, respiratory failure, hypotension and ischaemia. More delayed potential complications of TBI include hydrocephalus and post-traumatic epilepsy. What this means is that early management of TBI may require intense investigation and intervention by the emergency, trauma and neurosurgical teams. Much of the early spontaneous recovery seen after TBI is almost certainly due to resolution of temporary physiological changes, such as oedema (swelling) or raised intracranial pressure, which have caused functional disruption. The extent to which later recovery represents *restitution* of function, presumably via some form of anatomical reorganisation, or only *amelioration* through compensation and functional adaptation, remains unclear (see Ponsford, 2004 for a discussion). However, the focus of early rehabilitation is on adaptation.

In some ways, the acute end of neuropsychological rehabilitation for TBI is an uncomfortable place to start a practical guide for the clinician. Despite a considerable proliferation of papers and authoritative texts on rehabilitation, we are still relatively in the dark about optimal intervention in the acute stage. Where there is an evidence-base for good clinical practice, implementation can be difficult for logistical reasons. This chapter first sets out the role of the neuropsychologist in acute neuropsychological rehabilitation and then the context of acute work, and goes on to describe assessment and intervention of both in-patients and out-patients with a review of the evidence-base.

The Role of the Neuropsychologist

Acute neuropsychological rehabilitation is carried out in hospital settings with a wide range of clients. TBI patients are a heterogeneous group who frequently have complex needs, ranging from mild cases, where early information-giving and reassurance is important, to severe cases, where a specialist team working in relation to assessment and management is crucial. For the neuropsychologist in the acute setting, TBI patients constitute approximately 20 per cent of the case load, which also includes patients with stroke, brain tumours, epilepsy, dementia and movement disorders. Some neuropsychological skills are obviously transferable to this group, while others, such as training and expertise in recognising and managing post-traumatic amnesia or in meeting the challenges of the acute disinhibition and disorganised behaviour seen early post-head-injury, are more specific.

The British Psychological Society's Division of Neuropsychology document on rehabilitation services for adults with acquired brain injury clearly sets out the range of roles undertaken by clinical neuropsychologists, and these are equally applicable across the pathway of care. They include:

Assessment of cognitive functioning
Assessment of mood/emotion
Treatment/management of cognitive impairment
Treatment of mood disorder
Management of behaviour problems
Education for relatives/carers/other professionals on brain injury and its consequences
Research and audit e.g. evaluations of outcome of rehabilitation. (BPS DoN, 2005)

While one might argue that every head-injured patient should have the right to ready and timely access to neuropsychological input, the reality is that this is not always possible given the current level of demand on services, or indeed because the person may be discharged too rapidly for meaningful intervention. The main reasons for acute in-patient referral therefore tend to be problem based: distress on the part of the patient, their family or their key staff; disruptive, so-called 'challenging' or difficult-to-manage behaviour; assessment of the capacity to consent, usually to surgery; cognitive assessment, for example of oral comprehension or verbal memory which may have a direct bearing on management; or liaison with primary care or specialist neurorehabilitation centres. There is also a role in relation to the emergency and trauma departments where information and advice may be relevant; a number of people may go on to have cognitive problems, sufficient to interfere significantly with work and family life, even after mild head injury (Ponsford *et al.*, 2000). Cognitive assessment and intervention, whether mental health based or neuropsychological, are only part of acute working, and formulation, consultancy, liaison and information-giving are equally important roles.

The Context

Neuropsychologists in the UK working with people following TBI at their first point of contact with services, or soon after, are usually in a hospital-based regional neurosciences centre. These centres bring together specialists such as neurosurgeons, plastic and reconstructive surgeons and neurologists. The TBI work carried out in such units involves emergency investigation or treatment of very sick or at-risk patients. However, given the chronic and continuing lack of acute beds in the UK, resulting from a shortage of nursing staff, many brain-injured patients are never admitted to a specialist centre and have to be managed on trauma or orthopaedic wards at district general hospitals, or have to be discharged back to the referring hospital at the earliest opportunity. In addition, TBI patients who have been involved in road traffic accidents often have multiple complex injuries. This means that the head-injury component can be missed, or at best under-managed, and rehabilitation needs of the patient neglected. The neuropsychologist may have to visit patients at surrounding hospitals, or may lose a patient to follow-up because they are discharged to a different region. This is increasingly common given the current shortage of neuroscience intensive care unit beds in the UK, resulting in patients being taken for neurosurgical management long distances from their local service or the scene of the accident. Different models of care are beginning to be thought about and developed, with potential 'in-reach' support from neuropsychologists working in post-acute specialist regional inpatient neurological rehabilitation centres.

Patients who are admitted to a neurosciences centre for a longer stay are often struggling to come to terms with physical effects of the injury – learning to walk again, for example – and will not have had time to take on board the longer-term cognitive and psychological effects of their condition. The neuropsychologist may work closely with medical and nursing staff during admission but often needs to see the patient again on an out-patient basis when many of the acute medical features have settled and cognitive and emotional changes become much more relevant.

As neurorehabilitation team-working is less developed in the acute setting, considerable energy is required to maintain active lines of communication between specialties, and to ensure that neuropsychology input enhances rather than duplicates the work of colleagues in physiotherapy, speech and language therapy and occupational therapy. Support from these professions can be particularly helpful in mitigating some of the significant obstacles to establishing recommended therapeutic/behavioural interventions on acute medical wards. Introduction of the European Working Time Directive and increased use of agency staff have eroded consistency across shifts, which can impact negatively on implementation of programmes where response consistency is critical. Nursing staff may have limited training and time to invest in therapeutic interventions on the ward and, significantly, may not even see this as part of their remit, so that joined-up working with other professionals allied to medicine is key. In reality, much of the work is about subtly changing the culture and making small incremental adjustments, rather than wholesale introduction of complex behavioural programmes. This may be so particularly where young head-injured people are kept on an acute neurosurgical ward in an inappropriate environment too long, simply because of delays in finding (or funding) a more appropriate placement. Liaison with neurorehabilitation teams both locally and further afield is also key, and it is to be hoped that the emphasis on continuity of care emphasised in the *National Service Framework for Long Term Conditions* (Department of Health, 2005), together with proposed changes in commissioning, will strengthen this.

The patients

Patients can present with TBI at all ages and a good understanding of the developmental or life stage context is always important; however, head injury occurs predominantly in young adults, most commonly males, who may have limited education, an erratic work record and a forensic and/or drug history. Detailed comprehensive assessment needs to take account of any sensory-perceptual disturbance, any problems with movement or posture, any episodes of altered awareness, as well as premorbid medical/psychiatric history and current psychological status. This is important because head injury presents as a complex interplay of cognitive, emotional, behavioural and physical features. These interact with each other and may affect assessment or measurement of any one component. For example, if you are testing a patient's verbal memory by reading them a short paragraph and asking them to tell it back to you and they are suffering from tinnitus (ringing in the ears), then this may affect their attention, making the test less valid as a measure of verbal memory.

A 'whole person' approach to TBI, taking into account the context and significance of the experience, and of any continuing or persisting sequelae, is just as relevant at the acute end of rehabilitation as it is later on in the pathway of care. However, the neuropsychologist may be one of the few clinicians working at this level early on. An example of the relevance of context is illustrated by the case of a young man in his twenties who sustained a severe closed head injury as a van driver incurring a retrograde amnesia (loss of memory for the period immediately preceding the injury) of approximately eight years. During this time he had married his girlfriend and they had had two children. This meant that when his wife came on to the ward to visit him, he saw only a remote and casual partner with whom he had little shared experience, which obviously had massive implications for the rehabilitation process.

Medical context

Trainee psychologists are often surprised by what can seem an intimidating 'Casualty' or 'ER' type of environment in the acute setting, and probably our patients experience something of this too. Neuropsychologists need to be flexible in switching between a medical model, which allows them to communicate rapidly with medical colleagues, and more meaningful and ecologically valid psychological models which may have greater relevance when helping patients and their carers try to make sense of their experiences.

Joint working involves liaison with medical and nursing colleagues rather than the more sophisticated multidisciplinary teamwork which has evolved in post-acute and community rehabilitation settings. Where patients may be intubated and ventilated a crucial role is support of colleagues as well as of the patient's relatives and friends. However experienced and skilled the staff, the work can be stressful and time taken, for example to offer support to neurointensive care unit staff following death of a young head-injured patient, is another important component of the work.

Psychometric test results following head injury, as in any other area of neuropsychology, must be interpreted in the light of parallel investigations. The explosion in imaging techniques over the past 15 years has altered the role of neuropsychology. Computed tomography (CT) involves x-rays and is particularly good at detecting blood (e.g. a blood clot). Magnetic resonance imaging (MRI) exploits the different radio frequency signals produced by the protons in tissue molecules which are first lined up by a powerful magnet and then displaced by radio waves. CT and MRI allow us to look at the structural pathology of the brain-injured person. This means that neuropsychology is no longer so central to localisation of pathology but still crucial for identifying the functional correlates of the underlying brain pathology.

The evidence-base

There is now some clear evidence for the effectiveness of rehabilitation; see the National Institute for Clinical Excellence clinical guidelines on early management of head injury and the national clinical guidelines for *Rehabilitation following acquired brain injury* for helpful reviews (NICE, National Collaborating Centre for Acute Care, 2002; Royal College of Physicians and British Society of Rehabilitation Medicine, 2003; Royal College of Surgeons, 1999). There is also evidence emerging for its cost-effectiveness (Cardenas *et al.*, 2001). Early rehabilitation was found to be more effective in severe head injury in one American study (Cope & Hall, 1982); this retrospectively compared 16 and 20 severely brain-injured matched patients admitted to rehabilitation within one month of the injury versus more than a month after the injury. Patients admitted 35 days or more after injury required twice as much (multidisciplinary) acute rehabilitation even though both groups were comparable in initial disability and in outcome at two years.

Overall, the exact parameters of 'early' in the literature often vary, and there remains a need for more work to partial out the efficacy of neuropsychological/

cognitive rehabilitation within the acute setting. In general, TBI rehabilitation focuses on intervention in the areas of cognition, behaviour and social integration, and is therefore less amenable to rigorous scientific methods. Studies comparing functional outcomes in those given relatively early rehabilitation versus those not given rehabilitation are methodologically difficult but not impossible. Some studies that have been carried out are difficult to compare as they vary in so many parameters, including: pre-injury characteristics, site and severity of brain damage, time of injury to treatment, paradigm for matching, outcome measures, length/type/intensiveness of rehabilitation, etc. There is also, as elsewhere in the scientific literature, a practice of reporting only positive findings, and negative or equivocal results often do not emerge in the literature. Methodologically sound empirical research is obviously critical to advances in rehabilitation; Levine and Downey-Lamb (2002) have proposed a range of possible paradigms, and the role of meta-analysis is likely to be key.

Hall and Cope (1995) have subsequently reviewed two intensive care unit/trauma rehabilitation studies and seven acute rehabilitation programmes. There are certainly data from credible if limited studies in the USA which demonstrate that, when matched for initial severity of injury, those coming early to rehabilitation stay a significantly shorter number of days and are functioning significantly better (according to Disability Rating Score) than those admitted later, both at discharge and at two-year follow-up. In general, there are significantly demonstrable gains on functional measures after treatment, but not on cognitive measures. The over-arching conclusion of their review is that sufficient reliable and valid data do not yet exist to enable us to answer the question 'Does rehabilitation *really* work?', but that current evidence of the benefit of early rehabilitation, if not compelling, is at least indicative of a positive trend and worthy of future targeted research and audit.

The evidence-base for the more post-acute neuropsychological rehabilitation which may be carried out within an acute neurosciences centre, including in the domains of attention, memory, executive function and self-awareness and in relation to social and behavioural problems, is discussed in detail elsewhere (e.g. Ponsford, 2004). Evidence-based reviews of cognitive rehabilitation suggest that some of the most effective interventions are ameliorative or compensatory, such as training in the use of a memory notebook or in an external paging system such as *NeuroPage* (Cicerone *et al.*, 2000; Wilson *et al.*, 1997). Because of problems patients have in generalising skills, long-term gains have been demonstrated to require a focus on the real world and on skills normally performed by the person in everyday life (Seale *et al.* 2002).

In-patient Working

Identification and management of post-traumatic amnesia

The severity and length of impairment of consciousness is a critical indicator of the severity of injury. Following more severe head injury a person can be in coma for days, weeks or even months with reduced behavioural responsiveness to outside stimuli and internal drives. Following more mild head injury there may be only transient loss of consciousness followed by a period of 'concussion' with clouding of consciousness when the person is confused and disorientated for a time and subsequently has little or no recall of events from this period. This period of disruption of attentional and memory processes, including duration of loss of consciousness, until reinstatement of continuous day-to-day memory is termed *post-traumatic amnesia* (PTA) and is one of the best biological markers of severity of brain injury.

In practice, the neuropsychologist in a pressed neurosciences centre may not be involved with patients in coma or in that no man's land of wakeful unresponsiveness, persistent vegetative state. Indeed the evidence for acceleration of arousal or awareness via sensory stimulation programmes remains at best equivocal. However, there is a role for education and support of families at this time.

More pragmatically, the psychologist may need to be involved with patients still in PTA. PTA is obviously best assessed prospectively rather than retrospectively and there are various standardised instruments available (see Forrester *et al.*, 1994 for a review). At a very practical level, simply having familiarity with the phenomenon of PTA, and taking the time to assess *day-to-day* memory, can be enormously helpful when continuity of care is often unavoidably fragmented. Some junior medical staff are not aware that a patient in PTA may speak to them sensibly and appear perfectly lucid, yet be completely unable to recognise them the following day and have no recollection of what was said. Relatives, too, can be disconcerted and distressed when their loved one berates them for leaving them 'to rot in this bed', as one patient described it, when the family have in fact visited every day.

The key principles of managing a patient in PTA are essentially creating a safe but flexible environment, reducing stimulation, and gently working towards enhanced orientation (see Ponsford, 1995). Consistency, regular reassurance and avoiding making any early prognosis about recovery are also important components. This may naturally shade into management of the amnesic patient, once out of PTA. An orientation board, a visitors' book, a brief written statement of what has happened to preclude repetitive questioning, can all continue to be helpful.

Behavioural management

Agitation, disinhibition, wandering and other such behaviours are all common early features following significant TBI and are best managed with a combination of restructuring of the environment and application of basic behavioural principles via an 'antecedents/behaviour/consequences' analysis. Again, seeing one's loved one pulling out their tubes or swearing quite out of character can be upsetting for relatives. Education and explanation about these behaviours reflecting the person's reduced control over their own actions and being best ignored at this stage can be helpful. In practice, neurosciences nurses are in the main extremely experienced and skilled in managing such complex behaviours. The neuropsychologist is therefore usually only involved when the behaviour is disruptive and more difficult to ignore, or where the cognitive effects are contributing to the picture.

The following case highlights a number of the difficulties of acute neuropsychological rehabilitation. Namely, the fact that many of the people sustaining traumatic brain injury are by definition of no fixed address and lacking in appropriate social and physical networks of support. A forensic context of one kind or another is not unusual. There are often problems of co-existing sensory-perceptual disturbance or motor deficits, and/or cultural, social and educational constraints on psychometric assessment, which may require an intelligent case-by-case approach. It is often too early in the pathway of care for the patient to be able to take on board the full implications of the injury which they have sustained. Much of the work is therefore focused on ensuring that those caring for them, be they families or services, have a full awareness of the potential implications so that these can be monitored and appropriate intervention is sought and accessed as it becomes more relevant. The case also highlights the potentially distressing nature of the work, when often there are very real concerns about the social circumstances to which the, now highly vulnerable, brain-injured person is being required to return, and there is often very little the neuropsychologist can do about this harsh reality.

Case 2.1

Background

A 29-year-old man was referred by the trauma team three weeks after a serious head injury. He had fallen from a perimeter fence while attempting to escape from a detention centre for illegal immigrants. He was found unconscious and had sustained an open skull fracture. On arrival at a local district general hospital he was distressed, aggressive, vocal, and was bleeding from his right ear and had additional CSF leakage. A CT brain scan revealed a depressed left frontal skull fracture and an extra-dural haematoma (blood clot). He had a base of skull fracture along with various facial and vertebral fractures. He was transferred to the neurosciences centre and underwent neurosurgery in the early hours of the morning to elevate the depressed skull fracture and to evacuate the haematoma via a craniotomy (skull flap), and a right frontal intra-cranial pressure monitor was inserted. It was thought that he had lost the sight in his right eye and had impaired hearing in his right ear as a result of the head injury.

The reason for referral to neuropsychology was complex. In essence it was twofold. First, it reflected good practice in seeking to implement appropriate early assessment and management of a severe head injury. However, second, it was aimed at establishing the extent to which it was appropriate or ethical to discharge the patient, essentially back to custody. The trauma ward was, as usual, desperate for the bed; but there were concerns about the patient's capacity to understand and consent to the likely sequence of events.

It was not possible to obtain an accurate assessment of length of PTA as the patient was unable to detail his last memory before the accident nor when his memory subsequently became continuous. However, duration of loss of consciousness and evidence of skull fracture were sufficient to indicate that he had sustained a significant head injury.

Clinical presentation

The neuropsychologist first involved an Urdu translator and interpreter. This made it possible to establish that the patient was no longer in PTA as he had recall of events over the preceding days and weeks.

The patient presented as a shy and diffident man whose English was very limited. He was unable to give much of a history but a few essential details were elicited with the assistance of the interpreter. He had arrived in the UK four years earlier and had been unemployed during his stay in England. He came from the Punjab in India where he had worked as an agricultural labourer. He had left school at the age of nine and was illiterate in both Punjabi and English. He learned English only on coming to the UK. He stated that his family had been involved in a dispute with the police and he had been beaten up and his brother had been arrested and remained in prison. As an illegal immigrant, he feared deportation and believed he would suffer further physical abuse and possible imprisonment if he returned home.

Neuropsychological assessment

It was not possible to estimate premorbid intellectual function.

Current non-verbal intellectual functioning was assessed using Raven's Coloured Matrices as broadly 'average'. This test is considered to be relatively culturally fair and performance indicated unimpaired visuo-spatial function and non-verbal reasoning abilities.

He scored poorly on the Galveston Orientation and Amnesia Test, incorrectly giving his age, the day, date and month of the year. He was unable to talk about any important item of recent news.

Assessment of verbal memory was not possible owing to his limited English. However, on a short test of visual recognition memory his score was unimpaired, although this test had a low ceiling. His copy of a complex geometric figure was 'unscorable', as

Continued

were his immediate and delayed recall reproductions; this was thought to be due to his unfamiliarity with use of a paper-and-pencil task rather than to a specific memory or visuo-constructive deficits *per se*. Similarly, his reproduction of geometric shapes (revised Weschler Memory Scale) after a three-minute delay scored at below the first percentile.

On a simple naming test he was able to identify correctly the names of common objects.

On two categorical fluency tests (presented and performed in Punjabi) he scored at below the tenth percentile, and in describing a picture he was able to name only three features, but according to his interpreter, his spontaneous speech was fluent and error-free.

He was able to perform simple mental arithmetic correctly.

He made no errors on a 'go'/'no go' tapping task; this suggested no gross motor disinhibition.

Assessment was therefore severely constrained by the patient's limited English, low level of education and literacy, impaired vision and hearing and the forensic context of the situation. One can only guess at the likely levels of depression and anxiety given his situation; he admitted to being scared about being deported and the neuropsychologist felt that the extent to which he cooperated during assessment was questionable. Testing essentially made it possible to establish that he was out of post-traumatic amnesia, that his visual recognition memory and non-verbal reasoning were relatively unimpaired, that he was able to perform simple mental arithmetic and that his speech in Punjabi was fluent at interview.

Formulation and issues

Notwithstanding the restricted findings of the assessment, the neuropsychologist felt it reasonable to conclude that the patient had sustained a severe head injury from which some neurobehavioural sequelae would usually be expected. These might, for example, include problems with verbal expression, attention, memory and *possibly the appropriate self-regulation of behaviour*; but, for the contextual reasons mentioned, it could not be confirmed that these sequelae were present in this particular case.

An attempt was made to establish rapport with the patient with the aim of reducing anxiety and giving him a better understanding of his situation. However, he was really too frightened for this to be possible and instead access to a translator was set up to allow him to express his needs and be kept informed about his circumstances. Explanation and liaison both with the trauma ward and the detention centre were organised.

A second case highlights difficulties around the short time in which a patient remains in the acute setting and the need for focused work, including differential diagnosis and formulation, which does not render the patient inappropriately dependent but which allows referral on to local services, precluding the risk of loss to follow-up.

Case 2.2

Background

A 17-year-old girl was referred having sustained a significant head injury one week earlier. She had been a rear passenger on a joyriding motorbike. She had not been wearing a helmet and had been drinking. She had had a Glasgow Coma Scale (GCS) score of 3/15 at the scene of the accident and of 9/15 on arrival at the emergency department. This scale measures three aspects of consciousness, eye opening, verbal response and responsiveness of the body (e.g. to pain), and is often summarised as a score with a maximum of 15 (normal consciousness) and a minimum of 3 (severe coma). She had been seriously agitated and a general anaesthetic was required in order to do a routine CT brain scan. Scanning revealed a small extra-dural haematoma (clot) on the right side and she was transferred from her district general hospital to the neurosciences centre for evacuation of this. In addition she required fixation of a thoracic spine fracture.

Assessment and formulation

Referral was prompted by the patient's withdrawn and 'uncooperative' behaviour on the ward.

The neuropsychologist visited the patient twice a day over a period of a week in which time a supportive relationship was established in which the patient could express her distress appropriately and discuss more widely the difficulties in her life, including excess alcohol use and family conflicts. Relaxation and distraction techniques were also introduced to help her manage her panic attacks. At the time of admission she was living in a hostel having become estranged from her single-parent mother.

The patient felt the need to talk about intense feelings related to the belief that she was ugly, suggesting issues of low self-esteem. The neuropsychologist felt she had difficulty recognising, articulating and coping with these painful feelings and tended to cope by seeking external relief or escape, for example through alcohol or by

Continued

contemplating suicide. Much of the cognitive work focused on helping the patient recognise that these strategies left her difficulties largely unaddressed and created further problems for her, including the risk-taking behaviour such as that which had led to her accident.

Recommendations and issues

It was felt that, to some extent as a result of the 'crisis' of the road traffic accident, the patient was now highly motivated to deal with her emotional difficulties and alcohol use, though somewhat unhopeful about tackling them which needed to be addressed in any psychology therapy. Management therefore revolved around appropriate referral on to local mental health services to set up the therapy required to help her develop new emotional coping strategies in the context of managing her alcohol use and the underlying psychological issues.

Neuropsychological assessment

One might think that early psychometric assessment would be extremely valuable in helping predict recovery and plan management. However, in practice this is rarely the case (except in cases of mild head injury which are usually not admitted for any appreciable length of time). There are a number of reasons for this. Early post-trauma the cognitive picture may be changing very rapidly. Patients fatigue quickly and are often simply not well enough to generate valid and reliable test results. They may also still lack insight into any cognitive changes and pursuing this angle when they are struggling to come to terms with the physical and emotional sequelae can be unhelpful and feel slightly persecutory.

This is not to say that cognitive assessment is ruled out. It can sometimes be crucial to obtain a functional level of verbal memory or attention, or to check for a receptive language deficit, for example, which can result from a focal injury and where a deficit can be missed yet have a critical bearing on management. But, in general, testing is best kept to a minimum until the medical status is more stable (see below). What is appropriate is some documentation of status, and particularly estimated duration of PTA, and liaison on to the next point of care, hospital, neurorehabilitation centre or general practitioner, to try to ensure that the momentum for rehabilitation is maintained and referral back as an out-patient does actually happen if appropriate.

Out-patient Working

Out-patients seen at the acute end are essentially the 'walking wounded', that is the mild head-injury patient with a post-concussional syndrome which is taking time to resolve, or the moderately severe patient, perhaps where the cognitive sequelae are more disabling than was initially recognised, or where there are anger management issues. Such patients may be referred back by neurosurgeons, neurologists, trauma surgeons, psychiatrists and others, usually where the cognitive or emotional problem has only emerged late on, perhaps two to five or more years later.

The more severe cases with multiple disability are obviously best rehabilitated in a specialist regional in-patient neurological rehabilitation centre, or in a specialist centre in the independent sector for people with severe behavioural problems. This is because the scope at the acute end for shared work with other staff involved in the overall rehabilitation process is very limited. Hospital-based physiotherapy, occupational therapy (OT) and speech and language therapy (SALT) services have a limited remit to see out-patients. The neuropsychologist's role therefore tends towards that of case manager, and ingenuity is needed in tracking down other avenues of potential support local to the patient, such as a Job Centre-based work psychologist or colleagues in mental health. Medico-legal requests for assessment of severe cases of TBI pursuing compensation via a personal injury claim are often made of neuropsychologists at the acute end. Even in this non-clinical role there can be value in appropriate treatment or support recommendations, which may enable the person to obtain the required funding via their compensation claim.

The following case highlights two points relevant to rehabilitation in the acute setting. First, that the patient's recognition of how they may have changed since the head injury is two-thirds of the battle. Acknowledgement of, and adjustment to, what are effectively changes in the very core of one's being can be a painful and difficult process and certainly does not happen overnight. However, it is only when any changes have been recognised that the way is opened up for support and attempts at managing the change. Emotional support for the patient in building a new positive self-image is a central role for the neuropsychologist. Second, the fact is that rehabilitation is a very incomplete science. The neuropsychologist often feels helpless and impotent in the face of what may be very subtle but tangible impairments. Dysexecutive problems which undermine self-organisation may erode the patient's capacity to manage virtually every area of their life. Rehabilitation strategies do not generalise and therefore intervention is often necessarily limited by achieving only a handful of practical day-to-day solutions which the patient is unable to generalise.

Case 2.3

Background

A 31-year-old right-handed physiotherapist was referred with cognitive and emotional difficulties following a road traffic accident one year earlier.

There was no significant retrograde amnesia. She was cycling home from work when she was hit by a car. She was not wearing

Continued

a helmet and she was found by a passer-by at the roadside and admitted to a local hospital, confused and drowsy. During this time, she thought she could recall 'talking rubbish' and experiencing vomiting and headache. A CT brain scan was reported as showing no intracranial lesion and she was mobilised and discharged from hospital three days later. The Glasgow Coma Scale score was recorded as 13/15 for 48 hours. The severity of the head injury was unclear from her account. She believed that she was unconscious for about 15 minutes and the neuropsychologist inferred from the medical records and the account of her fiancé that the duration of post-traumatic amnesia was about 30 minutes, indicating that she had sustained a mild head injury.

She had been referred to a local neuropsychologist in the north of England in relation to her cognitive difficulties. However, she had been too distressed to complete any psychometric tests, although she had been seen for support and advice on a number of occasions. Following the road traffic accident, she had given up her job, as she planned to move to the south where her partner had begun work, and started a new job herself, again as a physiotherapist.

Clinical presentation

The patient complained of memory problems and excessive tiredness. Socially, she found it hard to be in a group and disliked noise. She was waking early in the mornings and worrying. She was inclined to be more weepy and irritable and had hit her partner on one occasion. She was no longer cycling and experienced considerable anxiety when driving, particularly when she observed a bicycle. She also reported some degree of word-finding difficulties. She denied any significant sensory-perceptual disturbance, motor deficit or any change in appetite but had experienced a decrease in libido and mildly disturbed sleep.

She was currently preparing for her wedding in Australia. She had little social support in the UK, apart from her fiancé. She clearly did not expect to be suffering any symptoms at this stage and had actually thought that she would be back at work a week after the accident, and throughout the year had been amazed that she was still having problems. During assessment she got extremely tired and was unable to complete the test. Her performance on the tests also distressed her.

Neuropsychological assessment

Overall performance on the Wechsler Adult Intelligence Scale III (WIAS-III) was mildly impaired against a background estimate of premorbid verbal ability in the 'average' range. The more crystallised verbal abilities were generally intact, with a decrease in attention and a very significant fall-off in processing speed.

Verbal and non-verbal anterograde memory scores were very severely impaired (2–3 standard deviations below the expected level). She could recall very little of a short story immediately after hearing it and did not retain the information over a 30-minute delay. Similarly, her performance on a list learning task was extremely poor. Immediate and delayed recall of complex geometric material was below the first percentile. Verbal fluency scores were significantly compromised in both category and initial letter paradigms.

Management and issues

Assessment after a putative mild closed head injury sustained in a road traffic accident had therefore revealed significant cognitive sequelae, reduced stamina and generalised anxiety. Although the neuropsychologist considered the test results as slightly unreliable because of fatigue, on the basis of test performance it was not thought surprising that the patient was experiencing day-to-day problems and had in fact done extremely well to return to work. The significant discrepancy between the history taken and the patient's current cognitive profile suggested that either she had sustained a more severe injury than was at first apparent, or the test results could not be considered a true reflection of her cognitive abilities in that her performance was being exacerbated by current functional and post-concussional factors. The most salient problem was a surprising lack of insight into the consequences of head injury on the part of the patient, almost to the point of denial. There was concern that what at first appeared as a stoical approach was in fact denial, undermining her recovery and adjustment needs.

Intervention was via six two-monthly appointments over the next year which took a very pragmatic approach. Information about recovery from head injury and anxiety reduction was targeted at specific examples from daily life recorded by the patient in a homework diary. Practical strategies for managing persisting difficulties were generated and discussed at sessions, implemented and then reviewed at the next session. In parallel with this work, the neuropsychologist sought to help the patient gradually

Continued

acknowledge and begin to adjust to what began to emerge as persisting changes in cognitive capacity and emotional response following the head injury. With the patient's permission, work also involved her fiancé and her line manager at work. Following the intervention, there were measurable gains in scores on a range of questionnaire measures; a reduction in recorded incidents of panic or some degree of episodic dyscontrol; and subjectively improved self-confidence and mastery in organising and managing herself both at work and in her home life. The gains, however, were limited, and the neuropsychologist remained concerned about the long-term viability of the marriage given that the patient's partner perceived her to be very different from the young woman to whom he had become engaged. Her capacity to work effectively and derive enjoyment and self-esteem from her job were also precarious. Difficulties at work were largely masked by the fact that she worked in the private sector in a setting where recruitment and retention was a problem and supervision and monitoring of her work were less than robust, yet a move to a different work environment might well have exposed the impairments which she was continuing to experience.

Neuropsychological assessment

The value of cognitive assessment is much more evident at this slightly later stage. It provides a means of relatively objective measurement of the person's impairments following TBI. An important part of the process can be the recognition that testing may or may not give the person insight into the fact that some of their mental faculties are not the same as they previously were. Crystallising out the areas of strength and weakness can contribute to understanding of difficulties occurring in daily living and can help generate appropriate management strategies.

As a result of diffuse axonal injury and the shearing effects of acceleration/deceleration forces giving rise to focal frontal and temporal damage, closed head injury tends to result in a characteristic array of cognitive impairments. These include problems with attention, learning and memory, reduced speed of information processing, restricted word fluency and executive deficits.

Executive function, which encompasses initiation, planning, self-monitoring, flexibility and goal-directed behaviour, may be difficult to assess exclusively by psychometric testing. In the test situation, the examiner is acting to some extent as the person's frontal lobes and problems of initiation, impulsivity and on-line processing may be less readily apparent. But as in any area of neuropsychological testing, collateral interview with a relative or friend from before the accident is an important adjunct to testing.

Recent work examining the nature of verbal memory deficits in people who have sustained a traumatic brain injury, compared to healthy controls, is consistent with impaired consolidation as the *primary* underlying memory impairment, rather than encoding or retrieval deficits (Vanderploeg *et al.*, 2001).

The universal general principles of psychometric assessment apply as in any other area of skilled neuropsychological testing, including a comprehensive clinical screening interview with review of past medical/psychiatric history and exclusion of any DSM-IV Axis 1 diagnoses, estimation of premorbid intellectual status, standardised sampling of a range of cognitive domains, and development and maintenance of rapport to preserve the patient's dignity and extract the maximum amount of information from the minimum of testing. A standardised battery of tests can be administered, but most neuropsychologists adopt a more flexible approach (Goldstein & McNeil, 2004), often using certain core tests plus other tests sampling specific cognitive domains as and when appropriate. The full written report should appropriately convey the clinical problem and its context, together with detailed description of the test results and findings and their interpretation, with a clear distinction between fact and observation and inference and interpretation. In relation to rehabilitation, the report can appropriately serve as a form of contract between the patient, their family or carers and the neuropsychologist, and so a goal-setting model may be helpful.

Interventions

Rehabilitative interventions in the acute setting can be tantalising and frustrating because a specialist tertiary neuroscience centre may serve a population of two to three million, many of whom live some distance away. Interventions are generally either neuropsychological rehabilitative procedures, or cognitive or behavioural treatments derived from mental health work.

Pragmatically, neuropsychological rehabilitative strategies tend to focus on palliative coping techniques (such as use of a watch with an alarm or digital display, sticky-backed notes, a diary, Filofax or personal organiser, routine) rather than on cognitive retraining. In truth, the evidence-base for both approaches remains less than robust. There are relatively few studies of *acute* rehabilitation, and those that exist are confounded by poor population definition and methodological limitations. Clinical experience bears out that subtle executive deficits can be crippling and undermine the capacity for retraining to generalise to other everyday situations.

The few studies which address the treatment of mild TBI all recognise the significance of emotional factors in recovery and emphasise the reduction of anxiety as a salient element in any intervention protocol (see King, 1997 for a review). For mild to moderate TBI, education and the reduction of anxiety are the most important components of treatments for patients suffering from post-concussional syndrome (PCS). PCS consists of an array of relatively minor but exceedingly troublesome and sometimes frightening symptoms, including some or all of the following: headache, dizziness, reduced tolerance to noise or light, tinnitus, visual disturbance, restlessness, insomnia, reduced speed of information processing, concentration and memory problems, fatigue, irritability, anxiety and depression. In many cases these symptoms resolve spontaneously over days or weeks. In some instances, however, the symptoms persist for months. Two recent large randomised controlled trials investigated whether providing early specialist follow-up for primarily mild and moderate head-injured patients affected outcome at six months post-injury. Results indicated that both social morbidity and severity of PCS were significantly reduced by predominantly psychological interventions in all but very minor head-injured patients (Wade *et al.*, 1997, 1998).

Not infrequently in acute clinical practice, one sees patients whose PCS symptoms persist beyond what would be expected given the known parameters of the severity of the TBI. Such cases are often extremely complex and interesting, and require skilled clinical acumen to fathom out and treat the aetiology. In essence, some of these cases represent more severe brain injury than may have at first been apparent – and certainly a CT brain scan reported as normal does not preclude subtle traumatic pathology. More often, the PCS symptoms are being maintained by a complex interaction with pre-existing psychological problems which have not previously been addressed and for which the brain injury somehow becomes a 'sounding board' (Lishman, 1988).

The final case illustrates that in clinical practice most cases are much more complex than the textbooks would lead you to believe. Management often requires a sensitive application of specialist neuropsychological skills together with more generic mental health skills and creative exploitation of the best available patient access to appropriate help.

Case 2.4

Background

A 26-year-old bank employee was referred nine months after a fall down a flight of stairs in her home for assessment of continuing problems with memory and concentration.

The exact circumstances of the fall were unclear as it was unwitnessed. It occurred late at night and it was thought that she had either slipped or had possibly been drinking which had affected her balance. Her housemate had heard the noise and found her at the bottom of the stairs. Duration of loss of consciousness was thought to be only transitory. She had headache and neck stiffness and vomited and was therefore taken to the local emergency department by her housemate. There were no neurological signs on assessment and she was kept for observation for the rest of the night and discharged the following morning.

She subsequently returned to the emergency department three weeks later with continuing concern about headache and a CT brain scan was performed which was reported as normal. In view of her continuing concerns she was referred by the duty consultant to a consultant neurosurgeon in the neurosciences centre. She was subsequently referred to neuropsychology for a routine out-patient appointment for assessment of memory and attentional problems, now some nine months post-head-injury.

Clinical presentation and assessment

The patient gave a very clear account of the sequence of events and subsequent problems experienced, which included a range of post-concussional symptoms, including headache, increased tiredness, irritability, reduced tolerance to noise, restlessness and disturbed sleep, concentration and memory problems, and anxiety.

Psychometric assessment revealed a generally good cognitive outcome with preserved intellectual function within the 'average' range on the WAIS-III and on tests of anterograde memory function, including story recall and list learning from the Adult Memory and Information Processing Battery, the Ray complex figure test and tests of category and phonemic verbal fluency. Virtually all tests were commensurate with age and estimated premorbid verbal calibre on the basis of current single word reading (National Adult Reading Test) and educational and occupational history. The only exceptions were mildly reduced performance on the digit symbol subtest of the WAIS-III and reversed digit span, suggesting mildly compromised auditory verbal 'working' memory.

More salient, however, than any cognitive sequelae from the head injury was a remote and emotionally brittle clinical presentation. Comprehensive clinical interview to provide the background and context for psychometric assessment routinely asked about significant life stressors in the preceding 12 months. Despite an extremely reticent account of past medical and psychiatry history, a recent overdose attempt was dropped into the interview as a recent life event. The context, motivation and psychological status resulting in this behaviour then obviously had to be explored. This essentially revealed a chronic post-traumatic stress disorder with all the cardinal features of hyperarousal, avoidance, intrusive imagery and emotional numbness, attaining a DSM-IV Axis 1 diagnosis, related to a violent sexual assault and rape while she had been on holiday with her parents several years earlier.

Psychological intervention and issues

Intervention was therefore aimed at treatment of the core post-traumatic stress disorder over a series of 10 weekly sessions. For the neuropsychologist in the acute setting, there is always a judgement

Continued

call about the appropriateness and cost-effectiveness of what might be deemed more generic mental health work. However, in this case, the neuropsychologist felt that treatment of the PTSD within a neurosciences context was appropriate, for two reasons. First, patients with PTSD are often highly resistant to speaking about the core trauma and engaging with treatment and, when the sufficient therapeutic trust and rapport have been established and the patient is motivated to begin to address the avoided issues, it does not seem appropriate to refer the patient elsewhere where they may go back to the bottom of a long waiting list. Second, in this case, the neuropsychologist felt that there might also be issues in relation to teasing out the symptoms arising from the PTSD from any sequelae of mild head injury.

In retrospect, this may not have been the correct decision in that the case turned out to be an extremely complex one in which the rape was in fact a sounding board for a core type II trauma of abuse in childhood. In the event, limited gains were attained, certainly in reducing the general level of anxiety and managing the suicidal behaviour. The post-concussional symptoms largely resolved and referral on to a specialist psychological service for abuse was organised, with work in the acute setting effectively acting as a holding operation until space became available within the specialist department.

Summary

Neuropsychological rehabilitation in the acute setting poses many of the same challenges as work in the post-acute and community settings. However, there are some important differences. The highly technical and medicalised context makes a shift in focus from the physical to the psychological perspective more difficult to achieve. Input needs to be flexible because of the heterogeneity and complexity of the client group. Early on, TBI patients are less ready to take on board the cognitive, emotional and behavioural consequences of their injury. Sensitive, measured early education of the family and loved ones may be equally important, particularly in helping to facilitate taking the long view: rehabilitation is a lifelong process. Generic clinical psychological skills derived from mental health working are necessary to complement specialist neuropsychological skills; and providing emotional support to enable the rebuilding of positive self-image is a central theme. Joint working is less highly developed in the acute setting and the neuropsychological input tends to be more 'stand alone', with liaison on to local services wherever they exist. Continually working to change the culture towards an ongoing focus on enabling and rehabilitating is essential. Much of the evidence for the efficacy of education and anxiety reduction in the acute stage is relatively robust, but further work is needed to elucidate other key components of *acute* neuropsychological rehabilitation which may contribute to enhanced long-term outcome.

Recommended Reading

McMillan, T.M. (2003). Neurorehabilitation services and their delivery. In B.A. Wilson (Ed.) *Neuropsychological rehabilitation: Theory and practice.* Abingdon: Swets and Zeitlinger.
A helpful summary chapter on the UK epidemiology and organisation of service delivery.

Ponsford, J. (Ed.) (2004). *Cognitive and behavioural rehabilitation: From neurobiology to clinical practice.* New York: The Guilford Press.
A comprehensive recent summary of the evidence base for rehabilitation organised by cognitive domain.

Turner-Stokes, L. & Wade, D. (2004). Rehabilitation following acquired brain injury: Concise guidance. *Clinical Medicine*, *4*(1), 61–65.
As the title suggests, this is a succinct summary of relevant recent BSRM guidance.

Wilson, B.A., Herbert, C.M. & Shiel, A. (2003). *Behavioural approaches in neuropsychological rehabilitation: Optimising rehabilitation procedures.* Hove: Psychology Press.
A helpful description of flexible and pragmatic techniques for remediation at all stages of the care pathway.

References

British Psychological Society Division of Neuropsychology (BPS DoN) (2005). *Clinical neuropsychology and rehabilitation services for adults with acquired brain injury.* Leicester: BPS.

Cardenas, D.D., Haselkorn, J.K., McElligott, J.M. & Gnatz, S.M. (2001). A bibliography of cost-effectiveness practices in physical medicine and rehabilitation: AAPM&R white paper. *Archives of Physical Medicine and Rehabilitation*, *82*(5), 711–719.

Cicerone, K.D., Dahlberg, C., Kalmar, K., Langenbahn, D.M., Malec, J.F., Bergquist, T., *et al.* (2000). Evidence-based cognitive rehabilitation: Recommendations for clinical practice. *Archives of Physical Medicine and Rehabilitation*, *68*, 111–115.

Cope, N. & Hall, K. (1982). Head injury rehabilitation: Benefits of early intervention. *Archives of Physical Medicine and Rehabilitation*, *63*, 433–437.

Department of Health (2005). *The national service framework for long-term conditions.* London: Department of Health.

Forrester, G., Encel, J. & Gefen, G. (1994). Measuring post-traumatic (PTA): An historical review. *Brain Injury*, *8*(2), 175–184.

Goldstein, L.H. & McNeil, J.E. (2004) *Clinical neuropsychology: A practical guide to assessment and management for clinicians.* Chichester: Wiley.

Hall, K.M. & Cope, D.N. (1995). The benefit of rehabilitation in traumatic brain injury: A literature review. *Journal of Head Trauma Rehabilitation*, *10*(1), 1–13.

King, N. (1997). Mild head injury: Neuropathology, sequelae, measurement and recovery. *British Journal of Clinical Psychology*, *36*, 161–184.

Levine, B. & Downey-Lamb, M.M. (2002). In P.J. Eslinger (Ed.) *Neuropsychological interventions: Clinical research and practice.* New York: The Guilford Press.

Lishman, W.A. (1988). Physiogenesis and psychogenesis in the 'post-concussional syndrome'. *British Journal of Psychiatry*, *153*, 460–469.

National Institute of Clinical Excellence (NICE) (2002). *Head injury: Assessment, investigation and early management of head injury in children and adult*. London: NICE.

Ponsford, J. (1995). *Traumatic brain injury: Rehabilitation for everyday adaptive living*. Hove: Psychology Press.

Ponsford, J. (Ed.) (2004). *Cognitive and behavioural rehabilitation: From neurobiology to clinical practice*. New York: The Guilford Press.

Ponsford, J., Willmott, C., Rothwell, A., Cameron, P., Kelly, A.M., Nelms, R., *et al.* (2000). Factors influencing outcome following mild traumatic brain injury in adults. *Journal of the International Neuropsychological Society*, *6*(5), 568–579.

Royal College of Physicians and British Society of Rehabilitation Medicine (2003). *Rehabilitation following acquired brain injury: National clinical guideline*. London: RCP, BSRM.

Royal College of Surgeons (1999). *Management of patients with head injuries. Report of a Working Party*. London: Royal College of Surgeons.

Seale, G.S., Caroselli, J.S., High, W.M. Jr., Becker, C.L., Neese, L.E., & Scheibel, R. (2002). Use of community integration questionnaire (CIQ) to characterize changes in functioning for individuals with traumatic brain injury who participated in a post-acute rehabilitation program. *Brain Injury*, *16*(11), 955–967.

Tennant, A. (2005). Admission to hospital following head injury in England: Incidence and socio-economic status. *BMC Public Health*. Retrieved 2 May 2007 from www.biomedcentral.com/1471–2458/5/21

Wade, D.T., Crawford, S., Wenden, F.J., King, N.S. & Moss, N.E.G. (1997). Does routine follow-up after head injury help? A randomized controlled trial. *Journal of Neurology, Neurosurgery and Psychiatry*, *62*, 478–484.

Wade, D.T., King, N.S., Wenden, F.J., Crawford, S. & Caldwell, F.E. (1998). Routine follow-up after head injury: A second randomized controlled trial. *British Medical Journal*, *65*, 177–183.

Wilson, B.A., Evans, J.J., Emslie, H. & Malinek, V. (1997). Evaluation of NeuroPage: A new memory aid. *Journal of Neurology, Neurosurgery and Psychiatry*, *63*, 113–115.

Vanderploeg, R.D., Crowell, T.A. & Curtiss, G. (2001). Verbal learning and memory deficits in traumatic brain injury: Encoding, consolidation and retrieval. *Journal of Clinical and Experimental Neuropsychology*, *23*(2), 185–195.

3

Post-acute In-patient Rehabilitation

Joanna Collicutt McGrath

Specific Aspects of This Situation

There are general principles of traumatic brain injury rehabilitation that apply across all settings and at all points in the history of the process. However, there are also some very specific considerations which arise from the context in which rehabilitation is delivered. This chapter is devoted to the practice of traumatic brain injury rehabilitation in an in-patient setting, where the patients have acquired their injuries relatively recently. These types of settings can range from highly specialist behavioural units for clients with very challenging behaviours through to small generic units attached to acute hospitals. Patients often progress from an acute hospital setting to an in-patient rehabilitation centre before receiving out-patient interventions, and finally long-term community rehabilitation.

This chapter will begin by noting some of the factors that distinguish this situation from acute hospital and long-term community or out-patient rehabilitation:

- It is likely that the onset of injury is relatively recent.
- It is likely that the brain injury is severe.
- There may be ongoing medical complications.
- There may be associated orthopaedic or soft tissue injuries.
- Rehabilitation is delivered by a multidisciplinary team of broad composition.
- The staff–patient ratio is relatively high.
- Treatment may be intense, and high demands are made of the patient.
- The rehabilitation unit is likely to be a regional specialist centre, which may be distant from the patient's home.

The *recency of the brain injury* may mean that the patient arrives at the unit still in, or only just beginning to emerge from, post-traumatic amnesia (PTA). Where the injury is severe this is a likely scenario even if transfer from the acute hospital occurs weeks or even months after the injury. As the patient emerges from PTA he or she has to make sense of an entirely novel situation. Where PTA has been of long duration the subjective situation of the patient effectively lags behind that of the professionals and, more importantly, family and friends. The patient may be expressing surprise, fear and shock on initially learning what has happened (the details of which he or she will only ever know from the accounts of others), whereas the family may already be experiencing a degree of grief and loss as they realise the implication of what has happened.

A person is said to have emerged from PTA when there is evidence that normal continuous memory has resumed. In fact, the clinical assessment of PTA presents something of a challenge. This is particularly so if the patient has been in PTA for an extensive period, raising the question of the distinction between prolonged PTA and a more permanent very severe memory impairment (Wilson *et al.*, 1999), or if the patient has problems with expressive language or comprehension of verbal material. Useful assessment tools include the Galveston Orientation and Amnesia Test (GOAT; Levin *et al.*, 1979); a visual recognition procedure (Fortuny *et al.*, 1980) which is useful for patients with limited speech and language skills; and the Wessex Head Injury Matrix (WHIM; Shiel *et al.*, 2000).

Approaches to managing patients in PTA will be discussed later in this chapter.

Of course, some patients may have emerged from PTA well before their admission to the rehabilitation unit. Nevertheless, the relative recency of their injury will mean that they too are dealing with a novel situation, and will be passing through a phase of rapid change and recovery of function. The unprecedented nature of the experience and the pace of change involved make their own demands, and are a particular challenge to self-confidence. However, at this early stage the uncertainty with regard to the future also leaves much room for hope in both the patient and the family, an emotion that is less evident at later stages of rehabilitation (see chapter 13).

Recent and severe brain injury is associated with *ongoing medical complications*. These may be neurological, such as late hydrocephalus or post-traumatic epilepsy (Jennet, 1975) that have not yet been effectively controlled. There may also be damage to the skull awaiting later neurosurgical repair. Chronic sub-dural haematomas may occur. Secondary effects of neurological damage may also have implications for medical treatment and care. For instance, muscle contractures may require treatment with botulinum toxin or even corrective surgery; or impaired swallow reflex may require insertion of a percutaneous endoscopic gastrostomy (PEG).

The patient may be recovering from *associated orthopaedic or soft tissue injuries* if the traumatic brain injury was sustained in a road traffic accident, fall or assault. Finally, the general effects of having been injured, having undergone surgery and having spent a period of time in hospital can make themselves felt. These may include under-nourishment, reduced cardiovascular fitness and susceptibility to complications such as infections or deep vein thrombosis.

These physical factors are usually far less of a problem for people with mild or moderate brain injuries, or for people who have sustained severe brain injuries some years earlier. They do, however, tend to dominate and can limit the early rehabilitation process, and are reflected in the composition of the *multidisciplinary team*. This team should consist of clinical neuropsychologists, family counsellors, neurologists(s), occupational therapists, physiotherapists, rehabilitation nurses, social workers or care managers, and speech and language therapists. There should also be easy access to a dietician, orthoptist, dentist and podiatrist, together with other medical and surgical specialisms, particularly neurosurgery and orthopaedic surgery. Links with voluntary groups such as Headway should also be established at this stage, if not before. As time since injury passes the role of these groups in supporting the patient, family and friends will become increasingly prominent, and the role of the medical and surgical specialists declines.

Intense therapy makes demands on patients who may be fatigued and who have until then experienced relatively low degrees of demand in a conventional in-patient setting. At this stage patients can appear unsure as to whether they should apply 'convalescence' or 'training' models to their rehabilitation. Behaviour problems (for instance defensive aggression, active or passive avoidance and escape) may emerge as the patient is required to engage in painful, tiring or frightening activities, or activities involving failure experience.

The in-patient rehabilitation unit may be a long way from the patient's home because these units offer a high degree of specialisation with low-volume throughput (McMillan & Greenwood, 1993). It is not cost-effective to disperse them too widely. Thus, a patient may be in a place where people speak in unfamiliar accents, support unfamiliar football teams, where he or she does not know the local area outside the unit, or even the local city centre (a consideration relevant to the teaching of community skills). Visits from family may be difficult because of work commitments, and travelling expense can sadly be a significant deterrent for families on lower income. Friends or children (see chapter 19) may feel uncomfortable about visiting a setting which is full of disabled or obviously damaged people. There is therefore a real danger of social isolation, separation from secure and familiar things, and consequent distress.

Goal Planning in Post-acute Rehabilitation

The particular combination of factors operating at the post-acute stage of TBI mean that in-patient rehabilitation has to be delivered via a tightly focused process of goal planning (McGrath & Davis, 1992; Wade, 1999a).

In this section it will be argued that rehabilitation should ideally be:

- patient centred *not* profession centred;
- participation/role based *not* impairment or activities based;
- interdisciplinary *not* multidisciplinary;
- goal directed *not* problem focused;
- individualised *not* programmatic.

The severity of the acquired cognitive problems, including PTA, together with the novelty of the situation, makes it highly likely that the patient will not have a good understanding of the issues involved. This also often applies to family members, who may have completely unrealistic expectations and ignorance of the functional consequences of severe brain injury, sometimes compounded by what they have been told by professionals in the acute hospital setting. The complexity of the problems involved requires a multidisciplinary team of professionals engaged in therapeutic activities in multiple domains. The in-patient environment can be alienating, resulting in poor engagement with therapy, and an overwhelming longing to return home.

This combination of factors can often lead to conflict. There is potential for conflict between the patient and the clinical team (for instance, the patient may wish to be at home, or may not see the point of certain therapies). There is a similar potential for conflict between the patient and/or the clinical team and family members. There is potential for conflict within the clinical team, where the pursuit of one therapeutic activity or goal may be detrimental to the achievement of another (for instance, active treatment of contractures by serial splinting may result in an increase in agitated behaviour when the patient is touched in other contexts). Unless there is a clear system for selecting and prioritising rehabilitation goals, decisions tend be made by the most powerful or vocal individuals (often a representative of a dominant profession, sometimes an assertive family member, rarely the patient).

However, such decisions can still be undermined or sabotaged by lack of cooperation from other members of the clinical team and, crucially, by lack of cooperation or outright resistance from the patient. While the origins of difficult or challenging behaviours in this group of patients are complex (see below), a frequent contributor is the mismatch between the wishes and expectations of the patient and those of others involved in his or her care. This will be compounded in situations where the patient has no voice, because of cognitive or communication problems arising directly from brain injury, or where the rehabilitation system does not allow the patient to have a voice (LaVigna & Donnellan, 1986, pp.22–24). Thus, the first task of rehabilitation is to enable the patient to express his or her point of view. The second task is to understand it, and to allow it to drive the planning and delivery of rehabilitation. *Grounding rehabilitation in the views of the patient* is ethically desirable, and enables fair arbitration in disputes within the multidisciplinary team, and between the multidisciplinary team and other interested parties.

Seeing the rehabilitation process from the point of view of the patient goes beyond merely consulting the patient about the details of particular therapy procedures. It involves:

- seeing the patient as a whole person;
- seeing disability in terms of its subjective impact;
- seeing the patient in his or her previous and future social and physical contexts.

These perspectives can be understood in terms of the World Health Organisation International Classification of Functioning, Disability and Health (World Health Organisation, 2002; Wade & Halligan, 2003). This is essentially a descriptive framework for talking about health conditions at a number of different levels: impairment, activity limitation and participation restriction. 'Impairment' is defined as a problem with a body structure and/or body function. 'Activity' is the carrying out of meaningful tasks, and is thus focused on behaviour. 'Participation' is involvement with life situations, and is focused on social role, position or relationships.

Problems at any of these levels occur in, and are affected by, personal, physical and social 'contextual factors'.

In terms of the WHO-ICF model these perspectives correspond most closely, though not completely, to the level of participation, and clearly also focus on contextual factors.

Multidisciplinary in-patient rehabilitation programmes by their nature work in opposition to this enterprise. First, the patient is partitioned into a set of functions, each defined in terms of the expertise of particular professions (cognition, communication, upper limb function, continence, mobility, etc. See critique by Kay & Silver, 1989, p.147). Second, rehabilitation culture is dominated by an emphasis on improving performance and promoting independence, with far less attention paid to subjective emotional states or the rebuilding of relationships (McGrath & Adams, 1999). Third, in-patient units are removed from the natural social and physical context of the patient, making generalisation of treatment gains after discharge a major issue (McGrath & Davis, 1992). Thus, real patient-centred practice is more counter-cultural in rehabilitation services than it might at first sight appear.

The rehabilitation team holds expert knowledge about the general effects of brain injury and, following appropriate assessment, about the specific pathology and impairments, and likely prognosis, of the patient. The patient holds expert knowledge about his or her feelings, immediate desires, and (unless there is an extensive retrograde amnesia) about his or her previous roles and values. Effective rehabilitation involves a marrying of these perspectives through constant negotiation and compromise, so that the goals set and the means by which they are achieved are acceptable to the patient, all members of the multidisciplinary team and, if possible, all other interested parties. This is a tall order, especially when the family dynamics are complex (Webster *et al.*, 1999).

Thus, the process of in-patient rehabilitation can be summarised:

1 Assessment of the patient's pathology, impairment, current abilities and future potential to carry out functional tasks.
2 Establishing the patient's motivating values, significant life roles and relationships, wishes, beliefs and expectations about rehabilitation.
3 Establishing the wishes, beliefs and expectations about rehabilitation of significant others (usually family members).
4 Taking all the above into account, setting team rehabilitation goals which are acceptable to all parties.
5 Carrying out therapeutic interventions and other activities directed towards the agreed goals.
6 Evaluating progress with respect to these goals.
7 Setting and achieving new goals in a similar way until discharge, and ensuring that the process is continued as necessary in the community or next placement.

Step 1 is usually carried out by each profession largely independent of the rest of the multidisciplinary team. This provides a useful range of perspectives on the patient's situation.

Step 2 is particularly challenging where the patient has significant impairments of cognition, speech and/or language. At the Oxford Centre for Enablement (formerly Rivermead Rehabilitation Centre), a structured interview is carried out by the patient's primary nurse in the second week of admission. This interview is based around the Rivermead Life Goals Questionnaire (Davis *et al.*, 1992 – see Appendix 3.1) and the Rivermead Patient's Expectations and Wishes Interview (McGrath *et al.*, 1995 – see Appendix 3.2). This procedure may take place over several hours in short bursts where the patient has problems with limited attention or fatigue. If the patient has communication problems the interview is facilitated by a speech and language therapist, sometimes using a pictorial version of the questions. It is possible to get some meaningful response to these questions from all but the most profoundly impaired patients.

Step 3 is vital, for instance sometimes revealing that a family or spouse is committed to continuing to live with the patient after discharge only on the condition that he or she has essentially returned to normal. It may also alert the team to major differences in expectations between the patient and family; for instance, the patient may be willing to take early retirement from work whereas the family may see return to work as the main goal of rehabilitation.

Interviews with family members who do not have cognitive impairment are less challenging than interviews with the patient, but it should be noted that family members have usually been exposed to months of severe stress, and may be dealing with major financial or other worries. A structured form, for instance the Rivermead Relative's Expectations and Wishes Interviews (Wade, 1999b – see Appendix 3.3), may help the process. Some relatives prefer to fill these forms out privately rather than go through a face-to-face interview.

Step 4, the setting of rehabilitation goals, is perhaps the most difficult step in the process. If the aims of the rehabilitation team are to be patient centred they should be set at the level of participation/role. (For instance, 'For X to have resumed his role of father to Y and Z'.) Such general aims need to be broken down into more specific objectives, which can be thought of a steps towards aims. (For a scheme to guide this process see Figure 3.1.) Where possible these should fulfil SMART conditions:

- Specific (including specifying which team members are involved);
- Measurable;
- Achievable;
- Relevant (to the aim);
- Timed.

These objectives are likely to straddle the areas of practice of different professions. For instance, 'For X to be able to play safely on the floor with Y in his own sitting room unsupervised' is likely to involve collaborative activity by a number of professions on the team. Thus, the practice involved moves beyond multidisciplinary parallel practice with intra-professional goal setting to include *interdisciplinary collaborative practice* (step 5) with inter-professional goal setting.

Steps 6 and 7 indicate that the whole process is recursive, with continual evaluation of progress towards goals, and setting more ambitious or more modest goals

LIFE GOALS AREA	ISSUES/QUESTIONS	ACTIVITIES/SKILLS INVOLVED
1. Residential & domestic	Where? (old home? new home? residential? nursing home?) Place available? Modifications needed? Other residents or family agree? Care Package?	• DADL (Domestic Activities of Daily Living) • PADL (Personal Activities of Daily Living)
2. Personal care	Control? Dignity? Privacy? Training/support of carers?	• PADL
3. Leisure, hobbies, interests	What are they? Physical accessibility? Alternatives or modifications available? Transport needs?	• Community skills • Specific skills • Social skills
4. Work	Job open? Modified Job available? What did job involve? Physical accessibility of work place? Transport needs?	• Community skills • Specific vocational skills • Social skills
5. Relationship with partner	Sexuality? Emotional role in relationship (e.g. listener, supporter)? Practical role in relationship (e.g. care giver, problem solver) Partner's feelings and intentions? Partner's needs?	• DADL • PADL • Community skills • Intimacy
6. Family life	Emotional role in family (e.g. listener, supporter)? Practical role in family (e.g. care giver, problem solver)? Children's needs? Other family member's needs?	• DADL • Community skills • Intimacy • Parenting skills
7. Friends	Access to the community? Role in relationships? Role in group?	• Community skills • Social skills
8. Religion or life philosophy	What is it? Reading/access to sacred writings Privacy and space for devotions Physical access to public worship or other group activities? Hospital chaplain?	• Community skills • Social skills • Specific skills
9. Finances	Benefits? Debts? Capacity?	• Community skills • Specific skills

Figure 3.1 Issues to consider when setting objectives in different life areas

dependent on this evaluation. This evaluation is carried out formally by the rehabilitation team, but it is also a vital component of the patient's psychological adjustment process as he or she seeks to make sense of what has happened and to build a new meaningful life (McGrath & Adams, 1999; Prigatano, 1999, pp.183–186).

What is usually referred to as 'discharge planning' should run through this process from the beginning. Even though the final place of discharge, the abilities and the care requirements of the patient may at first be uncertain, staff, patients, families and funding bodies need to be reassured that the patient is on his or her way somewhere. The precise arrangements for discharge will emerge gradually over the period of admission.

Because patients with traumatic brain injury have so many problems, it can be tempting to conceive rehabilitation as a process where these problems are enumerated and defined (with respect to a population norm) and whose aim is to return the patient to as near 'normal' in as many of these areas as possible. In contrast, the approach described above, which is *goal directed* as opposed to problem focused, asks the questions 'What is important to the patient?', 'Where does he or she want to get to?', 'What's getting in the way of this goal?' and then attempts either to remove the obstacles to the goal or to support the patient in redefining the goal (Carver & Scheier, 1990). This means that the goals for each patient will be *unique to that patient*, not programmatic or formulaic, and only those areas that are important to the patient need to be addressed by the team. These are the areas in which greatest cooperation is to be expected. For instance, independence in cooking may have no relevance or importance to a student who always ordered take-away food, but being able to use a telephone for this purpose is likely to be highly relevant. Achieving safe independent walking outside may not be good enough for a man whose main reason for walking outside is to exercise his dog who is his main life companion; dog-walking may have to form part of the physiotherapy programme.

The Role of the Clinical Psychologist in the Interdisciplinary Team

In a setting where interdisciplinary practice is crucial it would be unusual for a psychologist to work independently of other professionals. The role is one of supporting the patient and rehabilitation team in the achievement of mutually negotiated rehabilitation goals. This is achieved first through the functional analysis of behaviour (taking into account the patient's personal history, current situation, brain pathology and cognitive impairments), and second through the application of psychological interventions, if appropriate, usually in collaboration with, or indirectly through, other professionals. Sometimes the functional analysis or psychological formulation may indicate that 'do nothing' is the best option for a particular situation, and in such cases the role of the psychologist is to support other team members in living with a difficult decision.

The areas where the contribution of the clinical psychologist is most important are:

- the sharing of information about the nature and degree of cognitive impairment with the patient, family and team;
- the management of emotional distress in the patient, family or team (see chapters 13, 17 and 19);
- the management of problem behaviours in the patient or family (see chapter 10); and
- the management of cognitive disability in the patient (see chapters 6, 7, 8 and 9).

Adequate assessment in the areas of cognition and emotion is vital. This may be sufficient to give a good understanding of any problem behaviours that the patient is demonstrating. For instance, a patient who insisted that his room door be left open, and that his television be left on late at night playing at high volume, was discovered to be experiencing flashbacks to a very distressing period during his recovery in a neurosurgical unit. He was able to distract himself from these during the day, but was particularly troubled at night when he was alone. He was also afraid of falling asleep in case of nightmares. His rather concrete thinking style, underpinned by significant focal frontal lobe damage, had not enabled him to generate alternative coping strategies, or to take into consideration the needs of staff and other patients in the unit. His problem behaviours arose entirely from a combination of post-traumatic stress disorder and executive impairment.

Sometimes, however, further detailed assessment of problem behaviours is required, and this is discussed in the next section.

Assessment of cognition should be based on standardised neuropsychological tests and should aim to cover the domains of:

- memory;
- language;
- executive function;
- attention and speed of processing;
- visuo-spatial perception; and
- praxis.

The tests selected should be well grounded in neuropsychological theory, have good age-related norms, be in reasonably widespread use and be appropriate to the abilities of the patient.

In addition, while acknowledging their limitations in this group of patients, standard assessments of mood should be used where possible.

Direct observation of the patient, information from the family and from other members of the rehabilitation team are also important in gaining a full picture of the patient's functional abilities and behaviours in a range of settings.

Finally, in the assessment of emotional status in particular, it is of great importance to interview the patient if at all possible. While there is a good deal of evidence to suggest that patients with brain injury, especially injury to the right cerebral hemisphere, may have poor awareness of their acquired cognitive and behavioural problems (Bisiach *et al.*, 1986; Mizuno, 1991; Prigatano, 1994), there is some evidence that they are *more* aware of their subjective emotional state than are observers who attempt to infer this from the patients' overt behaviour. That is, patients with brain injury can experience significant levels of emotional distress which may not be evident in their behaviour and which they do not disclose unless directly questioned (McGrath, 1998). There appears to be a dissociation between the ability to experience emotion and the ability to monitor one's own emotional behaviour. In one study (McGrath, 1999), patients with focal right hemisphere lesions were found to be significantly poorer than patients with lesions in other brain areas at acknowledging the behavioural concomitants of their emotions, but even this group showed themselves capable of reporting the subjective aspects of their emotional state in some detail, and did not deny the presence of distressing emotions attributed to them by observers. Thus, it is always worth questioning the patient rather than relying solely on the report of others.

A good knowledge of the cognitive and emotional status of the patient, together with an understanding of his or her physical and social situation, gives a basis for *a formulation of his or her problems*, which should be shared with the rehabilitation team and, where appropriate, the patient and family. To be helpful, a formulation should have implications for intervention. For example, it is not helpful to explain irritable outbursts as the result of 'irreversible personality change, which is one known consequence of traumatic brain injury'. Rather, it is more helpful to examine the relationship between irritable outbursts and situations in which the patient experiences cognitive overload, pointing out that the threshold for cognitive overload is much lower in a patient with speed of processing or attentional problems. This second type of formulation has the advantage of giving a way into managing the problem, and also 'normalises' the behaviour because most people recognise the experience of becoming irritable when too many demands are placed on their attention. This in turn enables others to empathise with the patient's situation, rather than to distance themselves from it because it appears bizarre or strange.

Psychological formulations are the first step in the management of cognitive, emotional and behavioural problems. In this chapter the use of such formulations will be illustrated by describing a simple functional analytic approach to problem behaviours occurring in the post-acute in-patient rehabilitation setting. 'Problem behaviours' can be defined as anything that poses a challenge to those coming in contact with the patient, and may range from passivity and withdrawn behaviour, through socially inappropriate or rude remarks, through to outright physical threat or violence. Behaviours in such settings are often relatively easy to manage because they are recently acquired and have not yet had time to become firmly established, and because patients are relatively weak, immobile and dependent. However, post-acute units do not have the high levels of staffing characteristic of specialist behavioural units, and they are not locked. Thus, their ability to contain and manage extremely challenging behaviours is very limited.

The Behavioural Analysis Decision Tree

This procedure, represented schematically in Figure 3.2, has proved a useful tool for helping all members of the rehabilitation team at the Oxford Centre for Enablement think through the reasons why a patient may be behaving in a particular way,

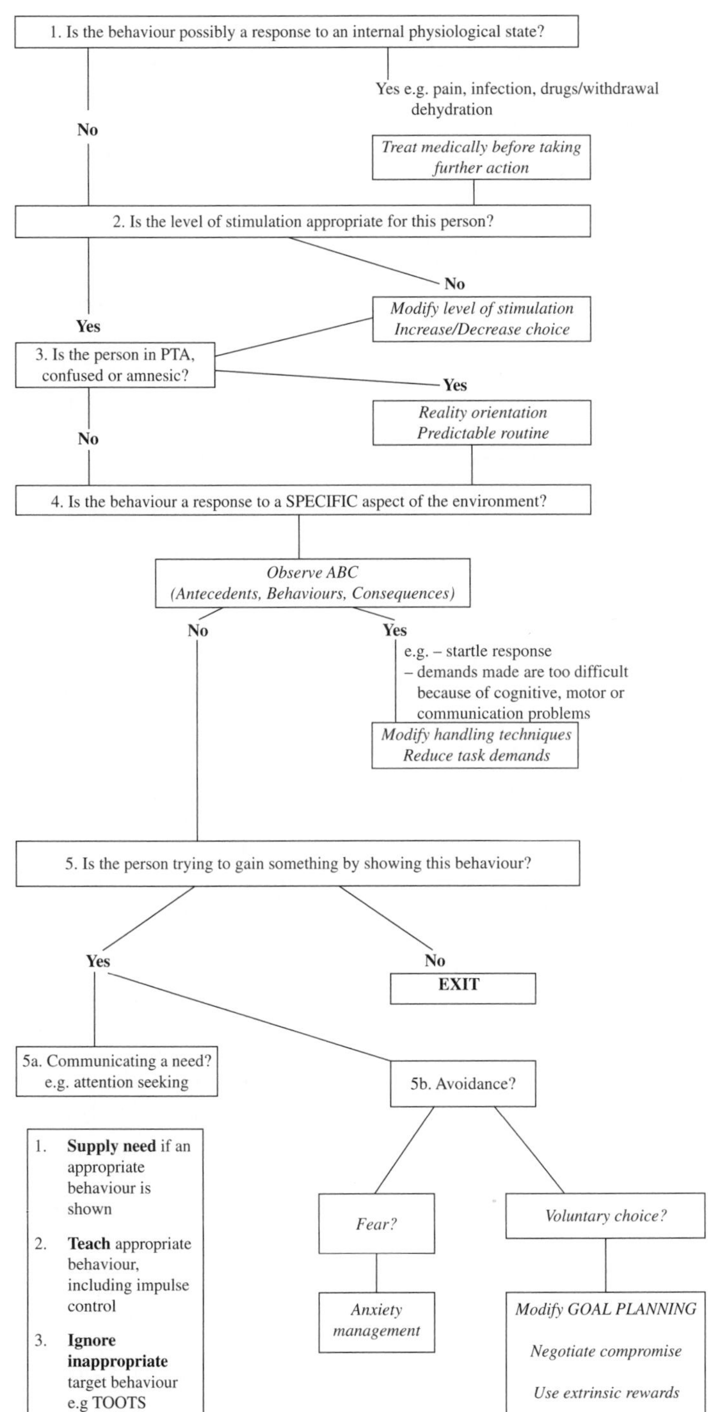

Figure 3.2 Behavioural analysis decision tree

and gives simple guidance as to the best practice for managing the situation. It provides an explicit and efficient process whereby team decisions on the management of problem behaviours can be agreed. It asks a series of questions to prompt further investigation or action.

Is the behaviour possibly a response to an internal physiological state?

This is often the simplest explanation of a problem behaviour. Even something as apparently trivial as constipation can be a cause of restlessness and irritability. In order to answer the question it is necessary to consider the medication history of the patient and other possible physiological factors which may be operating. Recording the frequency and/or intensity of the problem behaviour before intervening is desirable, in order to establish the degree of the success of the intervention. However, once staff are made aware that issues such as pain may be a problem it is often considered unethical to wait before beginning treatment.

Severe mental illness may also be relevant. Patients with traumatic brain injury are not immune from this (Bond, 1984; Lishman, 1987, pp.163–166), and their behaviour may be in part a response to psychotic experiences or profoundly low mood. In addition, post-traumatic epilepsy and primary drive disorders should be considered (Powell *et al.*, 1996). Effective medical control of such conditions may take some time to achieve. One advantage of in-patient units is that medication can be introduced and changed in a safe environment. While significant changes in medication are still taking place there is little point in introducing behavioural procedures other than the bare minimum needed to contain the problem behaviour, because it will not be clear whether any improvement achieved is related to the medication or to the behavioural approach. That is, the temptation to the 'belt and braces' approach should be resisted.

Is the level of stimulation appropriate?

In order to answer this question it is necessary to carry out some basic observations at different times in the patient's daily routine. People with recent brain injury are vulnerable to over-stimulation. This is related to the intensity, frequency and information content of environmental stimuli. Over-stimulation may be physical, for instance too much noise or light or other visual input. It may be social, for instance too many people talking at once, or using too many words. Simply turning off the radio, restricting the number of people present with the patient at any one time, the volume and amount of their speech, and the range of stimuli presented to the patient can effect a significant improvement in behaviour, for instance increasing task engagement or reducing irritability.

However, for some patients the general degree of stimulation is too *low*. They may be bored because there is insufficient activity in their programme, they have no visitors, they are in a featureless single room. Again, basic observation of the patient in different settings is important in establishing whether this is in fact the case. It is also important to remember that the appropriate level of stimulation for an individual is likely to change as the recovery process progresses, and therefore needs to be re-evaluated on a regular basis.

Is the person in PTA, confused (perhaps because of profound dysphasia or severe visual impairment) or amnesic?

These patients are particularly vulnerable to emotional distress because they have no resources to make sense of their situation. This distress can show itself in a range of problem behaviours. For instance, the person may attempt to leave the unit and return to home or work; constantly ask when he is going home; complain because he feels abandoned by family members; try to contact an ex-partner because he has forgotten that the relationship has ended; be very uncooperative with therapeutic activities because he has no understanding of their purpose and no recall of the therapists' identity; behave in a sexual manner to staff carrying out intimate care because he misreads the situation; try to walk using damaged limbs because he does not remember that they have been injured; enter other patients' rooms or get into their beds because he does not recognise his own room, etc.

In such cases orientation to the current situation is vital. There is some evidence that techniques of reality orientation can be applied to people with acquired brain injury (e.g. Godfrey & Knight, 1987; Harle *et al.*, 2003; Kaschel *et al.*, 1995). This should be carried out in whatever modality best suits the needs of the patient. Wall calendars, preferably with seasonal pictures, and accurate clocks and watches with dates should be available to all patients in this situation. In addition, a white-board in the bedroom with the details of the day, date and place, together with reassuring information, such as 'Today is Tuesday – you are going home for the weekend on Friday', is also useful *as long as its daily updating is explicitly built into the patient's programme*. The updating of such boards should take place early in the day, and the patient should participate in this process as much as he or she is able. For patients with visual impairment it is possible to use audiotapes in an analogous way. For patients with language impairment use can be made of symbols and pictures.

These patients also require orientating to the details of their own personal situation. This can be done using loose-leaf folders which should contain details of the history of the circumstances of the head injury, what happened in the early stages of recovery, why they are in the rehabilitation unit, what their current abilities are, what they have achieved so far, the identity of the key personnel involved in their care, what is happening to their loved ones, what their financial and employment situation is, and future plans including discharge planning. Text should be kept as simple as possible and supplemented by photographs.

These information folders have proved an invaluable therapeutic resource at the Oxford Centre for Enablement. Patients appear to gain pleasure from reading them together with a therapist or nurse. They give a content to conversation which might otherwise be lacking for people with very poor memory. They can be enormously reassuring, providing a means of reducing repetitive reassurance-seeking questions. Where patients are vulnerable to despair because they cannot remember therapeutic progress, visits from friends or trips out, the folders can be used to counter this, providing photographic evidence of progress, fun or achievements.

A highly structured, predictable daily timetable is also important in the management of these patients, as is training in route finding (using techniques such as errorless learning – see chapter 7), and the provision of material that makes their rooms personalised and thus recognisable.

Is the behaviour a response to a *specific* aspect of the environment?

Some behaviours are reactions to specific environmental events rather than the general aspects of the setting. This can be demonstrated by careful observation of the relationship between a behaviour and its antecedents. Simple '*ABC*' charts, which direct care staff can use to record the *antecedents*, target *behaviour* and its *consequences*, can provide information on stimuli that are associated with the onset of both undesirable and acceptable behaviours.

In addition to ABC charts, it is always useful to ask those directly working with a patient,

> 'What would you have to do to guarantee that X would show this behaviour now?'
>
> 'What would you have to do to guarantee that X would not show this behaviour now?'

Staff and or family members who have claimed that the behaviour occurs at random and is without meaning often surprise themselves by being easily able to give definite answers to these questions.

For instance, one patient who had been in prison at an earlier time in his life reacted by shouting if the staff working with him were male. Presumably they evoked memories of unpleasant experiences in prison. Another patient with left visual field loss and a degree of left-sided inattention startled and hit out when staff approached him from the left side to deliver personal care. Presumably they entered his field of vision/attention and intimate personal space effectively without warning.

In general, people respond with behaviour that could be described as irritated, frustrated or defensive when demands are made of them that are beyond their resources (LaVigna & Donnellan, 1986). Thus, in brain-injured patients undergoing rehabilitation a common antecedent of difficult behaviours is the demand (cognitive or physical) made by therapy. The behaviour may need to be managed by reviewing and modifying the therapeutic programme or approach. Information about the current cognitive abilities of the patient is clearly extremely important in informing this process. For instance, a patient with significant memory difficulties is not likely to respond well to a procedure in which he is required to learn by rote a complex sequence of actions for transferring into a wheelchair.

Is the person trying to gain something by showing this behaviour?

Often the behaviour is instrumental rather than merely reactive, or a behaviour that began as a reaction can take on instrumental characteristics. For instance, if a patient reacts to a painful procedure by screaming, she may learn over time that anticipatory screaming will lead to the procedure being postponed. Her naive reaction then becomes her (probably unconscious) learnt instrument of control.

Direct observation and the use of ABC charts, this time focusing on the relationship between the behaviour and its *consequences*, is again extremely important in formulating the problem.

Instrumental behaviour is maintained and increased by *positive reinforcement* (increasing the pleasant) or *negative reinforcement* (reducing the unpleasant).

Communicating a need? (positive reinforcement)

From the patient's point of view, positive reinforcement can be seen as the meeting of his or her needs. These needs or preferences vary from person to person, but a common need is for the attention or company of other human beings. This is such a ubiquitous human need that 'attention-seeking behaviour' can in no way be considered abnormal. In people with newly acquired brain injury, resident in a unit far from home, the need for company and reassurance may well increase, but the skills to seek it out effectively may have been significantly compromised. In addition, the ability to control impulses to swear or hit out when thwarted may be greatly reduced due to the direct effects of damage to frontal areas of the brain. A person seeking attention may call out, continually press the nurse call button, or make his or her presence felt around the ward nursing station or office. *In such cases the validity of the need and the right to express it has first to be acknowledged.* Then a managed way of addressing the need of the patient within the available resources, acknowledging duty of care to the patient and the safety of others, should be contrived. For instance, one-to-one sessions of conversation with a named person can be built formally into the patient's programme. This means that, for instance, if a nurse turns the patient away from the nursing office because she is busy with other duties, she can remind the patient that there is a session later in the day when he can discuss his concerns/share a joke etc. with an assistant psychologist. Secondly, the patient may need help in learning to express the need more acceptably. For instance, knocking on the nursing office door before entering, monitoring and reducing the frequency of his requests by use of a written or pictorial record/check list and clock. (These principles also clearly apply to people who are requesting things other than simple attention such as cigarettes.) Thirdly, *and only once the needs have been addressed and steps taken to teach appropriate means of achieving them*, the problem behaviour should be ignored. This may involve staff actually removing themselves from the presence of the patient for a short period of time ('Time Out On The Spot' – TOOTS).

It is important to bear in mind that approaches that involve removal of attention from the patient will only work if attention actually is rewarding to that person. For some patients removal of staff attention can be highly rewarding.

Sometimes staff need to remove themselves immediately from a situation because their physical safety is in question, usually in response to physical aggression by the patient. Staff safety is of course of paramount concern, but the management of a crisis by removing oneself from the patient should not be confused with the use of TOOTS as a component of a planned behavioural management programme.

Where any such programme is in place, however simple, it is important that written guidelines and face-to-face explanation are given to all staff involved so that a consistent approach can be maintained. The programme should also be discussed with the patient, where possible, to gain consent, and with family members. The success should be monitored by taking baseline measures of the target behaviour before the programme is introduced. The programme should be reviewed regularly with both staff and patient, bearing in mind that it may take a substantial amount of time for appropriate behaviours to become established (Wood, 1987) and for undesirable behaviours to reduce. However, one advantage of the post-acute stage is that there has been less time for problem behaviours to have become deeply fixed. They can be nipped in the bud.

Avoidance? (negative reinforcement)

Some behaviours achieve escape from, or avoidance of, certain activities (for instance, biting a physiotherapist in order to avoid doing sitting-to-standing exercises). The most common reason for avoiding activities is fear or anxiety. Again, as with attention-seeking, while the behaviour may be unacceptable, the fear which is behind it is often very understandable. This is a major issue in the rehabilitation of the person with traumatic brain injury, and is discussed in some detail in chapter 11. Where observations indicate that this is a significant contributor to the problem behaviour then the fear should be addressed using specific techniques (essentially modified cognitive behavioural therapy, see chapters 11 and 12).

Sometimes, however, a patient may attempt to escape or avoid an activity purely because she does not wish to participate. That is, she is expressing a voluntary choice. She should be given as much information as possible about the consequences of her choice so that it is an informed decision, and then should be supported in communicating this choice effectively. The goal-planning process described in this chapter enables the patient to do this. While her views must be respected, it is sometimes possible to negotiate a compromise, for instance increasing time in one activity which she enjoys contingent on her active participation in sessions which she finds less pleasurable.

At the end of the day the patient should have the final say as to whether or not he participates in rehabilitation activities, unless he has been formally assessed as lacking capacity to make decisions regarding his medical care. He has the right to make 'bad', or imprudent, choices that may not appear to be in his best interests (see, for instance, court case of Bird v. Lukie (1850) and the Department of Health document, 'No secrets', 2000). Useful questions to ask in such circumstances are:

> 'If X was living at home, attending as an out-patient, and kept missing appointments, would I feel comfortable about going to his house, entering his living room and physically bringing him to the unit?'
>
> 'If X could walk, and he just walked out of my session when he got fed up (rather than sitting in his wheelchair and swearing at me), would I have the right to stop him?'

Consideration of such questions can be a sobering exercise for rehabilitation professionals who believe that it is their duty to deliver a specified amount of therapeutic input to address particular impairments and disabilities.

Effectiveness of Post-acute Rehabilitation

Studies evaluating the effectiveness of cognitive rehabilitation in post-acute settings for people with traumatic brain injury are relatively sparse and often have significant methodological weaknesses. The cognitive rehabilitation programmes, however, which, according to current evidence, have the strongest outcomes are those that combine early intervention, compensatory strategies and supported employment (Carney *et al.*, 1999). Compensatory strategies appear to have demonstrable benefit in reducing everyday memory failures, minimising anxiety, increasing self-concept and improving interpersonal relationships. Similarly, behavioural approaches aimed at maximising skill acquisition and monitoring, including performance feedback and reinforcement, have a good evidence base (King & Tyerman, 2003). The best-evidenced forms of rehabilitation therefore are those which include educational, behavioural, psychotherapeutic and family approaches and which are delivered as part of a specialist interdisciplinary brain injury rehabilitation programme. It is these types of programmes that the *National Clinical Guidelines on Rehabilitation following Traumatic Brain Injury* (Royal College of Physicians and Society of Rehabilitation Medicine, 2003) most strongly advocate.

Conclusions

Post-acute in-patient rehabilitation poses significant challenges for a person with severe brain injury. The interaction between the cognitive, emotional, physical and behavioural consequences of their injury, coupled with the patient finding themselves in a highly alien environment, means that it is essential for the rehabilitation team to address a range of psychological issues. The use of systematic goal-planning procedures can help significantly in maintaining a client-centred focus and structure to the rehabilitation process. Ultimately it is of the utmost importance that the individuality and personhood of the patient are not lost as therapies and interventions are delivered and that whenever humanly possible the patient's wishes, hopes and goals take pre-eminence in decisions that are made on their behalf.

Recommended Reading

British Society of Rehabilitation Medicine and Royal College of Physicians (2003). *Rehabilitation following acquired brain injury; national clinical guidelines*. London: Royal College of Physicians.
National guidelines for service provision for patients with acquired brain injury, including post acute in-patient rehabilitation.

McGrath, J., Marks, J. & Davis, A. (1995). Towards interdisciplinary rehabilitation. Further developments at Rivermead Rehabilitation Centre. *Clinical Rehabilitation*, *7*, 346–355.

Reviews the development of an interdisciplinary approach to post-acute in-patient rehabilitation at Rivermead Rehabilitation Centre. It provides helpful details of the documentation and training initiatives used in their client-centred philosophy.

Prigatano, G. (1999). *Principles of neuropsychological rehabilitation*. New York: Oxford University Press.

An excellent introduction to the principles of neuropsychological rehabilitation with particular application to in-patient settings.

Wade, D. & Halligan, P. (2003). New wine in old bottles: The WHO ICF as an explanatory model of human behaviour. *Clinical Rehabilitation*, *17*, 349–354.

An editorial review of the strengths and weaknesses of the World Health Organisation's model of human behaviour. This has very practical applications to post-acute in-patient rehabilitation.

Useful Resources

Rivermead Lifegoals Questionnaire (see Appendix 3.1).
Rivermead Patient's Expectations and Wishes Questionnaire (see Appendix 3.2).
Rivermead Relative's Expectations and Wishes Questionnaire (see Appendix 3.3).
Directory of rehabilitation services for people with traumatic brain injuries, spinal cord injuries, orthopaedic injuries and burns (M.L. Paton & D.L. Hellawell, 1999) (see references).
UK Acquired Brain Injury Forum (UKBAIF) – www.ukabif.org.uk.

References

Bird v. Lukie (1850) 8 Hare 301.

Bisiach, E., Valler, G., Perani, D. Papagno, C. & Berti, A. (1986). Unawareness of disease following lesions of the right hemisphere: Anosognosia for hemiplegia and anosognosia for hemianopia. *Neuropsychologia*, *24*, 471–482.

Bond, M. (1984). The psychiatry of closed head injury. In D.N. Brooks (Ed.) *Closed head injury* (pp.148–178). Oxford: Oxford University Press.

Carney, N., Chesmet, R.M., Maynard, H., Mann, N.C., Patterson, P. & Helfand, M. (1999). Effect of cognitive rehabilitation on outcomes for persons with traumatic brain injury: A systematic review. *Journal of Head Trauma Rehabilitation*, *14*, 277–307.

Carver, C.S. & Scheier, M.F. (1990). Origins and function of positive and negative affect: A control process view. *Psychological Review*, *97*, 19–36.

Davis, A., Davis, S. Moss, N., Marks, J., McGrath, J., Hovard, L., *et al.* (1992). First steps towards an interdisciplinary approach to rehabilitation. *Clinical Rehabilitation*, *6*, 237–244.

Department of Health (2000). *No secrets: Guidance on developing and implementing multi-agency policies and procedures to protect vulnerable adults from abuse*. London: Department of Health.

Fortuny, L., Briggs, M., Newcombe, F., Ratcliff, G. & Thomas, C. (1980). Measuring the duration of post-traumatic amnesia. *Journal of Neurology, Neurosurgery, and Psychiatry*, *43*, 377–379.

Godfrey, H. & Knight, R. (1987). Interventions for amnesics: A review. *British Journal of Clinical Psychology*, *26*, 83–91.

Harle, T., Feyz, M., LeBlanc, J., Brosseau, J., Champoux, M-C, Christopher, A., *et al.* (2003). North Star Project: Reality orientation therapy in an acute care setting for patients with traumatic brain injury. *Journal of Head Trauma Rehabilitation*, *18*, 292–302.

Jennett, B. (1975). *Epilepsy after non-missile head injuries*. London: Heinemann.

Kaschel, R., Zaiser-Kaschel, H., Shiel, A. & Mayer, K. (1995). Reality orientation training in an amnesic: A controlled single case study. *Brain Injury*, *9*, 619–633.

Kay, T. & Silver, S.M. (1989). Closed head trauma: Assessment for rehabilitation. In M. Lezak (Ed.) *Assessment of the behavioral consequences of head trauma* (pp.145–170). New York: Alan R. Liss.

King, N.S. & Tyerman, A. (2003). Neuropsychological presentation and treatment of head injury and traumatic brain damage. In P.W. Halligan, U. Kischeau & J. Marshall (Eds.) *Handbook of clinical neuropsychology* (pp.487–505). Oxford: Oxford University Press.

LaVigna, G.W. & Donnellan, A.M. (1986). *Alternatives to punishment: Solving problem behaviours with non-aversive strategies*. New York: Irvington.

Levin, H., O'Donnell, V. & Grossman, R. (1979). The Galveston Orientation and Amnesia Test. *Journal of Nervous and Mental Disease*, *167*, 675–684.

Lishman, W.A. (1987). *Organic psychiatry*. Oxford: Blackwell.

McGrath, J. (1998). *Fear following brain injury*. Unpublished doctoral thesis, Oxford Brookes University.

McGrath, J. (1999). Self and observer awareness of emotions after brain injury. *Proceedings of the British Psychological Society*, *7*, 131 (abstract).

McGrath, J. & Adams, L. (1999). Patient-centred goal planning: A systemic psychological therapy? *Topics in Stroke Rehabilitation*, *6*, 43–50.

McGrath, J. & Davis, A. (1992). Rehabilitation: Where are we going and how do we get there? *Clinical Rehabilitation*, *6*, 255–235.

McGrath, J., Marks, J. & Davis, A. (1995). Towards interdisciplinary rehabilitation. Further developments at Rivermead Rehabilitation Centre. *Clinical Rehabilitation*, *9*, 320–326.

McMillan, T. & Greenwood, R. (1993). Models of rehabilitation programmes for the brain injured adult. *Clinical Rehabilitation*, *7*, 346–355.

Mizuno, M. (1991). Neuropsychological characteristics of right and left hemisphere damage: Investigation by attention tests, concept formation change test, and self-evaluation task. *Keio Journal of Medicine*, *40*, 221–234.

Powell, J., al-Adawi, S., Morgan, J. & Greenwood, R. (1996). Primary motivational deficits after brain injury: Effects of bromocriptine in 11 patients. *Journal of Neurology, Neurosurgery and Psychiatry*, *60*, 416–421.

Prigatano, G. (1994). Individuality, lesion location, and psychotherapy after brain injury. In A-L. Christensen & B. Uzzell (Eds.) *Brain injury and neuropsychological rehabilitation: International perspective* (pp.173–186). Hillsdale, NJ: Lawrence Erlbaum.

Prigatano, G. (1999). *Principles of neuropsychological rehabilitation*. New York: Oxford University Press.

Royal College of Physicians and British Society of Rehabilitation Medicine (2003). *National clinical guidelines on rehabilitation following traumatic brain injury*. London: Royal College of Physicians.

Shiel, A., Horn, S., Wilson, B., McLellan, D., Watson, M. & Campbell, M. (2000). The Wessex Head Injury Matrix (WHIM) main scale: A preliminary report on a scale to assess and monitor patients' recovery after severe head injury. *Clinical Rehabilitation*, *14*, 408–416.

Wade, D. (1999a). Goal planning in stroke rehabilitation: Why? *Topics in Stroke Rehabilitation*, *6*, 1–7.

Wade, D. (1999b). Goal planning in stroke rehabilitation: How? *Topics in Stroke Rehabilitation*, *6*, 16–36.

Wade, D. & Halligan, P. (2003). New wine in old bottles: The WHO ICF as an explanatory model of human behaviour. *Clinical Rehabilitation*, *17*, 349–354.

Webster, G., Daisley, A. & King, N. (1999). Relationship and family breakdown following acquired brain injury: The role of the rehabilitation team. *Brain Injury*, *13*, 593–603.

Wilson, B., Evans, J., Emslie, H., Balleny, H., Watson, P. & Baddeley, A. (1999). Measuring recovery from post-traumatic amnesia. *Brain Injury*, *13*, 505–520.

Wood, R.Ll. (1987). *Brain injury rehabilitation: A neurobehavioural approach*. London: Croom Helm.

World Health Organisation (2002). *Towards a common language for functioning, disability and health. ICF*. Geneva: World Health Organisation.

Oxford Centre for Enablement

Neurological Rehabilitation Service,
Windmill Road,
Oxford OX3 7LD

Tel: 01865-227600
Fax: 01865-227294

Rivermead Life Goals Questionnaire

Patient name:__________ Inter viewer name:__________ Date:__________

Various aspects and areas of life are given below. Please say how important each is to you, rating the importance of each:

0 = of no importance
1 = of some importance
2 = of great importance
3 = of extreme importance

Note:
The comments boxes are most important to us.

		Comments
My residential and domestic arrangements (where I live and who with) are:	0 1 2 3	
My ability to manage my personal care (dressing, toilet, washing) is:	0 1 2 3	
My leisure, hobbies and interests including pets are:	0 1 2 3	
My work, paid or unpaid, is: (or education if appropriate) is:	0 1 2 3	
My relationship with my partner (or my wish to have one) is:	0 1 2 3	
My family life (including with those not living at home) is:	0 1 2 3	
My contacts with friends and neighbours are:	0 1 2 3	
My religion or life philosophy is:	0 1 2 3	
My financial status is:	0 1 2 3	

Appendix 3.1 Rivermead Life Goals Questionnaire

Oxford Centre for Enablement

Neurological Rehabilitation Service,
Windmill Road,
Oxford OX3 7LD

Tel: 01865-227600
Fax: 01865-227294

Standards for Completion of the Life Goals Questionnaire

All patients are provided with a standard introduction to the Life Goals Process before the interview.

The Life Goals Questionnaire will be completed with every patient.

The Life Goals Questionnaire will be completed before the first Goal Planning Meeting and before every subsequent meeting.

The Life Goals Questionnaire will be completed with the patient on their own.

The interviewer's name will be completed and the date when the questionnaire was completed must be filled in.

Completed documentation will be filed in the patient's medical notes.

The information gathered will be presented at the Goal Planning Meeting.

There will be clear links between aims identified in the interview and aims of rehabilitation.

A member of staff who has met the patient before will complete the interview.

Appendix 3.1 *Continued*

Oxford Centre for Enablement

Neurological Rehabilitation Service,
Windmill Road,
Oxford OX3 7LD

Tel: 01865-227600
Fax: 01865-227294

Patient's expectations and wishes interview

Patient name:______________ Inter viewer name:______________ Date:______________

What **three things** are most important to you?
From Life Goals.

1.____________________
2.____________________
3.____________________

The following questions simply indicate suggested areas to consider.
Please adapt as necessary, and add anything else.

What are your main concerns that you would like us to consider?

What do you expect to be like in future, such as next year or when you leave here?

What makes your life enjoyable/meaningful/worthwhile?

What do you think your strong points are, what are you good at?

The planned review:

"Do you have any specific questions or issues you want discussed at the review?" (Prompt: "What would need to be discussed for it to be a helpful meeting for you"?)

"What involvement do you want for yourself and your relatives?"

Appendix 3.2 Rivermead Patient's Expectations & Wishes Questionnaire

Oxford Centre for Enablement

Neurological Rehabilitation Service,
Windmill Road,
Oxford OX3 7LD

Tel: 01865-227600
Fax: 01865-227294

Relative's expectations and wishes interview

Patient name:______________ Inter viewer name:______________ Date:______________
Name(s) and relationship(s) of relative(s) interviewed:______________________________________

What are your main concerns?

How have you been coping?

If patient is an in-patient: How long do you expect that s/he will be staying here?

In the future, such as next year or on leaving here:

What do you expect (your relative) to be like in future?
(Both in terms of abilities and how he or she will be as a person)

Do you anticipate any problems with the house/accommodation/living arrangements?

What support do you expect him/her to need, and who do you expect to be giving it?

Are you concerned about other immediate family members including children?

Is there anything else you think we should know about him/her or your situation?
(E.g. previous interests and characteristics, specific worries)

"Do you have any specific questions or issues you want discussed at the review?" (Prompt: "What would need to be discussed for it to be a helpful meeting for you"?)

"What involvement do you want for yourself and your relatives?"

Appendix 3.3 Rivermead Relative's Expectations & Wishes Questionnaire

Oxford Centre for Enablement

Neurological Rehabilitation Service,
Windmill Road,
Oxford OX3 7LD

Tel: 01865-227600
Fax: 01865-227294

Patient and Relative goals and expectations

Guidance for interviewer

The main reasons for undertaking the life goals questionnaire and structured interviews of the patient and relative(s) are to facilitate the rehabilitation process, ensuring that we identify the goals that motivate people and that we identify any unsuspected obstacles or areas of conflict as soon as possible.

The end product of the process should be an understanding of:

- The patient's main
  - concerns
  - motivating factors
  - hopes and expectations over next time period
- The relative's main
  - concerns
  - expectations
- Any other contextual factors that might facilitate or hinder rehabilitation

The forms provide a basis for the interviews, often helping both the interviewer and interviewee with the process. However it is important not to focus solely on obtaining 'scores' or answers to every question as written. It is vital to note both what is said and what is **not** said.

As the patients rate the importance of each area it may be useful to prompt/ask them how well that area is going for them (how satisfied they are) and whether they have any specific concerns.

Begin by reading through the information sheet with the patient-this provides a rationale for the questionnaire/interview and explains what will happen to the information collected.

Please offer the patient time to read though all the questions (either alone or with your support) and time to complete the questionnaire alone (if requested) before going through together.

Please consider timing and environmental factors (e.g. a quiet location, how well the patient is feeling, how tired the patient is feeling). Agree a time to complete the questionnaire and interview.

Please sign and date the Life Goals Questionnaire forms and place in the medical file.

Appendix 3.3 *Continued*

Oxford Centre for Enablement

Neurological Rehabilitation Service,
Windmill Road,
Oxford OX3 7LD

Tel: 01865-227600
Fax: 01865-227294

Patient and Relative goals and expectations

Guidance for patient or relative

The interview and questionnaire are to help us understand what things are most important to you in your life and what currently concerns you. This is so that our services can be tailored to your specific needs as far as possible. This information will be used to guide your treatment planning.

It is best if the forms are completed on your own, without any other family person around, so that you can say or write what you want. All answers are kept in strict confidence by us.

Some of the questions are quite difficult to answer. There is no correct or best answer. Please try to give the answers that seem best to you, that reflect your own wishes, opinions, or expectations.

A staff member here will support you with the forms, but you may choose to fill them in independently. If you choose to fill in the forms on your own you will be given the opportunity to discuss the answers with a staff member here who is known to you.

Please feel free to provide any additional information you think is important. The more you provide the better we will understand what you want from your rehab.

If you are going to complete these forms with someone here, we will always ensure that the person knows you well before doing it. And if you need help communicating this will be provided.

Appendix 3.3 *Continued*

4

Community Rehabilitation

Andy Tyerman and Nigel S. King

Introduction

Many people with traumatic brain injury (TBI) require specialist rehabilitation in the community, to promote recovery and to help them to manage residual difficulties and make positive adjustments. There are a variety of models of community rehabilitation after TBI, including community reintegration, milieu-based, community outreach, home-based, guided self-help and social support network approaches. In community-based rehabilitation the emphasis is usually on more extended activities of daily living, social integration and return to work or education. Interventions focus on enhanced participation, improved quality of life, psychological adjustment and carer stress (RCP/BSRM, 2003). In this chapter we use the term to refer to rehabilitation for people in the community, which focuses primarily on facilitating participation in life roles. (For a discussion of the nature and principles of community rehabilitation, see Barnes & Radermacher, 2003; Willer & Corrigan, 1994). This chapter focuses on psychological approaches to rehabilitation for people with TBI living in the community.

In the UK services for people with TBI in the past concentrated on acute care with all rehabilitation tending to diminish dramatically after six months, with little assistance in returning to an independent and productive role in society (Greenwood & McMillan, 1993; Murphy *et al.*, 1990). Without ongoing rehabilitation, many people are left languishing at home with no regular occupation or social life (Tyerman & Humphrey, 1988). This highlights the need for community rehabilitation to promote further recovery, to guide and support resumption of life roles and to facilitate personal, family, vocational and social adjustment.

'The lack of community support and care networks to provide ongoing rehabilitative care is the problem that emerged most strongly' in written evidence on head injury rehabilitation to the UK Select Committee on Health (2001). The lack of rehabilitation and long-term care available locally and the limited access to neuropsychology services are amongst the primary concerns of Headway (2003), the UK brain injury association. 'Active rehabilitation' of people with brain injury 'has a relatively low profile in Social Services with provision focused on continuing care after the initial stages of rehabilitation rather on continuing rehabilitation leading to social reintegration' (UKABIF, 2004). The Social Services Inspectorate (2003) concluded that '. . . generally speaking, services for people with acquired brain injury were under-resourced, under-developed and inappropriate to their needs, abilities and age'. The Select Committee on Health (2001) recommended that health authorities in the UK be required 'to provide rehabilitation in the community which includes the needs of neurologically disabled people who have a combination of physical and cognitive impairments'.

The *National Service Framework for Long-term Conditions* (NSF-LTC) (Department of Health, 2005) includes a specific quality requirement on 'Community Rehabilitation and Support'. This states that: 'People with long-term neurological conditions living at home are to have ongoing access to a comprehensive range of rehabilitation, advice and support to meet their continuing and changing needs, increase their independence and autonomy and help them to live as they wish.' The following 'evidence based markers of good practice' were identified:

1 There is improved access to community rehabilitation through:
   - flexible, individualised programmes of community rehabilitation and support which are focused on individual goals beyond basic daily care and promote participation in a full range of life roles;
   - interventions according to individual need may include:
     - rehabilitation and support centred on the person's home and environment;
     - holistic out-patient or day rehabilitation programmes.
2 Local multidisciplinary rehabilitation and support are provided in the community by professionals with the right skills and experience, and:
   - involve health and social services working together;
   - include access to specialist neurological expertise (e.g. neurorehabilitation, neuropsychology) to address the full range of practical and emotional challenges; and
   - are available in the longer term based on clinical need.
3 Providers of community rehabilitation and support services support people and their family members and carers to:
   - live with a long-term neurological condition;
   - develop knowledge and skills to manage their condition;
   - achieve a sense of well-being and make long-term psychological adjustments to altered personal, family and social circumstances; and
   - provide proactive intervention, where relevant, to maintain function and prevent deterioration as the condition progresses.

As such, the NSF-LTC requires provision of a comprehensive range of integrated community rehabilitation and support. This will require investment in specialist community rehabilitation services in the UK, including neuropsychological expertise. A number of 'evaluated examples of good practice' are summarised in a web-based Good Practice Guide (www.dh.gov.uk/long-termnsf). One such example, the Community Head Injury Service in Aylesbury, is outlined below. This chapter will review psychological approaches to community rehabilitation after TBI and provide an outline of this service example with a rehabilitation case example.

Psychological Approaches to Community Rehabilitation

The British Psychological Society (1989) has long advocated a community-based model of service provision for people with acquired brain injury. Whilst acknowledging the need for acute rehabilitation, specialist in-patient rehabilitation for the most severely injured and behavioural treatment units for those with marked behavioural disturbance, the heart of the model was a local day rehabilitation facility. It was envisaged that this would provide: out-patient assessment and advice; coordination of rehabilitation; treatment/retraining; an occupational/social outlet; and advice, training and support for families and professionals. The need for a range of other services (i.e. respite care, supported living, and work provision) was also stressed.

Since 1989 there has been some development of community-oriented brain injury rehabilitation services in the UK (Herbert, 2004; McMillan & Oddy, 2001), such as: the Head Injury Rehabilitation Centre, Sheffield (Body *et al.*, 1996); the Community Head Injury Service, Aylesbury (Tyerman, 1997); the Oliver Zangwill Centre for Neuropsychological Rehabilitation (Wilson *et al.*, 2000); the community outreach service at the Homerton Hospital, London (Powell *et al.*, 2002); and ICANHO – Suffolk Brain Injury Rehabilitation Centre (Gravell & Johnson, 2002). However, there remain to date very few evaluations of such services in the UK. A notable exception is the randomised controlled trial of the outreach service based at the Homerton Hospital, London. A small multidisciplinary team, led by a clinical neuropsychologist, provide individualised programmes on agreed short-term goals for clients at home or in other community settings. Compared with a control group (who received written information about alternative resources), participants receiving outreach support showed greater gains in independence and on two of six sub-scales of a community rehabilitation outcome scale (i.e. self-organisation and psychological well-being) (Powell *et al.*, 2002).

The development of community brain injury services in the UK has been limited. In a recent survey 23 per cent of health authorities in South-East England were found to have no community neurorehabilitation team (McMillan & Ledder, 2001). In the 35 teams identified it was estimated that there were fewer than 1.5 community team professionals for 4000–5000 persons with neurological disability and that only 3 per cent of the expected number of persons with disability after TBI were seen. Only two teams (6 per cent) specialised in cognitive impairment or personality change, the primary long-term effects of TBI. With the exception of the services of Headway and a small number of vocational and other community programmes, most provision in the independent and voluntary sectors is on an in-patient or residential basis. Headway provide a range of rehabilitation, leisure and social activities for people with brain injury on a one-to-one or group basis with some centres and branches also offering opportunities to develop independent living skills. In addition, a small number of people with TBI receive help from independent brain-injury case managers funded through compensation and insurance claims.

Whilst specialist services for people with TBI remain very patchy in the UK, there is an extensive range of health, Social Services, local council, education, employment, independent and voluntary services that have the potential to contribute to community rehabilitation and support of people with TBI and their relatives (see Figure 4.1). At present the value of the wide range of community support available is limited by a lack of inter-agency working and inadequate education and training on the nature and management of the effects of TBI, particularly cognitive and behavioural difficulties. The British Psychological Society (2005) stresses the need for an integrated network of services for people with TBI with clear care pathways (see chapter 1). A key role of the community brain injury team is to facilitate and support access to the full range of services in the community, as illustrated in Figure 4.1.

An awareness of neuropsychological difficulties is important for all community services involved in rehabilitation and support of people with TBI and their relatives. A working understanding of the nature and management of psychological needs is important not just for those directly involved in psychological assessment and treatment (e.g. clinical neuropsychologists) but for all members of the interdisciplinary rehabilitation team. Campbell (2000), for example, illustrates the importance of addressing cognitive and behavioural difficulties after TBI, both in integrated team assessment/goal planning and in the provision of physical therapy. The psychological difficulties experienced by people with TBI are many and varied and include:

- reduction in cognitive skills (e.g. attention, concentration, memory, speed of information processing, communication skills and executive functioning);
- loss of behavioural control (e.g. disinhibition, impulsivity, agitation, irritability, intolerance, short temper, aggressive outbursts, and mood swings);
- emotional impact (e.g. anger, frustration, fear, anxiety, depression and loss of confidence/self-esteem/self-belief); and
- difficulties in long-term psychological adjustment to neuropsychological and other disabilities and resultant changes in personal, family and social circumstances.

Neuropsychological rehabilitation

Key factors in neuropsychological rehabilitation for people with TBI living in the community include:

- the provision of a framework within which the person and family can make sense of the nature and effects of TBI;
- neuropsychological assessment to identify strengths and weaknesses, required management strategies and how these might best be implemented;
- sensitive feedback to promote understanding of particular difficulties and to focus attention on areas of strength and weakness in order to facilitate change;

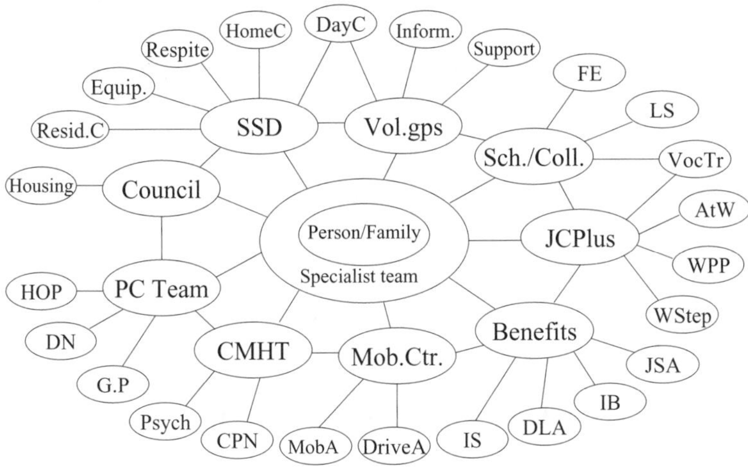

Key:

Council – Local Council	**Housing**	Housing
SSD – Social Services	**Resid.C.**	Residential care
	Equip.	Equipment & loans
	Respite	Respite care
	HomeC.	Home care
Vol. gps. – Voluntary groups	**Day C.**	Day care
	Inform.	Information
	Support	Support
Sch./Coll.– Schools/Colleges	**FE**	Further education
	LS	Learning support
	VocTr	Vocational training
JCPlus – Jobcentre Plus,	**AtW**	Access to Work provision
(Department for Work and Pensions)	**WPP**	Work preparation programme
	WStep	WORKSTEP (supported employment)
Benefits	**JSA**	Job Seeker's Allowance
	IB	Incapacity Benefit
	DLA	Disabled Living Allowance
	IS	Income Support
Mob. Ctr. – Mobility Centre	**DriveA**	Driving assessment
	MobA	Mobility assessment
CMHT– Community Mental Health Team	**CPN**	Community psychiatric nurse
	Psych.	Psychiatrist
PC Team – Primary Care Team	**GP**	General practitioner
	DN	District nursing
	HOP	Hospital out-patient (referral)

Figure 4.1 Community rehabilitation/support

- recommendations on levels of cognitive stimulation/activity appropriate to the person's needs at a particular stage of recovery or adjustment;
- development, evaluation and modification of strategies to help in managing cognitive, behavioural and emotional difficulties;
- assistance in returning to previous or alternative activities and in making psychological adjustment to altered circumstances; and
- availability of long-term support to respond to emergent long-term difficulties.

In developing community rehabilitation interventions clinical neuropsychologists have drawn on both neuropsychological and psychotherapeutic approaches. These are almost always inextricably linked and, whilst they will be outlined separately, they are rarely applied in this manner.

Neuropsychological interventions

There are at least four important general aspects of early rehabilitation: (i) engaging the person (and their family) in the rehabilitation process; (ii) facilitating the setting of realistic rehabilitation goals; (iii) facilitating the achievement of goals via coordinated interventions; and (iv) evaluating, reviewing and modifying goals over time. Successful engagement of a person (and their family) is often linked intrinsically to the collaborative development of realistic goals. It is common for the person (and their family), initially, to have unrealistic expectations about the extent and pace of goals that are achievable (e.g. complete cognitive recovery or return to full-time work within weeks or months of injury). These commonly need to be negotiated to allow for more time, a greater number of intervening steps or the inclusion of additional forms of support. Formal goal-planning procedures may help this process, although there is a need for evidence about how much they affect outcomes.

As previously noted (King & Tyerman, 2003), compensatory strategies most commonly used to manage neuropsychological difficulties fall under five broad headings:

i General cognitive strategies: e.g. using habits, routines and overlearned procedures; developing tidy environments; structuring daily activities; pacing activity and using breaks effectively; minimising distractions; minimising time pressures, unexpected events and 'busyness' in the environment; using a diary as an aide-memoire, a way of structuring time, an orientation device or as a means of overcoming initiation difficulties.
ii Memory strategies: e.g. using aides-memoire (i.e. diary, dictaphone, notes, etc.); developing photo or written journals; systemising storage of items with explicit labelling; maximising learning through errorless learning; using internal memory strategies and mnemonic devices; using behavioural principles to maximise learning of new skills; maximising use of spared implicit memory abilities.
iii Executive strategies: e.g. problem-solving training; monitoring techniques; maximising verbal mediation and 'self-talk'; breaking tasks down into their component parts; minimising unnecessary decision-making.
iv Behavioural management strategies: e.g. using specified feedback techniques for inappropriate social behaviours; maximising self-monitoring; video feedback; using behavioural therapy principles to shape, model and increase the frequency of appropriate social behaviours.
v Social skills strategies: e.g. teaching conversational skills in slowing, pacing, turn-taking and allowing 'thinking time'; teaching the social skills required for the person to be explicit about their problems and their required solutions; teaching others to use short sentences, high-frequency words and allowing extra time for the person to reply to questions; encouraging closed, multiple choice type questions rather than open-ended ones.

Psychotherapeutic interventions

Psychotherapeutic interventions are based largely on 'standard' approaches to psychotherapy from the adult mental health literature but with adaptations according to the person's specific neuropsychological impairments, as illustrated above. Cognitive behavioural therapy (CBT), in particular, has been advocated as a useful approach because many of its essential characteristics appear to be adaptable to people with brain injury. It is structured, educational, focused and collaborative and involves problem solving, behavioural training/rehearsal, stress awareness/management, concrete goal setting, combating maladaptive thoughts and improving self-awareness (Whitehouse, 1994). As noted previously (Tyerman & King, 2004), modified CBT approaches are typically used for problems with anger and irritability, generalised anxiety, social anxiety, phobic avoidance, post-traumatic stress symptoms and depression.

Psychodynamic approaches as well as the more Rogerian, non-directive approaches have been advocated, for example in facilitating the emotional acceptance of changes in personality and identity and long-term adjustment (interventions to facilitate adjustment are discussed in chapter 13). The value of group interventions should not be underestimated. These allow peer support, sharing of cognitive and emotional coping responses and an opportunity to provide formal education in an efficient way. They can be a very powerful and supportive means for developing insight and for exploring ways of minimising disability. Whilst some groups have an educational, skills or behavioural management focus (e.g. Malec *et al.*, 1993; Wilson *et al.*, 2000), others serve a broader psychotherapeutic function (e.g. Ben-Yishay & Lakin, 1989; Prigatano, 1986).

The integration of individual and group neuropsychological and psychotherapeutic approaches is critical to community rehabilitation after TBI. This is well illustrated in holistic neuropsychological rehabilitation programmes.

Holistic neuropsychological rehabilitation programmes

Holistic neuropsychological rehabilitation programmes offer 'integrated multimodal treatments' that emphasize improvement in self-awareness and acceptance alongside compensatory skills for coping with residual impairments and disabilities (Malec & Basford, 1996). Such programmes include: individual goal setting; holistic rehabilitation planning; neuropsychological orientation; 'therapeutic milieu'; outcome-oriented rehabilitation planning; intensive rehabilitation programme; and dedicated brain injury rehabilitation expertise (Trexler, 2000). The 'therapeutic milieu' model 'integrates systematically remedial and therapeutic elements aimed at ameliorating disturbances in the cognitive sphere, the interpersonal and social spheres, and the intra-psychic sphere, or the self' (Ben-Yishay, 2000). A few leading programme examples will be outlined.

A 'holistic, therapeutic milieu' day rehabilitation programme was developed in New York from 1978 (Ben-Yishay *et al.*, 1987). The Brain Injury Day Treatment Program provides rehabilitation in three phases: intensive remedial phase; guided work trials; and follow-up/maintenance. The intensive remedial phase comprises 'cycles' of 20 weeks' treatment (delivered 4 days per week, 5 hours per day) for groups of 10–12 trainees. The daily programme comprises an orientation session, interpersonal skills group exercise, individualised cognitive remedial training and 'community hour', plus weekly personal counselling, family counselling/group sessions, 'ad hoc crisis intervention' and/or clinical management; and 'mid-cycle and graduation parties'. 'Trainees' progress to a series of individual pre-work and/or actual work explorations, organised and supervised by a vocational counsellor, typically over three months, and are then assisted in finding a suitable work opportunity. Trainees receive follow-up vocational and maintenance support for indefinite periods after discharge. (See Daniels-Zide & Ben-Yishay, 2000.)

An early 'milieu-based' approach was also developed within the Neuropsychological Rehabilitation Program in Oklahoma. This focused on: awareness, acceptance and understanding; cognitive retraining; compensation skills; and vocational counselling (Prigatano *et al.*, 1984). This experience was built upon in the Adult Day Hospital for Neurological Rehabilitation in Arizona. This incorporates two programmes: Home Independence and Work/School Reentry. The service operates as a small therapeutic community with both individual and group-based sessions. This includes a 15-minute 'milieu' session, cognitive group, current events group, group psychotherapy, datebook group and relatives' group (Klonoff *et al.*, 2000, 2001).

An early European example is provided by the Centre for Rehabilitation of Brain Injury in Copenhagen where groups of 10–12 people with brain injury complete a programme of 'psychosocial rehabilitation' 6 hours per day, 4 days per week for 4.5 months. This comprised sessions of cognitive therapy, speech and language therapy and special education (where required), individual and group psychotherapy, physical exercise, family meetings and follow-up support. Positive outcomes are reported in terms of personal relationships, independence, work and social activities, with an independent study reporting that savings in public sector costs exceeded the cost of the programme (Teasdale *et al.*, 1993).

A UK example is provided by the Oliver Zangwill Centre for Neuropsychological Rehabilitation in Ely (Wilson *et al.*, 2000). Following multidisciplinary assessment and goal planning, up to 12 clients attend the programme for 4–5 months. This includes group programmes (cognitive strategy, understanding brain injury, community meeting, memory, problem solving, psychological support, discovery, independent living skills, current affairs and newsletter, relatives'/carers' group) plus individual sessions of speech and language therapy, occupational therapy, physiotherapy and psychological therapy. Individual work trials are set up by the client's programme coordinator.

Reviewing outcome research for holistic neuropsychological rehabilitation programmes, Trexler (2000) concludes that improved outcome has been demonstrated in terms of social, interpersonal and recreational integration, functional independence and vocational adaptation. Similarly, Diller and Ben-Yishay (2003) conclude that, whilst cost-effectiveness of such programmes is hard to demonstrate, some positive evidence is beginning to appear, for example positive outcomes in independent living and employment for the programme in Rochester, Minnesota, at an average cost of $21,377 per person (Malec *et al.*, 1993). However, such programmes require a large specialist staff team – the Center for Neuropsychological Rehabilitation in Indianapolis, for example, is staffed by 19 professionals – 4 neuropsychologists, 3 physical therapists, 5 occupational therapists, 3 speech therapists, 2 neuropsychology technicians, a social worker and a rehabilitation nurse (Trexler *et al.*, 2000).

Community brain injury services in the UK cannot provide such intensive programmes. However, there is evidence of the value of specific out-patient, outreach, behavioural management, home-based and guided self-help programmes (see Goranson *et al.*, 2003; Powell *et al.*, 2002; Feeney *et al.*, 2001; Pace *et al.*, 1999; Jacobs & DeMello, 1996; respectively). There is recent evidence from Australia that a community-based approach can be as effective in key outcomes (such as employment and independence) as more intensive centre-based out-patient services (Ponsford *et al.*, 2006). Within the Community Head Injury Service in Aylesbury, different components of rehabilitation are provided across a range of settings including community-based centre, home, local arts centre, workplace. This community rehabilitation service example will be outlined.

A Community Rehabilitation Service Example

The Community Head Injury Service (CHIS) in Aylesbury in the UK was set up in 1992 to provide assessment and rehabilitation for people with TBI and their families across Buckinghamshire and Milton Keynes, a population of around 700,000. The service operates under the umbrella of the Buckinghamshire Brain Injury Strategy. This sets out an integrated care pathway across the NHS, Social Services and Headway, implemented through a rehabilitation referral protocol and operational policy, supported by a county-wide professional training programme. The service network provides for coordinated access to both local and specialist county-wide services. Local rehabilitation services focus on early interventions to promote independence, whilst CHIS focuses on specialist programmes to address educational, cognitive, communication, emotional, occupational and family needs. The service aims to:

1 promote and maintain optimal recovery of function after brain injury; and
2 facilitate long-term personal, vocational and family adjustment.

Referrals/staffing

Up to 85 new referrals are received per annum from both acute sources (mainly medical consultants or brain injury clinical nurse specialists/therapists) and community sources (e.g. general practitioners (GPs), local rehabilitation teams, community mental health teams, Jobcentre Plus, Social Services and self/family). Referrals vary in terms of severity (from minor to extremely severe), time since injury (from a few days to over forty years post-injury) and presenting problems (from multiple and severe disability to single symptoms/issues). As such, whilst some clients require rehabilitation input over several years, others require specific short-term interventions. In other cases intervention is provided to maintain optimal outcome and prevent deterioration in those at high risk of personal, family or vocational breakdown.

The service is provided by an interdisciplinary rehabilitation team. The base staff establishment comprises occupational therapists (2.7 whole time equivalent (wte)), clinical neuropsychologists (2.4 wte including the Head of Service role), work placement consultant (1.0 wte), nurse specialist (0.4 wte), family specialist (0.4 wte), physiotherapist (0.2 wte), speech and language therapist (0.3 wte), medical consultant in neurorehabilitation (0.1 wte), technical instructor (1.0 wte) and assistant psychologist (0.5 wte). Clinical staffing (9.0 wte) is supported by administration and secretarial staff (2.0 wte). (A specialist brain injury care manager based within Social Services regularly also attends rehabilitation team meetings. Specialist neuropsychiatric input is available on a consultancy basis.)

Service structure

The service is structured around three linked programmes: core interdisciplinary rehabilitation programme (described below); Working Out, a brain injury vocational assessment and rehabilitation programme (described in chapter 15); and services for families and friends (described in chapter 18).

The aims of the core interdisciplinary rehabilitation programmes are as follows:

1 To provide information, advice and support for persons with brain injury and their families.
2 To assess rehabilitation, care and resettlement needs after brain injury.
3 To provide and coordinate rehabilitation programmes to optimise recovery, independence, participation and long-term adjustment.
4 To facilitate the restoration of an optimal quality of life for persons with brain injury and their families.

Initial assessment

New referrals to the rehabilitation team are seen for an initial assessment. This involves a detailed clinical and social history and profile of current problems, as perceived by the person and a relative or close friend. This routinely takes two hours, but longer for those with a complex course of recovery and/or long-standing injuries. The initial assessment (which is usually undertaken jointly by a clinical neuropsychologist or occupational therapist and another member of the team) includes structured interviews and rating scales, mostly developed from Tyerman (1987, 1999):

- Head Injury Background Interview Schedule;
- Head Injury Problem Schedule;
- Head Injury Semantic Differential;
- Hospital Anxiety and Depression Scale (Zigmond & Snaith, 1983); and
- Family Screening Assessment

The background interview is conducted jointly with the person and a relative or close friend. This starts with an exploration of personal, family, educational and occupational history, so that rehabilitation is anchored in the particular personal, family and social circumstances of the individual. It then proceeds to cover both past and current clinical history – including the nature of TBI, acute care, early difficulties, in-patient/out-patient rehabilitation, resettlement (e.g. return home, return to work, etc.), current situation and current issues. Questions are addressed mainly to the person with the injury, but the relative or close friend is encouraged to assist the person in recalling and explaining specific details (e.g. about early recovery), as well as to provide their own observations. (The background interview schedule is available from the first author.)

The second phase of initial assessment identifies the range of current difficulties through separate interviews with the client and a relative or close friend. A Head Injury Problem Schedule – comprising physical (14), sensory (5), cognitive (17), behavioural (6), emotional (6) and social (15) items – provides a profile of current problems as perceived by the person and relative. (The problem schedule is available from the first author.) A Head Injury Semantic Differential (described in chapter 13) provides an assessment of change in self-concept as viewed by the person and in personality/behaviour as perceived by family members. The Hospital Anxiety and Depression Scale provides a brief screen of the client's current emotional state. A brief Family Screening Interview (detailed in chapter 18), completed with the relative or close friend, provides an early assessment of the impact of the injury on the family.

After a brief recess to assimilate the information provided, further assessment and rehabilitation needs and proposed action are discussed with the person and the relative and any pressing needs addressed.

Team assessments/feedback

After discussion in a weekly rehabilitation team meeting, further assessments are arranged to meet specific individual needs. These may include: medical (consultant in neurorehabilitation); neuropsychological; occupational therapy; physiotherapy; speech and language therapy. Nursing care and home assessments are undertaken as required. (Those requiring social care assessments are referred to a specialist brain-injury care manager. When the major presenting issues are vocational people may be referred for a specialist vocational assessment on the Working Out Programme – see chapter 15).

A neuropsychological assessment is commonly undertaken. This is likely to include formal testing of cognitive skills such as general intellectual ability, memory, information processing and attention/executive function, plus other language, perceptual and spatial skills, as appropriate. (This may be supplemented by self or family rating scales to evaluate cognitive difficulties in daily life.) Parallel assessment of behaviour and emotional state is commonly undertaken, based on self, family and staff observation and ratings (see King & Tyerman, 2003). Neuropsychological assessment results are integrated with self and family reports and parallel assessments from other professionals in the rehabilitation team meeting before being fed back to the client and family member, preferably by the same staff members who completed the initial assessment.

Feedback of team assessments is undertaken in a structured format starting with a short debrief of the person on their experience of the assessment and family

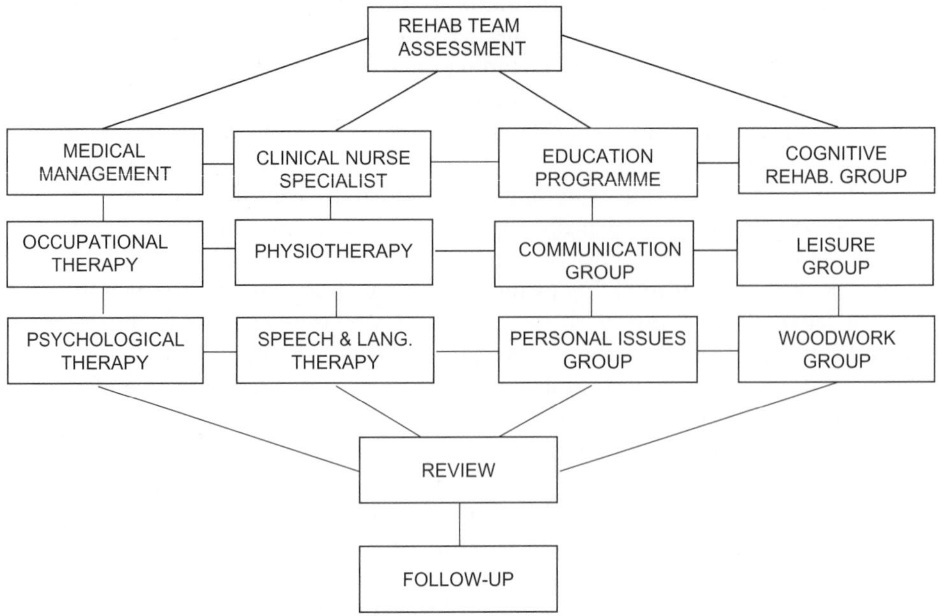

Figure 4.2 CHIS rehabilitation programmes

observations (e.g. of subsequent headache, fatigue, irritability, etc.). Prior to outlining the results it is helpful to set these in the context of TBI, time since injury and other issues identified on initial assessment. The rationale for and results of the team assessments are then outlined, reminding the client (and informing the relative) of the tasks and providing examples (as appropriate) of difficulties identified, making frequent cross-references to self and family reports. The short-term implications of the results are outlined, focusing on identified rehabilitation needs and recommendations. (In our experience it is best at this early stage to avoid confrontation with the client and relative that may risk engagement in rehabilitation – any discrepancies in views can be discussed further with the client and/or relative once a rehabilitation programme has been initiated.) The key outcome of the feedback session is agreement on an initial rehabilitation plan and overall goals. Ample opportunity is provided for questions and clarification.

Those requiring rehabilitation are offered a programme tailored to meet individual need (see Figure 4.2). Typically this includes a combination of individual therapy (within the centre, at home and/or in the community) and attendance at one or more of our specialist group programmes (see below). In parallel, family and friends may attend the relatives' educational programme, follow-up workshops and/or carer, couple or family counselling (as outlined in chapter 18).

Group programmes

Six group programmes are available to people on core rehabilitation programmes: brain injury educational programme; cognitive rehabilitation group; communication group; leisure and lifestyle group; personal issues group; woodwork group. (Care is taken not to invite people with mild TBI to groups if there a risk of fostering inappropriate attributions of secondary psychological problems to a primary neurological cause.)

Brain-injury educational programme

A series of 12 (90-minute) sessions provide information about the nature and effects of brain injury with sessions on physical/sensory, cognitive, communication, behavioural, emotional and family difficulties (as detailed in Figure 4.3). The majority of

TIME: 14.00–15.30 Wednesdays – weekly (Sept. – Dec. 2006)

CONVENOR: Consultant Clinical Neuropsychologist

PARTICIPANTS: People with acquired brain injury.

AIM: To increase understanding of the nature & effects of brain injury.

FORMAT: Talks, videotape examples, questions and discussion.

Programme – Presenters

1. Brain function & brain injury – Clinical neuropsychologist
   Outline of nature of brain function and how the brain is affected by a brain injury.
2. Physical & sensory difficulties 1 – Consultant in neurorehabilitation
   Outline of physical difficulties (e.g. weakness, poor balance/coordination, fatigue).
3. Physical & sensory difficulties 2 – Consultant in neurorehabilitation
   Outline of sensory difficulties (e.g. visual difficulties), headaches, fits & driving.
4. Cognitive difficulties 1. General – Clinical neuropsychologist
   Outline of common cognitive difficulties (e.g. memory, concentration, slow speed).
5. Cognitive difficulties 2. Executive – Clinical neuropsychologist
   Outline of executive difficulties (e.g. reasoning, planning, problem solving and insight).
6. Communication and social skills difficulties – Speech & language therapist
   Outline of difficulties in speech, swallowing, language and social skills.
7. Behavioural difficulties – Clinical neuropsychologist
   Outline of common behavioural changes (e.g. irritability, aggression & disinhibition).
8. Emotional changes – Clinical neuropsychologist
   Outline of common emotional changes (e.g. agitation, mood swings, low mood).
9. Vocational difficulties – Occupational therapist
   Outline of common difficulties in return to employment, education or training.
10. Leisure and social life – Occupational therapist
    Outline of difficulties in previous or alternative leisure and social activities.
11. Personal impact & adjustment – Clinical neuropsychologist
    Outline of personal impact and common difficulties in long-term adjustment.
12. Impact on family & friends – Clinical neuropsychologist
    Outline of the effects of brain injury on family & friends and family relationships.

Figure 4.3 CHIS Brain Injury Educational Programme

sessions are provided by a clinical neuropsychologist with a consultant in neurorehabilitation, occupational therapist and speech and language therapist contributing the remaining sessions. Most sessions follow a core format: a talk about the common difficulties in the specific topic area, illustrated by practical examples of how such difficulties affect people in daily life and supported by a summary handout; illustrative videotape example; and an opportunity for people to ask questions and share their own experiences. Clients currently being seen within the service are invited routinely. Some clients elect to attend a second series to assist them in retaining the information.

Cognitive rehabilitation group

This group runs weekly for 10 (120-minute) sessions and provides a focused programme for people experiencing difficulties with cognitive skills (e.g. memory, attention/concentration, executive, etc. – see Figure 4.4). The group combines information provision (e.g. on major areas of cognitive difficulties and management strategies), group discussion, brainstorming, group exercises, homework exercises and peer support. It generally runs on a 'closed group' basis but with the flexibility for new members to join the group later in the programme if practicalities and group dynamics allow. On completion of the group, individual follow-up sessions are arranged to address further needs. The group is typically led by a clinical neuropsychologist alongside another member of the team – usually an occupational therapist or speech and language therapist. The psychologist's role includes: providing psychoeducation; engendering a supportive group dynamic; facilitating group discussion; facilitating the exploration of emotional states associated with difficulties; maximising group dynamics to effect change; and overall coordination and evaluation of the programme. These roles are by no means the exclusive domain of the psychologist and many of them are taken on by the co-leaders of the group.

Personal issues group

The personal issues group focuses on behavioural and emotional effects of brain injury. With professional guidance and peer support, group members explore the nature and impact of TBI for themselves and their families. The group provides an opportunity for members to express their feelings, frustrations and worries about the effects of brain injury and help to cope emotionally with their new selves and circumstances. This group has usually been run by a clinical neuropsychologist supported by another member of the team. The format of this group is variable depending on needs at any given time. At times it has run on an open basis over a period of a year, on other occasions it has been more structured with prescribed topics (e.g. irritability, frustration, mood swings) and on one occasion as a specific anger management group. A planned topic for the group may be superseded by discussion of any pressing issues affecting a group member.

The other three groups are as follows:

- Communication group: This eight-session group led by the speech and language therapist is tailored to meet the specific communication needs of individual participants and aims to help them to develop their communication skills in everyday life.

PROGRAMME TITLE:	COGNITIVE REHABILITATION GROUP
AIMS:	• To educate clients about acquired brain injury, cognitive difficulties and how to best manage them; • To provide a supportive environment in which clients: – can share coping strategies – provide peer support – discuss experiences of managing impairments and practice / improve group communication skills; • To highlight clients' longer-term rehabilitation needs and promote insight and awareness as to how these might best be met.
PROGRAMME:	Workshop-style group with educational, brainstorming and peer support elements. Topics: 1. Introduction 2. Brain function and anatomy 3. Attention/concentration 4. Memory 1 5. Memory 2 6. Memory 3 7. Executive 1 8. Executive 2 9. Communication 10. Evaluation and feedback
LOCATION:	The Camborne Centre
FREQUENCY & LENGTH OF SESSION:	Weekly for 2 hours
PROGRAMME LENGTH:	10 sessions
LEAD THERAPISTS:	Clinical neuropsychologist and occupational therapist/speech & language therapist/clinical nurse specialist
PROGRAMME OPEN TO:	All clients attending the Community Head Injury Service. Clients with brain injury currently attending other services by referral and agreement.

Figure 4.4 CHIS Cognitive Rehabilitation Programme

- Leisure and lifestyle group: This eight-session group run by the occupational therapists assists people with brain injury to explore leisure and lifestyle options appropriate to their needs and to identify local opportunities to pursue on completion of the group, linking as appropriate with resources such as the local Headway group.
- Woodwork group: This group is run in a workshop in a local arts centre by occupational therapists and supervised by staff experienced in woodworking. The group provides practical assessment and development of physical and cognitive skills, as well as an opportunity to learn a new skill and complete an individual project.

Individual psychological therapy

Individual therapy provided by the rehabilitation team includes medical management, nursing care, occupational therapy, physiotherapy, speech and language therapy, as well as a broad range of psychological interventions. The latter include the following.

Brain-injury education/neuropsychological counselling

Building on assessment feedback, ongoing education and counselling are provided to enhance understanding of the psychological effects of brain injury and promote coping through detailed explanation, supportive counselling, joint monitoring of progress, promotion of insight/realistic expectations and resettlement advice/planning/support.

Cognitive rehabilitation/behavioural management

Linking with the cognitive rehabilitation group, the management of cognitive difficulties (e.g. in executive or memory function) includes explanation of cognitive function and impairment, strategies to help manage and compensate for skills difficulties, and ongoing advice and support in exploring alternative ways of organising tasks and limiting demands, for example in the workplace. Assessment and guidance on the nature and management of behavioural difficulties are commonly provided, often working closely with relatives. When major behavioural problems exist, liaison with the consultant in rehabilitation medicine and/or referral for specialist neuropsychiatric advice may be required. In extreme cases referral to a centre specialising in the management of severe behavioural problems may be required.

Psychological therapy/neuropsychotherapy

Individual psychological therapy commonly includes anxiety management, anger management, help with depression or post-traumatic stress, pain management, help with alcohol/drug abuse (or referral on to specialist services). Standard psychological treatment techniques are adapted to compensate for the cognitive constraints and to take into account any loss of emotional and behavioural control (see Tyerman & King, 2004). Specialist neuropsychotherapy is also available to assist people with TBI in addressing difficulties in making long-term psychological adjustments to altered personal, family and social circumstances (see chapter 13).

Family interventions

Family members are included routinely in initial assessments, feedback, rehabilitation planning, reviews and follow-ups. Family members are also provided with specialist advice and support in managing the effects of TBI and in coping with the impact of TBI on themselves and the family through specialist family services, including an educational programme, follow-up workshops and relationship counselling provided by clinical neuropsychologists and a family specialist (see chapter 18).

Review/follow-up

The rehabilitation programme is set up and monitored by an assigned key worker with general progress and specific goals reviewed in a rehabilitation team meeting. Progress is reviewed formally with the person and family at regular intervals with formal reassessment, as required. Following review some people require further rehabilitation, others are supported in moving forward (e.g. guided return to work), are referred to Working Out – brain-injury vocational rehabilitation programme (see chapter 15) or encouraged to join the local Headway group. After discharge we aim to see the person and primary carer routinely for follow-up to monitor progress. An open-door policy allows people to re-access the service to address any emergent long-term difficulties.

The integration of the above programmes will be illustrated through a case example.

Case 4.1: Example C

Background

At the time of her injury C was living with her husband and three young children and was expecting their fourth child. She was a full-time housewife, described by her husband as a 'brilliant mum, an earth mother'. She was reportedly in good health and family life was reported to be 'very settled' and 'very happy' prior to the injury.

C incurred multiple injuries including a severe TBI (GCS 7/15; PTA 5–6 weeks) in a road traffic accident (MRI scan: peri-ventricular abnormalities especially in frontal lobes). After an emergency Caesarean section C was admitted to intensive care (two weeks), surgical ward (two weeks) and maternity ward (four weeks). By nine weeks she had started to feed herself but had slow speech, poor concentration and 'a lack of emotion'. She was transferred to a rehabilitation unit where she seen briefly as an in-patient and then as a day-patient for eight weeks with follow-up occupational therapy and clinical psychology.

On return home C was assisted by daily support workers to care for the children and by a night-carer for the baby. Care support was discontinued at one year post-injury. Without this support C really struggled and became more tearful, aggressive and short-tempered, in spite of an enormous amount of support from her husband, mother and sisters. C was referred across county borders to the Community Head Injury Service in Aylesbury by her GP at 18 months post-injury.

Continued

Initial assessment

On initial assessment C remained totally reliant on family support with her mother staying 2–3 nights per week to help get the children up and to and from school/playschool. Whilst C's aggression and depression had improved in response to antidepressant medication prescribed by her GP, the family were very concerned about C's reduced parental skills, especially her lack of insight and safety awareness and her 'child-like' behaviour. C herself reported concerns about her memory, anger, relationship with the children, inappropriate behaviour/conversation (e.g. revealing personal details), word finding and a 'loss of mothering instincts'. C and her sister were interviewed separately about her current difficulties.

On the Head Injury Problem Schedule the difficulties reported by C are listed below – items with an asterisk denote additional difficulties reported only by her sister:

Physical: none + fatigue*.
Sensory: none.
Cognitive: general intellect, attention (distractibility), memory, word finding/selection + speed of processing*, planning/problem solving*, judgement*, awareness*.
Behavioural: irritability, aggression, disinhibition + frustration*, impulsivity*, passivity*.
Emotional: depression + mood swings*, anxiety*, loss of confidence*.
Social: reduced parental skills + personal and domestic independence*, strain on husband and mother*, concerns about children (reduced parental skills)*.

On the Head Injury Semantic Differential C rated herself very positively pre-injury but currently lower on 6 of 18 dimensions, notably so only in terms of being much more dependent. She was rated also very positively by her sister prior to injury but current ratings were much lower – down on 13 of 18 dimensions, notably in terms of being more unhappy, helpless, unstable, insensitive, incapable and dependent. On the Hospital Anxiety and Depression Scale C reported no significant anxiety or depression.

The value of a specialist initial assessment process is illustrated by her sister's comment: 'I went away feeling elated, it's the only way I can describe it because I actually felt as if somebody totally understood where we were coming from and the nightmare we had been through and, for me, I was just over the moon . . . The fact that you understood and you recognised that it was the head injury that was making her behave the way she was behaving. I was worried in case people wouldn't realise that and I knew that she needed help desperately still . . .'.

Rehabilitation team assessment

On neuropsychological assessment C presented with reduced 'social animation' and non-verbal communication and some disinhibition. She was noted to report very few difficulties apart from lack of concern over her difficulties such as awareness of social rules. She frequently referred to herself as like her husband's 'fifth child', reporting without concern how, if one of the children stuck their tongue out at her, she would stick her tongue back out at them. Formal testing confirmed significant cognitive difficulties, primarily of an executive nature, with concrete thinking, lack of initiation and reduced reasoning, planning and problem solving and self-monitoring. Reduction in attention, motor speed and verbal learning were also evident.

On occupational therapy assessment C was noted to be slightly disinhibited and to display executive difficulties with a suggestion of a reduction in spatial skills, hand – eye coordination and general speed of function. On speech and language assessment she was noted to have difficulties with 'topic fixation', in organising/verbalising her thoughts, in initiating conversations and in following complex verbal and written information. She also had some word retrieval problems.

Owing to the concern about the family situation C was visited at home by a specialist social worker and occupational therapist, in liaison with her local health visitor. This highlighted difficulties in managing her daily routine and in providing care and stimulation for the children, appearing restricted by reduced awareness and initiation but also unreliable memory. This resulted in safety concerns for the children, as well as herself. She remained dependent on ongoing prompting and direct help from her husband, mother and sisters.

The value of specialist team assessments and feedback was summed up by her husband: 'I said earlier on it was like living in a fog, well, when she came here it was like somebody had opened curtains in the fog and we walked through.'

Continued

Rehabilitation programme

C was offered a rehabilitation programme which comprised the following:

individual occupational therapy at home (twice weekly > weekly);

weekly cognitive rehabilitation group (weekly – 10 sessions);

personal issues group (weekly – ongoing);

brain injury educational sessions (weekly – 8 sessions);

family educational workshop programme (monthly – 6 half days);

individual psychological review consultations (occasional – ongoing).

The focus of rehabilitation was primarily on the management of executive difficulties and associated behaviour in the home, especially as a mother. Input by the occupational therapist focused on the establishment of a diary and coding system for routine daily activities, with prompts for hourly activity slots to address safety issues and promote domestic and parental skills. C found the cognitive group to be particularly useful as it linked well with the occupational therapy. Individual psychological input was provided to guide and support the occupational therapist in developing the diary system and in ongoing assessment/management of her behaviour.

C's husband and sisters found the relatives' educational workshops (see chapter 18) to be 'very helpful – it was actually explained to us what C was going through, what caused the problems C was having, with all the diagrams on the brain . . . meeting other families who were going through the same things . . . made it feel as through we weren't out there on our own . . . coming here we could actually sit down in a coffee morning situation and chat with other families having heard yourselves speak and it was brilliant. . . . it was like a rock being lifted off us, you know, a weight . . .'.

Over the next year C continued to receive weekly occupational therapy at home, developing a diary system and addressing domestic tasks such as meal planning, shopping, child care and emergency planning. (C was also assisted with computer skills, linked with home interventions.) This was supported by home visits by the family specialist and training sessions for family members provided by the occupational therapist and clinical neuropsychologist. C's husband and sisters continued to attend the relatives' follow-up workshops. C and her husband were also seen regularly for review. Liaison with Social Services and the health visitor over the children continued and information about C's difficulties was provided for the children's school.

During the year the diary system was consolidated, with C reported to be managing her executive and memory difficulties more effectively and functioning better at home, both in personal and domestic independence and in managing the children, for example getting the children off to school, planning an activity for the youngest child and picking the children up from school. C's sister observed that she was '"gelling" better with the children', although still 'robbed of motherhood'. Her husband remained optimistic, reporting how for the first time since her injury C had prepared for Christmas (e.g. sending out cards, buying presents for the children). However, whilst she had clearly benefited from the diary system, this had not generalised to new situations, nor had there been a return of safety awareness, planning, initiative or self-monitoring skills. Substantial difficulties remained, especially when there was any interruption to her normal daily routine. She continued to lack initiative and struggled to provide appropriate care for herself and the children, without prompting from her family.

On further review her husband voiced concerns about her ongoing difficulties in caring appropriately for herself and the children. It was reported that C still put herself at risk: leaving electrical appliances on; not monitoring/judging the temperature of bath water; lack of adherence to food hygiene; inability to anticipate physical hazards; impulsive buying/vulnerability to exploitation; and inappropriate behaviours (e.g. allowing the children to eat food in the supermarket before purchasing). She still required prompts to bathe, brush hair, clean teeth and wash her hands. The risks were magnified by a lack of safety awareness/judgement – she did not monitor, check or correct her actions reliably and could not sustain changes in her behaviour without supervision and prompting.

After nearly two years of sustained input and slow progress, C appeared to have reached a plateau, nearly four years post-injury. It was considered that ongoing supervision would be required to maintain progress, to ensure safety and to nurture her relationships with the children. As such, her husband reached the view, endorsed by the rehabilitation team, that the best option to ensure the well-being of C and the children would be for him to give up work to supervise her and care for the children. He was supported in this decision and in challenging and securing the benefit entitlements to enable him to do so.

Continued

Follow-up support

Once C's husband left work, the need for direct intervention in the home ceased. However, regular reviews were essential to support her husband, along with ongoing invitations to the relatives' follow-up workshops. He remained concerned about the risks of C's disinhibited behaviour and sought further assistance both in managing and in explaining her behaviour to others through an open letter. A subsequent letter was requested to address C's capacity to give informed consent. C continues to be reviewed annually. It is now eight years post-injury and the family situation continues to be much more settled, facilitated by her husband's ongoing supervision.

The experiences of C and her family highlight the need for specialist community rehabilitation to guide management and promote long-term personal and family adjustment. The need for joint working both within the specialist interdisciplinary team and also with local services (i.e. GP, health visitor, Social Services and the then Benefits Agency) was also highlighted. Specialist neuropsychological assessment, rehabilitation and advice played a critical role, both in working directly with C and her family and in supporting other members of the rehabilitation team.

Conclusions

Community rehabilitation services are essential for people with TBI, both in promoting optimal recovery and independence and in guiding and supporting long-term personal, family, vocational and social adjustment. Psychological approaches have a major contribution to make in the provision of community rehabilitation and support for people with neurological conditions, as required by the *National Service Framework for Long-term Conditions* (NSF-LTC; Department of Health, 2005). Given the prominence of cognitive and behavioural difficulties they have a particular contribution to make in community rehabilitation after TBI. To be fully effective neuropsychological expertise needs to be both integrated fully with the interdisciplinary brain-injury team and also available to other community services. Various models of community brain-injury rehabilitation have emerged over the past 20 years. We have reviewed a few specific programmes and outlined one service example, but encourage readers to research best practice across models and adapt this, as appropriate, to the local service context. There is an urgent need for further service development in the UK, combined with research to establish the most clinical and cost-effective community service models.

Based on our experience over the past 14 years, a specialist community TBI service (including integrated specialist vocational and family services) has worked well for the catchment area in Buckinghamshire and Milton Keynes (i.e. around

700,000 people). (The specialist programmes required would not be viable for a small health district, even if it were possible to recruit and train sufficient staff. Conversely, a regional catchment area would require excessive travel on the part of clients and staff.) As such, specialist community rehabilitation after TBI would seem to be most appropriately commissioned on a specialist collaborative basis within the framework of an integrated neuro-science, neurorehabilitation and social care pathway, as advocated in the NSF-LTC. Such services would be clinically viable, yet also responsive to variable local needs.

To be fully effective, community brain injury rehabilitation services need to forge close working links with a wide range of acute and community services: with acute hospitals, regional neuroscience and in-patient rehabilitation facilities to ensure appropriate referrals and smooth transfer of care; with local generic rehabilitation services to maximise use of limited resources; with local community mental health teams and/or the independent sector for those with severe behavioural difficulties; with Social Services to set up appropriate care and support packages; with local colleges for both special needs and mainstream courses; with Jobcentre Plus for provision of specialist vocational assessment and rehabilitation; with local Headway groups in the provision of information, support and specialist day care provision; and with local carers' groups in supporting families and friends. Working in partnership with these agencies, it is our experience that a specialist community rehabilitation service can address many of the needs of people with TBI and their families.

Recommended Reading

Barnes, M.P. & Radermacher, H. (2003). *Community rehabilitation in neurology.* Cambridge: Cambridge University Press.

Reviews models of disability and community rehabilitation for neurological conditions – includes chapters on outcome measures, research and a specific review of 'Neuropsychological rehabilitation in the community' by Klonoff and Lamb, pp.212–236.

British Psychological Society (2005). *Clinical neuropsychology and rehabilitation services for adults with acquired brain injury.* Leicester: British Psychological Society – Division of Neuropsychology.

Reviews the current state of services for people with acquired brain injury in the UK and obstacles to comprehensive services; outlines an updated model of service provision (including community services) and the role of the clinical neuropsychologist.

Christensen, A-L. & Uzzell, B.P. (2000). *International handbook of neuropsychological rehabilitation.* New York: Kluwer Academic/Plenum Publishers.

Edited book including chapters on acute management/recovery, neuropsychological assessment, neuropsychological rehabilitation – four general and nine specific chapters outlining programmes in the USA, South America and Europe including the Oliver Zangwill Center for Neuropsychological Rehabilitation (Wilson *et al.*, 2000).

Gravell, R. & Johnson, R. (2002). *Head injury rehabilitation: A community team perspective.* London: Whurr Publishers.

An account of community rehabilitation by a UK specialist TBI team. Introductory material followed by chapters on physical issues, cognition, behaviour problems, communication, vocational rehabilitation, psychosocial issues, families and carers.

Kreutzer, J.S. & Wehman, P. (Eds.) (1990). *Community integration following traumatic brain injury*. Baltimore: Paul H. Brooks Publishing.

Edited book (US authors): 19 chapters – sections on medical and physical aspects (3), cognitive/neuropsychological rehabilitation (3), specific aspects of rehabilitation in the community (4), vocational rehabilitation (3), family issues (3) and children's issues (2).

Useful Resources

www.dh.gov.uk/longtermnsf

The section of the Department of Health website on the National Service Framework for Long-term (Neurological) Conditions allows access to the specific Quality Requirement on 'Community Rehabilitation and Support'. The good practice guide includes examples of good practice for each requirement.

www.headway.org.uk

Headway, the brain injury association (UK), website provides information on the nature of TBI, local Headway groups and branches, the range of Headway publications and a list of personal injury solicitors in the UK.

References

Barnes, M.P. & Radermacher, H. (2003). *Community rehabilitation in neurology*. Cambridge: Cambridge University Press.

Ben-Yishay, Y. (2000). Postacute neuropsychological rehabilitation: A holistic perspective. In A-L. Chistensen & B.P. Uzzell (Eds.) *International handbook of neuropsychological rehabilitation* (pp.127–135). New York: Kluwer Academic/Plenum Publishers.

Ben-Yishay, Y. & Lakin, P. (1989). Structured group therapy for brain injury survivors. In D.W. Ellis & A-L. Christensen (Eds.) *Neuropsychological treatment after brain injury* (pp.271–295). Boston: Kluwer Academic.

Ben-Yishay, Y., Silver, S.M., Piasetsky, E. & Rattok, J. (1987). Relationship between employability and vocational outcome after intensive holistic cognitive rehabilitation. *Journal of Head Trauma Rehabilitation*, *2*, 35–48.

Body, R., Herbert, C., Campbell, M., Parker, M. & Usher, A. (1996). An integrated approach to team assessment in head injury. *Brain Injury*, *10*, 311–318.

British Psychological Society (1989). Working Party Report on *Services for young adult patients with acquired brain damage*. Leicester: British Psychological Society.

British Psychological Society (2005). *Clinical neuropsychology and rehabilitation services for adults with acquired brain injury*. Leicester: British Psychological Society – Division of Neuropsychology.

Campbell, M. (2000). *Rehabilitation for traumatic brain injury. Physical therapy practice in context*. London: Churchill Livingstone.

Daniels-Zide, E. & Ben-Yishay, Y. (2000). Therapeutic milieu day program. In A-L. Chistensen & B.P. Uzzell (Eds.) *International handbook of neuropsychological rehabilitation* (pp.183–193). New York: Kluwer Academic/Plenum Publishers.

Department of Health (2005). *The national service framework for long-term conditions*. London: Department of Health.

Diller, L. & Ben-Yishay, Y. (2003). The clinical utility and cost-effectiveness of comprehensive (holistic) brain injury day-treatment programs. In G.P. Prigatano & N.H. Pliskin (Eds.)

Clinical neuropsychology and cost outcome research: A beginning (pp.293–312). New York: Psychology Press.

Feeney, T.J., Ylvisaker, M., Rosen, B.H. & Greene, P. (2001). Community supports for individuals with challenging behaviour after brain injury: An analysis of the New York State Behavioural Resource Project. *Journal of Head Trauma Rehabilitation*, *16*, 61–75.

Goranson, T.E., Graves, R.E., Allison, D. & Frenieres, R.L. (2003). Community integration following multidisciplinary rehabilitation for traumatic brain injury. *Brain Injury*, *17*, 759–774.

Gravell, R. & Johnson, R. (2002). *Head injury rehabilitation: A community team perspective*. London: Whurr Publishers.

Greenwood, R.J. & McMillan, T.M. (1993). Models of rehabilitation programmes for the brain-injured adult. 1. Current provision, efficacy and good practice. *Clinical Rehabilitation*, *7*, 248–255.

Headway (2003). *Headways' response to Carers' and Users' Consultation on the National Service Framework for Long-term Conditions*. Nottingham: Headway, the brain injury association.

Herbert, C. (2004). Planning, delivering and evaluating services. In L.H. Goldstein & J. McNeil (Eds.) *Clinical neuropsychology: A practical guide to assessment & management for clinicians* (pp.367–383). Chichester: Wiley.

Jacobs, H.E. & DeMello, C. (1996). The Clubhouse model and employment following brain injury. *Journal of Vocational Rehabilitation*, *7*, 169–179.

King, N. & Tyerman, A. (2003). Neuropsychological presentation and treatment of head injury and traumatic brain injury. In P. Halligan, U. Kischka & J. Marshall (Eds.) *Oxford handbook of clinical neuropsychology* (pp.487–505). Oxford: Oxford University Press.

Klonoff, P.S., Lamb, D.G. & Henderson, S.W. (2001). Outcomes from milieu-based neurorehabilitation at up to 11 years post-discharge. *Brain Injury*, *15*, 413–428.

Klonoff, P.S., Lamb, D.G., Henderson, S.W., Reichert, M.V. & Tully, S.L. (2000). Milieu-based neurorehabilitation at the adult day hospital for neurological rehabilitation. In A-L. Chistensen & B.P. Uzzell (Eds.) *International handbook of neuropsychological rehabilitation* (pp.195–213). New York: Kluwer Academic/Plenum Publishers.

Malec, J.F. & Basford, J.R. (1996). Postacute brain injury rehabilitation. *Archives of Physical Medicine and Rehabilitation*, *77*, 198–207.

Malec, J.F., Smigielski, J.S., Depompolo, R.W. & Thompson, J.M. (1993). Outcome evaluation and prediction in a comprehensive-integrated post-acute out-patient rehabilitation program. *Brain Injury*, *7*, 15–29.

McMillan, T.M. & Ledder, H. (2001). A survey of services provided by community neurorehabilitation teams in South East England. *Clinical Rehabilitation*, *15*, 582–588.

McMillan, T.M. & Oddy, M. (2001). Service provision for social disability and handicap after acquired brain injury. In R.Ll. Wood & T.M. McMillan (Eds.) *Neurobehavioural disability and social handicap following traumatic brain injury* (pp.257–273). Hove: Psychology Press.

Murphy, L.D., McMillan T.M., Greenwood, R.J., Brooks, D.N., Morris, J.R. & Dunn, G. (1990). Services for severely head injured patients in North London and environs. *Brain Injury*, *4*, 95–100.

Pace, G.M., Schlund, M.W., Hazard-Haupt, T., Christensen, J.R., Lahsno, M., McIver, J., *et al.* (1999). Characteristics and outcomes of a home and community-based neurorehabilitation programme. *Brain Injury*, *13*, 535–546.

Ponsford, J., Harrington, H., Olver, J. & Roper, M. (2006). Evaluation of a community-based model of rehabilitation following traumatic brain injury. *Neuropsychological Rehabilitation*, *16*, 315–328.

Powell, J., Heslin, J. & Greenwood, R. (2002). Community based rehabilitation after severe traumatic brain injury: A randomised controlled trial. *Journal of Neurology, Neurosurgery and Psychiatry*, 72, 193–202.

Prigatano, G.P. (1986). Psychotherapy after brain injury. In G.P. Prigatano (Ed.) *Neuropsychological rehabilitation after brain injury* (pp.67–95). Baltimore: John Hopkins University Press.

Prigatano, G.P., Fordyce, D.J., Zeiner, H.K., Roueche, J.R., Pepping, M. & Wood, B.D. (1984). Neuropsychological rehabilitation after closed head injury. *Journal of Neurology, Neurosurgery and Psychiatry*, 47, 505–513.

RCP/BSRM (2003). *Rehabilitation following acquired brain injury: National clinical guidelines* (L. Turner-Stokes, Ed.). London: Royal College of Physicians/British Society of Rehabilitation Medicine.

Select Committee on Health (2001). *Third report: Head injury: Rehabilitation.* London: House of Commons.

Social Services Inspectorate (2003). *Independence matters: An overview of the performance of social services for physically and sensory disabled people.* London: Department of Health.

Teasdale, T.W., Christensen, A-L. & Pinner, E.M. (1993). Psychosocial rehabilitation of cranial trauma and stroke patients. *Brain Injury*, 7, 535–542.

Trexler, L.E. (2000). Empirical support for neuropsychological rehabilitation. In A-L. Christensen & B.P. Uzell (Eds.) *International handbook of neuropsychological rehabilitation* (pp.137–150). New York: Kluwer Academic.

Trexler, L.E., Eberle, R. & Zappala, G. (2000). Models and programs of the Center for Neuropsychological Rehabilitation: Fifteen years experience. In A-L. Chistensen & B.P. Uzzell (Eds.) *International handbook of neuropsychological rehabilitation* (pp.215–229). New York: Kluwer Academic/Plenum Publishers.

Tyerman, A.D. (1987). Self-concept and psychological change in the rehabilitation of the severely head injured person. Unpublished doctoral thesis. London: University of London.

Tyerman, A. (1997). Head injury: Community rehabilitation. In C.J. Goodwill, M.A. Chamberlain & C.D. Evans (Eds.) *Rehabilitation of the physically disabled adult* (2nd edn, pp.432–443). Cheltenham: Stanley Thornes.

Tyerman, A.D. (1999). Outcome measurement in a community head injury service. *Neuropsychological Rehabilitation*, 9, 481–491.

Tyerman, A. & Humphrey, M. (1988). Personal and social rehabilitation after severe head injury. In F.N. Watts (Ed.) *New developments in clinical psychology* (vol. 2, pp.189–207). Chichester: Wiley.

Tyerman, A. & King, N. (2004). Interventions for psychological problems after brain injury. In L.H. Goldstein & J. McNeil (Eds.) *Clinical neuropsychology: A practical guide to assessment & management for clinicians* (pp.385–404). Chichester: Wiley.

UKABIF (2004). *Mapping survey of Social Services provision for adults aged 16 years and over with acquired brain injury and their carers in England: Final report.* London: United Kingdom Acquired Brain Injury Forum.

Whitehouse, A.M. (1994). Applications of cognitive therapy with survivors of head injury. *Journal of Cognitive Psychotherapy: An International Quarterly*, 8(2), 141–160.

Willer, B. & Corrigan, J.D. (1994). Whatever it takes: A model for community-based services. *Brain Injury*, 8, 647–659.

Wilson, B.A., Evans, J., Brentnall, S., Bremner, S., Keohane, C. & Williams, H. (2000). The Oliver Zangwill Center for Neuropsychological Rehabilitation. In A-L. Chistensen & B.P. Uzzell (Eds.) *International handbook of neuropsychological rehabilitation* (pp.231–246). New York: Kluwer Academic/Plenum Publishers.

Zigmond, A.S. & Snaith, R.P. (1983). The Hospital Anxiety and Depression Scale. *Acta Psychiatrica Scandinavica*, 67, 361–370.

5

Residential Services

Andrew D. Worthington and Robert N. Merriman

Introduction

This chapter discusses specific issues likely to arise in the psychological management of head-injured adults living in residential settings. The term residential settings in this context refers to services which offer 24-hour care and support for adults, and includes residential rehabilitation centres and supported housing schemes offering longer-term support. In both instances such provision is available well beyond the conventional period of time for in-patient medical rehabilitation, and may be a lifelong commitment. In this chapter a brief historical note will serve by way of introduction to the concept of specific residential services for acquired brain injury, followed by a review of key issues in the design and development of such services. The management of important psychological issues in residential establishments is then discussed. Finally, the impact of legislation on service organisation and delivery is considered.

Why Residential Services for Traumatic Brain Injury?

Contemporary residential services for adults with acquired brain injury have been influenced by legislative and clinical factors. The prospects of lifelong institutional care for adults with severe neurological disability were altered significantly with the advent of the NHS and Community Care Act (Department of Health, 1990). In essence the onus shifted to Local Authorities to provide suitable services. Changes in funding streams and a reappraisal of how society should care for vulnerable adults meant an emphasis on supporting people to live at home, or at least in smaller residential schemes, in all but the severest cases. This emphasis on integration as opposed to separation has been given added impetus more recently to such an extent that, to some commentators, care in the community has become care *by* the community (Lewis, 1999). Even where community brain-injury teams exist they are often under-resourced and stretched beyond their means to cope adequately. This presents difficulties in ensuring safe and therapeutic management of adults with serious brain injury, a challenge resulting in the development of residential services in response. In recent years there has been an unprecedented growth of residential provision and supported housing in community locations. Although paid for by public money through statutory agencies, many of these services (for brain injury as for elderly care, mental health and learning disability) are now provided by the private and voluntary sectors. No figures are available for brain injury specifically, but the number of residential beds in Local Authority care homes since 1997 has reduced by over a third, while provision in the independent sector has increased by one-quarter. With regard to domiciliary support, Local Authority contact hours have fallen by 30 per cent and the overall number of all supported placements provided through the independent sector increased from 20 to 88 per cent in five years from 1999.

The second impetus for residential services came from the limitations of rehabilitation in medical settings. In-patient rehabilitation is traditionally undertaken in a medical facility, usually on a hospital site, within the same general atmosphere, eating the same food, and bound by the same rules and regulations as the rest of the hospital. The inadequacy of this model of rehabilitation for traumatic brain injury has been recognised for some time. For example, Eames (1989) stated: 'rehabilitation units for the head-injured should be developed separately from patients with other sorts of disorders, and should be located, as far as possible, away from hospitals'. Despite such sentiments there is little scope within the UK National Health Service for providing a more congenial setting, and the development of residential services for brain-injured adults has largely been undertaken within the independent sector (McMillan & Oddy, 2001; Wood, 1996). Initially these independent services focused only on the most severely behaviourally disturbed, starting with the Kemsley Unit at St Andrews Hospital, Northampton (Eames & Wood, 1985; see also Burke *et al.*, 1988 for a North American example). Such neurobehavioural units, as they are often known, are still few and far between. Examples include the Kemsley Unit at St Andrew's Hospital (Northampton), nearby Grafton Manor and its sister unit Elm Park in Colchester, and the Brain Injury Rehabilitation Trust facility, York House, in York. Other services, while still managing fairly difficult behavioural and cognitive disorder, provide a more community-oriented focus. The therapeutic advantages of this are considered below. Such services include West Heath House (Birmingham), Fenn House (Ely), Daniel Yorath House (Leeds), Thomas Edward Mitton House (Milton Keynes) and the Transitional Rehabilitation Unit (TRU) near Wigan. Residential services of this nature may be considered as transitional living centres (Goll & Hawley, 1989) or community integration units[1] to which one should also add a variety of residential facilities and housing schemes providing potentially lifelong support in numerous locations around the country. Where such services are interlinked, this can provide a model pathway of continuing care for adults with enduring needs. One such example is depicted in Figure 5.1 based upon the care continuum in Birmingham with which the first author is closely associated.

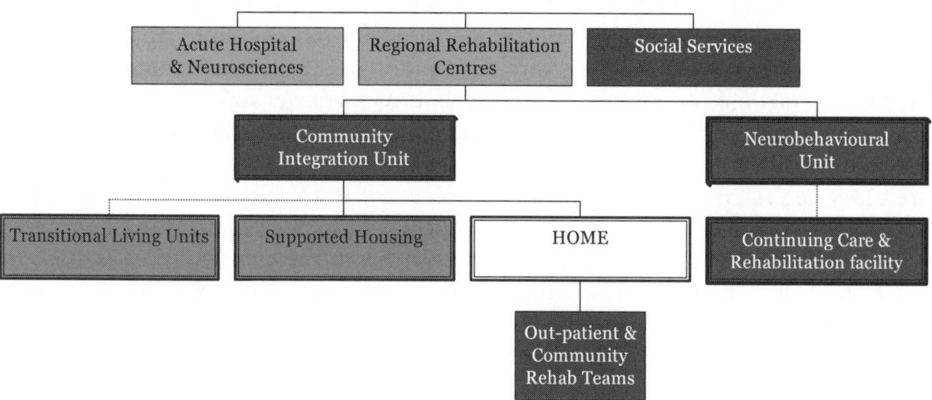

Figure 5.1 A continuum of non-hospital post-acute rehabilitation and support services (depicted by thick border) and their links with statutory services (depicted by thin border)

Neurobehavioural sequelae of traumatic brain injury

The value of residential services for brain-injured adults is inestimable, extending therapeutic support way beyond the conventional duration of medical rehabilitation. The reasons lie with the nature of neuropsychological and neuropsychiatric disorder after head injury. Particularly debilitating are the deficits of attention, working memory and executive skills that typically follow head injury and which can severely compromise a person's potential for independent living. The true nature of such deficits can be hard to appreciate in hospital settings owing to constraints on the assessment process (see Manchester *et al.*, 2004). The impact may be exacerbated by the presence of neuropsychiatric conditions, especially mood disorders, which may develop many months (occasionally years) after the original injury. It is therefore important that services for traumatic brain injury are constructed around the nature and time-course of such neurobehavioural deficits. Properly resourced residential settings can accommodate these difficulties and provide a long-term therapeutic environment through the development of an appropriate social milieu (Wood & Worthington, 2001a).

Community integration

Rehabilitation should aim to help people return to their communities. They should be equipped, as much as possible, with the social and practical skills needed to blend in with those communities. Certain skills, such as the ability to maintain personal hygiene, interact with one's peers and occupy one's time constructively, are widely accepted as valid steps towards these goals. However, views may differ about how such objectives should be pursued. For example, many a young adult recovering from a traumatic brain injury is discharged to the parental home under the misguided belief (shared by families and health professionals alike) that they are more likely to attain their independence this way. The alternative option of residential support is frequently considered to represent a more dependent state. Perhaps too, there is a sense that families are somehow failing their loved one if they countenance residential living too soon. Consequently, many admissions to residential facilities are made only when the domestic situation has broken down irretrievably.

Despite much debate as to how normative values of health should be established (De Wit *et al.*, 2000), the values and shared expectations of particular communities are often neglected. This is unfortunate because it is an important determinant of outcome. Essentially, it means that the values against which effective community integration should be judged are those derived from the communities themselves, not from a doctor or therapist who may not form part of the person's own community. This is especially relevant when setting goals for community integration with people from minority ethnic groups. Community integration is therefore a two-way process: the recovering brain-injured adult needs support to adapt back into the community, while the community at large need to be able to accommodate their brain-injured peers.

Issues in the Development of Post-acute Residential Services

Location, location

From a psychological perspective the most important question to ask is: does the proposed site reflect the kind of environment to which a client may one day return? One of the commonest reasons why supposed gains in rehabilitation do not transfer to a new setting when a person returns to a home of their own is the failure of the rehabilitation environment to reflect the client's own community (at least insofar as it would be desirable for them to return to a similar environment). The location of a new residential service is influenced by many factors but the needs of the potential residents must be given the priority they deserve. A building may be too small, too large, with inadequate communal space or insufficient private areas, too close to or too far from a main road. If these factors are not considered early on, the resultant service will be all the poorer and treatment outcomes will be affected.

Developing a team

Within a residential rehabilitation service teamwork is essential. The establishment will have a registered manager, who should have some relevant clinical experience, and the support team is often led by a clinical psychologist, sometimes an occupational therapist or, in supported housing, sometimes by a case manager. The clinical psychologist is an essential member of the team, as is an occupational therapist. These two professions must work alongside a complement of support workers or enablers who are responsible for day-to-day support. In a rehabilitation service other professions such as speech and language therapists and educational or employment specialists may assume a more pivotal role in the treatment process. Likewise, other professionals such as physiotherapists and medical specialists will be involved as appropriate but may not be regarded as central figures in a residential support team.

Team members, especially support workers, will have diverse backgrounds. The relevant training is often provided in-house, even for professional therapists, although there is now the possibility of obtaining certification in brain injury rehabilitation.[2] In this context, however, the traditional multidisciplinary approach of hospital rehabilitation wards is inappropriate. Instead, a greater blurring of roles is required, necessitating more joint working between professionals and non-professional support workers. This is the essence of a genuinely interdisciplinary team (Worthington, 2003a). The work is undoubtedly stressful and good support networks are crucial to effective team functioning. Team leadership is a matter of personal qualities as well as professional experience. No one profession has to provide the lead on all matters, but it is helpful if there is some clarity over roles. Perhaps most importantly, team leadership should be achieved with consensus from the other team members. Humility before one's colleagues is a useful asset.

Communications with other services

People living in residential services are usually under the medical care of a local GP, who is likely to have limited experience of traumatic brain injury. Consequently a lot depends on a good working relationship between the surgery and the residential service, so it is worth looking for a sympathetic medical practice. In addition, services should have access to the following specialist input:

- psychiatry – ideally with an interest in neuropsychiatry;
- rehabilitation medicine and/or neurology; and
- community dental, dietetic, chiropody and pharmacy services.

It may be possible to purchase psychology or psychiatric services on a retainer when not an intrinsic part of the team. Certainly this is worth considering as threats to placements often arise as a result of behavioural difficulties (see next section on psychological issues). However, involving other specialists on a restricted needs basis can be a mixed blessing. Therapists involved on an occasional or sessional basis (from primary care teams, hospitals or private agencies) may have little direct experience of traumatic brain injury and have minimal experience of teamwork outside their own discipline. The provider organisation does not have to buy in all necessary provision, as residents are entitled to access specialist NHS services. Here again, a good relationship with a local GP can ensure timely access to specialist medical opinion.

Designating goals

Behaviour is governed by goals and rewards, expectancies and attainment. It is therefore important that residential services operate according to an explicit system of constructive *goal-oriented* activity. Too often routine and regularity have replaced initiative and spontaneity, with the result that tasks are undertaken simply for their own sake. Of course structure and routine are important elements of an effective therapeutic environment for adults with brain injury, but one should not mistake routine for mindless repetition. Within a generic residential system there should still be opportunity to pursue individual client objectives, effectively a set of lifestyle goals. Like all goals, they should be clear and measurable and also directly related to increasing social participation. There can, and should, be a clear neuropsychological grounding to measures employed to enhance independence (Ylvisaker *et al.*, 2003). Goals should be agreed with clients but there may be therapeutic goals which a brain-injured individual with diminished self-awareness may not articulate. Other influences, such as religious beliefs, parental preferences and values inherent in the local community, may also need to be accommodated in the goal-planning process. The potential for conflict is clear and it may be important to involve family members and social care agencies in negotiations from the outset. Finally, whether or not they are in full agreement, clients should be given details of the goals underlying their rehabilitation, in whatever form they can understand.

Managing admissions and transfers

Requests for residential service provision tend to come from three principal sources: other healthcare providers, Social Services and solicitors (or their case managers). Other avenues include self-referral or via organisations like Headway. A pre-admission assessment is essential and proper evaluation of psychological and medical issues is paramount at this stage. Many potential clients will have been referred because previous placements have broken down, so it is important to investigate their clinical and social history, as well as the type of treatment and accommodation previously provided. One cannot overemphasise the importance of comprehensive risk assessment at this pre-admission phase, for which a detailed history is vital. Often referrals gloss over a pre-injury history of poor mental health, substance abuse, learning difficulty or conduct disorder. This may need further investigation – an injection of realism about what might be achieved is recommended at this early stage. People are generally thankful for sound realistic advice as to what rehabilitation might achieve.

While many brain-injured adults will at some stage leave residential services for their own homes, for others there will be no discharge as such, just a move along a continuum of supported residential placements of the kind illustrated in Figure 5.1. The timing of such transfers should reflect attainment of specific treatment goals, but must also be conducted in close communication with funding agencies and the client's family. Regrettably, a notional care pathway often fails to fulfil its potential owing to the absence of an appropriate move-on placement or contested funding issues (Worthington & Oldham, 2006). The resulting delays in meeting clients' needs appropriately are not only costly but can undermine their engagement with services. For clients needing long-term residential support the reactions of close family members need to be considered carefully. For example, many parents simply wish to grow old knowing that their son or daughter is settled and happy in residential care. Consequently it is not unknown for some families to oppose a move from a large residential establishment to a smaller supported house (despite this being an index of progress) because it introduces an element of uncertainty about a future they had previously considered secure.

Psychological Issues and Their Management

There are many intrapersonal and interpersonal difficulties to be addressed in supporting head-injured adults in community residence. For the sake of effective intervention, it is important to distinguish those problems that are directly related to the brain injury from secondary psychological or psychiatric disturbance.

Neuropsychological disabilities

Certain neuropsychological deficits after head injury can cause considerable social disability if they persist beyond the rehabilitation period. These can be considered in terms of five broad categories of neuropsychological disorder, each requiring specialist management.

Disturbances of arousal, awareness and orientation

Damage to basic physiological functions of arousal, subserving awareness and orientation can seriously limit participation in activities and disrupt behaviour. Such disturbances are characteristic of traumatic brain injury in the early phase. However, persistent disturbance of arousal, often associated with sleep problems, can have an impact on daily living many years after brain injury (Worthington & Melia, 2006). Instances of specific ventral or brain stem damage, sometimes with very diffuse cerebral insult such as hypoxia, can lead to highly dependent states. Persons with such a level of disability require close supervision, often in combination with extensive nursing care and physical assistance with basic care routines. In these instances consideration should always be given as to whether residential services are appropriate. There may be minimal engagement of the individual client in their care but basic quality of life can be significantly enhanced and involvement in basic decision making can be enhanced with communication aids. In cases where the clinical presentation is unlikely to improve, then long-term specialist care should be sought. Delivery of such support at home is often prohibitively expensive and frequently relies on dedicated family involvement. As an alternative to (often wholly unsuitable) nursing-home care, intermediate or 'slow-stream' support can be provided by specialist brain services in a cost-effective manner (Walker *et al.*, 1996). In some cases it may be difficult to manage such individuals on an open unit, and some degree of security is required, for example an alarmed door or a safe area of internal grounds.

Disturbances of attention, memory and learning

Another cause of severe disability is encountered in persons presenting with combined disorders of attention, learning and memory. This combination of deficits may occur in the absence of significant physical impairment, but nonetheless entails close monitoring and supervision. Again, these features are common to the early post-traumatic period, but severe attention disorder may also be prolonged and is often associated with failure to learn, and hence to benefit from rehabilitation. Persons with such disabilities often require residential services because of their inability to respond to classroom-based outpatient programmes and the demands placed upon carers at home. Such facilities need to provide a high staff ratio, as some personal and domestic activities require individual supervision to ensure sustained engagement with a task. The service needs to be highly structured, and modified to accommodate a person's inability to selectively attend to their environment. Nonetheless, it is usually possible for people to learn from experience, even without awareness, and in this process the development of a daily and weekly routine is paramount (Wood & Worthington, 2001b).

Disturbances of judgement and self-awareness

Many people who have suffered significant brain injury may, in time, make a reasonable intellectual recovery but remain handicapped in everyday life as a result of higher-level executive disorders (affecting, for example, planning, judgement and reasoning). As a result, many otherwise intelligent people are wholly unable to live without close supervision or support (Worthington, 2003b). Consider the case of Mr H, a former accountant, who sustained bifrontal cerebral contusions following a road accident. Two years later, his IQ was measured at 130, but he had lost his job and most of his friends, acquired extensive debts, been burgled, and his wife had left him. Yet despite feeling aggrieved at his 'bad luck' he steadfastly believed that there was an external cause for each of his misfortunes. He refused to consider that he was in any way different from the person he had been prior to his head injury. Such stories are not uncommon. Without family support, statutory care services are often ill-equipped to cope with such difficulties. Engagement with residential services is frequently only possible after a succession of disastrous personal mishaps. Even then, support staff may have difficulty establishing relationships with such adults who are often older than themselves, sometimes with high intellects, and who may never wholly accept that their residential placement is anything other than a temporary measure. Neuropsychological intervention is often critical in helping to sustain the placement and ensuring that rehabilitation is based on the growing evidence-base of effective therapies for people with executive difficulties (Worthington, 2005).

Disturbances of self control and mood regulation

By far the most common post-head-injury changes reported by relatives are those associated with disturbances of personality and behaviour (Connolly & O'Dowd, 2001; Devany *et al.*, 1995; Kreutzer *et al.*, 1994). Consequently, residential services are often populated by adults with some degree of behavioural dyscontrol or problems with regulation of mood. This is particularly common amongst persons who have suffered significant trauma to frontal or temporo-limbic brain regions for whom a propensity to disinhibited and impulsive acts of aggression is common. The behaviour of such persons is particularly susceptible to the external environment. The pattern for social interactions between residents is in part a function of the design of the building. The absence of factors like privacy, recognising the need for personal space, and noise level, together with the general feel of a building, can play an important part in the manifestation of these propensities. Where there is a high risk of aggression, safety is the most important issue in service design. Places where staff or clients could be 'boxed in' need to be modified; bedrooms need to be constructed to allow easy access in and out in an emergency; staff call-systems and sight lines need to be strategically developed. Environmental features need to be maintained to a high standard. Furnishings need to be robust but not devoid of homeliness; bedrooms and other private living space should afford the opportunity to be personalised.

Disorders of motivation

Disturbance of the normal drive, motivation and pleasure mechanisms causes some of the most misunderstood and difficult to manage problems arising from traumatic brain injury. The identification and classification of such dysfunctions is somewhat contentious; certainly there are varying degrees of organic motivational disorder, ranging from failure to show a normal affective response to a primary reinforcer such as food, to complex paradoxical behaviours which appear to be almost like game-playing (e.g. the maintenance of a regular catatonic-like state each morning which requires considerable effort to resist attempts to engage a person in getting dressed). Traumatic brain injury involving ventro-medial frontal regions may well produce an abulic syndrome, incorporating lack of volition and reduced aspontaneity (see chapter 10 by Worthington & Wood, this volume). Eames (1992) has suggested that the more pathological 'game-playing' behaviour is associated with very diffuse neuropathology, for example episodes of cerebral hypoxia or oedema, that can complicate a traumatic brain injury. There are few specific implications for the design of residential services for this group, but they are an important, albeit small, population because they tend to fare badly in rehabilitation. They often come to the attention of residential services after a succession of unsuccessful placements elsewhere. Presently there are no special units for these kinds of disorder, yet a conventional structured environment may exacerbate behaviour disorders of this nature, and reward-based therapeutic regimes may fail spectacularly. Verbal feedback methods that encourage a person to reflect on their behaviour may be counter-productive. A low-key largely non-confrontational approach is usually more successful in minimising escalations of behaviour that often contain a risk of self-harm.

Psychological disturbance and psychiatric disorders

The development of psychological or psychiatric disorders as a secondary response to brain injury can significantly undermine engagement with residential services. However, such 'diagnoses' have to be considered carefully according to context, given that the loss of autonomy which often follows a brain injury provokes understandable reactions, and it would be wrong to label all such responses as pathological. Nonetheless, three categories of psychological disturbance are common enough and sufficiently significant to warrant particular mention.

Anxiety disorders

Anxiety disturbance takes many forms but is often associated with loss, low self-esteem and anticipation of failure. Previous experiences can also play an important role in the development of anxiety. The very fact of placement within a residential service may act as a trigger for anxiety. A person may remain in their bedroom for days on end, or, conversely, repeatedly attempt to abscond. It is virtually impossible to support someone in day-to-day living unless the matter is addressed in some fashion. First, there are important environmental and resource issues that can minimise the impact of psychological distress. A building that affords privacy and personalisation, and that allows gradual exposure to the community at large, is clearly advantageous. This kind of benign therapeutic environment cannot be overemphasised in service planning, but it is all too often overlooked. In the more severe and persistent cases some form of psychological intervention is likely to be required. Medication should be used judiciously after brain injury, and should not be relied upon as a sole treatment for anxiety without consideration of non-pharmacological alternatives.

Depression

Affective disturbance often takes the form of low mood and irritability. The incidence of clinical depression after head injury is difficult to establish (Aloia *et al.*, 1995; Eames, 2001). There is some suggestion that brain injury is associated with increased incidence of depressive illness, but reactive depression is probably not as common as many people like to think. Premorbid history appears to be a significant factor (Fedoroff *et al.*, 1992). Where affective disorder is present, however, it is likely to result in disengagement from services, absconsion or non-compliance. More insidiously, there may be cause for concern about self-harm. For this reason, amongst others, storage and administration of medications and other hazardous substances (e.g. cleaning products) should be no less rigorous than in hospital, and registration authorities are rightly keen to ensure that this is the case. Similarly, other dangers inherent in the internal design of a building and access to and from the community require early identification followed by regular review through a risk assessment process.

Depression is easily misdiagnosed after brain injury as signs such as insomnia, loss of appetite, apathy and tearfulness can all have other causes. Where depression is suspected, other aetiological factors should be considered (e.g. loss of status, financial worries, estrangement from the family). Appropriate treatment requires an understanding of potentially confounding influences. General psychiatrists may over-diagnose depression after brain injury and an assessment by a neuropsychiatrist should be sought where there are particular concerns about diagnosis or management. If in doubt, an empirical trial of an antidepressant may be worthwhile but pharmacological intervention is rarely an adequate response and one should consider environmental and behavioural means to ameliorate the more alienating aspects of residential placements.

Adjustment disorder

It is often suggested that lack of awareness of one's deficits may protect individuals from depression. However, failure to acknowledge persistent disability can contribute to an equally debilitating adjustment disorder. The presence of a chronic adjustment disorder can be especially challenging for residential services as individuals come to resent staff. Activity programmes may be undermined by avoidance or non-compliance. Maladjustment can occur with depressive or anxious cognitions, and conduct disturbance, but is often misunderstood by inexperienced professionals who may attribute all such signs to the original brain injury. A good history is relevant here, with particular importance to any recent changes in behaviour. Advocates of psychotherapy with brain-injured persons are unlikely to find fertile ground, as residential services typically cater for people with significant cognitive impairment. Modified cognitive–behavioural interventions may be effective (Manchester & Wood, 2001) but expertise is scarce. Nonetheless, some form of ongoing psychological support should be sought, as failure to manage adjustment problems effectively risks undermining both the present endeavour and future placements.

Psychological Management in a Residential Setting

Psychological skills are not exclusive to professional psychologists. Indeed many residential support workers may have a particular aptitude for this kind of work. The key to effective psychological management is therefore to utilise each team member's skills in the most beneficial fashion. Consider the case of Elaine, a 33-year-old mother of three who suffered a head injury in a road accident one year previously. Elaine's concerns are with her primary school age children whom she misses terribly and never tires of telling people so. She does not regard her poor planning skills, impaired concentration and memory difficulties as having any bearing on her ability as a mother. Neither does she understand why her desire to tell people about her family arouses hostility in other residents. Her egocentric appraisal of events permits her to see herself as a perpetual victim and convinces her that she is getting no benefit from her placement in the rehabilitation facility. When she is told that she cannot return home she is understandably angry and upset. In such a case there is scope for psychological intervention on a number of levels. First, in terms of neuropsychological evaluation: is her memory getting any better, what is the longer-term prognosis? She may benefit from a demonstration and explanation of her cognitive deficiencies. Second, she may be able to improve her cognitive performance. She may be able to learn to use a diary to help plan her time, use a pager to prompt her memory, get into the habit of writing down what people tell her, switching off the television when the telephone rings and generally tackle only one thing at a time. She may find that her memory and organisational skills are more efficient and she is less irritable as a result. Third, she may benefit from cognitive–behavioural interventions, including behavioural experiments, to help her recognise the difficulties she has in coping with her children when they visit. This approach could be extended to incorporate graded home visits if a supported return home were viable. Fourth, she may need supportive therapy to help her come to terms with her residual disability and change of role. Finally, if a return home was realistic one could consider exploring the dynamics within the whole family unit in systemic fashion.

In order to carry out such a multifaceted intervention over time, the expertise of the clinical/neuropsychologist needs to be augmented by that of other members of the rehabilitation or residential support team. A support worker, for example, may complete structured observations of social behaviour, looking for signs of mood and cognitive disturbance. An occupational therapist may be involved in setting up practical tasks to test organisational skills, and arranging and evaluating home visits. If her own home was no longer appropriate to her needs, her social worker might be involved in supporting an application for rehousing. At times, input from an external agency is helpful, even mandatory. In Elaine's case any major concerns about her relationship with her children might lead to involvement of the child protection team under the auspices of the Protection of Children Act 1999 (POCA). If she and her husband were divorced the Court might appoint a welfare officer to supervise her access to the children. Elaine's support team would liaise with other agencies as dictated by the law, by risk assessments and in accordance with her rehabilitation goals. The composition of a residential support team varies depending on the service, so who does what is less important than identifying what needs to be done and distributing responsibilities effectively. This is the essence of role blurring mentioned above. In practice it is usually helpful to identify one individual to assume a coordinating role (such as a key worker) and one person, sometimes the same person, to act as principal liaison with other agencies.

Integration into the community

Contact with the family

Family involvement is difficult to achieve and maintain where commuting distances are prohibitive or the placement is long-term. Families may feel uncomfortable in maintaining close relationships and regular contact with their brain-injured relative, and indeed it may be impractical to do so. Yet perceived rejection by family and friends, together with loss of autonomy, may contribute to the development of depression or adjustment problems. Relationships between clients and their carers become critical. There is some evidence that interpersonal factors contribute to quality of life for recipients of support services (Marquis & Jackson, 2000). Residential staff also have a key role to play in maintaining good communications with core family members, and sustaining a semblance of family membership for those residents for whom it is an important part of their identity.

Risk from the community

Residential services are usually set near to or in the midst of local communities. Siting services in this manner is especially important for the learning and maintenance of independent living skills: people need to be exposed to the community at large. For instance, in this way a person can be helped to plan their weekly shopping, be supervised on public transport to the supermarket, be monitored in their budgeting and spending, be supported in social interactions and be assisted to prepare a meal on their return. Of course, this level of exposure also brings with it significant risks to vulnerable brain-injured residents. The risks inherent in community placements are various, including danger from traffic, from availability of alcohol and drugs (and perhaps sex), and from unscrupulous members of the community. In addition, there will be risks peculiar to each residential service, according to the nature of the client group and the local environment. Consequently, risk evaluation should be undertaken from the outset when commissioning a residential service. Additionally, assessments of key risks should be undertaken with each prospective resident. Aspects of a person's behaviour can be misinterpreted (for example, a resident with dysarthria or an ataxic gait may be mistakenly assumed by the public and police to be inebriated). The effectiveness of possible interventions to reduce such risks must be carefully considered before reaching a decision on admission.

Risk to the community

The opening of a new residential service in the heart of a busy community is often associated with a degree of concern, sometimes alarm, on the part of local residents and traders. This is almost always based on misunderstandings about the service, and very often reinforced by prejudice and ignorance about traumatic brain injury (Swift & Wilson, 2001). It is advisable to get to know the local community. Initial suspicion can be alleviated by having open days, or inviting community leaders in to talk about the service. Attitudes to the brain-injured can be softened by encouraging volunteer workers from the local community, and by supporting brain-injured clients to make use of local amenities.

Inevitably, some adults with brain injury may not be safe to leave their residence without a support worker in attendance, but this is usually for their own protection, rather than the risk they pose to the community. Nonetheless, one must not underestimate the fear and anger in a parent that can be provoked by an apparently innocent conversation that a client has with a passing child. This may represent a real, if manageable, risk to the community from clients who demonstrate behaviour that is clearly socially or sexually disinhibited. Responsible support staff will have anticipated this possibility and planned accordingly. They will also ensure that adequate steps are taken to minimise the risks associated with vulnerable brain-injured adults absconding from their place of residence. Nevertheless incidents do happen, and it is advisable to ensure there are sound 'missing persons' procedures in place. The local community needs to be reassured from time to time that the service is operating safely. In this context it is advisable to get to know, at a personal level, officers at the local police station (indeed there may be a vulnerable persons officer with this specific responsibility), who can be extremely helpful, both in finding missing persons and also in placating local residents should the need arise.

The Impact of Legislation on Service Organisation and Delivery

Legislation has had a large impact on the delivery of residential services, setting the parameters within which they operate and the standards to which they must conform. This has direct implications for the people that can be admitted and treated within a residential service. Those existing and forthcoming legislative initiatives with a direct bearing on the psychological management of adults with brain injury are briefly summarised below.

Care Standards Act 2000

The majority of residential services are registered under the Care Standards Act. Previously the regulating authorities were County Councils under the 1984

Registered Homes Act. The new Act, which came into force in 2002, stipulated a revised regulatory framework and introduced *National Minimum Standards for Care Homes*. The regulatory body was the National Care Standards Commission (NCSC) which was superseded in 2004 by the Commission for Social Care Inspection (CSCI). The principles of the Care Standards Act in setting minimum standards for quality of care remained in force. Unfortunately, there are no standards specific to brain injury and all services must adhere to a set of generic standards which are sometimes ill-suited to a complex disability like traumatic brain injury. This may change with time as the standards become refined. At the time of writing, the Department of Health have launched a consultation document setting out proposed changes to the regulatory framework for adult social care services. In 2008 CSCI (and its equivalent for independent hospitals, the Commission for Healthcare Audit and Inspection) will be replaced by a unitary body once more, the Healthcare Commission, who will regulate residential services. If the experience with CSCI is repeated, there will be a pressing need to educate the commission and inform individual inspectors about the particular needs of adults with traumatic brain injury.

Under existing legislation Registered Care Homes are not permitted to provide nursing care other than that which would be provided in the client's home, and therefore a close working relationship with primary healthcare teams is essential. Clients who are viewed as more challenging may require residence in a home currently registered under the aegis of an Independent Hospital. Within these terms it may be possible to admit clients under certain sections of the Mental Health Act (1983) if the registration applied for allows for the admission of clients with mental health problems. Other provisions of the Mental Health Act may be relevant for residential services, e.g. Guardianship Orders and Section 17 leave (conditions stipulated by the Act which allow a patient, currently liable to be detained in hospital, to be granted lawful leave of absence). The interested reader is referred to the Code of Practice or Mental Health Act Manual for further information.

Human Rights Act 1988

This has had a significant impact on the practice of rehabilitation, especially with regard to article 5 (affirming a right to liberty and freedom from unlawful detention) and article 8 (right to respect for privacy and family life). In particular, recent legal precedent from the European Court of Human Rights (the Bournewood judgment, 2004) has rendered unlawful any practices which, however well intentioned, could result in deprivation of a client's liberty, unless they are formally detained under the provisions of the Mental Health Act. As virtually all users of residential services will be informal patients, such services are at risk of placing their residents under de facto detention by limiting their freedom of movement in and out of the facility. This is the so-called Bournewood gap – the void between legally detained patients on the one hand and fully consenting clients on the other, into which fall many brain-injured adults who cannot give informed consent to their placement but fall short of meeting the criteria for formal detention under the Mental Health Act. Readers may be interested in the subsequent consultation process instigated by the Department of Health in an effort to establish a process that ensures residents' safety and well-being are maintained within the law (Department of Health, 2005a).

Protection of vulnerable adults

There is an additional legislative framework relating to the protection from abuse or exploitation of vulnerable adults. In March 2000 a government guidance paper 'No Secrets' was issued under section 7 of the Local Authorities Social Services Act (1970) requiring inter-agency collaboration in developing local policies and procedures for protecting vulnerable adults, and giving Social Services a coordinating role. Managers and clinicians will find their local Protection of Vulnerable Adults (POVA) team a helpful source of advice in managing a range of difficulties with vulnerable residents. Their involvement when abuse is suspected or known is mandatory. The Care Standards Act (2000) also requires the Secretary of State to retain a Protection of Vulnerable Adults (POVA) Register of persons deemed unsuitable to work with vulnerable adults, which includes work in residential services.

Mental Capacity Act 2005

Where possible, admission to residential services should be undertaken with the informed consent of the client. Failure to obtain (and document) consent to admission may leave a service open to criticism and potential legal proceedings. If a person is unable to give consent, every effort should be made to ensure that all parties with an interest in the person's welfare (e.g. psychologist, social worker, family, Receiver) are in agreement with the planned admission. Once admitted, further consideration may need to be given to a person's capacity to consent to specific procedures and activities. This is a complex issue which is particularly pertinent for brain-injured clients who may well have impaired reasoning and judgement, and be unaware of their vulnerabilities. There are certain recognised legal tests of capacity (Lush, 2001) but the Mental Capacity Act and its ensuing code of practice will provide a new framework for assessing capacity and managing responsibilities on behalf of a person deemed to lack capacity. Regrettably, the Act does not provide a statutory role for clinical psychologists but they are likely to be called upon increasingly to provide evidence in support of a person's mental capacity or lack thereof.

Mental Health Bill

At the time of writing the proposed Mental Health Bill has not become law, but if there is a new Mental Health Act, depending on its eventual form, it may have significant implications for the role of clinical psychologists and the management of psychological disorders in residential settings. Under the terms of the existing Mental Health Act (1983), residential services can accommodate detained persons under a Section 17 leave arrangement, and those under a Guardianship Order. Currently responsibility for their care rests with a responsible medical officer, though this may change with new legislation.

National Service Framework for Long-term Conditions 2005

After a disappointing response from the government to the Health Select Committee inquiry into head-injury rehabilitation (Department of Health, 2001) came the

National Service Framework (NSF) for long-term conditions (Department of Health, 2005b). The NSF is one of several similar initiatives intended to provide a basis over the next 10 years for improvements in quality of health and social care. It has much to commend it so far as it enshrines good practice, but the NSF comes with no new money and is concerned with a wide range of different conditions such as Parkinson's disease and cerebral palsy. It has been given a cautious welcome after attempts to secure a service framework specific to acquired brain injury failed. Only time will tell whether this document proves to have any lasting impact on the landscape of rehabilitation services for traumatic brain injury.

Evaluating Residential Services

Service evaluation takes many forms, incorporating the audit and inspection responsibilities of external agencies, measurement of clinical outcomes and cost-effectiveness. All providers of residential services should have in place procedures for effective clinical governance. Unfortunately, despite commendable regional initiatives to improve standards (e.g. South Thames Brain Injury Rehabilitation Association, 2000), there is no nationally recognised accreditation of rehabilitation facilities in the UK and the national minimum standards for residential services are those established for residential care homes rather than rehabilitation facilities.

There is a body of literature, much of it from North America, testifying to the benefit of post-acute residential programmes for traumatic brain injury. Summaries can be found in Cope (1995), High *et al.* (1995), Mazaux and Richer (1998) and the National Institutes of Health consensus paper (NIH, 1999). Methodological and ethical constraints prevent the use of controls and randomised allocation to residential services, though randomisation can be used to evaluate specific techniques within a service. Comparison of outcomes across services is difficult because many studies do not provide sufficient information about their programmes or their clinical populations to establish parity (Glenn *et al.*, 2005).

To date, attempts to evaluate the cost-effectiveness of rehabilitation have been crude. It would be wrong to consider treatment which aims to get people back to work (and paying tax) as necessarily more cost-effective and for many more severely injured persons this is unrealistic. Rehabilitation can lead to productive lifestyles and improvements in quality of life. Changes in living status can be translated into cost savings (Ashley *et al.*, 1990) and there is evidence to suggest that this monetary gain can be increased with transitional placements prior to eventual discharge (McLaughlin & Peters, 1993). Wood *et al.* (1999) evaluated a community integration programme on two sites and demonstrated significant changes in accommodation and occupation following residential rehabilitation. Gains were evident well beyond the period when most spontaneous recovery might be expected, but projected savings in care costs were greatest for persons admitted within two years of injury. Treatment costs were omitted from this study but have been included in a more recent multi-site evaluation by the first author (Worthington *et al.*, 2006) confirming that cost-savings can be made even for persons admitted five or more years after injury, though the largest financial benefits are made where rehabilitation is commenced within one year of injury.

Conclusion

This chapter has attempted to provide the reader with an overview of key aspects of the design and delivery of residential services for traumatic brain injury. Legislation is having an increasing impact on residential services and it is therefore vital that clinicians, managers and the regulating authorities work hand in hand to understand one another's roles and develop effective means of rehabilitation and support. Clinicians and managers must keep abreast of legislative changes that are likely to affect how services are delivered, adapting practices accordingly.

Throughout the chapter we have raised issues which are of relevance for effective psychological intervention. A number of documents have been produced previously, recommending particular forms of service provision (summarised in Herbert, 2004), but nationally service development has been patchy (see McMillan, 2003). Residential services in particular have been poorly served by such documents, which tend to focus on hospital and community provision. The British Psychological Society's Working Party report on services for young adults with brain injury (British Psychological Society, 1989) recommended residential services for managing behaviour disturbance and long-term supported living. No specific recommendations were forthcoming from the government-funded National Traumatic Brain Injury Study (Centre for Health Service Studies, University of Warwick, 1998). Moreover, recent guidelines from the British Society of Rehabilitation Medicine (BSRM, 2003) perpetuate the dichotomy between hospital-based rehabilitation (including post-acute care) and community support on an out-patient or domiciliary basis. This prevailing somewhat medicalised view stands contrary to the evidence. Rather than being squeezed out by hospital services at one end and community rehabilitation at the other, residential services for traumatic brain injury have been expanding significantly in the past decade. There is now a clear range of such services, from standalone neurobehavioural facilities, through residential rehabilitation units offering community integration programmes, to 'continuing rehabilitation' centres offering lifelong support and numerous supported housing schemes throughout the country.

Notes

1 A term introduced by the first author in relation to West Heath House on its inception. This may be the first time the term was used in relation to a specific facility, though the notion of a community integration rehabilitation programme has been adopted for many years.

2 Since September 2005 the Psychology Department at the University of Swansea has offered a certificate, diploma and MSc degree in brain injury rehabilitation.

Recommended Reading

Eames, P., Turnbull, J. & Goodman-Smith, A. (1989). Service delivery and assessment of programs. In M. Lezak (Ed.) *Assessment of the behavioural consequences of head trauma* (pp.195–214). New York: Alan R. Liss.

This is an excellent chapter, in an otherwise rather dated book, which has not been surpassed in addressing key issues in the dynamics of a rehabilitation team.

Muir-Giles, G. & Clark-Wilson, J. (1999). *Rehabilitation of the severely head injured adult: A practical approach* (2nd edn). Cheltenham: Stanley Thornes.
This book provides a very practical overview of behaviourally based intervention methods in practical contexts, combining psychological and functional perspectives to good effect.

Wesolowski, M.D. & Zenicus, A.H. (1994). *A practical guide to head injury rehabilitation. A focus on post-acute residential settings.* New York: Plenum Press, 239pp.
This North American book covers an extensive range of issues likely to be encountered in post-acute residential settings, including treatment planning and team working.

Wood R.Ll. & McMillan, T.M. (2001). *Neurobehavioural disability and social handicap following traumatic brain injury.* Hove: Psychology Press, 315pp.
This book contains excellent chapters on key aspects of post-acute rehabilitation, including challenging behaviour, psychological therapy, mental capacity and service development.

References

Aloia, M.S., Long, C.J. & Allen, J.B. (1995). Depression among the head-injured and non-head-injured: A discriminant analysis. *Brain Injury*, *9*, 575–583.

Ashley, M.J., Krych, D.K. & Lehr, R.P. (1990). Cost/benefit analysis for post-acute rehabilitation of the traumatically brain-injured patient. *Journal of Insurance Medicine*, *22*, 156–161.

British Psychological Society (1989). *Services for young adults with acquired brain damage.* Leicester: British Psychological Society.

British Society of Rehabilitation Medicine/Royal College of Physicians (2003). *Rehabilitation following acquired brain injury: National clinical guidelines* (L. Turner-Stokes, Ed.). London: RCP/BSRM.

Burke, W.H., Wesoloswki, M.D. & Guth, M.L. (1988). Comprehensive head injury rehabilitation: An outcome evaluation. *Brain Injury*, *2*, 313–322.

Connolly, D. & O'Dowd, T. (2001). The impact of different disabilities arising from head injury on the primary caregiver. *British Journal of Occupational Therapy*, *64*, 41–46.

Cope, D.N. (1995). The effectiveness of traumatic brain injury rehabilitation: A review. *Brain Injury*, *9*, 649–670.

Department of Health (1990). *NHS and Community Care Act.* London: HMSO.

Department of Health (2001). *Government response to the Health Select Committee: Inquiry into head injury rehabilitation.* Norwich: The Stationery Office.

Department of Health (2005a). *Bournewood Consultation: The approach to be taken in response to the judgment of the European Court of Human Rights in the 'Bournewood' case.* London: Department of Health.

Department of Health (2005b). *The National Service Framework for Long-term Conditions.* London: Department of Health.

Devany Serio, C., Kreutzer, J.S. & Gervasio, A.H. (1995). Predicting family needs after brain injury: Implications for intervention. *Journal of Head Trauma Rehabilitation*, *10*, 32–45.

De Wit, G.A., Busschbach, J.J.V. & De Charro, F.Th. (2000). Sensitivity and perspective in the valuation of health status: Whose values count? *Health Economics*, *9*, 109–126.

Eames, P. (1989). Head injury rehabilitation: Towards a 'model' service. In R.Ll. Wood & P. Eames (Eds.) *Models of brain injury rehabilitation* (pp.49–58). London: Chapman & Hall.

Eames, P. (1992). Hysteria following brain injury. *Journal of Neurology, Neurosurgery and Psychiatry, 55*, 1046–1053.

Eames, P. (2001). Distinguishing the neuropsychiatric, psychiatric and psychological consequences of acquired brain injury. In R.Ll. Wood & T.M. McMillan (Eds.) *Neurobehavioural disability and social handicap following traumatic brain injury* (pp.29–45). Hove: Psychology Press.

Eames, P.G. & Wood, R.Ll. (1985). Rehabilitation after severe head injury: A follow-up study of a behaviour modification approach. *Journal of Neurology, Neurosurgery and Psychiatry, 48*, 613–619.

Fedoroff, J.P., Starkstein, S.E., Forrester, A.W., Geisler, F.H., Jorge, R.E., Arndt, S.V. *et al.* (1992). Depression in patients with acute traumatic brain injury. *American Journal of Psychiatry, 149*, 918–923.

Glenn, M.B., Rotman, M., Goldstein, R. & Selleck, E. (2005). Characteristics of residential community integration programs for adults with brain injury. *Journal of Head Trauma Rehabilitation, 20*, 393–401.

Goll, S. & Hawley, K. (1989). Social rehabilitation: The role of the transitional living centre. In R.Ll. Wood & P. Eames (Eds.) *Models of brain injury rehabilitation* (pp.142–163). London: Chapman & Hall.

Herbert, C. (2004). Planning, delivering and evaluating services. In L.H. Goldstein & J.E. McNeil (Eds.) *Clinical neuropsychology: A practical guide to assessment and management for clinicians* (pp.367–383). Chichester: Wiley.

High, W.M., Boake, C. & Lehmkuhl, L.D. (1995). Critical analysis of studies evaluating the effectiveness of rehabilitation after traumatic brain injury. *Journal of Head Trauma Rehabilitation, 10*, 14–26.

Kreutzer, J.S., Gervasio, A.H. & Camplair, P.S. (1994). Patient correlates of caregivers' distress and family functioning after traumatic brain injury. *Brain Injury, 8*, 211–230.

Lewis, J. (1999). The concept of community care and primary care in the UK: The 1960s to the 1990s. *Health and Social Care in the Community, 7*(5), 333–341.

Lush, D. (2001). Understanding and assessing capacity. In R.Ll. Wood & T.M. McMillan (Eds.) *Neurobehavioural disability and social handicap following traumatic brain injury* (pp.91–103). Hove: Psychology Press.

Manchester, D., Priestley, N. & Jackson, H. (2004). The assessment of executive functions: Coming out of the office. *Brain Injury, 18*, 1067–1081.

Manchester, D. & Wood, R.Ll. (2001). Applying cognitive therapy in neurobehavioural rehabilitation. In R.Ll. Wood & T.M. McMillan (Eds.) *Neurobehavioural disability and social handicap following traumatic brain injury* (pp.157–174). Hove: Psychology Press.

Marquis, R. & Jackson, R. (2000). Quality of life and quality of service relationships: Experiences of people with disabilities. *Disability and Society, 15*(3), 411–425.

Mazaux, J.M. & Richer, E. (1998). Rehabilitation after traumatic brain injury in adults. *Disability and Rehabilitation, 20*, 435–447.

McLaughlin, A.M. & Peters, S. (1993). Evaluation of an innovative cost-effective programme for brain injury patients: Response to a need for flexible treatment planning. *Brain Injury, 7*, 71–75.

McMillan, T.M. (2003). Neurorehabilitation services and their delivery. In B.A. Wilson (Ed.) *Neuropsychological rehabilitation. Theory and practice* (pp.271–291). Lisse, The Netherlands: Swets & Zeitlinger.

McMillan, T.M. & Oddy, M. (2001). Service provision for social disability and handicap after acquired brain injury. In R.Ll. Wood & T.M. McMillan (Eds.) *Neurobehavioural disability and social handicap following traumatic brain injury* (pp.257–273). Hove: Psychology Press.

National Institutes of Health (NIH) (1999). Rehabilitation of persons with traumatic brain injury. *Journal of the American Medical Association*, *282*, 974–983.

National Traumatic Brain Injury Study (1998). *National Traumatic Brain Injury Study: Summary of report.* Warwick: Centre for Health Services, University of Warwick.

South Thames Brain Injury Rehabilitation Association (2000). *User's guide to minimum standards for post acute brain injury rehabilitation.* Tadworth: South Thames Brain Injury Rehabilitation Association.

Swift, T.L. & Wilson, S.L. (2001). Misconceptions about brain injury among the general public and non-expert health professionals: An exploratory study. *Brain Injury*, *15*, 149–165.

Walker, W.C., Kreutzer, J.S. & Witol, A.D. (1996). Level of care options for the low-functioning brain injury survivor. *Brain Injury*, *10*, 65–75.

Wood, R.Ll. (1996). Ten years of post acute brain injury rehabilitation (a view from the independent sector). *Personal Injury*, *3*, 203–211.

Wood, R.Ll., McCrea, J.D., Wood, L. & Merriman, R.N. (1999). Clinical and cost effectiveness of post-acute neurobehavioral rehabilitation. *Brain Injury*, *13*, 69–88.

Wood, R.Ll. & Worthington, A.D. (2001a). Neurobehavioural rehabilitation: A conceptual paradigm. In R.Ll. Wood & T.M. McMillan (Eds.) *Neurobehavioural disability and social handicap following traumatic brain injury* (pp.107–131). Hove: Psychology Press.

Wood, R.Ll. & Worthington, A.D. (2001b). Neurobehavioural rehabilitation in practice. In R.Ll. Wood & T.M. McMillan (Eds.) *Neurobehavioural disability and social handicap following traumatic brain injury* (pp.133–155). Hove: Psychology Press.

Worthington, A. (2003a). Out on a limb? Developing an integrated rehabilitation service for adults with acquired brain injury. *Clinical Psychology*, *23*, 14–18.

Worthington, A.D. (2003b). The natural recovery and treatment of executive disorders. In P.W. Halligan, U. Kischka & J.C. Marshall (Eds.) *Handbook of clinical neuropsychology* (pp.322–339). New York: Oxford University Press.

Worthington, A. (2005). Rehabilitation of executive disabilities: Effective treatment of relayed disabilities. In P.W. Halligan & D.T. Wade (Eds.) *Effectiveness of rehabilitation for cognitive deficits* (pp.257–267). New York: Oxford University Press.

Worthington, A., Matthews, S., Melia, Y. & Oddy, M. (2006). Cost-benefits associated with social outcome from neurobehavioural rehabilitation. *Brain Injury*, *20*, 947–957.

Worthington, A. & Melia, Y. (2006). Rehabilitation is compromised by arousal and sleep disorders: Results of a survey of rehabilitation staff. *Brain Injury*, *20*, 327–332.

Worthington, A. & Oldham, J.B. (2006). Delayed discharge from brain injury rehabilitation. *Clinical Rehabilitation*, *20*, 79–82.

Ylvisaker, M., Jacobs, H. & Feeney, T. (2003). Positive supports for people who experience behavioural and cognitive disability after brain injury. *Journal of Head Trauma Rehabilitation*, *18*, 7–32.

Part II

Cognitive Rehabilitation

6

Communication Difficulties

Pat McKenna and Claire Willson

Introduction

Communication is a far-reaching term to cover not only the tools of words and sentences used in spoken and written language, but also the use of voice, intonation gesture, facial expression and body stance in 'extralinguistic' non-verbal interactions. It also includes the meta-level understanding that takes place in interpersonal relationships in the workplace, between colleagues, friends, family and intimates. Communication is the glue that binds people within a healthy functional social network. As such, good communication is fundamental to the well-being of individuals.

In terms of brain function, communication reflects a huge array of very complex linguistic and extralinguistic functions. Following severe and very severe traumatic brain injury, there are very often significant alterations in communication skills, sometimes at the level of words and sentences, often within extralinguistic, non-verbal skills and nearly always at the meta-level of relationships. The duration and severity of difficulty will vary with the severity of traumatic brain injury from mild through to moderate, severe and very severe.

There have been major breakthroughs in our understanding of brain function over the past 30 years which have revealed organisational principles which are counterintuitive and provoke much controversy among researchers, not least in the field of language and communication. In this context, notions of informed rehabilitative practice must be tempered by an awareness that we are still feeling our way and rehabilitation is still exploratory and experimental. We should be tentative rather than authoritative in our pronouncements on 'how to do it'. As yet, we do not have a global systematic roll-out of programmes but small innovative ideas based on our gradual discoveries of how communication works.

This chapter will provide an overview of our current understanding of how the brain organises and delivers our multiple means of communication and its associated neuro-anatomical correlates; the effects of traumatic brain injury on communication in terms of the types and range of communication difficulties seen after traumatic brain injury; and the interventions used in rehabilitation programmes to address these issues.

In the spirit of adventure that defines good rehabilitation, the interventions described here illustrate individualised, creative programmes both to assess and treat language and communication difficulties.

The Functional Organisation of Communication in the Brain

Non-verbal communication

There is an evolutionary order to our acquisition of communication and language skills seen in our phylogenetic development (i.e. as a species) and which is also echoed in the ontogenetic order of acquisition (i.e. in the development of the child). As a species, we communicated in non-verbal mode long before we acquired spoken language, and are probably far more accurate in using it than we are in using words and sentences to communicate. Non-verbal communication consists of eye contact and facial expression, gestures, particularly unconscious ones, body language in the way one moves, stands, sits in relation to others and also the qualitative use of voice (intonation) as opposed to the literal content of words and sentences. It is certainly more powerful in conveying emotional intent than words. For example, the speaker who is very angry but uses placatory words, or is fearful but uses bold words, or is indifferent but uses kind words will provoke, at the least, confusion, and at most, disbelief, in the listener.

Non-verbal communication is mostly an unconscious process which is probably why it has taken so long to reach our collective neuropsychological awareness in research, assessment or tests. It has, however, long been recognised in speech and language therapy in terms of 'prosody', that is, the intonation, stress and rhythm used in uttering words and sentences. Box 6.1 gives an example of the power of prosody in adding both affective and linguistic meaning to an utterance.

Box 6.1 Example of the power of prosody to convey affective and linguistic meaning

'Give me the book' =

'***Give*** me the book' (stop waving it about, hanging onto it, procrastinating . . .) conveys irritation

'Give ***me*** the book' (don't give it to them, they won't look after it . . .) conveys beseeching

'Give me the ***book***' (not the papers or the pen or the packaging . . .) conveys neutral clarification, or impatience

In keeping with most aspects of non-verbal communication, prosody is thought to be very heavily dependent on right hemisphere functioning. As with aphasia batteries, tests of non-verbal functioning focus on comprehension rather than self-expression simply because the correct response is a known quantity whereas self-expression is very idiosyncratic and difficult to assess in terms of being correct or wrong. The Right Hemisphere Language Battery (Bryan, 1995), the Brief Inventory of Communication and Cognition (Burns, 1997) and the Conversational Analysis Profiles for People with Aphasia (Whitworth *et al.*, 1997) are some of the few tests which specialise in screening for the comprehension of the figurative use of language focusing particularly on the implicit meaning contained in words and sentences. These include the understanding of metaphor, humour and prosody with a small foray into the purely non-verbal aspects of communication in discourse analysis, a qualitative exercise.

A more recent test, The Awareness of Social Inference Test – TASIT (McDonald *et al.*, 2002), uses video material to specifically test for comprehension of non-verbal communication. We have found this to be a useful tool to adapt and trial for treatment as it has two versions. The first can be used for assessment and then as material for re-education with the second as reassessment following treatment. The test uses actors conveying increasingly complex emotions and social interactions. The first part consists of emotional evaluation, with parts 2 and 3 requiring social inferences of intentions, attitudes and meanings of the speakers.

All the more basic aspects of non-verbal communication are thought to be particularly dependent on right hemisphere functions and are seen to be disrupted in right hemisphere pathology. Beyond this, however, there is no fine mapping of these functions in terms of brain–behaviour correlates.

Verbal communication

Verbal communication involves words and sentences, which, in the light of our growing understanding of cerebral organisation, translates into *semantics* (content words) and *syntax* (the rules of grammar). There is much evidence to show that this dichotomy has its counterpart in distinct cerebral systems in the brain (e.g. Garrard *et al.*, 2004).

Semantics

The verbal semantic system is composed of all those things in the world for which human primates have produced a verbal label. In terms of individual acquisition, we develop first visual and then verbal representations of the objects in our physical environment, and it seems to be easier to acquire labels for animals and fruits and vegetables before artificial objects (e.g. McKenna & Parry, 1994). Later we acquire labels for movements ('jumping', 'running') and then labels for abstract concepts ('pleasure', 'ability'). All these memory representations are without time coordinates, and are just 'known' without recourse to how and when acquired. They form our general knowledge stock and personal vocabulary and include the names of colours, body parts, facts of arithmetic, and all the scholastic knowledge-base of facts as well as the names of places and people that come to make up our world. This vast knowledge-base has come to be known as the semantic memory system.

Warrington's (1975) seminal paper first provided clinical evidence for the circumscribed existence of a dedicated semantic memory system in the brain by describing three patients with semantic dementia whose semantic memory systems were impaired while other linguistic processes, visual perception and general intellectual functioning were intact. The 'agnosia' (loss of meaning) was purely for those words and concepts which make up the vocabulary and knowledge-base. While the individuals could see something clearly and even draw it or recognise that the object was the same from diverse angles and consequently completely different percepts, they no longer knew what the thing was (though they might recognise it as familiar). This is now well documented in many cases of acquired brain injury and especially in patients with semantic dementia (e.g. Hodges *et al.*, 1992; Snowden *et al.*, 1989).

Warrington developed her theory for category-specific and modality-specific organisation within the semantic memory system based on clinical investigations (Warrington, 1981). With her colleagues, she later showed that within the semantic memory system, those things that make up the natural world of animals, plant life and fruits and vegetables can dissociate from those things that make up the technical environment of artificial objects, so that patients can lose knowledge about things within one category but not the other (e.g. Warrington & McCarthy, 1983; Warrington & Shallice, 1984).

Similarly, in considering the difference between visual recognition of an object (knowing what scissors are for, when you *see* them) and verbal comprehension of an object (understanding the word 'scissors' when you *hear* it), patients may lose the representation derived by one modality but not the other (McCarthy & Warrington, 1986). Furthermore, this effect can be restricted to *a circumscribed category*. For example, McCarthy and Warrington (1988) describe a patient who had a difficulty restricted to animals which he could identify by sight but not by name. Following TBI, category and modality effects can sometimes be seen in the earlier stages of recovery, but for the most part they are transient or sufficiently slight to have low priority for the client and family in the longer-term rehabilitation programme.

A similar dissociation for abstract and concrete vocabulary was first noted by Warrington (1975). More recently, Crutch and Warrington (2005) have provided evidence to show that the organisational structure of abstract vocabulary is intrinsically different from the organisation of concrete vocabulary, as revealed by the pattern of breakdown in agnosic patients.

There has been much research, debate and controversy in clinical and academic departments internationally on the subject of the category-specific organisation of the semantic system and this has now been incorporated into the relatively new area of cerebral localisation using highly developed neuroradiological equipment to observe brain activity in non-injured subjects or to delineate areas of damage in neurological patients. So far, the dominant hemisphere is accepted as the seat of the linguistic aspects of communication and the left temporal lobe appears critical for semantic functioning (for an overview see McKenna & Warrington, 2000).

Following traumatic brain damage, it is common for individuals to have a degraded knowledge-base. In rehabilitation practice, we have found that students in school or higher education are particularly vulnerable and often need to revisit academic areas of study that were well known beforehand. When this is compounded by episodic memory problems and executive difficulties, the expectation of catching up and continuing with studies without support is usually unrealistic. Similarly, the effect of reduced efficiency in semantic functioning following traumatic brain injury is seen in more demanding naming tests where the items are graded in difficulty, such as the Graded Naming Test (McKenna & Warrington, 1983), a test composed of 30 black-and-white drawings of objects to name, and the Category-Specific Names Test (McKenna, 1997), a test composed of 120 coloured photographs of fruits and vegetables, animals and objects. Though no overt dysphasia or word-finding difficulties are evident, in our experience people in the earlier stages of recovery from TBI commonly score below the tenth percentile and often below the first percentile. With more focal damage to the left temporal lobe subserving the semantic system, the individual may have an associative agnosia and have lost basic knowledge about the objects. An example of such difficulties is provided in Case 6.1 by QL, whose TBI produced a focal area of damage in the left temporal lobe and who had lost much of her knowledge of animals and some of fruits and vegetables, with comparative sparing of artificial objects.

We are now beginning to appreciate that many more people have subtle loss of knowledge which would previously have been interpreted as an executive difficulty. For instance, one patient who appeared overwhelmed by the size of a supermarket picked up a peach as an ingredient in making a tomato-based sauce for spaghetti. Another patient in preparing a sauce began chopping an onion in crude hunks with the skin still intact, and chopped a green pepper with the stalk, seeds and pith included. As these errors were restricted to foodstuffs which the individuals had used premorbidly in cooking, they may well reflect impaired semantic functioning or a degraded semantic knowledge-base.

Syntax

Syntax is a more technical term for grammar and refers to the words that give sentence structure. It includes function words (e.g. 'the', 'of') and smaller units called morphemes which are the non-semantic parts of verbs and content words (e.g. '***was*** run***ning***', book***s***) and the rules of word order that dictate the meaning (e.g. 'the cat chased the dog'/'the dog chased the cat', 'the dog was chased by the cat'/'the cat was chased by the dog'). Syntax seems to have evolved to allow a verbal carriage to convey to others a description of the interaction of things (semantic representations) over space and time. Very little is understood about the cerebral organisation of syntax apart from the critical role of an area in the left frontal region for language production, and syntax in particular. Topographically this is Broadman's area 44/45, also known as Broca's area. Focal damage here results in telegrammatic, halting speech with comparatively rich semantic vocabulary but no grammar. Content words can be produced without syntax. For example, 'table . . . water . . . floor . . . spill' might be produced for 'I have just spilt some water on the table and it's gone onto the floor'. Pure or gross forms of these syndromes are not particularty associated with TBI but these landmark syndromes can help to understand how language is organised. Furthermore, elements of them can begin to be detected in milder form following TBI and become most evident when the client is cognitively overloaded.

Case 6.1: Category-specific agnosia in a patient, QL, following traumatic brain injury

- **History:** TBI following horse-riding accident, causing subarachnoid haemorrhage and left cerebellar, left temporal and left parietal haematomas. In spite of being highly articulate, QL had episodic and semantic memory deficits including moderately impaired ongoing memory for events and an agnosia which was selectively poorer for animals. QL had lost a little of the schema of animal kingdom knowledge but particularly the links between this schema and individual animals.
- **Examples:**
  Thought
  - a badger could fly;
  - a hippopotamus could be eaten and could be tamed;
  - whales usually eat what people put out for them, like vegetation and nuts, usually in man-made circuses and can be trained;
  - a rhinoceros could be tamed;
  - an eagle is a bird that sings, goes into the garden and eats bird food;
  - a hedgehog is good for breeding, can make clothes and can make them do things, used for knitting.

  Whereas:
  - Confetti: paper that's cut in a point way into V . . . and used at weddings and throw over bride and groom.
  - Whisk: electric instrument you put things in. Can cut apart, mix 2 liquids together.
  - Tambourine: musical instrument. Rounded one side on it and made of muslin and round rings. If you bash it, it will make a noise.
  - Hand grenade: bomb – blow up. Cause injury and shatter things. Makes a noise.
  - Binoculars: look through and enlarge what you're looking at. Can be writing on paper and then enlarged or drawing . . .

QL was able to improve her knowledge with daily practice, but there was no lasting effect once the practice stopped, and the efficacy of remediating semantic deficits is still to be ascertained. QL also had marked difficulties in episodic memory retention, so this double deficit may have contributed to her difficulty in regaining this knowledge. The degree of linkage in these processes is still being mapped.

Crutch and Warrington (2003) have very recently provided evidence to suggest a critical role for abstract vocabulary in fuelling sentence production. They describe a non-TBI patient who had a significant word-finding difficulty for concrete, but not abstract, word vocabulary and whose performance on simple naming tests was halting and very impaired. In striking contrast, his pragmatic communication (i.e. social conversation) was normal, fluent and competent and his word-finding difficulty was not detectable. When presented with naturalistic pictures and photographs, they showed that he was able to describe these effectively but when shown the traditional pictures used in naming therapy, which are crowded with things, he became dysphasic. This tantalising finding makes phylogenetic sense in that abstract vocabulary is undoubtedly a second-level conceptual development and closer sequentially to sentence production in the timescale of our development. Difficulties in monitoring speech output and self-expression are not uncommon following traumatic brain injury and these new findings may help us understand the consequent difficulties that some of this client group have with the more abstract levels of thinking and in monitoring verbal output, which may be reduced to simple concrete statements on one hand or rambling and circuitous on the other.

Comprehension and expression in verbal communication

It is again very instructive to consider childhood development to understand the development of our verbal skill. Children can first understand many words and easy sentences when listening to adults. However, it takes enormous effort and a considerably longer time before their attempts at short utterances can be understood. It is helpful to emphasise the close association between the semantic memory system and cerebral operations involved in comprehension. It echoes the natural order of acquisition in understanding before speaking, and acquiring semantics (first visual then verbal) before syntax. The auditory cortex (Heschl's gyrus) sits compactly in the fold between the superior temporal gyrus and angular gyrus and, on the left, is best placed to cascade to the semantic system. Lesions adjacent to this area lead to difficulties in comprehension and semantics and often produce the fluent but meaningless verbal outpourings characteristic of Wernicke's aphasia.

In the dysphasic population, it is far more common to have more severe difficulties in self-expression compared to understanding spoken language. In TBI this is also reflected in the very common incidence of dysarthria (a difficulty in articulation affected by a weakness or paralysis in the muscles for speaking) and dyspraxia (when the programmes for the coordination of the muscles used for speech break down). Where this is particularly poor, the individual may require a communication aid such as an alphabet chart or a keyboard system (e.g. see section on using an alphabet chart).

Literacy

Literacy refers to reading and writing and is subserved by cerebral functioning within the left parietal lobe. Literacy is a subsidiary and secondary form of language expression and is therefore heavily dependent on spoken language. Thus, if spoken language is severely disrupted then the ability to communicate in written mode will usually mirror this, in terms of the content of the written message. However, it is possible for literacy skills and spoken language to dissociate. Furthermore, where deficits are restricted only to systems subserving literacy, it is possible to be able to read but not write, or vice versa. However, very often following traumatic brain injury, the ability to read for *meaning* is impaired though the basic mechanical skills of reading and writing are intact. This can also be compounded by a further difficulty in the fine visual tracking needed to scan prose as many people have subtle difficulty with binocular vision following traumatic brain injury. Reduced cerebral resources are taken up with the lower sensory levels of the reading and writing activity with consequent impairment to the higher-level functions involved in encoding and decoding for meaning.

Executive function in communication

The preceding sections have demonstrated the complexity of the *basic* skills of non-verbal and verbal communication. However, bringing these skills to bear in everyday situations of home, work and social life to communicate effectively is a far more complex process. It is here that many people living with acquired brain injury experience huge difficulty and distress. While the automatic skills of social niceties, and intellectual discourse, give an appearance of normal, even impressive, interpersonal competence at first meeting, over time an inability to maintain and develop relationships becomes apparent as family, work or social relations break down. Often people and their families will need much support in on-line maintenance of communication and understanding.

Normal human development in these areas is still relatively embryonic and getting it wrong (conflict, miscommunication and stress) is as 'normal' as getting it right (harmony) within interpersonal relationships. However, this is probably one of the most difficult challenges for human adults, and relies almost entirely on frontal lobe functioning – areas of the brain which are particularly vulnerable in traumatic brain injury. Working with people who have suffered a traumatic brain injury highlights the amazing complexity in normal social intercourse and the easy loss of societal contact and confidence with even a little depletion or impairment of executive skills.

Normal emotional, cognitive and social processes are amazingly complex and consequently faults in these processes such as occurs following frontal lobe damage are still little understood, but can be easily conceptualised as faults in the 'stop, start and change mechanisms'. In social exchanges, fast-rising anger, impatience or anxiety cannot be stopped or changed, leading to further breakdown in communication. Passivity, lack of awareness of turn-taking, reduced ability to understand idioms, absurdities and sarcasm, poor topic maintenance and lack of initiative can make the relationship one-sided. Inability to think flexibly can cause rigidity and obsessionality to replace spontaneity and rationality, and egocentricity to replace empathy and altruism. More subtly still, a sudden, unexpected behaviour in an otherwise consistent predictable pattern, like the virus in the computer, can cause chaos and confusion in interpersonal life.

TBI and Communication

Though any pure dysphasic syndrome can occur as a result of TBI, this is comparatively rare. These syndromes include Broca's aphasia (characterised by loss of syntax, particularly in self-expression, making speech telegrammatic), Wernicke's aphasia (where speech is plentiful but without meaning as semantics are affected) or the transcortical aphasias (characterised by a partial disconnection between comprehension and production). Syndromes affecting reading (dyslexia) and writing (agraphia) can also occur. These forms of focal linguistic impairments will be intensively addressed by programmes and methods provided by specialist communication professionals.

However, the near-universal difficulties in communication following the more severe forms of TBI occur as a result of generalised damage throughout the cortex and particularly the frontal systems. They represent the computational interactions of impaired basic skills of language, perception, memory, thinking and organisation and affect both intellectual operations and social functioning. For instance, Adolphs *et al.* (2000) found that damage to the right somatosensory-related cortices together with the amygdala and right visual cortices can give rise to emotion-perception deficits. Reduced self-awareness and perception of others, disinhibition, reduced processing and memory of events and themes, and problems understanding subtleties in conversation are only some of the common issues faced by individuals with traumatic brain injury. There is an ever-changing kaleidoscope of ways in which the creative act of communication can break down following TBI which cannot be encapsulated by a set number of descriptive labels. However, the following interventions describe and address means to help overcome some of these difficulties.

Communicating with people in the early stages of recovery from TBI

Though it is the long-term communication difficulties which have dominated the rehabilitation literature on traumatic brain injury, there are important communication issues for the patient in the immediate and earlier stages of recovery which need to be addressed by the care team.

Low levels of awareness and the early stages of recovery

Many people recovering from severe head injury will have been in a coma for days or weeks in an intensive care unit and a high-dependency unit within the acute setting of a hospital before being transferred to a rehabilitation unit. Typically, the family will have experienced the shock of possible bereavement but will now be euphorically optimistic as a result of transfer to a rehabilitation unit. For most families, it is an alien idea that a person and their brain are in many ways one and the same, and the lay concept of a brain is that it bestows lesser or greater degrees of intelligence or is like a modem through which the person (who is intact somewhere) communicates with the world. Families often expect a clear moment of awakening or a gradual daily, weekly or monthly rise in level of awareness until the person arrives back again in their entirety. In reality there is no guarantee during this time that the next stage of awareness will occur. The most honest advice to the family at this time is to emphasise the wait-and-see principle but it is fair to say there is nearly always improvement, but how much and how far is different for each individual. This allows the necessary hope that the family need, and gives them time to adjust to a period of not knowing what may happen next, and for the therapist to gently educate the family in the concepts of brain functioning.

During these early days, the individual may well engage in primitive behaviours which can be misinterpreted as awareness or conscious attempts to communicate. Those areas of the brain which govern the earliest stages of our evolution in terms of basic survival and primitive behaviours are also the best protected in an injury to the head. Thus the deepest centres that govern the autonomic nervous system and cranial nerves may be on auto pilot, with no awareness on the part of the individual. Such individuals may orient to noise, open and shut their eyes, track a moving object or person, grimace, yawn, etc. If the patient is deeply unresponsive, the occupational therapists and speech and language therapists may harness a coma battery to stimulate and screen for smell, sight, sound and touch, on a regular regime throughout the day or week (depending on staffing levels). The next area of evolutionary development within the brain, the limbic system, governs primitive drives such as fear, aggression, hunger, thirst and sexual behaviour. Without an understanding of the social context, many patients at this level of functioning will repulse or attack, in an instinctive, primitive response, anyone who interferes with their bodies. Resistance to nursing care and physiotherapy is very common at this stage and can intensify with the dawning of awareness.

Good psychological approaches are central to the care of the patient and the family at this stage. One is to interact verbally, visually and physically as gently as possible. At this stage, individuals are also hypersensitive to stimulation, which can be extremely irritating, particularly in auditory or tactile mode. People talking, especially in a loud voice, or many people talking at once can agitate people at this stage of recovery. It is very common for them to be supersensitive to touch, which may provoke high tone, spasm or severe pain. Nursing care requires a balancing act in auditory, visual and tactile communication between reducing the stimulation (only one of the nurses handling the patient should speak, and do so softly) and making visual and physical contact gently, with warning, and as slowly as possible. In an ideal world the same nursing team should work with a designated patient as, even without conscious awareness, a relationship appears to build based on predictability of contact. The nurse should approach well within the patient's visual field and, following a small delay, with a gentle greeting and, again with a small delay, begin touch. The same technique can be used by family and visitors. The patient may be unable to move, unable to lay down autobiographical memory, unable to process speech and be prey to bodily sensations which may well include pain. This fragility needs very skilled handling in these early stages of recovery from traumatic brain injury. It is important to gently explain and pre-warn the patient of what you are about to do, even if verbal comprehension is impaired, as the non-verbal aspects of communication will signal reassurance and individual words may connect. This is especially important for physically invasive procedures.

The next stage of awareness reflects the primacy of vision in our development as the individual really does begin to observe the environment and watches people first, objects later. Similarly, patients will hear and listen long before beginning to speak. At this stage of recovery, it is important to introduce an orientation sheet which bears the simple message that the patient is in hospital recovering from an accident and that memory is still weak. The message should also be reassuring. A typical sheet is demonstrated in Figure 6.1.

October 2005

TOM

Welcome to Rookwood Hospital, Cardiff.

You had an accident and knocked your head. Your memory is still not working properly yet so you may feel a bit confused. You will feel better soon.

Your mum visits every day about 4.00 pm.

Figure 6.1 Typical orientation sheet for use with patients in early stages of recovery from traumatic brain injury

This should be written or typed in very large, very bold print and should be in a visible location by the bedside and, if the patient can read, within reach. Rehabilitation staff and family should use it regularly with the patient and it should always be repeated in exactly the same verbal form. This is because the patient will then learn the message via the semantic system even if the episodic system is unreliable. It will be learned much like a poem or prayer and the patient will easily be able to recite it automatically once prompted. This provides a way for patients to reorient themselves even when everything still feels dreamlike.

Impassivity in the early stages of recovery from acquired brain injury

Very often, patients in early stages of recovery will have an impassive expression which will often continue indefinitely without intervention. If ignored, staff and family will unwittingly reinforce a lack of non-verbal communication. Though this can result from cerebral or cranial nerve damage, it most often seems to be a simple result of being in an extended period of coma, during which time facial muscles are immobile. Green *et al.* (2004) suggest that patients with recently acquired TBI are also impaired in the ability to perceive emotions in faces even without focal injury to those areas known to subserve face perception. During the slow early period of re-entry into the world, staff, family and friends make total allowance for this lack of non-verbal communication and do not give the negative feedback which would normally be instant in the premorbid state. With very little practice, individuals can again smile, grimace, screw their noses, raise their eyebrows and blow out their cheeks but may still need constant prompting to use these muscles in social interactions and to smile in greeting. On one occasion, months after a head injury, a young patient, Mavis, was interacting socially with the multidisciplinary team when one member of staff told a joke. Everybody laughed with the exception of Mavis and, when questioned, she agreed that she found it very funny. When informed that she wasn't actually smiling she immediately produced a very genuine and expansive grin. It was a powerful example of how automatic this mode of communication generally is, and how easy it can be to reawaken it in people recovering from head injury. Some years later, this patient is a regular attendee at Headway and noted for her animation and engagement in social interaction, not least for her non-verbal communication. Often, patients will also need to be reminded to use the automatic verbal greetings in saying hello and goodbye until this becomes again an automatic, unconscious process.

Use of an alphabet chart

It has been estimated that as many as two-thirds of the people who suffer a severe head injury have some form of dysarthria as a consequence of damage to the speech centres or apparatus (Murdoch & Theodoros, 1999). This can be so severe as to render the patient anarthric (unable to produce speech), or unintelligible. Even with slow and restricted movement, the ability to spell out a word is immeasurably empowering for someone whose ability to move is severely restricted and who cannot speak. Sometimes the person can be encouraged to scan and indicate (e.g. with a nod or blink) a letter on an alphabet chart as the therapist moves their finger along letters. Similarly, asking the person to think of a three-letter word and spell it out on a simple, quickly devised, alphabet chart maximises the reader's ability to deduce the word and reduces the load on the writer's physical and cognitive resources. When movement is so restricted and the activity very new, the exercise can be facilitated by asking for a particular category, e.g. 'a three-letter animal'. The 'eureka' climax is worth a lot for both writer and reader (especially when 'owl' emerges instead of the expected 'cat' or 'dog'). The pace should be gentle and dictated by the stamina of the patient. The format should include a yes/no code, which can be on the chart or in words or other symbols, or can be conveyed by blinking or gesture depending on the movement range of the patient. When there is very little contribution on the part of the patient, the therapist may need to be a little brave in guessing and reflecting the thoughts and feelings of the patient as well as reassuring, and do most of the talking; this also applies when the individual is very restricted in their ability to affirm what the clinician is saying by facial expression or other form of overt communication. Over time it is possible to see great fluency in the use of an alphabet chart when working with someone whose diction and movement are severely restricted. Quick shorthand methods evolve – numbering lines, separating vowels, letters standing for whole words. These earlier, slower stages in communication have invariably proved to have been highly valued by the individual and provided a strong platform for a therapeutic alliance, not least because they signalled patience, reassurance and faith in the individual's ability to eventually communicate. Speech and language therapists are experts in devising and producing more developed and professional alphabet and communication charts and can also access a variety of communication aids, including litewriters which speak aloud the message typed by the patient.

Addressing longer-term communication difficulties

Though long-term sequelae seen after traumatic brain injury can include the very specific focal difficulties as outlined above in verbal and non-verbal communication, the types and range of communication difficulties which are very common occur at the level of complex social interaction, where the summation of verbal and non-verbal communication interact with executive functioning. This reflects in part an overall reduction in cognitive resource as a result of the global nature of the injury to the brain and in part more selective damage to executive function subserved by the frontal lobes which are particularly vulnerable in traumatic brain injury.

Addressing the psychological repercussions of aphasia, dyspraxia and dysarthria

How individuals respond to sudden loss of ability to use words and sentences depends on many factors other than the change itself. For the multidisciplinary team, it is important, first, to consider and assess the premorbid personality of individuals and pre-existing configurations of, among other things, family, friends and work in formulating programmes of treatment. Language and communication are, after all, only a few of many threads in the texture of an individual's existence. Most often the cognitive changes are not selective to language and communication but may involve impairment in visual perception, memory or the executive system, with concomitant changes to intellectual, social or emotional capacity. It is essential to have a good understanding of the status of all these other areas of cognition, and monitor changes within them to time interventions appropriately. Clinicians have to work from the perspective of the individual patient, building on cognitive and emotional strengths to reinforce self-esteem and forge partnerships to decide which approach is best suited to rehabilitation. The actual remediation of aphasic symptoms may be least relevant to best outcome.

In aphasia, symptoms are immediate, overt and tangible and, as such, may be readily catastrophised by individuals, family and friends, who may all feel that the only solution is to regain the power of speech. Speech and language therapists can provide expert programmes of remediation where this is appropriate. In contrast, subtle deficits in the executive system usually go unnoticed at first by individuals, family and friends but, without specialist intervention, can cause havoc in many aspects of that individual's life. In many ways, it can be easier for an individual to cope with a circumscribed loss of language than a difficulty which is only apparent in stages over a protracted length of time and which is difficult to understand.

Addressing non-verbal communication difficulties

Non-verbal communication is a particularly pertinent aspect of behaviour after traumatic brain injury. For instance, Bara *et al.* (2001) showed that, in a group of 30 people who had sustained a closed head injury, extralinguistic communication was systematically more difficult for them than linguistic communication and this was revealed in a particular difficulty with the meta-level inferences of language in irony and deceit compared to simple and complex acts. This difficulty was due not to the analysis of words and sentences but to the extralinguistic context whereby the words and sentences are rendered ironic or deceitful. Even slight disruption to its smooth running produces magnified effects for interpersonal interactions in all areas of an individual's life, and, without recognition and intervention, can result in a downward spiral of isolation and depression.

As non-verbal communication is a predominantly unconscious process, the patient is often unaware of any deficits they may have. Patients with impairment in these areas of functioning tend to be slightly or distinctly off key in turn-taking in conversation, in making or dropping eye contact appropriately and in using and interpreting facial expressions. Some people may have a tendency to talk to thin air, particularly if the listener is on their left, making no eye contact at all, and the monologue may need to be interrupted to establish a dialogue. Alternatively, eye contact may be overlong and the person may stare. The rules of natural distance may be flouted and the individual may appear to stand menacingly close. Where the unconscious and automatic skills of social interaction ends and the higher-level executive behaviours of social intercourse begin is difficult to disentangle, especially as our awareness and research into non-verbal communication is in its infancy. Fortunately, the rehabilitation treatment is the same for both and is described next in the section on working with executive deficits in communication.

Addressing executive deficits in communication

The executive systems are heavily involved in effective communication, particularly in non-linguistic or pragmatic form. Difficulties in following the social and cultural rules of communication can be common experiences associated with executive dysfunction and may be exclusive of aphasia. For example, some may have good grammar, articulation and semantics, but lack social judgement in their interaction. Pragmatic communication (applied to actual social situations) or social skill deficits have been shown to be more evident in TBI clients compared with orthopaedic controls, with poor appropriateness, effort and initiation reported (Bond & Godfrey, 1997; Godfrey *et al.*, 1993). In Bond and Godfrey's (1997) study, TBI participants were noted to prompt less in conversation and spoke for longer than controls. Other research findings suggest that these individuals have difficulty finding words and expressing themselves clearly, particularly if they also have dysarthria (Wong *et al.*, 2005). Such difficulties are likely to reduce the frequency of social relationships and result in over-reliance on family contact; with implications for increased familial stress and breakdown.

Judd (1999) has separated communication pragmatics into six areas:

1 **Non-verbal behaviour:** Typical non-verbal impairments can include misjudgements of gestures, of physical proximity, of eye contact or of voice volume.
2 **Turn-taking:** Managing the flow and timing of conversation can be difficult, particularly if there is a lack of insight or self-monitoring. In such cases the person may fail to allow others to comment, interrupt conversations or have problems initiating speech. For observers, the extent of the individual's capabilities and understanding might be overlooked if judged solely on the

quality of the interaction. John, a young gentleman with anoxic brain damage, was referred to our community rehabilitation service for rehabilitation with a focus on improving his limited understanding and expression. Assessment revealed significant initiation difficulties in speech and action, but intact semantic knowledge. Through rehabilitation friends and family members were encouraged to allow a 20- to 30-second time lapse following a question as a means of providing him with enough time to process and respond. A significant increase was subsequently noted in his inclusion in general conversation.

3 **Topic maintenance**: Other pragmatic communication difficulties can include managing the structure of a conversation or conveying the point of the conversation. For those with attention difficulties, external and internal distractions can interfere with the flow of thoughts, resulting in detours from the main focus, usually characterised as jumping from one topic to the next. Some individuals tend to convey all information with little or no structure and lose salient points. Perseveration and confabulation are very common with these difficulties.

   Receptive processing is also affected. Many individuals are unable to sustain attention long enough to process all the details provided; they cannot prioritise information or they jump to conclusions based on the limited information they have processed. Some describe the ease of one-to-one communication, particularly in quiet environments, but struggle to process conversation in group situations, especially in noisy situations such as pubs. This is because they are not able to filter out unwanted stimuli, nor track a conversation across many voices.

4 **Social appropriateness**: Damage to the orbital frontal regions is associated with social interaction difficulties including impulsivity, self-centredness and lack of empathy. Clients with these symptoms are often described by family or friends as self-absorbed and lacking any understanding of the needs of others. In conversation, these individuals discuss topics that relate only to themselves, have difficulty turn-taking in conversation and fail to ask others their opinions. Individuals with damage to these systems also respond inappropriately, have difficulty understanding humour and find it hard to pick out the subtleties in conversation (e.g. unable to respond to hints or non-verbal cues). Often people with traumatic brain injury find it hard to recognise when they make inappropriate and insensitive comments.

5 **Conversational repair**: Typically the individual is unable to correct mistakes made in conversation.

6 **Cohesiveness of narrative**: For some individuals, there is an ability to convey the general topic of conversation, but ideas within the dialogue seem somewhat disjointed.

Communication style

Confusion and frustration are common emotions experienced by individuals following TBI, and are often associated with misinterpretation of demands and poor understanding of concepts. As therapists, it is important to adapt communication style and presentation of ideas in therapy to reduce feelings of inadequacy and ineffectiveness from both parties; the client and therapist. When working with individuals with any form of language difficulty, it is important to ensure the client understands what you are trying to convey.

Reduced cognitive capacity and slowed processing are experiences shared by many individuals with brain injury. For some it takes a longer period of time to comprehend information and thus respond in an appropriate time, making conversations appear disjointed or giving the impression that the individual does not understand what is being said. Assessing the client's optimum speed of processing is essential for enhancing communication, and often involves the speaker slowing down the pronunciation of words, leaving gaps between words and ensuring time for the individual to respond.

In addition, there is a chance of overwhelming the client by providing too much information or making concepts too complex. An individual's capacity to process information may fluctuate according to several factors, including time of day, environment, people present, illness, fatigue and other stressors. Tailored treatment programmes focused on optimising the individual's capacity to process information might include limiting the length of session and never going beyond three or four pieces of information at any one time.

Disorders of attention can also impede comprehension and expression. As external factors can distract an individual trying to attend to a target conversation, clinicians need to consider modifying the environment in order to enhance comprehension. For example, turning off the television or radio, diverting telephone calls, ensuring lighting is appropriate, restricting noise or conversation from others and closing blinds or curtains. Providing a clear structure within a therapy session with regular prompts can also help re-orientate the client back to the focus of the task. Sometimes attention problems can be exacerbated by intrusive anxious thoughts, which might be helped with relaxation therapy or other therapeutic techniques such as mindfulness (which builds up the ability to focus on what is happening in the immediate present together with the ability to disengage as a calm observer).

Thinking about word use and content is essential. A thorough assessment by a speech and language therapist will provide detailed information about the types of words an individual might understand, including difficulties with syntax and problems recognising words outside the immediate context. Using concrete ideas and familiar words can help convey information more effectively. Professionals need to be aware of limiting jargonised phrases or words that have little or no meaning to the client. In addition, applying cultural and age-specific language sensitively not only helps the person express themselves in their own words, but can strengthen the therapeutic relationship.

Treatment Approaches

Over the past few years, there has been a move away from treatments based on remediation of specific communication impairments with uniform packages to developing more tailored strategies that consider individual patterns of impairment. These client-centred models have highlighted the importance of appropriate and meaningful goals, with a focus on a balance between the clinical setting and real-life experiences and contexts (Snow & Ponsford, 1995). This is particularly pertinent for community rehabilitation if, following a period of cocoon-like convalescence at home, the individual fails to re-engage with pre-existing family roles. At this point, the individual and/or family may be anxious to revisit the issue of prognosis. With gentle support from therapists, they begin to understand that recovery is not a linear progression to 'normality' and that the restitution of communication skills is possibly less relevant than learning the use of compensatory skills in communication.

While the treatment of communication problems has typically fallen within the domain of speech and language therapy (e.g. with programmes targeted at impairments associated with dysphasia, dyslexia, dyspraxia, articulatory dysfunction, laryngeal and velopharyngeal dysfunction), there is now a greater emphasis on applying collaborative interdisciplinary team approaches to communication difficulties experienced by individuals with TBI. Professionals involved should work jointly with a shared goal, allowing role overlap and liaising regularly to evaluate goal outcome. For example, occupational therapists might have an overview of communication needs within a vocational setting and, with support and consultation from the communication specialist, enable a programme to improve integration in the workplace.

Before any therapeutic work can begin, factors including age, gender, culture, educational background, occupational experiences, support systems and interests need to be assessed in order to facilitate the formulation of client-centred goals. Such factors are likely to heavily influence treatment suitability and efficacy. Clients and supporting individuals will need to be active participants, with professionals collaborating regularly with all involved.

Developing skills in communication pragmatics

Case 6.2 provides a case illustration of focal difficulties in non-verbal communication and how intervention can prevent the spiral of social isolation.

Formal assessment tools for evaluating social skills like the Fear of Negative Evaluation Scale and Social Avoidance & Distress Scale (Watson & Friend, 1969) can help identify pragmatic difficulties. Social skills therapy might include supporting the client to use more eye contact, monitor the volume of their voice, use smiles and apply appropriate gestures. Audiotape, videotape and mirrors can also be useful methods to highlight specific communication problems, particularly where there is a discrepancy between internal representation and external behaviour. Observation of interaction styles in everyday life, television programmes or films provides concrete examples for many clients. Another technique developed by Ylvisaker and Feeney (2000) encourages individuals to consider a person they admire (e.g. actor, politician, teacher) and assume their characteristics to help in social skills, in self-confidence and self-assertion.

As most people adapt their interaction according to whom they are communicating with, it is important to emphasise the various topics of conversation, nuances and non-verbal interactions that might be more suitable in one situation compared with another. Making conversation specific to the people included can help to maximise and maintain relationships. This might involve engaging the listener's attention by using their name in conversation, although this should be done cautiously as excessive use could have a negative effect. Similarly, helping the person to learn specific information in relation to the person they are talking to, e.g. their interests, family life and recent events, can help to develop positive relationships

Case 6.2: A case example of specific difficulties in non-verbal communication

Edward was a man in his early 30s who had sustained a head injury which resulted in a right hemisphere infarct visible on radiological investigation and memory problems. No other neurological symptoms were evident. He had developed a social life which was centred on alcohol, and had fallen downstairs when ejected from a flat after a drinking session. He had no friends and his behaviour was somewhat confused, and the referring community team thought he would respond to a period of in-patient rehabilitation. On arrival at the ward, his behaviour was found to be bizarre and, in the absence of overt pathology, discomforting. On first meeting, Edward was anxious and described needing to get back to his flat to sort out his affairs, but on questioning there was very little to manage in his life, he had no flat and had been living in rough lodgings. He stared and stood too close to people and he had no idea how to give voice to his anxiety and social confusion. Instead, he would talk disjointedly and perseveratively. In interview with Edward and his family, it became clear that Edward had had two previous head injuries, one while still a teenager when he came off a motorbike, and was unconscious for a short while. The second was in his 20s when he was assaulted. Edward appeared to recover physically from these incidents but his social history had spiralled downwards. In spite of a high IQ, Edward had not been able to negotiate social mores and had little social insight, had displayed sudden unpredictable behaviour and was vulnerable to predatory characters. In the rehabilitation unit, Edward would turn up to departments at all times of day, and once was found in the ward office using the phone, and on another insisted on washing his clothes through the night in preparation for his family's visit the following day.

Edward responded extremely well, first to gentle re-education in the normal rules of turn-taking, and eye contact. Exercises in controlling monologues included immediate cessation if the listener lifted their hand. Gradually this was generalised to stopping if the listener dropped eye contact or moved restlessly. It was also important to change roles. Later, role play with three people was introduced; Edward very quickly picked up the cues and his social skills rapidly improved. Similar exercises in using voice to convey emotions in role play were used. Eventually, staff came to trust that his odd behaviour was neither intentional nor menacing and began giving him positive guidance and feedback. Edward grew in confidence and social skills, was able to experience belonging within the social network of the hospital and developed very positive relationships with staff. He was eventually placed in a foster home, and had a good measure of independence, although he required lifelong gentle supervision and support.

that don't feel one-sided. Such approaches can allow the person to become more familiar with individual speech patterns and approaches (e.g. knowing that Bob says 'hello my love' as a greeting to everyone rather than as an expression of his love towards me).

The TASIT, already described (see page 115) can be used as a test for identifying non-verbal communication difficulties, including poor recognition of facial expression, social inference, innuendo and prosody. It can also be used as a therapeutic tool in the early stages of therapy to help individuals monitor and learn subtle interactional cues as well as develop problem-solving skills without having to use these *in vivo*. The material presented can also provide ideas for role play before techniques are applied to social situations.

An individual's memory functioning will have a significant impact on retention of information presented in conversation. Clients unable to remember previous discussions might repeat a topic over and over again without realising, often leaving the listener bored or irritated (Body & Parker, 2005). In these situations the client might be empowered to ask 'Have I said this before?' Strategies to aid memory retention might include teaching the individual to summarise information, or doing this for them at the end of a conversation, and recording these summaries on audiotape or videotape allows the client a chance to recap between sessions as they might have forgotten or misinterpreted comments, which can later be discussed. It is helpful to start any session with a short summary and recap of the previous session before introducing new information.

Developing the use of gestures, drawing or communication boards recommended by speech and language therapists can provide other means of communication if verbal expression is poor. Some clients might require input to help develop confidence in using new communication methods, and assertiveness training can also be very effective in encouraging clients to ask others to slow down, repeat instructions or give them time to respond.

Group interventions can help to reinforce or consolidate techniques covered in one-to-one sessions. Acknowledging shared experiences or hearing advice from people who have been in a similar situation can reduce feelings of being alone with the problem. Indeed, when there is an atmosphere of group support, individuals might feel more confident in practising communication strategies and expressing ideas. However, clear inclusion criteria are essential when selecting individuals for group treatment, as the nature and severity of some cognitive deficits may make individual therapy more appropriate.

Following brain injury many people experience reduced social contact with friends or work colleagues, often as a result of communication difficulties. Increased isolation and fewer social opportunities can lead to reduced self-confidence and reluctance to practise communication techniques acquired in rehabilitation. With encouragement and support some individuals embrace the opportunity to develop new social interests, subsequently developing new networks. It is worth exploring Headway (national headquarters in Nottingham), the national support system for people with acquired brain injury and their families.

Symptoms associated with psychological problems, including depression, psychosis and anxiety, can often be misinterpreted in relation to speech and communication deficits observed following traumatic brain injury. Factors like poor eye contact, initiation difficulties, apathy and odd or inappropriate patterns of speech need to be assessed in detail to ensure that the individual is diagnosed accurately and treated appropriately. For instance, a client might be referred for speech therapy when they are actually depressed. Alternatively, poor non-verbal expression can be interpreted as depression and mistreated with medication. In many cases both are present and this creates its own problems, especially when emotional distress cannot be expressed in either words or facial expression. One lady who experienced a brain injury following a fall was unable to cry and would laugh as a means of expressing emotion. In the early stages, she felt she wasn't taken seriously by family members or professionals when reporting feelings of depression or anger. Encouraging her to point to pictures of facial expressions helped others understand how she was really feeling. In addition, family and friends were educated not to rely on tone of voice or facial gestures as a representation of her mood.

Working with families is essential to facilitating the best environment for improving communication skills (Togher *et al.*, 2004). This might include advice about slowing the speed of conversation, regulating tone and volume, talking one at a time, speaking in simple terms, keeping sentences short, refraining from using innuendos and giving the person time to respond. Being aware that the person may misinterpret subtleties of language and confuse meaning might help others refrain from using subtle or sarcastic language. Specific training for family members as conversation partners can be addressed using the SPPARC training package (Lock *et al.*, 2001). Developing a rapport with family members is also essential in aiding discussion about coming to terms with changes in the client's communication, clarifying expectations and helping them to adjust appropriately. Moreover, involvement in prompting and supporting the individual in their use of recommended strategies can help to build a better bond with the client. Case 6.3 provides a case illustration of intervention to help re-establish working relationships within the family.

Snow and Ponsford (1995) emphasise the importance of a close liaison with social networks, particularly family members, in the development of a shared ownership and increased understanding.

Conclusion

This chapter has outlined the current understanding of how language and communication systems are organised in the brain; how these systems are affected following traumatic brain injury; and how this understanding has impacted on our treatment approaches in rehabilitation practice. In particular, the content of communication extends far beyond words and sentences and tackling the pragmatics of communication is most relevant for people living with TBI. Furthermore, communication needs change over time in the recovery course which starts in the intensive care unit, continues into the acute and sub-acute units of inpatient care and finally in the extended, lifelong period in the community. Emphasis is given to a client-centred, creative and experimental approach which we feel is intrinsic to the individual needs of clients and is the essence of successful rehabilitation. For longer-term care, the community rehabilitation of individuals with TBI must take into account that their needs change within an idiosyncratic timescale. The length and intensity of professional input is dictated by this individual need which may well outlast any prescribed course of rehabilitation.

Case 6.3: Example of social-executive difficulties in communication

Jerry is a forty-year-old man who sustained a severe frontal lobe injury following a fall. As well as experiencing verbal memory problems, decision-making difficulties and occasional aggressive outbursts, Jerry had great difficulty adapting the content of his conversation to the setting. When meeting people he would talk in depth about the food he had eaten that day or repeat stories about his past that he had recounted many times before, even if they had no relevance to the conversation. Many of his friends and the professionals around him stated that he was never interested in them as a person. However, Jerry was aware that his social network had reduced and that people responded differently to him since his head injury.

Some of the work conducted with Jerry involved helping him to gather specific pieces of information about key individuals in his life and learn to associate this information with the person. He also learnt to categorise this information according to the setting he was in. As Jerry has good visual memory he was able to envisage a chest of drawers in his mind, storing visual images for specific people and situations in each drawer. When meeting a person, he would visualise opening the appropriate drawer and asking them questions about themselves or the context. Jerry's wife subsequently reported that he was far less egocentric and their communication was a more mutual experience. Furthermore, he no longer returned home from shopping with goods that only related to his personal needs, but could remember the items for the rest of the family.

Acknowledgements

We are particularly indebted to Sarah Gwilliam, Speech and Language Therapist with the Community Brain Injury Team, for her very helpful comments on this chapter.

Recommended Reading

Judd, T. (1999). *Neuropsychotherapy and community integration: Brain illness, emotions and behaviour*. New York: Kluwer Academic/Plenum Publishers.
Excellent overview of treatments with good examples of experimental approach.

McKenna, P. (2004). Disorders of language and communication. In Laura H. Goldstein & Jane E. McNeil (Eds.) *Clinical neuropsychology: A practical guide to assessment and management for clinicians* (pp.165–184). Chichester: Wiley.

This chapter provides a more detailed account of the organization of language and communication.

Powell, T. (2004) *Head injury: A practical guide*. Wilmslow: Speech Mark Publishing. Most popular book for people and families coping with brain injury.

Snow, P., & Ponsford, J. (1995). Assessing and managing changes in communication and interpersonal skills following TBI. In J. Ponsford (Ed.), *Traumatic brain injury rehabilitation for everyday adaptive living* (pp.33–64). Hove: Lawrence Erlbaum Associates.

References

Adolphs, R., Damasio, H., Tranel, D., Cooper, G. & Damansio, A. (2000). A role for somatosensory cortices in the visual recognition of emotion as revealed by three-dimensional lesion mapping. *Journal of Neuroscience*, *20*, 2683–2690.

Bara, B.G., Cutica, I. & Tirassa, M. (2001). Neuropragmatics: Extralinguistic communication after closed head injury. *Brain and Language*, *77*, 72–94.

Body, R. & Parker, M. (2005). Topic repetitiveness after traumatic brain injury: An emergent, jointly managed behaviour. *Clinical Linguistics and Phonetics*, *19*(5), 379–392.

Bond, F. & Godfrey, H.P.D. (1997). Conversation with traumatically brain-injured individuals: A controlled study of behavioural changes and their impact. *Brain Injury*, *11*, 319–329.

Bryan, K. (1995). *The Right Hemisphere Language Battery* (2nd edn). London: Whurr Publishers.

Burns, M. (1997). *Brief inventory of communication and cognition*. San Antonio, TX: Psychological Corporation Publishers.

Crutch S.J. & Warrington, E.K. (2003). Preservation of propositional speech in a pure anomic: The importance of an abstract vocabulary. *Neurocase*, *9*, 465–481.

Crutch S.J. & Warrington, E.K. (2005). Abstract and concrete concepts have structurally different representational frameworks. *Brain*, *128*, 615–627.

Garrard, P., Carroll, E., Vinson, D. & Vigliocco, G. (2004). Dissociation of lexical syntax and semantics: Evidence from focal cortical degeneration. *Neurocase*, *10*, 353–362.

Godfrey, H.P.D., Partridge, F.M., Knight, R.G. & Bishara, S. (1993). Course of insight disorder and emotional dysfunction following closed head injury: A controlled cross-sectional follow-up study. *Journal of Clinical and Experimental Neuropsychology*, *15*, 503–515.

Green, R.E.A., Turner, G.R. & Thompson, W.F. (2004). Deficits in facial emotion perception in adults with recent traumatic brain injury. *Neuropsychologia*, *42*, 133–141.

Hodges, J.R., Patterson, K., Oxbury, S. & Funnell, E. (1992). Semantic dementia. Progressive fluent aphasia with temporal lobe atrophy. *Brain*, *115*, 1783–1806.

Judd, T. (1999). *Neuropsychotherapy and community integration. Brain illness, emotions and behaviour*. London: Kluwer Academic/Plenum Publishers.

Lock, S., Wilkinson, R., Brian, K., Maxim, J., Edmondson, A., Bruce, C. *et al*. (2001). SPPARC (Supporting Partners of People with Aphasia in Relationships and Conversations). *International Journal of Language and Communication Disorders*, *36*, 25–30.

McCarthy, R.A. & Warrington, E.K. (1986). Visual associative agnosia: A clinico-anatomical study of a single case. *Journal of Neurology, Neurosurgery and Psychiatry*, *49*, 1233–1240.

McCarthy, R.A. & Warrington, E.K. (1988). Evidence for modality-specific meaning systems in the brain. *Nature*, *334*, 428–430.

McDonald, S., Flanagan, S. & Rollins, J. (2002). *The Awareness of Social Inference Test (TASIT)*. Oxford: The Psychological Corporation, Harcourt Assessment.
McKenna, P. (1997). *Category Specific Names Test*. Hove: Psychology Press Associates.
McKenna, P. & Parry, R. (1994). Category specificity in the naming of natural and man-made objects: Normative data from adults and children. *Neuropsychological Rehabilitation*, *4*, 255–281.
McKenna, P. & Warrington, E.K. (1983). *Graded Naming Test*. Cambridge: Cambridge Cognition.
McKenna, P. & Warrington, E.K. (2000). The neuropsychology of semantic memory. In L.S. Cermak (Ed.) *Memory and its disorders* (vol. 2, pp.355–382); F. Boller & J. Grafman (Eds.) *Handbook of neuropsychology* (2nd edn). Amsterdam: Elsevier.
Murdoch, B.E. & Theodoros, D.G. (1999). Dysarthria following traumatic brain injury. In S. McDonald, L. Togher, & C. Code (Eds.) *Communication disorders following traumatic brain injury* (pp.211–234). Hove: Psychology Press.
Powell, T. (2004). *Head injury: A practical guide*. Winslow: Speech Mark Publishing.
Snow, P. & Ponsford, J. (1995). Assessing and managing changes in communication and interpersonal skills following TBI. In J. Ponsford (Ed.) *Traumatic brain injury rehabilitation for everyday adaptive living* (pp.33–64). Hove: Lawrence Erlbaum Associates.
Snowden, J.S, Goulding, P.J. & Neary, D. (1989). Semantic dementia: A form of circumscribed cerebral atrophy. *Behavioural Neurology*, *2*, 167–182.
Togher, C., McDonalds, S., Code, C. & Grant, S. (2004). Training communication partners of people with traumatic brain injury: A randomised control trial. *Aphasiology*, *18*(4), 313–335.
Warrington, E.K. (1975). The selective impairment of semantic memory. *Quarterly Journal of Experimental Psychology*, *27*, 635–657.
Warrington, E.K. (1981). Neuropsychological studies of verbal semantic systems. *Philosophical Transactions of the Royal Society. London B. Biological Science*, *295*, 411–423.
Warrington, E.K. & McCarthy, R. (1983) Category specific dysphasia. *Brain*, *106*, 859–878.
Warrington, E.K. & Shallice, T. (1984) Category specific semantic impairments. *Brain*, *107*, 829–854.
Watson, D. & Friend, R. (1969). Measurement of social evaluative anxiety. *Journal of Consulting and Clinical Psychology*, *33*, 448–457.
Whitworth, A., Perkins, L. & Lesser, R. (1997). *Conversational Analysis Profiles for People with Aphasia (CAPPCA)*. London: Whurr Publishers.
Wong, Y.T., Kent, R.D., Duffy, J.R. & Demois, J.E. (2005). Dysarthria associated with traumatic brain injury: Speaking rate and emphatic stress. *Journal of Communication Disorders*, *38*(3), 231–260.
Ylvisaker, M. & Feeney, T. (2000). Reconstruction of identity after brain injury. *Brain Impairment*, *1*, 12–28.

7

Memory Problems

Barbara A. Wilson, Jonathan J. Evans and W. Huw Williams

Introduction

This chapter is concerned with memory problems experienced by people who have sustained a traumatic brain injury (TBI). After a discussion about the nature of human memory, post-traumatic amnesia (a temporary state) is considered. Typical and less common memory difficulties likely to be faced by people with TBI are reviewed and links are established between these problems and underlying pathology. Methods for the assessment of memory functions are addressed and suggestions made for the management and rehabilitation of memory problems. The chapter concludes with a brief reference as to who should carry out memory rehabilitation and where this should take place.

The Nature of Human Memory

Although we tend to talk about memory as if it were one skill, function or system (e.g. 'I have a terrible memory' or 'she has a photographic memory'), memory is, in fact, comprised of several skills, systems or functions working together. The number of these subdivisions and their roles depend on the model or classification system used to explain or interpret memory functioning. One can consider memory in terms of the length of time information is stored, the type of information to be remembered, the stages involved in remembering, recall and recognition, explicit and implicit memory, and retrograde and anterograde memory. These classifications are not mutually exclusive, but simply different dimensions to consider when talking about memory.

Time-dependent memory

Thinking about memory in terms of the length of time information is stored has been greatly influenced by the Working Memory model of Baddeley and Hitch (1974). This model subdivides memory into three main types depending on both time-based and conceptual differences. The first system, *sensory memory*, is a brief and rather literal trace resulting from a sensory (e.g. visual or auditory) event, probably lasting no longer than 250 milliseconds. This is the system we use to make sense of incoming sensory perceptions. As most people with a damaged sensory memory system would present with perceptual or language disorders, we would not normally think of them as having memory problems.

The second system, *working memory*, is considered to have two main components or functions. The first of these is short-term or immediate memory and lasts for several seconds. This period of time can be extended to several minutes if the person is rehearsing or concentrating on the information to be remembered. Unlike sensory memory, information in working memory has already undergone substantial cognitive analysis, so it is typically represented in meaningful chunks such as words or numbers. We use this system when looking up a new telephone number and holding on to it long enough to dial.

The second component of working memory is a hypothetical construct called the *Central Executive*. This can be conceived of as an organiser, controller or allocator of resources. The Central Executive enables us to do two different tasks at the same time (such as drive a car and listen to the radio). Sufficient resources are allocated to each task. If, however, an unexpected or demanding situation occurs on the road we may need to turn off the radio as all our resources are required to deal with the unexpected or demanding situation.

The third system in the Baddeley and Hitch (1974) model is *long-term memory* which encodes information in a reasonably robust form and can last for decades. Although there are differences in memory for things that happened five minutes ago and five years ago, these differences are less clear-cut than those between the sensory (quarter of a second) and the immediate (few seconds) memory systems. The following terms can be used to differentiate between time periods in long-term memory: (i) *delayed* memory, which refers to memory for information presented in the last few minutes, (ii) *recent* memory, which refers to memory over the past few days or weeks, and (iii) *remote* memory, which refers to memory over several years.

All the systems described so far refer to memory for information or events that have already occurred, i.e. retrospective memory. Frequently, however, we need to remember to do something in the future such as pay an electricity bill, or buy a loaf of bread on the way home from work. This system is known as *prospective memory*, i.e. remembering to do something at the right time (e.g. 'At 8 pm I must 'phone my friend'), or within a certain time period (e.g. 'By the end of today I must send that letter'), or when a certain event occurs ('When I pass the post box I must post the letter to my bank'). Many complaints from memory-impaired people are concerned with failures of prospective memory.

Type of information to be remembered

Remembering what the word 'telephone' means, remembering whether you fed your cat this morning and remembering how to ride your bicycle all involve different memory systems and can be differentially affected by damage to the brain. Knowing that 'telephone' means an instrument used to speak to people some distance away involves semantic memory. Semantic memory refers to knowledge about the world, e.g. that Paris is the capital of France, and that a giraffe has a long neck. It is also concerned with the meanings of words, with social customs and how things look, feel, taste and smell. Most memory-impaired people do not forget this type of information, although they may have difficulty adding to their store of semantic knowledge. For example, they may be unable to learn new words or abbreviations coming into the language since the onset of their memory problems.

Remembering whether or not you fed your cat involves episodic memory. Episodic memory represents what most of us would think of as memory because it refers to a specific episode that has been experienced and can be recalled. So remembering what you ate for lunch today, or when you last paid your telephone bill, or what you read a few minutes earlier, are all examples of episodic memory. This system is frequently damaged in people with organic memory impairment and is often the most noticeable characteristic of people with memory problems.

Remembering how to ride a bicycle involves procedural memory. This is the system used for learning new skills. Many people with memory problems show normal or nearly normal procedural memory even though they may have no conscious recollection of carrying out the task before. For example, some very amnesic people have learned to type, use a computer or even play the piano, despite their amnesia. They may, however, have no idea *how* they learned such skills.

Stages involved in remembering

Typically there are three stages involved in remembering, namely encoding, storage and retrieval. Encoding refers to the registration stage or getting information into memory. Storage refers to the maintenance of information in the memory store, and retrieval refers to the stage of extracting or recalling the information when it is required. After an injury to the brain, any or all of these stages can be affected. People with attention problems may have difficulty registering or encoding information, some kinds of brain injury may lead to storage problems and many memory-impaired people have retrieval deficits.

Recall and recognition

Recall and recognition are two of the main ways we remember information. Recall involves actively finding the information to be remembered. Summarising what you have read in this chapter so far would involve recall. In some situations, however, we do not need to recall the information but to recognise it. You might, for example, have difficulty recalling the face of a friend, i.e. getting a clear picture of the face in your mind, but you would probably have no problem recognising that friend at a meeting. Most memory-impaired people find recall harder than recognition, although often both systems are affected. Some people have problems with both verbal and visual recall and recognition while others might have problems in only one of these modalities.

Explicit and implicit memory

In many situations we need to consciously recall information, i.e. we need to have explicit recollection of an event. If you were asked what happened in the football match last night and could give an account of this, you would be using explicit memory to provide the account. If, on the other hand, you were asked how you learned to ride a bicycle, you may not be able to recall this yet could easily demonstrate how to ride a bicycle. This information is implicit – you do not need to recall how, when or where you learned in order to demonstrate the skill. Like procedural memory, implicit memory is usually intact or relatively intact in people with organic memory impairment.

Retrograde and anterograde memory

Following a brain injury people typically have a gap in their memory functioning from before the insult. This is known as retrograde amnesia. This gap is very variable. It may be for as little as a few seconds or minutes or as much as several decades. In the first few hours, days or weeks following a traumatic brain injury, the length of retrograde amnesia may shrink, so, for example, a person with a head injury may come out of coma and fail to recall anything that has happened in the past two years, i.e. the duration of retrograde amnesia in this example is two years. Gradually the period may shrink until most memories up to a week or so before the accident may eventually be recalled. The final retrograde amnesia in this case will be one week. Retrograde amnesia is usually less of a problem and less handicapping than anterograde amnesia which refers to memory difficulties dating from the time of the brain injury.

Post-Traumatic Amnesia

Post-traumatic amnesia (PTA) can be defined as 'a period of variable length following closed head trauma during which the patient is confused, disoriented, suffers from retrograde amnesia, and seems to lack the capacity to store and retrieve new information' (Schacter & Crovitz, 1977, p.151). Most people who have sustained a TBI have a period of PTA. PTA is a useful index of the severity of brain damage (McMillan *et al.*, 1996): it is one of the best predictors of recovery (Haslam *et al.*, 1994; Russell, 1971); it enables us to monitor recovery from brain injury; and is often used to make decisions about discharge from hospital and referral to rehabilitation services (Wilson, Evans *et al.*, 1999).

As almost all people in PTA have problems with orientation questions (about time and place) and have difficulty retaining information; measures of PTA typically include orientation and memory questions, e.g. the Galveston Orientation and Amnesia Test (Levin *et al.*, 1979) and the Westmead Post-traumatic Amnesia Scale

(Shores *et al.*, 1986). People with chronic memory impairment, however, also have difficulty with orientation and memory questions, yet most of these would not be considered to be in PTA.

In an attempt to clarify the characteristics of people in PTA, Wilson and colleagues carried out a pilot study in which four groups were compared on a number of tests of memory and attention (Wilson *et al.*, 1992). The first group consisted of people in PTA, the second comprised people who had sustained a head injury with chronic memory impairment, in the third group were people with a pure amnesic syndrome and the fourth group contained people who had sustained orthopaedic injuries with no head injury or organic memory difficulties. Results from this study indicated that people in PTA showed a much wider range of deficits than people with chronic memory impairment or with the amnesic syndrome. PTA does not appear to be solely a disorder of memory and orientation but includes slowing of cognitive functioning and motor speed, poor retrieval from semantic memory and a higher frequency of errors on a semantic processing task. A more detailed study of how people recover from PTA was carried out by Wilson, Evans *et al.* (1999). The results suggested that cognitive recovery is a gradual process rather than an all-or-nothing phenomenon. This study also made several suggestions about tests to include when assessing recovery from PTA. These will be referred to later in the section on assessment.

Characteristics of Memory Impairment

The typical picture of someone with memory problems after TBI is for that person to have (a) difficulty learning and remembering most kinds of new information, (b) a normal or nearly normal immediate memory (i.e. to be able to hold on to information for a few seconds), (c) a period of retrograde amnesia which may range from a few seconds to several years, (d) unimpaired semantic memory functioning for facts and knowledge acquired prior to the head injury, and (e) adequate implicit memory (i.e. remembering without conscious awareness). Someone with a pure amnesic syndrome will show these characteristics in isolation, with other cognitive functions remaining intact. This is not often the case after TBI, however, as most people with a head injury will have additional cognitive problems such as attention difficulties, word-finding problems and general slowing of thinking or processing of information. Whether or not these additional cognitive problems are present, the typical picture of a memory-impaired person is someone whose immediate memory is reasonably normal, who has difficulty remembering after a delay or distraction, who finds new learning difficult, who remembers things that happened some time before the accident better than things that happened a short time before and who has no loss of memory for his or her personal identity.

An example of a young man with memory problems following TBI is Carl, seen recently at the Oliver Zangwill Centre for Neuropsychological Rehabilitation in Ely, Cambridgeshire. Carl sustained a severe head injury in a road traffic accident when he was 21 years of age. He was in coma for 4 weeks and had a PTA of 2–3 months. Of average intellectual ability, Carl had some attentional and fluency deficits. He had a retrograde amnesia of several years and could not remember much of his earlier life except that he was a fan of Manchester United Football Club. Despite a good immediate memory, his anterograde memory was poor, he forgot conversations, could not remember what he had been doing and what he was about to do. He became socially withdrawn, refusing to go out because he could not remember what he had said or what people said to him. He also became obsessive about checking things, for example whether he had locked the back door and whether he had his wallet, his keys and his mobile phone with him. He responded well to a rehabilitation programme that focused on his emotional, social and cognitive problems.

Less common manifestations of memory disorders

Although the majority of people with memory problems following TBI will fit the picture described above, there are other manifestations of memory disorders that may be encountered every now and again. For example, one can find people who have deficits in the memory system that holds information for a few seconds. This system can be subdivided into the *phonological loop* (the system we use when dialling a new telephone number and in dealing with other short-term phonological tasks) and the *visuo-spatial sketchpad* (VSSP) (analogous to the 'mind's eye', a temporary system used in creating and manipulating visual images).

Although relatively rare, patients with phonological loop deficits have been reported. Luria *et al.* (1967) described two patients who had sustained head injuries to the left temporal lobe. Both showed defective repetition of auditory-verbal sequences such as phonemes, digits and words. Furthermore, both improved with visual presentation. Warrington and Shallice (1969) described a patient, KF, with an impairment of auditory-verbal short-term memory (for further review see Vallar & Papagno, 1995). One of the main everyday problems faced by people with a phonological loop deficit is difficulty learning new vocabulary (see e.g. Baddeley *et al.*, 1988) and difficulty comprehending sentences in tasks where word order is crucial. Deficits in the visuo-spatial sketchpad are also much rarer than the episodic memory deficits that follow TBI – but a number have been reported (Farah, 1984; Wilson, Baddeley *et al.*, 1999). The latter case is that of a sculptress with systemic lupus erythematosus (SLE), an auto immune disorder. She had a number of everyday problems – for example she complained of difficulty dressing herself because she could not 'see' what clothes and colours went together. She was expecting her first grandchild and although pleased about this, could not 'see' herself holding the baby. She reported that her 'mind's eye was faulty', she could not hold on to things or relate one thing to another. One of the most dramatic changes was in her sculptures. Prior to the episode, her pieces were full of detail and realistic. Afterwards they were lacking in detail and very abstract.

Another kind of memory deficit that one should be aware of is a deficit of semantic memory, i.e. loss of knowledge about the world. Damage to the semantic memory store, or impaired access to that system, may result from brain injury. People may have a general impairment of semantic memory in which they lose knowledge both for the meanings of words and for what things look like, and this is true for both manufactured and living things; or they may have a selective semantic memory impairment. KG, for example, a head-injured woman reported in Wilson (1997a), had a general semantic memory impairment with anomia, reduced fluency, impaired single-word comprehension and impoverished general knowledge. Furthermore, she showed deficits on both manufactured and living items. It is also possible to see patients with selective loss of knowledge of what things look like (e.g. Davidoff & Wilson, 1985). Warrington (1975) suggests that visual object agnosia (the failure to recognise objects despite adequate eyesight, language and naming ability) is due to a deficit of the visual semantic memory system (for further review of agnosia see Ratcliff & Newcombe, 1982). Some patients show a selective impairment of living versus non-living items. Warrington and Shallice (1984) first demonstrated that there are category-specific deficits, with some patients able to recognise non-living but not living items. The opposite has also been described, i.e. people who can recognise living but not non-living objects (Hillis & Caramazza, 1991). Wilson (1997a) reported four patients with semantic memory problems; two had sustained a severe head injury and two had survived herpes simplex viral encephalitis. All showed greater impairment with living items, possibly because living items are more similar to one another than non-living items (Gaffan & Heywood, 1993). People with semantic memory deficits are likely to have problems recognising objects in the real world, problems expressing themselves and they may be considered to be globally intellectually impaired because of the errors they make.

In recent years there has been a considerable interest in semantic dementia, a term coined by Snowden *et al.* (1989) and studied in some detail by Hodges and his colleagues (Hodges *et al.*, 1995; Hodges, Patterson *et al.*, 1992). Patients with semantic dementia show a progressive deterioration of the semantic memory store associated with damage to the temporal neocortex. The four patients described by Wilson (1997a) have stable, non-progressive conditions, although in many ways they are similar to the people studied by Hodges and his colleagues. There are age differences, of course, and Wilson's patients had more severe episodic memory problems. Semantic memory loss may be more widespread among TBI patients than previously recognised. If neuropsychologists are not routinely assessing for such deficits, they may be missed.

We discussed retrograde and anterograde amnesia earlier, and noted that most people with memory impairments have a gap in their memory prior to the insult. In general, the anterograde memory difficulties are more handicapping than the retrograde problems. There are a few people, however, who appear to have normal or minimally impaired anterograde memory functioning together with severe retrograde amnesia. Kapur (1993) provides a good review of the topic. Hodges (1995) says that severe retrograde amnesia with relatively mild or no anterograde amnesia appears to be exceedingly rare. Indeed, there was, until recently, doubt about the very existence of the syndrome owing to the fact that it is associated with psychogenic or functional amnesia (Evans *et al.*, 1996). There are, however, a few well-documented cases of organic brain damage associated with isolated retrograde amnesia (Evans *et al.*, 1996). One of the first of these cases was a 36-year-old man who had sustained an open head injury (Goldberg *et al.*, 1981). Initially this man had both retrograde and anterograde deficits but over several years his anterograde deficits resolved, leaving him with a 20-year dense retrograde amnesia for both public and autobiographical events.

Patients with retrograde amnesia appear to be able to 'relearn' autobiographical facts, although they seem to have no 'emotional memory' for these. One of our head-injured clients, for example, 'knew' she had been to India on holiday and had been to medical school because she had been told these things and her adequate anterograde memory enabled her to retain this information. In herself, however, she had no feeling of familiarity for these memories.

Relating pathology to memory impairment

The temporal and frontal lobes are crucially involved in human memory. Both these structures are frequently damaged following a TBI. Kapur (1988) says the temporal and basal frontal regions are the most common sites of cerebral contusion in closed head injury. Within the temporal lobes, the medial areas including the left and right hippocampal areas are particularly important for adequate memory functioning. The principal role of these areas is for the acquisition of new factual knowledge (Tranel & Damasio, 1995) and disruption of this function can have devastating consequences for everyday life. These areas are also highly important for episodic, explicit memory and damage results in anterograde amnesia. People with bilateral hippocampal damage may be densely amnesic (see, e.g., Wilson *et al.*, 1995).

If other brain structures are unaffected then these people will have a pure amnesic syndrome (Baddeley, 1999; Scoville & Milner, 1957). Although it is possible to see this syndrome following TBI, such cases are relatively uncommon and are more frequently associated with encephalitis, surgical damage, bilateral posterior cerebral artery infarction and other conditions (see, e.g., Kapur, 1988; Lishman, 1998). TBI, as mentioned earlier, tends to be associated with more widespread, diffuse damage and thus with additional cognitive problems.

Within the frontal lobes there are several systems involved in memory. Some argue that they have an indirect rather than a direct role on memory and exert their influence through processes such as attention, encoding and problem solving (see Tranel & Damasio, 1995 for a discussion). What is clear is that memory disorders associated with damage to the frontal lobes are different from those that occur with medial temporal lobe damage. People with TBI can, of course, have both kinds of problems. Memory problems associated with frontal lobe damage include poor prospective memory, inability to judge how recently or how frequently something has happened, confabulation, i.e. believing something has happened that did not happen, and poor retrieval problems in linking various components of a memory together so that mismatching may occur, i.e. components from different memories may be incorrectly linked together. Markowitsch (1998) discusses different types of memory problem associated with particular anatomical sites. Some believe that the left temporal lobe is particularly involved with encoding information and the right with the retrieval of information (see, e.g., Shallice *et al.*, 1994; Tulving *et al.*, 1994). In short, people with typical episodic anterograde memory deficits are likely to have lesions in and around the hippocampal area. Those with confabulation, poor attention or encoding, poor retrieval and prospective memory difficulties are likely to have frontal lobe damage. Working-memory deficits are also associated with frontal lobe lesions (Goldman-Rakic & Friedman, 1991). Working memory is used to bridge temporal gaps, i.e. hold on to information long enough to make responses to stimuli or events (Tranel & Damasio, 1995), and this appears to be a function of the dorsolateral frontal lobe. There would appear to be several lesion sites that may give rise to phonological loop deficits, including the left basal frontal, parietal and superior temporal areas. The right occipital, parietal and prefrontal areas appear to be involved in visuo-spatial sketchpad deficits. Baddeley (1999) says that the left perisylvian area in the parietal lobe is associated with storage and the frontal area is associated with articulatory rehearsal components as far as the phonological loop is concerned, with four areas of the right hemisphere associated to VSSP performance, namely the occipital area for vision, the parietal area for spatial processing and two areas in the right frontal area for control processes.

Semantic memory deficits are associated with damage to the lateral temporal neocortex, with the hippocampal areas being relatively unaffected (Graham *et al.*, 1997). All four of Wilson's (1997a) patients with semantic memory deficits had temporal lobe damage with either unilateral left or bilateral lesions.

Procedural memory appears to depend on the basal ganglia and cerebellar regions (Markowitsch, 1998; Tranel & Damasio, 1995). Although most people with TBI show normal procedural learning (Wilson *et al.*, 1996), it is possible to see the reverse, i.e. relatively normal episodic memory but impaired procedural learning. This occurs in patients with cerebellar damage and can also be seen in patients with Parkinson's disease or Huntington's disease when the basal ganglia is affected and the medial temporal lobes are unaffected. Procedural memory is one aspect of implicit learning. Other aspects such as verbal and perceptual priming are not dependent on these areas. Instead the cortex is more involved. Implicit memory is not a unitary system (Wilson *et al.*, 1996).

Both recall and recognition memory functions are typically impaired in the amnesic syndrome, although memory impairment following frontal lobe damage may result in much poorer recall than recognition. Because such patients are likely to have poor retrieval skills, tasks involving recognition reduce the need to implement a retrieval strategy – the choices are present and do not require retrieval. As stated earlier, the right frontal lobe is believed to play a role in retrieval of information (Shallice *et al.*, 1994; Tulving *et al.*, 1994). Deficits of recall may follow both temporal hippocampal and frontal lobe damage.

Retrograde amnesia is believed to result from lesions in different areas of the brain from anterograde amnesia. Medial temporal lobe structures are responsible for anterograde memory and anterolateral temporal lobe areas, especially on the right, are thought to be critical for retrieval of retrograde factual knowledge (Calabrese *et al.*, 1996; Jones *et al.*, 1998).

Another recent paper by Eslinger (1998) argues for both left and right temporal lobe involvement in autobiographical memory, which is one component of retrograde memory but with more severe impairment following bilateral damage. He suggests that left temporal lobe lesions result in the impairment of factual personal knowledge but not in deficits of autobiographical incidents, whereas bilateral temporal lobe damage causes extensive autobiographical impairments. Furthermore, although bilateral frontal lobe damage also resulted in severe impairment, this was because of disorganised retrieval.

Finally, what can be said about the pathology underlying PTA? As the length of PTA reflects the severity of the brain injury, such patients are likely to have a diffuse closed head injury but, in particular, are likely to have brain stem damage with consequent disruption of the reticular activating system. This is the most likely cause of their earlier coma and poor arousal (Wilson, Evans *et al.*, 1999).

Assessment of Memory Functioning

Assessments are carried out in order to answer questions, and the nature of each question will determine the assessment procedures or tools employed. If we are interested in theoretical aspects of memory we are likely to use different assessment procedures from those we use when answering clinical questions (Mayes, 1995). Readers of this chapter are more likely to be interested in clinical questions. Clinically, memory assessment is part of a broader cognitive assessment usually carried out by a neuropsychologist. As well as understanding the strengths and weaknesses of aspects of memory functioning, we need to know the strengths and weaknesses of other cognitive functions such as general intellectual ability, language, perception, thinking, speed of information processing, attention, problem solving and so forth.

As far as memory is concerned, some of the important questions we need to answer are:

- Does this person have an organic memory deficit?
- To what extent are the memory problems due to attention, language, perceptual or other deficits?
- Is this score in the impaired range?
- How does this person score compare with scores of other people in the same age range or with the same diagnosis?
- Are the memory deficits restricted to certain kinds of material such as verbal or visual material?
- What is the nature of the memory deficit (i.e. is immediate memory normal; recall and recognition equally affected; does this person have normal implicit memory; is semantic memory unimpaired?)

These and similar questions can, on the whole, be answered with standardised tests. There are adequately normed, reliable and valid tests to answer each of the above questions. Such tests, however, are not good at answering questions that are more concerned with the impact of memory problems on everyday life. This is partly because these tests do not take into account factors such as motivation, personality, premorbid lifestyle, family support and so forth and partly because they do not approach these questions directly. Standardised tests tend to be more concerned with the structure of memory rather than the manifestation of memory difficulties in natural situations. Thus they are not particularly helpful in answering questions such as:

- What everyday problems are faced by this person with memory difficulties?
- How does the memory-impaired person cope with or react to these problems? (Also, how do family members/health-care staff/colleagues etc. cope or react?)
- What problems cause particular concern to the client and the family?

- Can this person return to school/work/driving etc?
- Are the problems exacerbated by anxiety and/or depression?

These questions require a more behavioural or functional approach such as direct observation (either in real-life settings or in analogue or role-playing situations) or through information gained from checklists, rating scales, diaries or questionnaires (usually completed by relatives and health-care staff as the person with memory problems may be unable to remember the extent and severity of the difficulties encountered in real life). Wilson (1999, ch. 3) describes several of these behavioural memory assessments in some detail.

Although everyday problems and questions about treatment are best answered through behavioural assessment or direct observation, it is possible to make standardised tests more relevant to real-life situations (Hart & Hayden, 1986). For example, one can make standardised tests more like real-life tasks. The Rivermead Behavioural Memory Test (RBMT; Wilson *et al.*, 1985) is such a test. Administered and scored like any other standardised test, the test items comprise tasks analogous to real-life situations such as remembering an appointment, remembering to deliver a message and learning a new route. This test and its successor, The Rivermead Behavioural Memory Test – Extended (RBMT-E; Wilson, Clare *et al.*, 1999) (a more difficult version of the original) have proved to be good at predicting (a) everyday problems following brain injury (Wills *et al.*, 2000; Wilson *et al.*, 1989), (b) independence (Wilson, 1991a) and (c) employability (Schwartz & McMillan, 1989). As well as information obtained from the behavioural or functional measures described above, we need supplementary information from other sources to include problems that need tackling in rehabilitation.

Not every person referred for memory assessment requires testing in great detail. If the question one is trying to answer is very specific, such as 'Does this person have evidence of an organic memory deficit?', then one of the existing screening tests such as the Wechsler Memory Scale – Revised (Wechsler, 1987), Wechsler Memory Scale III (Wechsler, 1997) or the Adult Memory and Information Processing Battery (AMIPB; Coughlan & Hollows, 1984, 1985) would probably be sufficient. The Wechsler Memory Scales grew out of the original Wechsler Memory Scale (Wechsler, 1945) which was designed to be a 'rapid, simple and practical memory examination' (p.3) to detect organic memory impairment. One big disadvantage of the Wechsler scales is that they do not have alternative or parallel versions so it is more difficult to interpret results if one wants to regularly reassess. One does not know whether any change is due to improvement or to practice effects. Wilson, Watson *et al.* (2000) consider the effects of repeated assessments (particularly with regard to memory) on people with and without brain injury. The AMIPB was designed to help clinicians detect and evaluate memory impairment, i.e. decide whether or not the scores on the subtests are in the abnormal range. This test has two versions. The RBMT mentioned earlier has four parallel versions and the RBMT-E has two parallel versions.

Frequently testers will need a more thorough and fine-grained memory assessment, particularly for people one sees for rehabilitation when a detailed picture of memory strengths and weaknesses is required. One structure we follow is outlined in Table 7.1 (see Wilson, 1996 for a more detailed discussion).

Once again, however, these tests would not tell us much about the memory-impaired person's ability to perform everyday tasks, or about the main concerns of

Table 7.1 Assessment of memory functioning: What aspects to assess

1 Immediate memory	(a) verbal			(digit span)
	(b) visual			(visual span)
2 Delayed	(a) verbal		– recall	(story recall)
			– recognition	(word recognition)
	(b) visual		– recall	(recall of designs)
			– recognition	(face recall)
3 New (episodic) learning	(a) verbal			(verbal paired associate learning)
	(b) visual			(visual paired associate learning)
4 Procedural or implicit learning	(a) motor			(visuo-motor tracking)
	(b) verbal			(stem completion)
	(c) visual			(fragmented pictures)
5 Remote memory	(a) autobiographical			(Autobiographical Memory Interview)
	(b) retrograde amnesia			(Famous Events/ Famous Faces)
6 Prospective memory	(a) remember to do things at a given time			(from RBMT)
	(b) remember to do things within a certain interval			
	(c) remember to do things after a certain time interval			
7 Orientation	(a) for time	}		(from Wechsler Memory Scale – Revised)
	(b) for place			
	(c) for person			
8 Semantic memory	(a) verbal	}		(see Hodges, Salmon *et al.*, 1992)
	(b) visual			

the person or the family, or which problems to select for treatment. Wilson (1999) presents several case studies illustrating how information from standardised and behavioural assessments is combined to help plan treatment.

Assessment of people in PTA requires a different approach because of their distractibility and poor attention. The two main published tests of PTA are the Galveston Orientation and Amnesia Test (Levin *et al.*, 1979) and the Westmead PTA Scale (Shores *et al.*, 1986). However, Wilson, Evans *et al.* (1999) recommended several tests for determining whether or not someone was in PTA owing to the fact that PTA is not restricted to deficits in memory and orientation. They recommended five types of tests in addition to orientation, namely (1) simple reaction time, (2) semantic processing (from the Speed and Capacity of Language Processing test (SCOLP;

Baddeley, Emslie, & Nimmo-Smith, 1992), (3) backward digit span, (4) a visual recognition test, and (5) a word list learning test.

The management and rehabilitation of memory problems

Some understanding of the natural recovery of memory functioning following TBI is required when one engages in intervention or management strategies. Wilson (1991a, 1998) considers recovery of memory and other cognitive functions following brain damage and recognises that people with TBI may do better, i.e. show more recovery in the long term than people with other conditions such as encephalitis and anoxia. Nevertheless, many factors other than diagnosis come into play in determining recovery. These include age, duration of coma and length of PTA. Full discussion of this topic is beyond the scope of this chapter but see Robertson (1999), Robertson and Murre (1999) and Wilson (1991a, 1998) for more detail.

Although some recovery of memory functioning can be expected in the months following TBI, people with memory impairment and their relatives should not be led to believe that significant improvement can occur once the period of natural recovery is over. This does not mean that nothing can be done to help. Distress can be reduced, problems can be avoided, people can be taught to compensate for their difficulties, and health staff or family members can help people with memory difficulties to learn more efficiently.

One of the simplest therapeutic procedures to reduce stress in people with TBI and their families is to provide information. Some people fear that memory problems are an indication that they are going crazy; many experience anxiety and depression; fatigue and social isolation are also commonly encountered. Some people will be satisfied with a simple explanation or reassurance that these feelings are common, others will require detailed explanations. Anxiety management techniques, cognitive behaviour therapy strategies, psychotherapy and participation in memory groups may reduce anxiety, depression and social isolation (see Wilson, 1995, 1999 for further discussion of these issues).

Written information is particularly helpful, not only for people with memory problems who are unlikely to remember oral information, but also for their families who may have difficulty retaining explanations, especially if they are under stress when listening to these explanations.

In addition to the reduction of stress, anxiety and depression, there are more practical things to be done. For those people with very severe and widespread cognitive deficits, the best way to help may be to modify or restructure their environments so they can cope without a memory. For example, providing cookers, lights and other pieces of electrical equipment that turn themselves off after a certain interval circumvents the need to remember to turn them off. Labelling rooms, cupboards and drawers avoids the need to remember which room is which or where socks, jumpers and underwear are kept. Signposts can be used to direct people to the bedroom or bathroom, and positioning objects (e.g. clipping a notebook to a belt) so they cannot be forgotten are other environmental adjustments to reduce or avoid the load on memory. Sometimes a particular piece of behaviour or repetition of a question, story or joke can be avoided by identifying a 'trigger' or an antecedent that elicits this behaviour. Thus, by eliminating the 'trigger' one can avoid the repetitious behaviour. For example, one young head-injured man, Michael, is in PTA at the time of writing. If staff say to him 'How are you today?', he always replies 'Just getting over my hangover'. If staff simply say 'Good morning', however, he replies 'Good morning', so the repetitious comments about his supposed hangover (and no doubt he feels like he has a hangover) can be avoided.

Modification or restructuring of the environment means that problems due to memory impairment can be avoided. The origins of this approach can be found within the field of behaviour modification, especially in the area of severe learning disability (Murphy, 1987). Despite being, at times, an effective and rapid way of reducing problems, this approach does not always work. For example, people have to be able to understand the labels and the signposts; some repetitious behaviours are not triggered by external events and the notebook clipped to a belt is no good if it is never used. In addition, one has to be aware of possible ethical considerations of an environment that is too restrictive. So, it might be possible to avoid any demands on memory by placing someone in an environment where every move is supervised by a staff member, leaving the person with memory problems completely unable to exercise any choice. Like other psychiatric and psychological methods of management, environmental control is open to abuse. Nevertheless, there is little doubt that for some people with severe and widespread cognitive impairments, environmental restructuring or modification is the best chance of having some degree of independence.

Compensating for memory problems is probably one of the best strategies for improving quality of life for people with TBI and significant memory impairment. The approach adopted here is to try to find an alternative means to achieve a goal. This idea can be traced back to Zangwill (1947) when he discussed his principle of compensation, and is also similar to Luria's (1963) principle of functional adaptation, i.e. if you cannot achieve something one way, try to find an alternative way to achieve the goal. In memory rehabilitation, compensation is often achieved through the use of external memory aids such as diaries, organisers, computers, tape recorders, lists, wall charts and so forth. Although most people without memory problems use such external aids, efficient use involves memory so the very people who need them most often have the greatest difficulty using them. It is possible to (a) find aids that are easy to use, (b) spend time teaching the use of aids, (c) use aids that were employed prior to the onset of the brain damage and (d) use a mixture of the above solutions.

There is no doubt it is possible for some people with significant memory problems to use a complex system of external memory aids. JC, for example, a very amnesic young man, spent 10 years developing a sophisticated compensatory system (Wilson, JC *et al.*, 1997). Others may do well with specialised teaching (Kime *et al.*, 1996). Sohlberg and Mateer (1989) describe one method of teaching the use of compensatory memory books, and Wilson and Watson (1996) discuss a practical framework for understanding compensatory behaviour in people with organic memory impairment. Wilson (2000) expands this theme further to include compensation for cognitive deficits other than memory.

Two of the major problems faced when trying to persuade people to use external memory aids are: first, that they think it is cheating to use an aid, or that it will slow down any natural recovery; and second, that they forget to use the aid. The first problem can usually be overcome by discouragement of these misconceptions and by demonstration of the fact that most people (including the neuropsychologists, doctors and therapists engaged in rehabilitation) use external aids; it is normal and sensible to do so and there is neither evidence nor reason to believe such use will slow down any recovery. This discouragement, explanation and reassurance will probably need to be repeated and demonstrated several times.

The second and bigger problem, of forgetting to use the aids, usually needs more careful and structured input. Those needing to learn how to use new aids may do better with uncomplicated ones that do not require complicated programming. Wilson (1991a) found that people seen for memory rehabilitation were more likely to be using compensatory strategies 5 to 10 years later than they were during or at the end of rehabilitation, despite the fact that much of the rehabilitation emphasised the use of such aids. Furthermore, people using six or more strategies or aids were significantly more likely to be independent (defined as living alone or in paid employment or in full-time education) than those using five or less. The numbers of people using each kind of compensatory aid/strategy can be found in Wilson (1995). The most popular were writing notes, mental retracing of events (an internal strategy), using wall calendars/wall charts and writing lists.

One simple aid that we have been evaluating in Cambridge since 1994 is NeuroPage®, a portable paging system designed in California by Treadgold, the engineer father of a young man who sustained a severe head injury, working together with Hersh, a neuropsychologist (Hersh & Treadgold, 1994). NeuroPage® uses a computer, linked by a modem and telephone to a paging company. The scheduling of reminders or messages for each individual is entered into the computer and from then on no further human interaction is necessary. On the appropriate date and time NeuroPage® automatically transmits the message to the paging company, which transmits the information to the individual's pager (e.g. 'Take your medication', 'Today is ——', 'Feed the dog' and 'Check your diary').

One major advantage of NeuroPage® is that the system avoids many of the difficulties faced by people with memory impairments when they try to use a compensatory strategy. The pager either emits a sound or vibrates when a message is coming through, so there is no need to remember to look, or to enter the message (families and therapists usually telephone in once a week with the messages that need to be sent); the pager is usually considered to be prestigious so there is no embarrassment at having to use an aid; it is simple to use, being controlled by one button easy to press even by those with motor difficulties (Wilson, Evans *et al.*, 1997).

Pilot studies and case studies showed the marked benefit of the system, and, more recently, a large randomised control study involving a crossover design has been carried out confirming the benefits of NeuroPage® for helping people manage everyday tasks (Wilson *et al.*, 2001). Of 200 people originally referred from throughout the United Kingdom, 143 completed all stages of the study. Each had one or more of the following: memory, planning, attention or organisation problems. Most had sustained a traumatic head injury or a stroke. The crossover design ensured all people received a pager at some stage. Following a two-week baseline, participants were randomly allocated to treatment (pager) or waiting list. Those with the pager were sent reminders for seven weeks and were monitored for the last two weeks of this period. Those on the waiting list were also monitored for the last two weeks of this seven-week period. At the end of this time, those with the pagers returned them and those on the waiting list were given pagers for a further seven weeks. Both groups were monitored for the last two weeks of this period. Thus there were three assessment periods, baseline, six and seven weeks post-baseline and 13 and 14 weeks post-baseline.

More than 80 per cent of those who completed the 16-week trial were significantly more successful in carrying out everyday activities such as self-care, self-medication and keeping appointments when using the pager in comparison with the baseline period. For the majority of these, significant improvement was maintained when they were monitored seven weeks after returning the pager.

Although NeuroPage® is simple and effective, the messages have to be sent from a central station and participants cannot enter their own messages. In an attempt to overcome this disadvantage, particularly for less handicapped people needing more control over their lives, Rogers *et al.* (2000) investigated pocket computers as memory aids. An electronic memory aid was developed consisting of a diary and a notebook that enabled links to be made between diary entries and pages in the notebook. The memory aid was specifically designed to limit the demands made on memory by providing cues on the interface. This reduced the amount of learning required. The memory aid was implemented on two machines differing in how the text was entered. One machine used a keyboard and the other a touch pen. The success of the aid was evaluated both with respect to people's ability to use it and their willingness to use it over a two-month period. A pilot study with 10 people aged between 21 and 53 years showed that all were able to use the diary on both machines after only two training sessions. The frequency of use suggested a bi-modal distribution between high and low users. The high frequency users tended to prefer the keyboard machines while the low frequency users either had no preference or preferred the touch-pen machine. This suggests that it is possible to teach memory-impaired people to use pocket computers and that individual styles have to be taken into account.

Computers have, of course, been used in rehabilitation for a number of years. In the past, one of their main uses was in the provision of exercises or drills in attempts to improve cognitive functioning (see Wilson, 1997b for a discussion). Computers as communication aids for people with speech and language problems are well established. Computers have been used as task guidance systems and as cognitive prostheses (Bergman & Kemmerer, 1991; Kirsch *et al.*, 1987). More recently, virtual reality systems are proving useful in cognitive rehabilitation (Brooks *et al.*, 1999; Rizzo *et al.*, 1997; Rose *et al.*, 1996). There is little doubt that technology is here to stay and the benefits of computerised and other technological systems are likely to increase in the future.

Although environmental adaptations and external aids can be of great help to people with memory problems, it is unlikely that they will me*et all* their needs. There are occasions when new information needs to be learned and taken on board. One obvious example is learning the names of people with whom one comes into contact regularly. These names can, of course, be written down and even paired with a photograph or description, but it is socially embarrassing to expect people to wait while you hunt through your book or organiser to find the name. One often needs to be able to retrieve the name sufficiently quickly to greet the person in an appropriate manner. Consequently, some aspects of memory rehabilitation are typically concerned with the facilitation of new learning. There are several ways to achieve this, including the use of mnemonics, spaced retrieval and errorless learning.

Mnemonic systems are those that enable people to organise, store and retrieve information more efficiently. Sometimes the term 'mnemonics' is used to refer to anything that helps people to remember, including external memory aids. Usually, however, the term is used for methods involving mental manipulation of material. For example, in order to remember how many days there are in each month, most people use a mnemonic. In the United States of America and the United Kingdom this is typically the rhyme 'Thirty days hath September, April, June and November . . . ' and so forth. In other parts of the world people use their knuckles and the dips in between to remember the long and the short months, or else they have different suffixes and prefixes to distinguish them. Every country using our calendar system appears to have a mnemonic for remembering the long and the short months. Mnemonics are also frequently employed to learn notes of music, colours of the rainbow, cranial nerves and other ordered material.

Mnemonics can be employed to help people with memory impairments learn new information (see Wilson, 1987 for a whole series of studies using a variety of mnemonics). It is usually best for the psychologist, therapist or carer to work out the mnemonic (perhaps together with the memory-impaired person) and work through this together. People with TBI often find it difficult to devise their own mnemonics and forget to employ the mnemonics or to use them spontaneously in novel situations. This is not always the case (Kime *et al.*, 1996) as some people can be taught to use them in new situations. The real value of mnemonics, however, is that they are useful for teaching new information to people with memory difficulties, and they almost always lead to faster learning than rote rehearsal (Clare *et al.*, 1999; Moffat, 1989; West, 1995; Wilson, 1987). Clare *et al.* (1999) employed a combination of strategies, including a visual mnemonic, spaced retrieval and errorless learning, to re-teach the names of people at a social club to a man with Alzheimer's disease.

Spaced retrieval (also known as expanding rehearsal) is another method to improve or enhance learning. In this procedure information to be taught is first presented, then tested immediately while it is still held in immediate memory, tested again after a very brief delay, then after a slightly longer delay and so on. The retention interval is gradually increased. This is a form of distributed practice, i.e. distributing the learning trials across a period of time rather than massing them together in one block. Distributed practice is a more efficient learning strategy than massed practice (Baddeley, 1999). This phenomenon has been known since the 1930s (Baddeley & Longman, 1978; Lorge, 1930). In 1978 Landauer and Bjork employed this method for name learning and from that time spaced retrieval/expanding rehearsal has been used in memory rehabilitation (Camp, 1989; Landauer & Bjork, 1978; McKitrick & Camp, 1993; Moffat, 1989; Schacter *et al.*, 1985). Although many of the published studies describe work with people with dementia, spaced retrieval has been used with people with TBI and other non-progressive conditions (Wilson, 1989b).

There are other strategies from the field of study techniques (e.g., Robinson, 1970) and learning disability (e.g., Yule & Carr, 1987) that have been successfully adapted in cognitive rehabilitation for people with TBI (Glasgow *et al.*, 1977;

Wilson, 1991b). Perhaps one of the most important techniques is that of 'errorless learning', first described in 1963. It has recently become one of the most important components of memory rehabilitation.

Errorless learning is a teaching technique whereby people are prevented, as far as possible, from making mistakes while they are learning a new skill or acquiring new information. Instead of teaching by demonstration, which may involve the learner in trial and error, the experimenter, therapist or teacher presents the correct information or procedure in ways that minimise the possibility of erroneous responses. For example, someone learning names might be given pictures of faces and names underneath. Then, on subsequent trials, less of the name is given (from 'Jonathan' to 'Jonath–' to 'Jon——'), eventually to no name.

There are two theoretical backgrounds to investigations of errorless learning in people with organic memory impairment. The first is the work on errorless discrimination learning from the field of behavioural psychology, first described by Terrace in the 1960s (Terrace, 1963, 1966). Terrace was working with pigeons and found it was possible to teach pigeons to discriminate a red key from a green key with a teaching technique whereby the pigeons made no (or very few) errors during learning. Furthermore, the pigeons learning via errorless learning were reported to show less emotional behaviour than the pigeons who learned with trial-and-error-learning.

Sidman and Stoddard (1967) soon applied errorless learning principles to children with developmental learning difficulties. They were able to teach these children to discriminate ellipses from circles. Others soon took up the idea (e.g. Cullen, 1976; Jones & Eayrs, 1992; Walsh & Lamberts, 1979).

Cullen (1976) believed that if errors were made during learning it was harder to remember just what had been learned. He also pointed out that more reinforcement occurred during errorless learning as only successes occurred, never failures. To this day, errorless learning is a frequently used teaching technique for people with developmental learning difficulties.

The second theoretical impetus came from studies of implicit memory and implicit learning from cognitive psychology and cognitive neuropsychology (e.g. Brooks & Baddeley, 1976; Graf & Schacter, 1985; Tulving & Schacter, 1990; and many others). Although it has been known for decades that memory-impaired people can learn some skills and information normally through their intact (or relatively intact) implicit learning abilities, it has been difficult to apply this knowledge to reduce the real-life problems encountered by people with organic memory deficits.

Glisky and colleagues (Glisky & Schacter, 1987; Glisky *et al.*, 1986) tried to capitalise on intact implicit abilities to teach people with amnesia computer terminology using a technique they called 'the method of vanishing cues'. Despite some successes, the method of vanishing cues involved considerable time and effort both from the experimenters and the people with amnesia. Implicit memory or learning, on the other hand, does not involve effort as it occurs without conscious recollection. This, together with certain other anomalies seen during implicit learning (such as the observation that in a fragmented picture/perceptual priming procedure, if an amnesic patient mislabels a fragment during an early presentation, the error may 'stick' and be repeated on successive presentations), led Baddeley and Wilson (1994) to pose the question 'Do amnesic patients learn better if prevented from making mistakes during the learning process?'. In a study with 16 young and 16 elderly control participants, and 16 densely amnesic people, employing a stem completion procedure, it was found that every one of the amnesic people learned better if prevented from making mistakes during learning.

Baddeley and Wilson (1994) believed errorless learning was superior to trial and error because it depended on implicit memory. As the amnesic people could not use explicit memory effectively, they were forced to rely on implicit memory. This system is not designed to eliminate errors, so it is better to prevent the injection of errors in the first place. In the absence of an efficient episodic memory, the very fact of making an incorrect response may strengthen or reinforce the error.

Errorless learning principles were quickly adopted in the rehabilitation of memory-impaired people. Wilson *et al.* (1994) described a number of single case studies in which amnesic people were taught several tasks such as learning therapists' names, learning to programme an electronic organiser and learning to recognise objects. Each participant was taught two similar tasks in an errorful or an errorless way. In each case errorless was superior to errorful learning. Wilson and Evans (1996) provided further support for these findings. Squires *et al.* (1996) taught a man with amnesia to use a notebook with an errorless learning procedure. The same group (Squires *et al.*, 1998, 1997) found that errorless learning procedures enabled amnesic people to learn novel associations, and to acquire word processing skills. More recently, these principles have been used successfully with people with Alzheimer's disease (Clare *et al.*, 1999, 2000).

Hunkin *et al.* (1998) believed that errorless learning capitalised on the impoverished, residual, explicit memory capacities. Further investigations in Cambridge (Page *et al.*, 2006) suggest that implicit memory is the stronger of the two explanations.

When to begin memory rehabilitation

As far as we know, there is no time when it is too late to begin memory rehabilitation. Is there a time when it is too early? Again, we do not really know the answer, although the general consensus of clinical opinion seems to be 'begin as early as possible'. Obviously, we cannot carry out memory rehabilitation with people in coma, although it is certainly possible to promote the best possible conditions for optimal recovery and thus be ready for cognitive rehabilitation after coma. We also know that people in coma can learn simple tasks (Shiel *et al.*, 1993). We have seen earlier that people in PTA can learn (Wilson, Evans *et al.*, 1999) and one of the patients in the errorless learning study by Wilson *et al.* (1994) was in PTA. He certainly benefited more from errorless than errorful learning when taught the names of people in the hospital and other everyday information such as the name of the ward. Most people receiving memory rehabilitation in our rehabilitation wards and centres will be beyond this stage and however long post-insult, can almost certainly benefit from therapy programmes (see Wilson, 1999 for examples).

The rehabilitation needs of individuals will differ depending on the severity of the memory impairment, the extent of other deficits, the length of time that has elapsed since the brain injury, the preferences of the individual and the family, the particular life circumstances and the resources available.

Who should provide memory rehabilitation

The process of rehabilitation should not be restricted to one professional group. Neuropsychologists, clinical psychologists, speech and language therapists and occupational therapists are the groups most often involved in the United Kingdom. Ideally, these work together in an interdisciplinary way, running groups as well as being involved in individual sessions (Wilson, Evans *et al.*, 2000), but in some circumstances only one professional group is available to do this, perhaps with opportunities for discussion and/or supervision by colleagues from their own and other professions. One important point to note, however, about rehabilitation is that it should not be restricted to professionals – whatever their profession. McLellan (1991) argued that rehabilitation is a two-way, interactive process – a partnership between people with the problems, their relatives and professionals. Nor should rehabilitation be restricted to one setting: successful programmes have been carried out in rehabilitation centres, on patient wards, out-departments, nursing homes, the individual's own home and other settings. It is up to us to solve the problems facing us and our clients, to be imaginative, to set appropriate goals in negotiation with clients and families and to adjust to changing needs.

Case 7.1: Mark

Mark was in his early thirties and was a very successful international property underwriter for a large insurance company. On a mountain biking holiday in Switzerland he fell 1000 feet down a mountain. He was airlifted to a specialist hospital in Switzerland. He had suffered a severe head injury, having been in a coma for one week, and experienced post-traumatic amnesia of one week. CT scan showed diffuse axonal injury, oedema, small deep midline haemorrhages and a sub-dural haematoma. The haematoma was evacuated via a burr hole. He had a tracheostomy for 10 days. He contracted subsequent illnesses of meningitis, pneumonia and septicaemia. He was transferred to London for treatment at an acute rehabilitation centre. He was ataxic and agitated. He needed two people to help him stand from a sitting position. Good physical recovery was made, but he had ongoing cognitive problems.

At nine months post-injury he was admitted to The Oliver Zangwill Centre for Neuropsychological Rehabilitation. He was referred for help with memory, attention and planning problems. He was described as lacking initiative compared to his premorbid personality. He had some insight into his difficulties but did not appreciate the nature and extent of his memory problems and the

Continued

potential impact of such impairments on his work. He noted he had difficulty 'time-stamping' his memories. Because Mark had been assessed numerous times before coming to the Oliver Zangwill Centre, he was given only a short neuropsychological assessment at the centre. He was on the low average to above average range on a general cognitive test. He was above average on a measure of pre-injury functioning. His memory was assessed as being poor. He had particular problems with memory, together with some mild executive deficits.

With the rehabilitation team, Mark set some specific goals for his programme, which lasted 20 weeks, the first 10 weeks being intensive (i.e. 5 days per week) and the second 10 weeks being divided between home, work and the rehabilitation centre. The goals for his programme were (1) to develop an awareness of his strengths and weaknesses in a written form consistent with his neuropsychological profile and describe how any problems would impact on domestic, social and work situations; (2) to identify whether he could return to his previous employment; (3) to manage his financial affairs independently; (4) to demonstrate competence in negotiation skills as rated by a work colleague; (5) to develop a range of leisure interests. To achieve these goals Mark engaged in a programme which consisted of both group work (e.g. Understanding Brain Injury Group, Memory Group, Planning/Problem Solving Group) as well as work with individual team members.

There were many elements to Mark's programme, but one of the most critical was helping him cope with memory difficulties. His insight into these problems was achieved by education about the nature of memory and the problems that may exist after brain injury (through Understanding Brain Injury Group and Memory Group). He was given feedback from the results of the standardised assessments. He was asked (prompted and monitored) to keep a diary of memory errors. He was asked to consider his work role and to identify the demands on memory that are made as part of his work. He developed better insight into his difficulties, which had a 'downside' in that he began to feel low as he became less confident that he would be able to return to work. However, the rehabilitation team supported him in developing a set of strategies designed to compensate for the problems. He has adopted these strategies successfully. He uses a large diary for appointments and 'things to do'. He began to use a computer 'contacts' card system for recording relevant information about brokers who came to him with business. He also learned to use mnemonic strategies for remembering people's names and other information. Mark recognised that the ability to judge risk effectively was the essence of his premorbid success as an underwriter, and that his ability to do this depended upon picking up on and remembering pieces of information about locations (e.g. earthquake zones), companies etc. that might present a risk. To compensate for his memory in relation to this issue, he developed a database of information about insurance risks (i.e. details of major losses/disasters compiled from the Lloyds list of such losses), in order to keep up to date with information, to which he could refer when assessing risk associated with new business. Many of these strategies might be used by the non-memory-impaired underwriter, but Mark had previously been successful without any of them. For this reason he had to go through the process of appreciating the nature of his difficulties, accepting the need for memory aids, implementing strategies and evaluating their value. There was a risk of Mark developing depressive symptoms when faced with developing his insight. Managing the emotional component of his rehabilitation involved psychological support though group sessions and occasional individual support (for more on emotion, mood and rehabilitation see Williams *et al.*, 2003a, 2003b).

Critical to Mark's successful return to work was, we believe, a programme of stepwise increases in the level of work responsibilities. Initially he shadowed other underwriters, who would ask him for his views on business offered to them by brokers. Next he undertook 'minimal risk' business such as insurance renewals. Next he was able to make underwriting decisions, but these had to be checked by his manager. Finally he was given full underwriting authority.

This staged approach was necessary for a variety of reasons. It allowed his manager to develop confidence in Mark's judgement in a high-risk business. It enabled Mark to develop his confidence. It also allowed time for Mark to learn to apply the strategies he had developed to compensate for memory problems.

Seven months after commencing his rehabilitation programme, Mark was reinstated on the company payroll and four years later he remains employed. He continues to use the strategies he learned, which he reports are absolutely necessary to his success at work. By being in work he contributes to the cost of his rehabilitation through the tax he pays on his salary and through the tax his company pays as a result of Mark's success in his work. By being in work, welfare costs are also saved. Not all patients undertaking rehabilitation are in a position to make such clinical or financial gains. While it might seem unethical to judge the value of rehabilitation by its cost-effectiveness, cases such as Mark's illustrate that rehabilitation can be both clinically and cost effective.

Summary and Conclusions

This chapter has emphasised that memory should be regarded as a multifunctional cognitive system that can be understood in a number of ways. We can consider the length of time information is stored, the type of information being stored, the stages involved in remembering, whether information is recalled or recognised, whether explicit or implicit recollection is required, or whether memories date from before or after neurological insult.

Most memory-impaired people have difficulty learning and remembering new information; they have a normal, or nearly normal, immediate memory span but have problems remembering after a delay or distraction, and they usually have a period of retrograde amnesia that may range from minutes to decades. Less common memory disorders include semantic memory impairment and immediate verbal or visuo-spatial deficits. The temporary state of PTA is also considered.

Although restoration of memory functioning is unlikely to occur in the majority of people whose memory impairments follow neurological insult, there is, nevertheless, much that can be done to reduce the impact of disabling and handicapping memory problems and foster understanding of the issues involved. These include: dealing with emotional sequelae such as anxiety and depression, which are often associated with organic memory impairment; environmental modifications that can enable very severely impaired people to cope in their daily lives despite lack of adequate memory functioning; teaching how to use external memory aids to help compensate for memory difficulties; and the employment of errorless learning principles to improve the learning ability of memory-impaired people.

The chapter concludes with a brief discussion about who should provide memory rehabilitation and recommends that (a) several professional groups can provide this, preferably working together if circumstances allow; and (b) rehabilitation should be a partnership between the person with memory problems, the family and health-care professionals. A case illustration where a young man was enabled to return to gainful employment using compensatory systems is described.

Recommended Reading

Baddeley, A.D. (1994). *Your memory: A user's guide*. London: Penguin.
This book provides a practical and user-friendly overview of how human memory systems operate.

Baddeley, A.D., Kopelman, M.D. & Wilson, B.A. (Eds.) (2004). *Handbook of memory disorders for clinicians* (pp.757–784). Chichester: Wiley.
This book offers an authoritative review of the key areas of research and development in the field of memory.

Campbell, R. & Conway, M.A. (1995). *Broken memories: Case studies in memory impairment*. Oxford: Blackwell.

This book explores some of the unusual and disabling disturbances of memory or knowledge to which people have fallen prey through brain disease or accident.

Clare, L. & Wilson, B.A. (1997). *Coping with memory problems: A practical guide for people with memory impairments, relatives, friends and carers*. Bury St Edmunds: Thames Valley Test Company.
This book is written especially for the friends and relatives of people with memory problems to help them cope with practical everyday difficulties manifested by those with severe memory impairment.

Wearing, D. (2005). *Forever today: A memoir of love and amnesia*. London: Doubleday.
This book is written by the wife of a man with extremely severe amnesia following encephalitis. It tells his story with great warmth, love, humour and insight.

Wilson, B.A. (1999). *Case studies in neuropsychological rehabilitation*. New York: Oxford University Press.
This book describes the assessment and treatment of twenty people with non-progressive brain injury. Each chapter contains a personal account by the patient and/or a relative. It won the British Psychological Society's book award for 2003.

Useful Resources

There are several booklets available for clients and families including:

- *Memory problems after head injury* (Wilson, 1989a), written for the National Head Injuries Association (now The Brain Injury Association);
- *Managing your memory* (Kapur, 1991), a self-help manual for improving memory skills;
- *Coping with memory problems* (Clare & Wilson, 1997), a practical guide for people with memory impairments, their relatives, friends and carers;
- A useful reference on the topic of self-help and support groups for people with memory problems and their carers is Wearing (1992).

Also see the UK-based websites for charities in brain injury: www.headway.org.uk and www.encephalitis.info/.

References

Baddeley, A.D. (1999). *Essentials of human memory*. Hove: Psychology Press.
Baddeley, A.D, Emslie, H., & Nimmo-Smith, I. (1992). *The speed and capacity of language processing*. Bury St Edmunds: Thames Valley Test Company.
Baddeley, A.D., & Hitch, C. (1974). Working memory. In C.H. Bower (Ed.) *The psychology of learning and motivation* (vol. 8, pp.47–89). New York: Academic Press.
Baddeley, A.D., & Longman, D.J.A. (1978). The influence of length and frequency on training sessions on the rate of learning to type. *Ergonomics*, *21*, 627–635.
Baddeley, A.D., Papagno, C., & Vallar, G. (1988). When long-term learning depends on short-term storage. *Journal of Memory and Language*, *27*, 586–595.
Baddeley, A.D., & Wilson, B.A. (1994). When implicit learning fails: Amnesia and the problem of error elimination. *Neuropsychologia*, *32*, 53–68.

Bergman, M.M., & Kemmerer, A.C. (1991). Computer-enhanced self sufficiency: Part 2. Uses and subjective benefits of a text writer for an individual with traumatic brain injury. *Neuropsychology*, *5*, 25–28.

Brooks, B.M., McNeil, J.E., Rose, D.F., Greenwood, R.J., Attree, E.A., & Leadbetter, A.G. (1999). Route learning in a case of amnesia: A preliminary investigation into the efficacy of training in a virtual environment. *Neuropsychological Rehabilitation*, *9*, 63–76.

Brooks, D.N., & Baddeley, A. (1976). What can amnesic patients learn? *Neuropsychologia*, *14*, 111–122.

Calabrese, P., Markowitsch, H.J., Durwen, H.F., Widlitzek, H., Haupts, M., Holinka, B. *et al.* (1996). Right temperofrontal cortex as critical locus for the ecphory of old episodic memories. *Journal of Neurology, Neurosurgery and Psychiatry*, *61*, 304–310.

Camp, C.J. (1989). Facilitation of new learning in Alzheimer's disease. In G. Gilmore, P. Whitehouse & M. Wykle (Eds.) *Memory and aging: Theory, research and practice* (pp.212–225). New York: Springer.

Clare, L., & Wilson, B.A. (1997). *Coping with memory problems: A practical guide for people with memory impairments, relatives, friends and carers*. Bury St Edmunds: Thames Valley Test Company.

Clare, L., Wilson, B.A., Breen, E.K., & Hodges, J.R. (1999). Errorless learning of face–name associations in early Alzheimer's disease. *Neurocase*, *5*, 37–46.

Clare, L., Wilson, B.A., Carter, G., Breen, K., Gosses, A., & Hodges, J.R. (2000). Intervening with everyday memory problems in dementia of Alzheimer type: An errorless learning approach. *Journal of Clinical and Experimental Neuropsychology*, *22*, 132–146.

Coughlan, A.K., & Hollows, S.E. (1984). Use of memory tests in differentiating organic disorder from depression. *British Journal of Psychiatry*, *145*, 164–167.

Coughlan, A.K., & Hollows, S. (1985). *The adult memory and information processing battery (AMIPB)*. Leeds: A.K. Coughlan, St James University Hospital.

Cullen, C.N. (1976). Errorless learning with the retarded. *Nursing Times*, 25 March.

Davidoff, J., & Wilson, B.A. (1985). A case of associative visual agnosia showing a disorder of pre-semantic visual classification. *Cortex*, *21*, 121–134.

Eslinger, P.J. (1998). Autobiographical memory after temporal lobe lesions. *Neurocase*, *4*, 481–495.

Evans, J.J., Breen, E.K., Antoun, N., & Hodges, J.R. (1996). Focal retrograde amnesia for autobiographical events following cerebral vasculitis: A connectionist account. *Neurocase*, *2*, 1–11.

Farah, M.J. (1984). The neurological basis of mental imagery: A componential analysis. *Cognition*, *18*, 245–272.

Gaffan, D., & Heywood, C.A. (1993). A spurious category-specific visual agnosia for living things in normal human and nonhuman primates. *Journal of Cognitive Neuroscience*, *5*, 118–128.

Glasgow, R.E., Zeiss, R.A., Barrera, M. Jr., & Lewinsohn, P.M. (1977). Case studies on remediating memory deficits in brain-damaged individuals. *Journal of Clinical Psychology*, *33*, 1049–1054.

Glisky, E.L., & Schacter, D.L. (1987). Acquisition of domain-specific knowledge in organic amnesia: Training for computer-related work. *Neuropsychologia*, *25*, 893–906.

Glisky, E.L., Schacter, D.L., & Tulving, E. (1986). Computer learning by memory impaired patients: Acquisition and retention of complex knowledge. *Neuropsychologia*, *24*, 313–328.

Goldberg, E., Antin, S.P., Bilder, R.M. Jr., Gerstman, L.J., Hughes, J.E., & Mattis, S. (1981). Retrograde amnesia: Possible role of mesencephalic reticular activation in long-term memory. *Science*, *213* (18 Sept.), 1392–1394.

Goldman-Rakic, P.S., & Friedman, H.R. (1991). The circuitry of working memory revealed by anatomy and metabolic imaging. In H.S. Levin, H.M. Eisenberg, & A.L. Benton (Eds.) *Frontal lobe function and dysfunction* (pp.72–91). New York, NY: Oxford University Press.

Graf, P., & Schacter, D.L. (1985). Implicit and explicit memory for new associations in normal and amnesic subjects. *Journal of Experimental Psychology: Learning, Memory and Cognition*, *11*, 501–518.

Graham, K.S., Becker, J.T., & Hodges, J.R. (1997). On the relationship between knowledge and memory for pictures: Evidence from the study of patients with semantic dementia and Alzheimer's disease. *Journal of the International Neuropsychological Society*, *3*, 534–544.

Hart, T., & Hayden, M.E. (1986). The ecological validity of neuropsychological assessment and remediation. In B. Uzzell & Y. Gross (Eds.) *Clinical neuropsychology of intervention* (pp.21–50). Boston: Martinus Nijhoff.

Haslam, C., Batchelor, J., Fearnside, M.R., Haslam, S.A., Hawkins, S., & Kenway, E. (1994). Post-coma disturbance and post-traumatic amnesia as nonlinear predictors of cognitive outcome following severe closed head injury: Findings from the Westmead Head Injury Project. *Brain Injury*, *8*, 519–528.

Hersh, N., & Treadgold, L. (1994). NeuroPage: The rehabilitation of memory dysfunction by prosthetic memory and cueing. *NeuroRehabilitation*, *4*, 187–197.

Hillis, A.E., & Caramazza, A. (1991). Category-specific naming and comprehension impairment: A double dissociation. *Brain*, *114*, 2081–2094.

Hodges, J.R. (1995). Retrograde amnesia. In A.D. Baddeley, B.A. Wilson, & F.N. Watts (Eds.) *Handbook of memory disorders* (pp.81–107). Chichester: Wiley.

Hodges, J.R., Graham, N., & Patterson, K. (1995). Charting the progression in semantic dementia: Implications for the organisation of semantic memory. *Memory*, *3*, 463–495.

Hodges, J.R., Patterson, K., Oxbury, S., & Funnell, E. (1992). Semantic dementia: Progressive fluent aphasia with temporal lobe atrophy. *Brain*, *115*, 1783–1806.

Hodges, J., Salmon, D.P., & Butters, N. (1992). Semantic memory impairment in Alzheimer's disease: Failure of access or degraded knowledge? *Neuropsychologia*, *30*, 301–314.

Hunkin, M.M., Squires, E.J., Parkin, A.J., & Tidy, J.A. (1998). Are the benefits of errorless learning dependent on implicit memory? *Neuropsychologia*, *36*, 25–36.

Jones, R.D., Grabowski, T.J., & Tranel, D. (1998). The neural basis of retrograde memory: Evidence from positron emission tomography for the role of non-mesial temporal lobe structures. *Neurocase*, *4*, 471–479.

Jones, R.S.P., & Eayrs, C.B. (1992). The use of errorless learning procedures in teaching people with a learning disability. *Mental Handicap Research*, *5*, 304–212.

Kapur, N. (1988). *Memory disorders in clinical practice*. London: Butterworths.

Kapur, N. (1991). *Managing your memory. A self help memory manual for improving everyday memory skills*. Available from the author at the Wessex Neurological Centre, Southampton General Hospital, Southampton.

Kapur, N. (1993). Focal retrograde amnesia in neurological disease: A critical review. *Cortex*, *29*, 217–234.

Kime, S.K., Lamb, D.G., & Wilson, B.A. (1996). Use of a comprehensive program of external cuing to enhance procedural memory in a patient with dense amnesia. *Brain Injury*, *10*, 17–25.

Kirsch, N.L., Levine, S.P., Fallon-Krueger, M., & Jaros, L.A. (1987). The microcomputer as an 'orthotic' device for patients with cognitive deficits. *Journal of Head Trauma Rehabilitation*, *2*, 77–86.

Landauer, T.K., & Bjork, R.A. (1978). Optimum rehearsal patterns and name learning. In M.M. Gruneberg, P.E. Morris & R.N. Sykes (Eds.) *Practical aspects of memory* (pp.625–632). London: Academic Press.

Levin, H.S., O'Donnell, V.M., & Grossman, R.G. (1979). The Galveston Orientation and Amnesia Test. A practical scale to assess cognition after head injury. *Journal of Nervous and Mental Disorders*, *167*, 675–684.

Lishman, W.A. (1998). On: Cerebral beriberi (Wernicke's encephalopathy). *Journal of Psychosomatic Research*, *44*, 631–632.

Lorge, I. (1930). Influence of regularly interpolated time intervals upon subsequent learning. Quoted in Johnson, H.H., & Solso, R.L. (1971) *An introduction to experimental design in psychology: A case approach*. New York: Harper & Row.

Luria, A.R. (1963). *Recovery of function after brain injury*. New York: Macmillan.

Luria, A.R., Sokolov, E.N., & Klimkowski, M. (1967). Toward a dynamic analysis of memory disturbances with lesions of the left temporal lobe. *Neuropsychologia*, *5*, 1–11.

Markowitsch, H.J. (1998). Cognitive neuroscience of memory. *Neurocase*, *4*, 429–435.

Mayes, A.R. (1995). *Human organic memory disorders*. Cambridge: Cambridge University Press.

McKitrick, L.A., & Camp, C.J. (1993). Relearning the names of things: The spaced-retrieval intervention implemented by a caregiver. *Clinical Gerontologist*, *14*, 60–62.

McLellan, D.L. (1991). Functional recovery and the principles of disability medicine. In M. Swash & J. Oxbury (Eds.) *Clinical neurology* (pp.768–790). Edinburgh: Churchill Livingstone.

McMillan, T.M., Jongen, E.L., & Greenwood, R.J. (1996). Assessment of post-traumatic amnesia after severe closed head injury: retrospective or prospective? *Journal of Neurology, Neurosurgery & Psychiatry*, *60*, 422–427.

Moffat, N. (1989). Home based cognitive rehabilitation with the elderly. In L.W. Poon, D.C. Rubin, & B.A. Wilson (Eds.) *Everyday cognition in adulthood and late life* (pp.659–680). Cambridge: Cambridge University Press.

Murphy, G. (1987). Decreasing undesirable behaviours. In W. Yule & J. Carr (Eds.) *Behaviour modification for people with mental handicaps*. London: Croom Helm.

Page, M., Wilson, B.A., Shiel, A., Carter, G., & Norris, D. (2006). What is the locus of the errorless-learning advantage? *Neuropsychologia*, *44*, 90–100.

Ratcliff, G., & Newcombe, F. (1982). Object recognition: Some deductions from the clinical evidence. In A.W. Ellis (Ed.) *Normality and pathology in cognitive functions* (pp.147–171). New York: Academic Press.

Rizzo, A.A., Buckwalter, J.G., & Neumann, U. (1997). Virtual reality and cognitive rehabilitation: A brief review of the future. *Journal of Head Trauma Rehabilitation*, *12*, 1–15.

Robertson, I.H. (1999). Theory-driven neuropsychological rehabilitation: The role of attention and competition in recovery of function after brain damage. In D. Gopher & A. Koriat (Eds.) *Attention and performance XVII: Cognitive regulation of performance: Interaction of theory and application* (pp.677–696). Cambridge, MA: The MIT Press.

Robertson, I.H., & Murre, J.M.J. (1999). Rehabilitation after brain damage: Brain plasticity and principles of guided recovery. *Psychological Bulletin*, *125*, 544–575.

Robinson, F.P. (1970). *Effective study*. New York: Harper and Row.

Rogers, N., Wright, P., Hall, C., Wilson, B.A., Evans, J., & Emslie, H. (2000). *The development of a simplified pocket computer memory aid for use by people with non-progressive memory impairment*. Abstract presented at the Twenty-Third Annual International Neuropsychological Society Mid-Year Conference (Brussels, Belgium, July 2000).

Rose, F.D., Attree, E.A., & Johnson, D.A. (1996). Virtual reality: An assistive technology in neurological rehabilitation. *Current Opinion in Neurology*, *9*, 461–467.

Russell, W.R. (1971). *The traumatic amnesias*. London: Oxford University Press.

Schacter, D., & Crovitz, H. (1977). Memory function after closed head injury: A review of the quantitative research. *Cortex*, *13*, 105–176.

Schacter, D.L., Rich, S.A., & Stampp, M.S. (1985). Remediation of memory disorders: Experimental evaluation of the spaced-retrieval technique. *Journal of Clinical and Experimental Neuropsychology*, *7*, 79–96.

Schwartz, A.F., & McMillan, T.M. (1989). Assessment of everyday memory after severe head injury. *Cortex*, *25*, 665–671.

Scoville, W.B., & Milner, B. (1957). Loss of recent memory after bilateral hippocampal lesions. *Journal of Neurology, Neurosurgery and Psychiatry*, *20*, 11–21.

Shallice, T., Fletcher, P., Frith, C.D., Grasby, P., Frackowiak, R.S.J., & Dolan, R.J. (1994). Brain-regions associated with acquisition and retrieval of verbal episodic memory. *Nature*, *368*, 633–635.

Shiel, A., Wilson, B.A., Horn, S., Watson, M., & McLellan, L. (1993). Can patients in coma following traumatic head injury learn simple tasks? *Neuropsychological Rehabilitation*, *3*, 161–176.

Shores, E.A., Marosszeky, J.E., Sandman, J., & Batchelor, J. (1986). Preliminary validation of a clinical scale for measuring the duration of post-traumatic amnesia. *The Medical Journal of Australia*, *144*, 596–572.

Sidman, M., & Stoddard, L.T. (1967). The effectiveness of fading in programming simultaneous form discrimination for retarded children. *Journal of Experimental Analysis of Behavior*, *10*, 3–15.

Snowden, J.S., Goulding, P.J., & Neary, D. (1989). Semantic dementia: A form of circumscribed cerebral atrophy. *Behavioural Neurology*, *2*, 167–182.

Sohlberg, M.M., & Mateer, C. (1989). Training use of compensatory memory books: A three-stage behavioural approach. *Journal of Clinical and Experimental Neuropsychology*, *11*, 871–891.

Squires, E.J., Aldrich, F.K., Parkin, A.J., & Hunkin, N.M. (1998). Errorless learning and the acquisition of word processing skills. *Neuropsychological Rehabilitation*, *8*, 433–449.

Squires, E.J., Hunkin, N.M., & Parkin, A.J. (1996). Memory notebook training in a case of severe amnesia: Generalising from paired associate learning to real life. *Neuropsychological Rehabilitation*, *6*, 55–65.

Squires, E.J., Hunkin, N.M., & Parkin, A.J. (1997). Errorless learning of novel associations in amnesia. *Neuropsychologia*, *35*, 1103–1111.

Terrace, H.S. (1963). Discrimination learning with and without 'errors'. *Journal of Experimental Analysis of Behavior*, *6*, 1–27.

Terrace, H.S. (1966). Stimulus control. In W.K. Honig (Ed.) *Operant behaviour: Areas of research and application* (pp.271–344). New York: Appleton-Century-Crofts.

Tranel, D., & Damasio, A.R. (1995). Neurobiological foundations of human memory. In A.D. Baddeley, B.A. Wilson & F.N. Watts (Eds.) *Handbook of memory disorders* (pp.27–50). Chichester: Wiley.

Tulving, E., Kapur, S., Craik, F.I., Moscovitch, M., & House, S. (1994). Hemispheric encoding/retrieval asymmetry in episodic memory: Positron emission tomography findings. *Proceedings of the National Academy of Sciences of the USA*, *91*, 2016–2020.

Tulving, E., & Schacter, D.L. (1990). Priming and human memory systems. *Science*, *247*, 301–306.

Vallar, G., & Papagno, C. (1995). Neuropsychological impairments of short-term memory. In A.D. Baddeley, B.A. Wilson & F.N. Watts (Eds.) *Handbook of memory disorders* (pp.135–165). Chichester: Wiley.

Walsh, B.F., & Lamberts, F. (1979). Errorless discrimination and fading as techniques for teaching sight words to TMR students. *American Journal of Mental Deficiency*, *83*, 473–479.

Warrington, E.K. (1975). The selective impairment of semantic memory. *Quarterly Journal of Experimental Psychology*, *27*, 635–657.

Warrington, E.K., & Shallice, T. (1969). The selective impairment of auditory verbal short-term memory. *Brain*, *92*, 885–896.

Warrington, E.K., & Shallice, T. (1984). Category specific semantic impairments. *Brain*, *107*, 829–854.

Wearing, D. (1992). Self help groups. In B.A. Wilson & N. Moffat (Eds.) *Clinical management of memory problems* (2nd edn, pp.271–301). London: Chapman and Hall.

Wechsler, D. (1945). A standardised memory scale for clinical use. *Journal of Psychology*, *19*, 87–95.

Wechsler, D. (1987). *The Wechsler Memory Scale – Revised*. San Antonio, TX: The Psychological Corporation.

Wechsler, D. (1997). *Wechsler Memory Scale III*. San Antonio, TX: The Psychological Corporation.

West, R.L. (1995). Compensatory strategies for age-associated memory impairment. In A.D. Baddeley, B.A. Wilson & F.N. Watts (Eds.) *Handbook of memory disorders* (pp.481–500). Chichester: Wiley.

Williams, W.H., Evans, J.J. & Fleminger, S (2003a). Assessment and management of anxiety disorders in acquired brain injury. *Neuropsychological Rehabilitation – Special Issue*, *1*, 133–148.

Williams, W.H., Evans, J.J. & Wilson, B.A. (2003b). Neurological rehabilitation for post-traumatic stress symptoms after traumatic brain injury. *Cognitive Neuropsychiatry*. *8*(1), 1–18.

Wills, P., Clare, L., Shiel, A., & Wilson, B.A. (2000). Assessing subtle impairments in the everyday memory performance of brain injured people: Exploring the potential of the Extended Rivermead Behavioural Memory Test. *Brain Injury*, *14*, 693–704.

Wilson, B.A. (1987). *Rehabilitation of memory*. New York: The Guilford Press.

Wilson, B.A. (1989a). *Memory problems after head injury*. Nottingham: National Head Injuries Association.

Wilson, B.A. (1989b). Designing memory therapy programmes. In L. Poon, D. Rubin, & B. Wilson (Eds.) *Everyday cognition in adult and later life* (pp.615–638). Cambridge: Cambridge University Press.

Wilson, B.A. (1991a). Long term prognosis of patients with severe memory disorders. *Neuropsychological Rehabilitation*, *1*, 117–134.

Wilson, B.A. (1991b). Behaviour therapy in the treatment of neurologically impaired adults. In P.R. Martin (Ed.) *Handbook of behavior therapy and psychological science: An integrative approach* (pp.227–252). New York: Pergamon Press.

Wilson, B.A. (1995). Management and remediation of memory problems in brain-injured adults. In A.D. Baddeley, B.A. Wilson, & F.N. Watts (Eds.) *Handbook of memory disorders* (pp.451–479). Chichester: Wiley.

Wilson, B.A. (1996). Assessment of memory. In L. Harding & J.R. Beech (Eds.) *Assessment in neuropsychology* (pp.135–151). London: Routledge.

Wilson, B.A. (1997a). Semantic memory impairments following non progressive brain damage: A study of four cases. *Brain Injury*, *11*, 259–269.

Wilson, B.A. (1997b). Cognitive rehabilitation: How it is and how it might be. *Journal of the International Neuropsychological Society*, *3*, 487–496.

Wilson, B.A. (1998). Recovery of cognitive functions following non progressive brain injury. *Current Opinion in Neurobiology*, *8*, 281–287.

Wilson, B.A. (1999). *Case studies in neuropsychological rehabilitation*. New York: Oxford University Press.

Wilson, B.A. (2000). Compensating for cognitive deficits following brain injury. *Neuropsychology Review*, *10*, 233–243.

Wilson, B.A., Baddeley, A.D., Evans, J.J., & Shiel, A. (1994). Errorless learning in the rehabilitation of memory impaired people. *Neuropsychological Rehabilitation*, *4*, 307–326.

Wilson, B.A., Baddeley, A.D. & Kapur, N. (1995). Dense amnesia in a professional musician following herpes simplex virus encephalitis. *Journal of Clinical and Experimental Psychology*, *17*, 668–681.

Wilson, B.A., Baddeley, A.D., Shiel, A., & Patton, G. (1992). How does post traumatic amnesia differ from the amnesic syndrome and from chronic memory impairment? *Neuropsychological Rehabilitation*, *2*, 231–243.

Wilson, B.A., Baddeley, A.D., & Young, A.W. (1999). LE, a person who lost her 'mind's eye'. *Neurocase*, *5*, 119–127.

Wilson, B.A., Clare, L., Baddeley, A.D., Cockburn, J., Watson, P. & Tate, R. (1999). *The Rivermead Behavioural Memory Test – Extended Version.* Bury St Edmunds: Thames Valley Test Company.

Wilson, B.A., Cockburn, J., & Baddeley, A.D. (1985). *The Rivermead Behavioural Memory Test.* Bury St. Edmunds: Thames Valley Test Company.

Wilson, B.A., Cockburn, J., Baddeley, A.D., & Hiorns, R. (1989). The development and validation of a test battery for detecting and monitoring everyday memory problems. *Journal of Clinical and Experimental Neuropsychology*, *11*, 855–870.

Wilson, B.A., Emslie, H.C., Quirk, K., & Evans, J. (1999). George: Learning to live independently with NeuroPage®. *Rehabilitation Psychology*, *44*, 284–296.

Wilson, B.A., & Evans, J.J. (1996). Error free learning in the rehabilitation of individuals with memory impairments. *Journal of Head Trauma Rehabilitation*, *11*, 54–64.

Wilson, B.A., Evans, J., Brentnall, S., Bremner, S., Keohane, C., & Williams, H. (2000). The Oliver Zangwill Centre for Neuropsychological Rehabilitation: A partnership between health care and rehabilitation research. In A-L. Christensen & B.P. Uzzell (Eds.) *International handbook of neuropsychological rehabilitation* (pp.231–246). New York: Kluwer Academic/Plenum Publishers.

Wilson, B.A., Evans, J.J., Emslie, H., Balleny, H., Watson, P.C., & Baddeley, A.D. (1999). Measuring recovery from post traumatic amnesia. *Brain Injury*, *13*, 505–520.

Wilson, B.A., Evans, J.J., Emslie, H., & Malinek, V. (1997). Evaluation of NeuroPage: A new memory aid. *Journal of Neurology, Neurosurgery, and Psychiatry*, *63*, 113–115.

Wilson, B.A., Green, R., Teasdale, T., Beckers, K., Della Sala, S., Kaschel, R. *et al.* (1996). Implicit learning in amnesic subjects: A comparison with a large group of normal control subjects. *The Clinical Neuropsychologist*, *10*, 279–292.

Wilson, B.A., JC, & Hughes, E. (1997). Coping with amnesia: The natural history of a compensatory memory system. *Neuropsychological Rehabilitation*, *7*, 43–56.

Wilson, B.A., & Watson, P.C. (1996). A practical framework for understanding compensatory behaviour in people with organic memory impairment. *Memory*, *4*, 465–486.

Wilson, B.A., Watson, P.C., Baddeley, A.D., Emslie, H., & Evans, J.J. (2000). Improvement or simply practice? The effects of twenty repeated assessments on people with and without brain injury. *Journal of the International Neuropsychological Society*, *6*, 469–479.

Yule, W., & Carr, J. (Eds.) (1987). *Behaviour modification for people with mental handicaps.* London: Croom Helm.

Zangwill, O.L. (1947). Psychological aspects of rehabilitation in cases of brain injury. *British Journal of Psychology*, *37*, 60–69.

8

Visual-perceptual and Spatio-motor Disorders

Andrew D. Worthington and M. Jane Riddoch

Introduction

Disorders of visual perception and spatio-motor deficits present some of the greatest challenges in rehabilitation, requiring both specialist knowledge and therapeutic creativity from a range of disciplines. This may include not just clinical psychology and occupational therapy but also neurology, neuro-ophthalmology, rehabilitation engineering and disability employment advisers. Recognising the contribution of different disciplines for both assessment and rehabilitation is essential for a potentially debilitating perceptual disorder. In everyday life we take for granted our ability to perform highly complex perceptuo-spatial judgements. We can recognise objects from different viewpoints and under different viewing conditions (e.g. bright sunlight or shadow). We can readily recognise black-and-white photographs even when colour may be the most salient feature of the object (e.g. an orange). We are able to reach accurately and quickly to objects in the environment, and to pick them up appropriately. We can manipulate objects in order to achieve a desired end (e.g. angling a tennis racquet appropriately in order to hit a ball). We can use the physical properties of objects to achieve a desired goal – even if the object was not specifically designed for that purpose (e.g. using the heel of a shoe to hammer a nail into the wall). Our impression of a coherent visual world of sensation, perception and action arises from integration of information processing in separable neural pathways. The distinction between input streams for different visual dimensions such as colour, form, stereo depth and motion perception provides a framework for understanding the breakdown in our otherwise coherent perceptual world, and which can result in selective impairments in perceiving some of the basic features that make up objects, such as their form, colour and motion.

Understanding how perceptual impairments arise after brain injury also requires an appreciation of the effects of trauma. Traumatic brain injury results in characteristically diffuse lesions of cortical neurons and white matter tracts with involvement of subcortical brain structures as a result of mechanical rotational forces. Even patients with cerebellar damage and no identifiable cerebral injury may show visuo-spatial deficits on examination (Molinari *et al.*, 2004). While focal insults, such as localised haemorrhage, often occur after trauma, pathology is usually widespread throughout the brain. Consequently, visual processing efficiency is reduced, with the result that it takes longer to identify stimuli after brain injury (Mattson *et al.*, 1994). This is an important point for understanding functional consequences in the real world. Perception under time constraints may be poor, despite no apparent deficit on untimed tasks. In addition, where insight is preserved, the debilitating loss of a facility like visual perception frequently has psychological implications. Consequently, disorders of specific cognitive functions like visual perceptual processing typically occur in the context of generalised neuropsychological dysfunction and emotional sequelae. Unfortunately for the clinician seeking to navigate their passage through the rocky waters of perceptual rehabilitation, there is no guiding light. One might ask, for instance, why there is no section on the treatment of perceptual disorders in Sohlberg and Mateer's (2001) influential text on cognitive rehabilitation. The answer in part is because perceptual deficits are notoriously difficulty to treat. Very often the most effective form of therapy is helping the person to live with the disorder, rather than aiming to treat it. It is no coincidence that a recent book devoted to reviewing the evidence-base for rehabilitation of cognitive disorders (Halligan & Wade, 2005) does not contain a single chapter devoted exclusively to the treatment of perceptual deficits. In contrast, this chapter will attempt to outline a structured approach to the assessment and treatment of disorders of visual perceptual processing. However, because they rarely occur in isolation after a head injury, skilled investigation and rehabilitation requires an appreciation of other cognitive and behavioural factors that might influence the presentation of the deficit. Moreover, visuo-spatial disorders are complex, and yet most standard neuropsychological test batteries provide only cursory examination of perceptual functioning. Clinicians are often unsure how to select more specialised tests or how to interpret them. This chapter will present an overview of principal perceptuo-spatial disorders in terms of their neurological basis, their clinical presentation and functional implications.

Theoretical Models of Visual-perceptual and Spatio-motor Disorders

Mindful that 'without a clear and unifying conceptual structure it is hard to organise a rational assessment approach' (Beaumont & Davidoff, 1992, p.115), some attempt will be made to provide the clinician with a pragmatic theoretical framework (though no single model encompasses all the disorders reviewed). One such model is provided in Figure 8.1. It is based upon the idea that vision results from processing via a number of modular (i.e. separable) sub-systems, which, when combined in a hierarchical fashion, give rise to object recognition (e.g. Marr, 1982). This general principle that vision involves a set of separable hierarchically organised processes is particularly helpful in understanding how visual processes may break

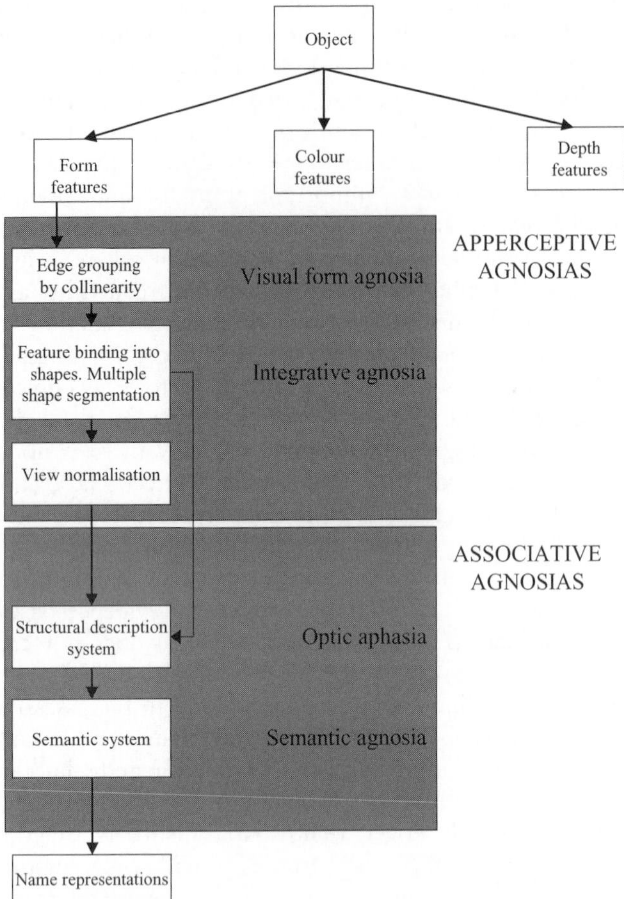

Figure 8.1 A theoretical framework for investigating visual perceptual disorders

down following brain damage, because assessment can be devised for the different levels of visual processing. The most elaborate example of this approach is the BORB or Birmingham Object Recognition Battery (Riddoch & Humphreys, 1993). This test provides clinicians with a range of structured tasks useful in assessing components of visual perception as illustrated in Figure 8.1.

The Functional Neuroanatomy of Visual-perceptual and Spatial Processing

There is substantial functional segregation in the visual pathways from the retina onwards (Zeki, 1993), with two distinct cortical pathways projecting from the occipital lobes to the temporal and parietal lobes respectively. There is a broad consensus that the temporal lobes (the ventral processing pathway) contain cells that code 'what' an object is, whilst the parietal lobes (the dorsal pathway) contain cells that code 'where' it is (Ungerleider & Mishkin, 1982), and indeed how it might mediate the control of goal-directed actions (Milner & Goodale, 1995).

Damage to the dorsal pathway often causes impairments in spatial analysis and orientation. The additional involvement of anterior brain regions after traumatic brain injury tends to result in disorders reflecting the interaction between perception and action. Examples of such spatially mediated problems include the inability to reach accurately to visually presented targets (optic ataxia); the inability to construct objects with their constituent elements in the correct spatial relationships to each other (constructional apraxia); and the inability to gesture the use of visually presented objects (apraxia). In addition, disorders such as the failure to process information from one side of space (unilateral neglect) may be associated with lesions of the dorsal pathway.

Lesions of the ventral visual pathway affecting regions outside the primary visual cortex (the so-called extrastriate visual areas) can lead to perceptual problems in deriving some of the basic dimensions of visual stimuli. This includes their colour (achromatopsia), their depth, or their form (apperceptive agnosia). Where damage implicates the later stages of this visual processing pathway, the resulting disorders reflect the involvement of other brain structures such as the temporal lobes. Examples of disorders resulting from interruption to later stages of the ventral visual pathway are optic aphasia and associative agnosia. We now focus on some of the issues involved in the initial assessment of visuo-perceptual and spatio-motor disorders before focusing on the different disorders associated with lesions of the two visual pathways.

Initial Assessment of Visuo-perceptual and Spatio-motor Disorders

A thorough assessment of cognitive functioning is necessary to provide an accurate appreciation of the nature of any deficit. This should incorporate detailed neuropsychological investigation and behavioural observations of the individual's performance on real-life tasks. Where there may be scope for a restorative approach to rehabilitation then clearly an accurate formulation of the problem is necessary in order to focus on the impaired processing. However, even if it is felt that the damage is so severe that any restitution of function will be negligible, a specific diagnosis is often a comfort to the individual as it can help them to understand why they are no longer able to engage in simple activities of everyday living and may help the therapist to focus on procedures to help compensate for the deficit.

There is a range of standard tests useful for investigating perceptual and spatial functioning. Most routine clinical tests are reviewed by Lezak (1995) and Spreen and Strauss (1998). Additional normative data for selected tests is provided by Mitrushina *et al.* (1999). A useful clinical screening tool for many (but not all) of the disorders associated with lesions of the dorsal and ventral pathways is the Visual Object and Space Perception Battery (VOSP; Warrington & James, 1991). It consists of a number of subtests designed to distinguish disorders of visual perception from disorders of space processing. However, there are some problems associated with using VOSP with clients with traumatic brain injury in that many of the subtests are also sensitive to the effects of frontal lobe lesions (e.g. impulsiveness, perseveration, poor perceptual reasoning and judgement). Consequently, care must be taken in its interpretation.

Disorders of Vision

A brief note is required concerning the potential confounding effects on visual perception of visual disturbance. Transient visual disturbance, including double vision (diplopia), restriction of visual fields and poor visual scanning, is often associated with traumatic brain injury, due to damage to the oculomotor apparatus and visual pathways (Mishra & Digre, 1996). The term post-trauma vision syndrome has been suggested to encompass this constellation of typical features (Padula & Argyris, 1996). It is important to correctly identify and try to remedy any early stage visual processing deficit. Failure to carry out proper evaluation can lead to misdiagnosis and many futile therapy hours. This can have significant implications for everyday living, not least in whether people can return to driving (Priddy *et al.*, 1990; Strano, 1989).

Brain injury can produce positive perceptual disturbances, as well as losses. Another common feature of visual disturbance after traumatic brain injury is the occurrence of visual perseverations and visual illusions. This includes after-images that may obscure real objects, perception of multiple images of the same object (polyopia) and persistence of a visual image from a few minutes to an hour or more (palinopsia). While most of these phenomena are caused by damage to visual pathways, they can take on the form of complex hallucinations. These may occur in the context of epilepsy or cortical visual loss and often resolve spontaneously (Kolmel, 1993). Nevertheless, the experiences can be extremely distressing and are easily misdiagnosed. Similarly, perceptual disturbances associated with altered bodily representations such as visuo-spatial neglect can lead to anomalous beliefs (sometimes known as 'somatoparaphrenia'). This should be considered in cases of visual neglect and hemiplegia (Halligan *et al.*, 1995; Worthington & Beevers, 1996).

There are a number of interventions which can be explored for people with so-called low vision and other consequences of early-stage visual processing disorders, including light-filtering lenses for photophobia (Jackowski *et al.*, 1996) and patches for double vision (Politzer, 1996). Several of these are reviewed by Kerkhoff (2003). However, treatment outcome is variable and the value of in-patient programmes specifically designed to treat visual disorder has been questioned (Schlageter *et al.*, 1993). Visual stimulation, for example, can temporarily reduce visual field loss around the margins (Zihl & Von Cramon, 1979) but does not lead to sustainable benefit, any functional improvement arising spontaneously, which may be augmented with repetitive training (Poggel *et al.*, 2001), or from compensatory interventions such as prisms (Streff, 1996). If deficits persist beyond six months, then some form of intervention should be considered. Often a combination of measures will be required to treat a multitude of deficits (see case study by Ludlam, 1996).

Disorders of Primary Visual Processing

Loss of colour perception (achromatopsia)

Selective loss of the ability to see colours (achromatopsia) leaves a person seeing the world in black and white and shades of grey (Humphreys & Riddoch, 1987). The disorder is one of colour *perception* and not just recognition (e.g. associating red with a post box) or naming. Perceptual tests of colour include the Farnsworth–Munsell 100-hue test (Farnsworth, 1943), the Ishihara Test (Ishihara, 1982) and City University Colour Vision Test (Fletcher, 1998). However, these do not assess the patient's *knowledge* of colour, which requires a more extensive battery (see Davidoff, 1991).

Impaired depth perception

Impairments affecting all aspects of depth perception (both monocular and binocular) have long been reported in patients with bilateral occipital-parietal damage (Holmes & Horrax, 1919; Riddoch, 1935; Valkenberg, 1908). Such patients describe the world as if it is two-dimensional (Riddoch, 1917). The impairment usually occurs in combination with other perceptual deficits and can render the afflicted person clumsy and unable to coordinate behaviours such as reaching, throwing and judging distance.

Apperceptive Disorders

The neurologist Lissauer first distinguished visual recognition deficits resulting from damaged perceptual processes from those following damage to stored memories, giving these deficits the labels apperceptive and associative agnosia (Lissauer, 1890). This distinction, though conceptually debatable, still has some clinical utility. In both instances, however, basic sensory processing should be intact. Apperceptive agnosia takes many forms according to which aspect of visual processing is damaged.

Deficits of form perception

The edges of objects are perceived by grouping together elements on the basis of their similarity. This allows the boundaries of an object to be distinguished from the background and from other nearby or overlapping shapes. 'Form agnosia' is an impairment in identifying such boundaries between objects, or internal regions in an object (such as the eyes in a face) (Efron, 1968; Milner *et al.*, 1991). Visual form agnosia is associated with extrastriate occipital lesions (Heider, 2000). Patients with this condition are unable to identify or to copy line drawings of common objects or even simple geometric shapes. However, while the processing of size, orientation and shape may be particularly impaired, other abilities such as colour, brightness and movement discrimination may be preserved (Efron, 1968). Assessment should include discrimination between shapes (Efron, 1968), between figure and ground (see the initial subtest of the VOSP (Warrington & James, 1991) and tests of simple visual discriminations (such as differences in length, size etc. as in the Cortical Vision Screening test (James *et al.*, 2001) or the first four tasks in the BORB (Riddoch & Humphreys, 1993).

Integrative agnosia

Some authorities argue that there is a separate stage of processing which involves grouping together separate features of an object into a coherent shape. Deficits here result in the so-called 'integrative agnosia' (Humphreys *et al.*, 1992; Riddoch & Humphreys, 1987). A good clinical assessment of feature binding can be obtained with overlapping figures tasks (Riddoch & Humphreys, 1993) where the person has to group elements of different objects with others of the same object.

View normalisation

Following the derivation of shape, view normalisation is the next stage of perceptual processing, permitting a perception of object constancy despite differences in viewing conditions (e.g. usual and unusual views). Thus an upright chair, and same chair knocked over, will be perceived as being the same object despite the different patterns of retinal stimulation. Disruption to invariant object recognition typically follows right hemisphere damage (Warrington & Taylor, 1973) involving inability to match critical features across viewpoints (Warrington & James, 1986) or changes in the principal axis of the object (Humphreys & Riddoch, 1984).

Assessment of perceptual constancy using BORB (Riddoch & Humphreys, 1993) requires matching a conventional view of the object with its unusual view.

A rather different procedure is followed in VOSP (Warrington & James, 1991) where the patient is assessed on the amount of rotation from an extreme foreshortened view that is necessary to allow identification of the object (Figure 8.2).

Associative Agnosias

The ability to recognise features of the visual world is influenced by knowledge about objects, their uses and appearances. Deficits in visual recognition can be caused by disruption to these processes following a traumatic brain injury, principally as a result of posterior left hemisphere damage. Although there is no consensus on classifications for associative agnosias, we first discuss two kinds of impairment here which follow from the model in Figure 8.1: (a) problems in linking knowledge about visual form to knowledge about objects, and (b) deficits in accessing stored knowledge about object identification and function. Two other agnosic disorders, pure alexia and prosopagnosia, are also described though they lie outside the model represented in Figure 8.1.

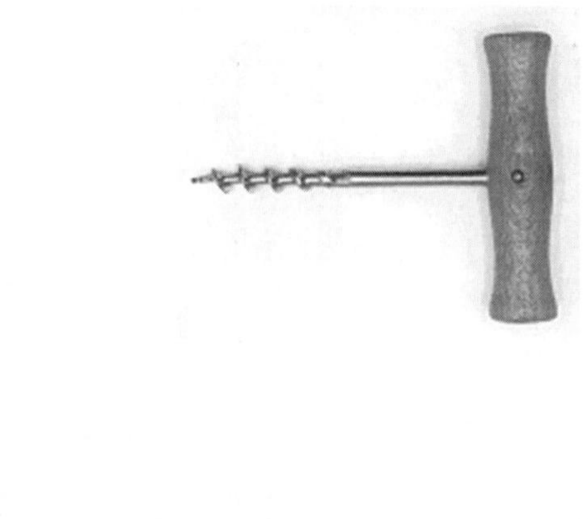

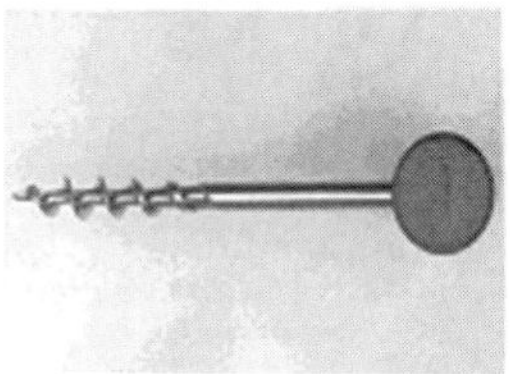

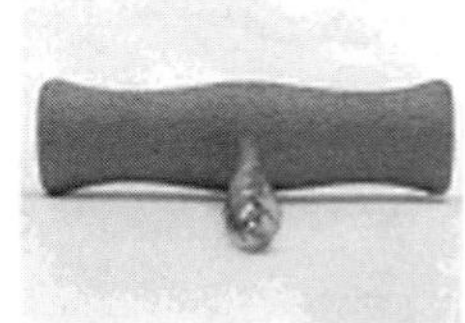

Figure 8.2 Example of Unusual views test

Disorders in linking knowledge about visual form to knowledge about objects

In severe cases traumatic brain injury can produce gross deficits of object recognition. Experience suggests that this is more common where there is evidence of bilateral posterior cerebral involvement. A person with such a disorder is unable to discriminate between objects or recognise real objects from non-objects (Hillis & Caramazza, 1991; Sheridan & Humphreys, 1993; Stewart *et al.*, 1992). A similar task is depicted in Figure 8.3, where the objective is to distinguish the real animal from the made-up animal. JB, who suffered a left parieto-occipital lesion as a result of a road traffic accident (Riddoch & Humphreys, 1987), could distinguish between real and non-real objects (object decision) but was impaired at judging from vision which two of three objects would be used together (e.g. hammer, nail, spanner). This problem with matching objects based on their functional associations was modality specific; when given the name of the objects JB carried out the same task with ease. Thus JB was impaired at accessing knowledge about object use from vision but was able to use knowledge about the appearance of objects in order to perform the object decision task. Riddoch and Humphreys proposed that this reflected a distinction between access to stored structural descriptions for objects and access to stored semantic information (specifying functional and associative knowledge).

Knowledge about object shape can be assessed using subtests from the VOSP (Warrington & James, 1991) and BORB (Riddoch & Humphreys, 1993). The

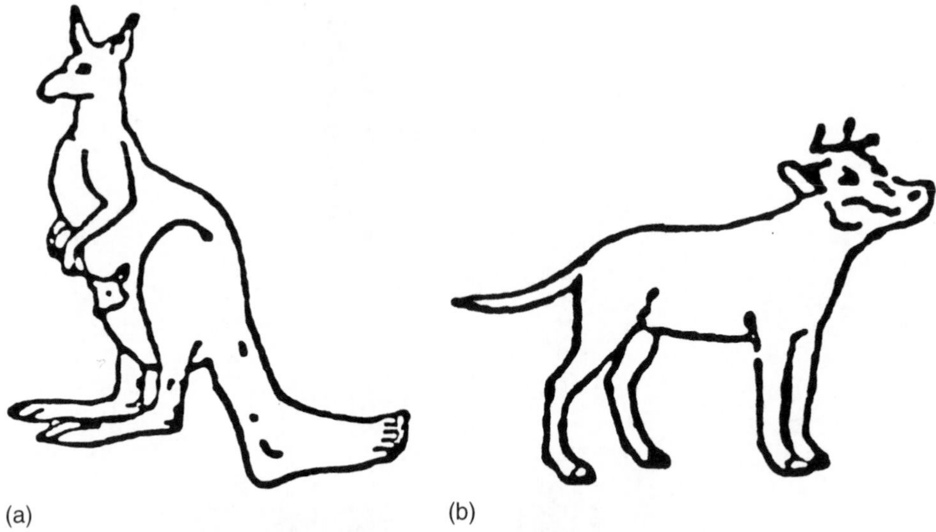

Figure 8.3 Examples of real vs. non-real discrimination stimuli

procedures used in the two batteries are rather different. In BORB patients are presented with either real or unreal pictures of animals or tools and simply have to decide whether that item could exist in real life or not. In VOSP an odd-man-out task is used. A silhouette of a real object is presented together with three silhouettes of non-objects. The task is to determine which silhouette depicts the real object. Artefacts are used as target items, and these are often rotated slightly in depth giving a rather distorted view of the object.

Deficits in accessing stored knowledge about object structure and function

In addition to failure to recognise objects because of a difficulty in mapping from structural descriptions to semantics, recognition problems can also be caused by a selective semantic deficit. In such patients recognition (and naming) problems may be expected even with verbal descriptions of the functional properties of objects, as well as when objects are presented visually. Nevertheless, using object decision tasks it can be shown that patients retain knowledge of object structure (Sheridan & Humphreys, 1993; Stewart *et al.*, 1992). Tests of object naming may also reveal poor recognition of objects. According to the model in Figure 8.1, name retrieval operates following access to semantic knowledge, indicating that access to some forms of semantic information is deemed necessary. The evidence that object naming can proceed non-semantically is weak (Hodges & Greene, 1998, though see Brennen *et al.*, 1996). Clinicians should also be aware that inability to name objects presented visually can occur despite preservation of naming with tactile object presentation, and the ability to mime object use. The basis for this so-called 'optic aphasia' is disputed, but its co-occurrence with associative agnosia is well documented. Cases caused by traumatic brain injury have been reported by Costlett and Saffran (1992), Wilson (1999) and Riddoch and Humphreys' (1987) case JB described above.

Pure alexia

Alexia is the inability to read despite normal comprehension and writing (alexia without agraphia). Individuals with pure alexia therefore cannot easily read their own handwriting, and may spell out difficult words in letter-by-letter fashion. Apperceptive deficits resulting from ventral stream dysfunction may contribute to the problem (Farah, 1990) but pure alexia is generally considered to be a form of associative agnosia, affecting verbal material in the visual modality. Many pure alexic patients also show object agnosia, though the two disorders are dissociable. Individuals have adequate visual perception of letters and words (i.e. no apperceptive deficit) but appear to have problems in recognising words from constituent letters (Patterson & Kay, 1982).

Prosopagnosia

Faces are a highly unusual class of visual stimuli, and the processing of facial information can break down selectively or in combination with other perceptual problems after traumatic brain injury. The term prosopagnosia to describe face-processing impairments was introduced by Bodamer in 1947 (Ellis & Florence, 1990, have translated the original paper). People with prosopagnosia can generally match faces from different views and discriminate between different faces, but have difficulty in recognising faces (Ellis, 1992). More recent conceptualisations (e.g. Bruce & Young, 1986) have distinguished between processing of visual and other features of the face, thereby suggesting a taxonomy for prosopagnosic impairments (e.g. McNeil & Warrington, 1993). Cases have also been reported involving loss of the ability to recognise a variety of animal species too, including birds, cows, sheep and horses. Right hemisphere damage appears to be sufficient to cause the disorder (Landis *et al.*, 1986), which Damasio *et al.* (1982) suggest arises from disruption to the ventral stream. Cognitive models of face processing have also proved heuristic in some of the more unusual misidentification syndromes that can accompany traumatic brain injury (Breen *et al.*, 2000). It is important for clinicians to recognise that poor recognition of once familiar faces after a head injury may not always be a sign of memory loss. For example, Burgess *et al.* (1996) reported a young man whose delusional misidentification of nursing staff after a head injury was confounded by face recognition problems.

Assessment of prosopagnosia has been influenced by cognitive models of face processing. The Cortical Vision Screening Test (James *et al.*, 2001) has a subtask sensitive to basic facial feature analysis. Memory for faces can be tested using Warrington's (1984) Recognition Memory Test, while the Facial Recognition Test (Benton *et al.*, 1983) is sensitive to perceptual constancy across different views. Familiar face recognition can be tested with photographs of famous faces and family members. Person identification requires comparison of face recognition with the ability to identify people from other sources of information such as their voice.

Disorders of Spatial Processing

There are a number of disorders of spatial analysis of which the clinician should be aware. Some are common though often occur in mild form, while others are comparatively rare but severely debilitating when they occur.

Motion perception

The selective impairment of motion perception (akinetopsia) is a rare disorder. It has been most comprehensively studied in a woman with severe bilateral damage to the middle temporal gyrus and the adjacent part of the occipital gyri together with subcortical damage affecting lateral occipital and occipito-parietal white matter (Zihl *et al.*, 1983). The critical areas of damage producing this devastating disability are unclear but the effects are apparent in all aspects of everyday life whether making a cup of tea, understanding facial expressions and speech, or crossing the road safely.

Orientation perception

Perception of orientation may also occur selectively, but is usually observed in combination with other apperceptive deficits, and is believed to result from disruption to the dorsal stream pathway which is involved in recognising object shape, and probably preparation for action (Milner & Goodale, 1995). Impaired perception of orientation is typically associated with damage to the right hemisphere (Umiltà *et al.*, 1974), and is commonly assessed using the line orientation test of Benton *et al.* (1978). The multiple-choice format of this test, however, means that many head-injured patients with impulsive, perseverative or problem-solving difficulties may perform poorly without a selective spatial-processing deficit.

Visual disorientation

The neurologist Gordon Holmes (1918) is credited with some of the earliest reports of visual disorientation after head injury. He recorded problems in visually localising the position and distance of objects in soldiers who had suffered gunshot wounds to posterior brain regions. This condition, reported in association with difficulties perceiving multiple items in a scene (simultanagnosia), and problems in visually guided action (optic ataxia), represents the cardinal features of so-called Balint's syndrome (De Renzi, 1996; Hecaen & De Ajuriaguerra, 1954). The conditions are dissociable, however, and the validity of the syndrome is dubious (Rizzo, 1993), though the defects are all caused by extensive destruction of parieto-occipital regions. Spatial localisation can be assessed by asking patients simply to count stimuli on a page (see VOSP). Omission of features when describing complex visual scenes may reveal simultanagnosia, though the disorder may also be apparent in reading difficulties (and needs to be distinguished from the unilateral omissions characteristic of visuo-spatial neglect – see below). Furthermore, Farah (1990) suggested that damage to the dorsal stream produces a simultanagnosia characterised by the piecemeal quality of perception of single object, in contrast to ventral simultanagnosia which typically causes problems in perception of multiple objects. Wilson (1999) describes a case of so-called dorsal simultanagnosia in a young woman following a severe traumatic brain injury sustained in a road traffic accident. As a result of extensive practice she was able to re-learn the names of everyday objects. However, the improvement was largely confined to treated stimuli and did not generalise to other objects, thus illustrating one of the major limitations with interventions based upon paired-associate learning, as opposed to training people on compensatory strategies. More successfully, Zihl (2000) reported a complex intensive training regime that enhanced visual fixation and localisation resulting in improved object recognition in everyday life.

Visuo-spatial neglect

Unilateral neglect may result from lesions to either right or left hemisphere of the brain, but is typically more severe and longer lasting following right-side lesions (usually in the parieto-temporal region). The disorder can occur in tactile and auditory modalities but is most readily diagnosed as a deficit of visual attention. In everyday life a person may only eat the food from one side of the plate, may bump into the side of doorways, miss out words on one side of text, or make errors when reading individual words.

Assessment of visual neglect requires investigation of the kinds of omissions patients tend to make. In this respect a robust distinction is found between a tendency to omit items to the left (or occasionally the right) side of space, versus a propensity to omit the left (occasionally the right) portions of stimuli across the visual field. Interestingly, there are a few reports of individuals with unilateral *left* hemisphere or bilateral lesions who neglect different sides of space according to the task (Cubelli *et al.*, 1991; Riddoch *et al.*, 1995b). The bilateral nature of lesion distribution after traumatic brain injury suggests that the presentation of visual neglect after head injury may present in complex form.

Particularly noteworthy in this context is the differentiation of perceptual neglect from motor neglect. The former is suggested by inability to attend to one side of space. Motor neglect, in contrast, occurs as either a total absence of movement or delayed inception, slowed execution and/or reduced amplitude of movement in one hemispace. Incidentally, the distinction usually made between the behavioural manifestation of a deficit as contralateral or ipsilateral to the lesions site is less helpful after traumatic brain injury, and the clinician is advised to report the phenomenon as they see it. Tasks sensitive to both kinds of neglect can be found in the Behavioural Inattention Test (Wilson *et al.*, 1987). Behavioural observation of neglect in everyday life can also be useful and semi-structured scales have been devised for this purpose (Azouvi *et al.*, 1996; Zoccolotti & Judica, 1991).

Standard assessment of visual fields may not reliably distinguish between visual neglect and visual field loss (especially homonymous hemianopia). The Balloons Test (Edgeworth *et al.*, 1998) is a visual search task which attempts to do this by contrasting the subject's ability to find a target defined in terms of the *presence* and *absence* of a feature. Edgeworth and Robertson argue that performance should not differ on these two search tasks if the patient has a field loss –

similar numbers of targets should be missed both in the feature-present and feature-absent searches. However, a patient with unilateral neglect may be expected to perform more poorly on the feature-absent task since it is a more attentionally demanding search task.

The evidence base for treatment of perceptuo-spatial disorders is almost exclusively based on visual neglect (Worthington, 1995a). There is now a burgeoning literature on rehabilitation strategies for visual neglect (Robertson & Halligan, 1999). Techniques have focused on providing visual cues, the stimulation of the neglected side of space (hemispheric activation) and active or passive stimulation of a limb in the neglected hemispace (so-called limb activation) (see review by Robertson & Halligan, 1999). There is a theoretical argument for using right-sided cueing to alleviate left neglect (Delis *et al.*, 1985; Halligan & Marshall, 1994) based on a distinction between left hemisphere focal attention and right hemisphere global attention systems (Humphreys & Riddoch, 1994; Worthington & Young, 1996). More recently, Wilson and Manly (2003) reported an improvement in self-care in a man with visual neglect 2½ years after a traumatic brain injury, using an auditory cue in a procedure known as sustained attention training.

Disorders of Constructional–Motor Skills

Integration of perceptual and spatial information is crucial to being able to carry out effective visually-guided action. The disorders of visual perception and spatial analysis reviewed above are often sufficient to compromise this process. In addition, traumatic brain injury frequently involves damage to frontal brain regions which can result in disorders of perceptually based action, even in the absence of pure perceptual deficits.

Optic ataxia

Optic ataxia is an unusual but striking disorder resulting in an impaired ability to generate reaching and grasping movements to objects. This may affect one hand or both hands. Lesions restricted to one hemisphere are sufficient to cause optic ataxia, in which cases patients misreach to objects located in the visual field contralateral to their lesion (Ratcliff & Davies-Jones, 1972). Misreaching (which is worse under conditions of no visual feedback) is sometimes confounded by poor hand and finger posturing. The 'reach' component of optic ataxia may be assessed by asking the patient to reach to pre-set locations on the table top on both left and right sides and measuring the degree and direction of inaccuracy. To assess the grasp component patients should be asked to reach for and to grasp an object held by the examiner – a small object will require greater coordination by the patient than a larger one. Assessment of performance in both central and peripheral vision should be made. Non-clinical studies have shown that the brain's ability to programme movements to improve accuracy of reaching and grasping can be influenced by instructions (Fisk & Goodale, 1989). This has obvious implications for therapy but the potential has not been systematically investigated.

Constructional apraxia

Constructional apraxia is a problem in the spatial aspects of a task (such as drawing, or constructing or arranging blocks and objects) in the absence of limb apraxia (Kleist, 1912). It is usually associated with parietal lobe damage (De Renzi, 1982), that is, impairments of the dorsal visual stream. Some authors have argued that the nature of the constructional deficit will differ according to whether the lesion is posterior (parieto-occipital), where the deficit seems to involve the analysis of spatial relations, or anterior (frontal), where the disorder seems to reflect a deficit in movement planning. Problems with construction may be apparent in copying tasks in two dimensions (e.g. the Rey Complex Figure), or on three-dimensional constructional tasks such as the Block Design subtest of the WAIS-III (Wechsler, 1991). Patients with many different deficits (e.g. planning, attention, self-monitoring) have problems with these tasks, however, and it may be necessary to explore a diagnosis of constructional apraxia further (see Benton *et al.*, 1978).

Apraxia

Skilled voluntary actions are performed by the execution of engrams or 'memories' of motor commands and their accompanying proprioceptive sensations. These are normally activated automatically in response to current situational and environmental cues. However, intentional control is necessary to perform actions to instruction or in circumstances when behaviour must be modified due to novel demands. Impairment in the execution of skilled voluntary movements which could not be accounted for by paralysis was first termed 'apraxia' by Steinthal (1871). The definition was later extended to state that limb apraxia is a disorder of skilled movement not caused by elementary motor deficits such as weakness, akinesia, chorea, ataxia, tremor or motor deficits (Geschwind, 1975).

Three main types of dyspraxia have been described: ideational dyspraxia, ideomotor dyspraxia and limb-kinetic dyspraxia, loosely based on distinctions made between conceptual and production action systems (Roy & Square, 1985). The conceptual system contains knowledge of object use and function, and relates to knowledge about meaningful and familiar gestures. The production system includes information about action motor programmes and their instantiation into skilled motor performance (see Figure 8.4).

Ideational dyspraxia

Ideational dyspraxia is thought to represent a disorder of the conceptual system and is characterised by impaired knowledge of the meaning or purpose of actions. A person so afflicted will use objects inappropriately (e.g. combing their hair with a pen) or make errors when a sequence of movements is necessary (e.g. the component steps in making a cup of tea) where steps may be omitted, or implemented in the incorrect order (De Renzi & Luchelli, 1988; Ochipa *et al.*, 1989). In a neuropsychological model of limb praxis developed by Rothi and colleagues (see Rothi & Heilman, 1997), ideational dyspraxia results from damage to action semantics (including knowledge of the functions of tools and objects), resulting in a deficit in

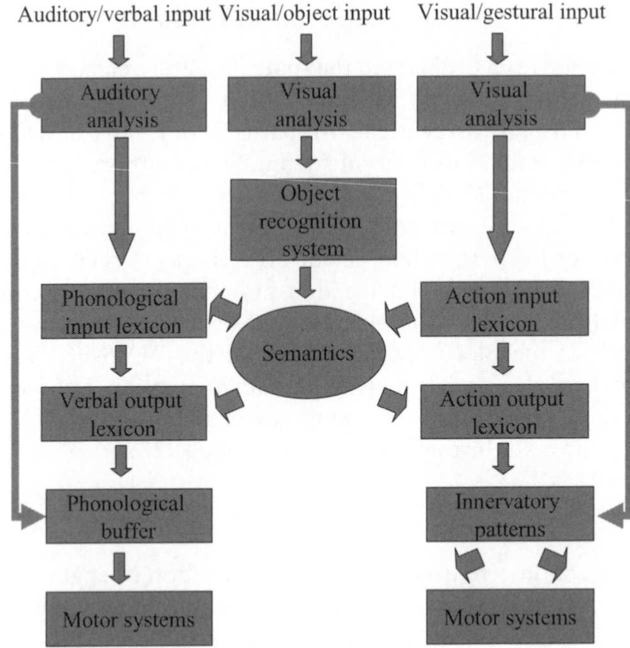

Figure 8.4 An information processing model of apraxia

knowing 'how' to use tools (Buxbaum *et al.*, 2000). Liepmann (1920) proposed that ideational apraxia resulted from lesions of the left parieto-occipital junction, but a number of cases have been reported with frontal lobe damage (De Renzi & Luchelli, 1988). Impairments of complex action characteristic of ideational apraxia can occur after closed head injury (e.g. Buxbaum *et al.*, 1995; Schwartz *et al.*, 1998), but appear to be less purely perceptually based than similar problems after unilateral brain damage, and may be consequent upon decrements in general-purpose information-processing resources (Buxbaum *et al.*, 1998).

Ideomotor apraxia

In ideomotor dyspraxia stored knowledge about the meaning of actions is thought to be preserved, but there is an inability to execute this knowledge appropriately so that the shape, order and spatial features of the movement are distorted. Generally, the patients perform well in naturalistic environments but demonstrate the impairment when asked to pantomime gestures and especially when asked to imitate gestures performed by an examiner. Recent evidence suggests that the long-term prognosis for ideomotor apraxia is poorer in association with frontal brain lesions than posterior lesions (Basso *et al.*, 2000). Some patients with frontal lobe lesions may have difficulty in performing action sequences (such as making a cup of tea) whilst having intact knowledge and recognition of the individual objects used in the task. Such a deficit is known as action disorganisation syndrome (see Humphreys

& Forde, 1998; Schwartz *et al.*, 1991). Schwartz and Buxbaum (1997) have argued that disruption to everyday tasks may arise as a consequence of a double impairment in the underlying procedural substrates for action (or action schemas) and in executive control processes that might otherwise compensate for such difficulties. These authors speculated that such a disorder is most likely to occur in association with diffuse pathology like dementia or traumatic brain injury. The Naturalistic Action test (Schwartz *et al.*, 2002) is a structured investigative tool for action disorganisation. Rehabilitation interventions for action disorganisation have been suggested by Worthington (2003).

Limb-kinetic dyspraxia

Like ideomotor apraxia, limb-kinetic dyspraxia is thought to represent disorders of the production system (Rothi & Heilman, 1997). Limb-kinetic dyspraxia is thought to represent a disturbance of innervatory patterns. Blasi *et al.* (1999) describe the characteristic features of limb-kinetic apraxia as: intact knowledge of tool function and use; intact gesture recognition; the deficit is consistent whatever task the patient is asked to perform (i.e. imitating gestures, gesture to verbal command, demonstrating object use both with and without objects) and interferes with daily activities; errors are due to clumsiness and slowness of movement. In the case of unilateral lesions, the impairment is shown contralateral to the lesion site. Movement difficulty is more marked distally than proximally.

Assessment of apraxia

Apraxia is a heterogeneous disorder. The taxonomy presented above is not without its problems, and clinical assessments remain crude (Tate & McDonald, 1995). A number of different tests for apraxia have been described in the literature:

1 gestural abilities on verbal command;
2 gesture imitation;
3 miming; and
4 action sequences.

Imitating gestures may be assessed by the Imitating Gestures Test (De Renzi *et al.*, 1980). This test requires patients to perform 24 arm–hand movements. Each item is classified according to three dimensions: (i) finger movement versus whole hand–arm movement; (ii) holding a position versus carrying out a motor sequence; and (iii) symbolic versus meaningless gestures.

Rehabilitation of Spatio-motor and Perceptual Disorders

Effective management of perceptual and spatio-motor disorders requires first and foremost generic clinical skills to respond to the potential psychological effects that can be associated with any disabling cognitive disorder (including a need for education and emotional support). If nothing else, this can help alleviate some of the distress associated with perceptual disorder. However, how much better it would be if we could intervene to improve perceptual functioning or at least ameliorate the consequences of dysfunction.

Most rehabilitation studies for perceptual disorders have been undertaken with people who have suffered strokes. Their relevance for the treatment of traumatic brain injury is limited by the unilateral nature of brain injury after stroke, and the posterior localisation of the lesion in many of the cases reported. A second limitation, given the conceptual basis for understanding perceptual disorder expounded in the present chapter, is that intervention studies are frequently conducted without recourse to any theoretical analysis. Treatment is usually undertaken on an empirical basis, with training methods bearing an intuitive rather than theoretically plausible relation to the underlying deficit, which itself is typically under-specified (e.g. Hawkins & Gadsby, 1991). Often no benefit of treatment is observed (Edmans & Lincoln, 1991), though such studies rarely make it into print. Even when some improvement is noted it is difficult to identify the mechanism responsible. Thus Young *et al.* (1983) described a programme in which participants with neglect or scanning problems (diagnosed from a solitary cancellation task) received training in cancellation, visual scanning or block design. Those receiving more training did better and made modest improvements on some paper-and-pencil tasks and reading. Remarkably, the treatment was given only two months after brain injury. The authors noted, with belated hindsight and understatement, 'whether or not these [really quite modest] treatment effects represent a real increase in performance which would otherwise not have occurred by the time the maximum recovery period was over, remains a question' (Young *et al.*, 1983, p.211). Gordon *et al.* (1985) reported sustainable gains from a more comprehensive perceptual retraining programme but this was also an empirical rather than theoretically motivated trial, with poor characterisation of the participants beyond the presence of a right hemisphere lesion and left visual neglect.

Over a decade ago, Humphreys and Riddoch (1994) stated 'there have been remarkably few cognitive neuropsychological studies of visual rehabilitation, and those that have been carried out have, to date, shown little success'. In our view the absence of an explicit theoretical framework has impeded the progress of rehabilitation for perceptual deficits. Even when intervention is unsuccessful, a conceptual analysis can offer insights into the therapeutic process. For example, Riddoch and Humphreys (1992) reported a head-injured man who suffered bilateral occipital and right frontal damage in the context of pre-existing temporal lobe epilepsy. He had severe difficulties in recognising visually presented objects (especially animate objects), in drawing them from memory and describing their visual attributes. Although he was able to learn visually based definitions (e.g. that a male lion has a furry mane around his head), this did not help him recognise objects visually. It appeared that such verbal knowledge did not translate into improved visual representations of objects. It was hypothesised that his degraded visual knowledge was activated automatically (and frequently inaccurately) when he saw an object and remained unaffected by his improved verbal knowledge of object appearance.

Despite the benefits of designing rehabilitation programmes around well-formulated theories of the component stages of cognitive abilities, many clinicians have been slow to convert. The reasons for this are numerous, including time constraints on assessment, limited availability of materials and inaccessibility of much of the literature. It has been argued that simply observing a patient's functional behaviour may be sufficient to point the way to appropriate rehabilitation but trial-and-error approaches are never the most efficient form of intervention and rarely enrich an understanding of a problem.

Another difficulty is that cognitive models may be under-specified in some areas (Caramazza & Hillis, 1993). There have been attempts to tailor assessment packages so that the time spent evaluating performance is reduced but in some circumstances this may not prove possible. Ongoing evaluation of therapy is also important, since, with almost any condition, some degree of spontaneous recovery occurs and it is necessary to distinguish the effects of therapy from the effects of natural recovery. We report below the case of a young man who suffered a severe head injury after being hit by a dust cart when he was aged eight years. MGM (Francis *et al.*, 2001) had severe visual perceptual difficulties (apperceptive agnosia), aspects of associative visual agnosia, and an impaired verbal memory. In his case, detailed and prolonged assessment was necessary to establish levels of impairment in a number of different cognitive areas. The outcome of a successful therapy programme for MGM depended on identification of the level of visual processing deficit (given his visual agnosia), awareness of his memorial ability, and knowledge of the processes underlying word recognition.

Case 8.1: Agnosic alexia

MGM suffered a severe traumatic brain injury in a road accident at the age of eight years which resulted in a severe visual agnosia and impaired visual and verbal memory. Prior to his head injury, MGM had had a normal development, and was able to read and write at a level consistent with his age. Following the injury, MGM was educated at special needs schools for 11 years. He was referred for a detailed cognitive assessment when aged 19. His particular wish was to be able to learn to read, although all prior attempts (both 'look and say' and letter sounding) had been marked with failure. At the time of referral, MGM was able to recognise only four letters. On assessment it was shown that he had some problems in perceiving letters (he made some errors when asked to match a target letter with an identical letter in an array of distractor letters; performance became more impaired when the target letter differed from its match and the distractor letters in terms of font). He also had an impaired visual memory, so that while he was reasonably good at copying visually presented letters, his performance deteriorated if the target was removed and he had to wait 10 seconds prior to drawing the shape from memory. Therapy focused on both MGM's visuo-perceptual and memory impairments. The numbers of items used in a test session were small, and further letters were introduced once

Continued

these items had been learned. Therapeutic tasks stressed letter shape (in particular, targeting the most salient visual feature of the letter (for instance, lower case 'b' was described as 'having a right big bottom'!)). Alliteration (big bottom) or rhyme was also used to facilitate verbal memory. The treatment was effective, and after five months MGM averaged between 20 and 23 of 26 letters correct per therapy session. Importantly, MGM was able to generalise from letter recognition to word reading (which was impossible prior to therapy); he was able to read 80 per cent of three-letter words (even though there had been no attempt to address word reading during therapy). Reading was accomplished by MGM assigning phonemes to the letters he had identified and thus sounded out the target word. Francis *et al.* (2001) argue that the cognitive neuropsychological approach was the significant factor underlying MGM's achievement. The detailed prior assessment enabled the locus of MGM's difficulties to be identified, and treatment appropriately targeted. He had been subject to less focused approaches for the prior 11 years without success.

Rehabilitation of a case of visuo-spatial neglect

Probably the most emphatic example of how cognitive approaches to assessment can lead to the development of effective intervention is the rehabilitation of visual neglect (see Robertson & Halligan, 1999). As described above, visuo-spatial neglect is usually defined as a failure to attend to contralesional stimuli. This defect is often defined in behavioural terms (a person may fail to respond to visual, auditory and/or tactile stimuli). The primary goal of assessment is therefore to identify the particular circumstances where neglect is shown (for example, is it primarily perceptual or motor in nature? Does it relate to a particular modality of stimulus presentation?). Visuo-spatial neglect is commonly regarded as a disorder of attention, since cueing to the affected side can result in a dramatic improvement in performance (Halligan *et al.*, 1991; Riddoch & Humphreys, 1983). The effects of cueing may be optimised if the modality of the cue and the modality of the task are congruent. Thus reading responds well to visual cues (Riddoch *et al.*, 1995a; Worthington, 1996) while a motor cue is more effective than a visual cue in written spelling (Riddoch *et al.*, 1995a). Cueing has also been shown to be more effective when self-initiated (e.g. the patient making a small movement with the contralesional limb) than if it is passive (e.g. the therapist moving the contralesional limb) (see Robertson & North, 1992, 1993). However, while cueing may significantly reduce neglect, the effects are often short-term, with little effect on everyday life (Halligan *et al.*, 1992; Seron *et al.*, 1989). Robertson and colleagues have attempted to address this problem by attempting to encourage the orientation of attention to contralesional space (by the use of a visual cue such as the patient's contralesional arm) together with attempts to increase generalised arousal (by training the patient to place the limb immediately adjacent to the area of current activity – such as the left side of a book when reading, placing the limb in the bowl when washing).

Treatment effects in cases of visuo-spatial neglect tend to be restricted to tasks similar to those used during training with no generalisation to other tasks, and the effects of training tend to dissipate rapidly with time. One of the factors underlying poor carry-over may be the failure to address the non-lateralised attentional deficit (i.e., lowered levels of arousal) which may result from right hemisphere lesions. Robertson (1994) has argued that cueing should be combined with strategies directed at increasing general arousal levels and has demonstrated significant effects of doing so in a number of different studies (Robertson *et al.*, 1995; Robertson & Cashman, 1991; Robertson *et al.*, 1997; Robertson & North, 1993).

Robertson *et al.* (1992) describe severe visuo-spatial neglect in a man who sustained a traumatic brain injury falling down stairs. His baseline performance was assessed on a number of different activities (including letter cancellation and reading) over a period of time. Performance was stable, indicating that spontaneous recovery had probably reached a plateau. Robertson *et al.* (1992) trained the patient to use his left arm as a visual cue. In order to enhance general arousal, the patient was encouraged to position the arm (using the right hand) so that it was within view during all his daily activities. In order to encourage their patient to learn this strategy, he was instructed by a psychologist for an hour a day for 11 days; in addition, nursing staff and occupational therapists reinforced this strategy when he was involved in activities on the ward or in therapy sessions. A clear improvement in the baseline measures was observed. Robertson (1994) argues that a learning strategy of this sort will be effective when generalised arousal or vigilance is low.

Conclusion

Perceptual and spatial disorders can cause severe disability after traumatic brain injury. A selective visual perceptual disorder such as a loss of colour vision may substantially affect the quality of life (much of our enjoyment of food is associated with the richness and variety of its colours). Spatial disorders have the potential to render even simple tasks difficult, such as walking through doorways (Tromp *et al.*, 1995), and may completely exclude people from more complex activities like driving (Brouwer & Withaar, 1997). The diversity and complexity of visual perceptual and spatial disorders means that accurate identification of problems is difficult, even for clinicians with experience of brain injury. Unilateral lesions are often sufficient to cause such disorders, and a history of intracranial haemorrhage or secondary haematoma after traumatic brain injury should alert the clinician to this possibility. The problems are often confounded, however, by generalised cognitive dysfunction, co-existing arousal, motivational and affective problems, additional motor impairments and (possibly) behavioural difficulties. Each of these in turn may be exacerbated by impaired perception. These factors make the accurate identification of perceptuo-spatial disorders both an important and a necessary prerequisite to a comprehensive rehabilitation programme. Patterns of perceptual disturbance after brain injury have been influential in the development of conceptual models of perceptuo-spatial processing. Clinicians should be able to use these models to guide task selection, or in post-hoc fashion to interpret test results, with the selection of some tests being influenced by the interpretation of the results of others previously administered. Detailed neuropsychological assessment should be augmented by observation of performance on everyday tasks as much as possible. The aim of treatment, after all, is reduction of functional disability, not improved test scores.

Therapy should be designed with evaluation in mind, and clinicians should be familiar with basic methods of structuring interventions for individual cases. An accessible introduction to single-case designs for therapists was provided by Worthington (1995b). The limitations of any specific treatment lead most commentators to recommend a hybrid approach to rehabilitation, employing both restorative and compensatory methods (Anderson, 2002). Furthermore, the importance of affective as well as cognitive factors in determining treatment efficacy should not be overlooked. Therapists will doubtless have their own examples, but Gianutsos and Matheson (1987) reported one head-injured man with hemiparesis and homonymous hemianopia, who turned his head right around to view any approaching female, oblivious to the potential dangers awaiting him as he continued walking. However, as demonstrated in the case of MGM, a cognitive approach to rehabilitation is not incompatible with the need facing most clinicians to take into account complex co-existing deficits.

Recommended Reading

Kerkhoff, G. (2000). Neurovisual rehabilitation: Recent developments and future directions. *Journal of Neurology, Neurosurgery and Psychiatry*, *68*, 691–706.

A useful summary of currently available techniques for improving visual function. Focuses predominantly on disorders of early stage visual processing.

Robertson, I.H. & Halligan, P.W. (1999). *Spatial neglect: A clinical handbook for diagnosis and treatment*. Hove: Psychology Press.

A comprehensive guide for practitioners to understanding and assessing manifestations of visuo-spatial neglect. Also includes a wide range of potential treatment techniques. A little dated but yet to be surpassed.

Wilson, B.A. (1999). *Case studies in neuropsychological rehabilitation*. New York: Oxford University Press, 384pp.

A very accessible set of case studies which includes four examples of rehabilitation of visuo-spatial deficits. Provides useful examples of the relationships between pathology, cognitive testing and everyday disabilities.

Zihl J. (2000). *Rehabilitation of visual disorders after brain injury*. Hove: Psychology Press.

A good reference book on a wide range of visual and perceptual disorders. Although technical in places, there are many good examples of compensatory, restoration and substitution approaches to rehabilitation.

References

Anderson, S.W. (2002). Visuoperceptual impairments. In P.J. Eslinger (Ed.) *Neuropsychological interventions* (pp.163–181). New York: The Guilford Press.

Azouvi, P., Marchal, F., Samuel, C., Morin, L., Renard, C., Louis-Dreyfus, A., *et al.* (1996). Functional consequences and awareness of unilateral neglect: Study of an evaluation scale. *Neuropsychological Rehabilitation*, 6, 133–150.

Basso, A., Burgio, F., Paulin, M. & Prandoni, P. (2000). Long-term follow up of ideomotor apraxia. *Neuropsychological Rehabilitation*, 10, 1–13.

Beaumont, G. & Davidoff, J. (1992). Assessment of visuo-perceptual dysfunction. In J.R. Crawford, D.M. Parker & W.W. McKinlay (Eds.) *A handbook of neuropsychological assessment* (pp.115–140). Hove: Lawrence Erlbaum.

Benton, A.L., Sivan, A.B., Hamsher, K. de S., Varney, N.R. & Spreen, O. (1983). *Contributions to neuropsychological assessment: A clinical manual*. New York: Oxford University Press.

Benton, A.L., Varney, N.R. & Hamsher, K.D. (1978). Visuospatial judgement: A clinical test. *Archives of Neurology*, *35*, 364–367.

Blasi, V., Labruna, L., Soricelli, A. & Carlomagno, S. (1999). Limb-kinetic dyspraxia: A neuropsychological description. *Neurocase*, *5*, 201–211.

Breen, N., Caine, D. & Coltheart, M. (2000). Models of face recognition and delusional misidentification: A critical review. *Cognitive Neuropsychology*, *17*(1/2), 55–71.

Brennen, T., Danielle, D., Fluchaire, I. & Pellat, J. (1996). Naming faces and objects without comprehension. *Cognitive Neuropsychology*, *15*, 93–110.

Brouwer, W.H. & Withaar, F.K. (1997). Fitness to drive after traumatic brain injury. *Neuropsychological Rehabilitation*, *7*(3), 177–193.

Bruce, V. & Young, A. (1986). Understanding face recognition. *British Journal of Psychology*, *77*, 305–327.

Burgess, P.W., Baxter, D., Rose, M. & Alderman, N. (1996). Delusional paramnesic misidentification. In P.W. Halligan & J.C. Marshall (Eds.) *Method in madness: Case studies in cognitive neuropsychiatry* (pp.51–78). Hove: Psychology Press.

Buxbaum, L.J., Schwartz, M.F., Coslett, H.B. & Carew, T.G. (1995). Naturalistic action and praxis in callosal apraxia. *Neurocase*, *1*, 3–17.

Buxbaum, L.J., Schwartz, M.F. & Montgomery, M.W. (1998). Ideational apraxia and naturalistic action. *Cognitive Neuropsychology*, *15*, 617–643.

Buxbaum, L.J., Veramonti, T. & Schwartz, M.F. (2000). Function and manipulation of tool knowledge in apraxia: Knowing 'What for' but not 'How'. *Neurocase*, 6, 83–97.

Caramazza, A. & Hillis, A. (1993). For a theory of remediation of cognitive deficits. *Neuropsychological Rehabilitation*, *3*, 217–234.

Costlett, H.B. & Saffran, S. (1992). Disorders of higher visual processing: Theoretical and clinical perspectives. In D.I. Margolin (Ed.) Cognitive neuropsychology in clinical practice (pp.353–404). New York: Oxford University Press.

Cubelli, R., Nichelli, P., Bonito, V., De Tanti, A. & Inzaghi, M.G. (1991). Different patterns of dissociation in unilateral neglect. *Brain and Cognition*, *15*, 139–159.

Damasio, A.R., Damasio, H. & Van Hoesen, G.W. (1982). Prosopagnosia: Anatomic basis and behavioural mechanisms. *Neurology*, 32, 331–341.

Davidoff, J. (1991). *Cognition through colour*. Cambridge, MA: MIT Press.

Delis, D.C., Robertson, L.C. & Balliet, R. (1985). The breakdown and rehabilitation of visuo-spatial dysfunction in brain-injured patients. *International Journal of Rehabilitation Medicine*, *5*, 132–138.

De Renzi, E. (1982). *Disorders of space exploration and cognition*. Chichester: Wiley.

De Renzi, E. (1996). Balint-Holmes' syndrome. In C. Code, C-W. Wallesch, Y. Joanette & A.R. Lecours (Eds.) *Classic cases in neuropsychology* (pp.123–143). Hove: Psychology Press.

De Renzi, E. & Luchelli, F. (1988). Ideational apraxia. *Brain*, *111*, 1173–1185.

De Renzi, E., Motti, F. & Nichelli, P. (1980). Imitating gestures: A quantitative approach to ideomotor apraxia. *Archives of Neurology*, *37*, 6–10.

Edgeworth, J.A., Robertson, I.H. & McMillan, T.M. (1998). *The Balloons Test.* Bury St. Edmunds, UK: Thames Valley Test Company.

Edmans, J.A. & Lincoln, N.B. (1991). Treatment of visual perceptual deficits after stroke: Single case studies on four patients with right hemiplegia. *British Journal of Occupational Therapy*, *54*, 139–144.

Efron, R. (1968). What is perception? *Boston Studies in Philosophy of Science*, *4*, 137–173.

Ellis, H.D. (1992). Assessment of deficits in facial processing. In J.R. Crawford, D.M. Parker & W.W. McKinlay (Eds.) *A handbook of neuropsychological assessment* (pp.141–150). Hove: Lawrence Erlbaum.

Ellis, H.D. & Florence, M. (1990). Bodamer's (1947) paper on prosopagnosia. *Cognitive Neuropsychology*, *7*, 81–105.

Farah, M.J. (1990). *Visual agnosia.* Cambridge, MA: MIT Press.

Farnsworth, D. (1943). Farnsworth–Munsel 100-hue and dichotomous test for colour vision. *Journal of the Optical Society of America*, *33*, 568–578.

Fisk, J.D. & Goodale, M.A. (1989). The effects of instructions to subjects on the programming of visually directed reaching movements. *Journal of Motor Behaviour*, *21*, 5–19.

Fletcher, R. (1998). *The City University Colour Vision Test.* Windsor: Keeler.

Francis, D.R., Riddoch, M.J. & Humphreys, G.W. (2001). Treating agnosic alexia complicated by additional impairments. *Neuropsychological Rehabilitation*, *11*, 113–145.

Geschwind, N. (1975). The apraxias. *American Scientist*, *63*, 188–195.

Gianutsos, R. & Matheson, P. (1987). The rehabilitation of perceptual disorders attributable to brain injury. In M.J. Meier, A.L. Benton & L. Diller (Eds.) *Neuropsychological rehabilitation* (pp.202–241). Edinburgh: Churchill Livingstone.

Gordon, W.A., Hibbard, M.R., Egelko, S., Diller, L., Shaver, M.S., Lieberman, A., *et al.* (1985). Perceptual remediation in patients with right brain damage: A comprehensive program. *Archives of Physical Medicine and Rehabilitation*, *66*, 353–359.

Halligan, P.W., Donegan, C.A. & Marshall, J.C. (1992). When is a cue not a cue? On the intractability of visuospatial neglect. *Neuropsychological Rehabilitation*, *4*, 283–293.

Halligan, P.W., Manning, L. & Marshall, J.C. (1991). Hemispheric activation vs spatiomotor cueing in visual neglect: A case study. *Neuropsychologia*, *29*, 165–176.

Halligan, P.W. & Marshall, J.C. (1994). Right sided cueing can ameliorate visual neglect. *Neuropsychological Rehabilitation*, *4*, 63–73.

Halligan, P.W., Marshall, J.C. & Wade, D.T. (1995). Unilateral somatoparaphrenia after right hemisphere stroke: A case description. *Cortex*, *31*, 173–182.

Halligan, P.W. & Wade, D.T. (Eds.) (2005). *Effectiveness of rehabilitation for cognitive deficits.* New York: Oxford University Press.

Hawkins, S. & Gadsby, M. (1991). Perceptual-motor deficit: A major learning difficulty. *British Journal of Occupational Therapy*, *54*, 145–149.

Hecaen, H. & De Ajuriaguerra, J. (1954). Balint's syndrome (psychic paralysis of visual fixation) and its minor forms. *Brain*, *77*, 373–400.

Heider, B. (2000). Visual form agnosia: Neural mechanisms and anatomical foundations. *Neurocase*, *6*, 1–12.

Hillis, A. & Caramazza, A. (1991). Category-specific naming and comprehension impairment: A double dissociation. *Brain*, *114*, 2081–2094.

Hodges, J.R. & Greene, J.D.W. (1998). Knowing about people and naming them: Can Alzheimer's disease patients do one without the other? *Quarterly Journal of Experimental Psychology*, *51A*, 121–134.

Holmes, G. (1918). Disturbances of visual orientation. *British Journal of Ophthalmology*, *2*, 449–468, 506–516.

Holmes, G. & Horrax, G. (1919). Disturbances of spatial orientation and visual attention with a loss of stereoscopic vision. *Archives of Neurology and Psychiatry*, *1*, 385–407.

Humphreys, G.W. & Forde, E.M.E. (1998). Disordered action schema and action disorganisation syndrome. *Cognitive Neuropsychology*, *15*, 771–811.

Humphreys, G.W. & Riddoch, M.J. (1984). Routes to object constancy: Implications from neurological impairments of object constancy. *Quarterly Journal of Experimental Psychology*, *36A*, 385–415.

Humphreys, G.W. & Riddoch, M.J. (1987). *To see but not to see: A case of visual agnosia.* London: Lawrence Erlbaum.

Humphreys, G.W. & Riddoch, M.J. (1994). Attention to within-object and between-object spatial representations: Multiple sites for visual selection. *Cognitive Neuropsychology*, *11*, 207–241.

Humphreys, G.W., Riddoch, M.J., Quinlan, P.T., Donnelly, N. & Price, C.A. (1992). Parallel pattern processing and visual agnosia. *Canadian Journal of Psychology*, *46*, 377–416.

Ishihara, S. (1982). *The series of plates designed as a test for colour blindness.* Tokyo: Kanehara.

Jackowski, M.M., Sturr, J.F., Taub, H.A. & Turk, M.A. (1996). Photophobia in patients with traumatic brain injury: Uses of light-filtering lenses to enhance contrast sensitivity and reading rate. *Neurorehabilitation*, 6, 193–201.

James, M., Plant, G.T. & Warrington, E.K. (2001). *Cortical Vision Screening Test.* Bury St Edmunds: Thames Valley Test Company.

Kerkhoff, G. (2003). Recovery and treatment of sensory perceptual disorders. In P.W. Halligan, U. Kischka & J.C. Wade (Eds.) *Handbook of clinical neuropsychology* (pp.125–146). New York, Oxford University Press.

Kleist, K. (1912). Der gand und der gegenwärtige stand der apraxie-forschung. *Ergebnisse der Neurologie und Psychiatrie*, *1*, 342–452.

Kolmel, H.W. (1993). Visual illusions and hallucinations. In C. Kennard (Ed.) *Bailliere's clinical neurology* (pp.2, 243–264). London: Bailliere Tindall.

Landis, T., Cummings, J.G., Christen, L., Bogen, J.E. & Imhof, H.G. (1986). Are unilateral right posterior cerebral lesions sufficient to cause prosopagnosia? Clinical and radiological findings in six patients. *Cortex*, *22*, 243–252.

Lezak, M.D. (1995). *Neuropsychological assessment* (3rd edn). New York: Oxford University Press, 1026pp.

Liepmann, H. (1920). Apraxie. *Ergebnisse der Gesamten Medizin*, *1*, 516–543.

Lissauer, H. (1890). Ein fall von seelenblindheit nebst einem beitrage zur theorie derselben. *Archiv für Psychiatrie und Nervenkrankheiten*, *21*, 222–270.

Ludlam, W.M. (1996). Rehabilitation of traumatic brain injury associated with visual dysfunction. *Neurorehabilitation*, 6, 183–192.

Marr, D. (1982). *Vision.* San Francisco: W.H. Freeman.

Mattson, A.J., Levin, H.S. & Breitmeyer, B.G. (1994). Visual information processing after severe closed head injury: effects of forward and backward masking. *Journal of Neurology, Neurosurgery and Psychiatry*, *57*, 818–824.

McNeil, J.E. & Warrington, E.K. (1993). Prosopagnosia: A face specific disorder. *Quarterly Journal of Experimental Psychology*, *46A*, 1–10.

Milner, A.D. & Goodale, M.A. (1995). *The visual brain in action.* Oxford: Oxford University Press.

Milner, A.D., Perrett, D.I., Johnston, R.S., Benson, P.J., Jordan, T.R., Heeley, D.W., *et al.* (1991). Perception and action in 'visual form agnosia'. *Brain*, *114*, 405–428.

Mishra, A.V. & Digre, K.B. (1996). Neuro-ophthalmologic disturbances in head injury. In M. Rizzo & D. Tranel (Eds.) *Head injury and post-concussion syndrome* (pp.201–225). New York: Churchill Livingstone.

Mitrushina, M.N., Boone, K.B. & D'Elia, L.F.D (1999). *Handbook of normative data for neuropsychological assessment*. New York: Oxford University Press, 531pp.

Molinari, M., Petrosini, L., Misciagna, S. & Leggio, M.G. (2004). Visuospatial abilities in cerebellar disorders. *Journal of Neurology, Neurosurgery and Psychiatry*, *75*, 235–240.

Ochipa, C., Rothi, L.J.G. & Heilman, K.M. (1989). Ideational dyspraxia: A deficit in tool selection and use. *Annals of Neurology*, *1989*, 190–193.

Padula, W.V. & Argyris, S. (1996). Post trauma vision syndrome and visual midline shift syndrome. *Neurorehabilitation*, *6*, 165–171.

Patterson, K.E. & Kay, J. (1982). Letter-by-letter reading: Psychological descriptions of a neurological syndrome. *Quarterly Journal of Experimental Psychology*, *29*, 307–318.

Poggel, D.A., Kasten, E., Muller-Oehring, E.M., Sabel, B.A. & Brandt, S.A. (2001). Unusual spontaneous and training induced visual field recovery in a patient with a gunshot lesion. *Journal of Neurology, Neurosurgery and Psychiatry*, *69*, 236–239.

Politzer, T.A. (1996). Case studies of a new approach using partial and selective occlusion for the clinical treatment of diplopia. *Neurorehabilitation*, *6*, 213–217.

Priddy, D.A., Johnson, P. & Lam, C.S. (1990). Driving after severe head injury. *Brain Injury*, *4*, 267–272.

Ratcliff, G. & Davies-Jones, G.A.B. (1972). Defective visual localisation in focal brain wounds. *Brain*, *95*, 49–60.

Riddoch, G. (1917). Dissociation of visual perception due to occipital injuries, with especial reference to the appreciation of movement. *Brain*, *40*, 15–57.

Riddoch, G. (1935). Visual disorientation in homonymous half-fields. *Brain*, *58*, 376–382.

Riddoch, M.J. & Humphreys, G.W. (1983). The effect of cuing on unilateral neglect. *Neuropsychologia*, *21*, 589–599.

Riddoch, M.J. & Humphreys, G.W. (1987). Visual object processing in optic aphasia: A case of semantic access agnosia. *Cognitive Neuropsychology*, *4*, 131–185.

Riddoch, M.J. & Humphreys, G.W. (1993). *BORB: The Birmingham Object Recognition Battery*. Hove: Lawrence Erlbaum Associates.

Riddoch, M.J., Humphreys, G.W., Burroughs, E., Luckhurst, L., Bateman, A., & Hill, S. (1995a). Cueing in a case of neglect: Modality and automaticity effects. Cognitive *Neuropsychology*, *12*, 605–621.

Riddoch, M.J., Humphreys, G.W., Luckhurst, L., Burroughs, E. & Bateman, A. (1995b). 'Paradoxical neglect': Spatial representations, hemisphere-specific activation and spatial cueing. *Cognitive Neuropsychology*, *12*, 569–604.

Rizzo, M. (1993). 'Balint's syndrome' and associated visuospatial disorders. In C. Kennard (Ed.) Bailliere's clinical neurology: Visual perceptual defects (pp.415–437). London: Bailliere Tindall.

Robertson, I.H. & Halligan, P.W. (1999). *Spatial neglect: A clinical handbook for diagnosis and treatment*. Hove: Psychology Press.

Robertson, H., Tegnér, R., Tham, K., Lo, A. & Nimmo-Smith, I. (1995). Sustained attention training for unilateral neglect: Theoretical and rehabilitation implications. *Journal of Clinical and Experimental Neuropsychology*, *17*, 416–430.

Robertson, I. (1994). The rehabilitation of attentional and hemi-attentional disorders. In M.J. Riddoch & G.W. Humphreys (Eds.) *Cognitive neuropsychology and cognitive rehabilitation* (pp.173–186). Hove: Lawrence Erlbaum Associates.

Robertson, I. & Cashman, E. (1991). Auditory feedback for walking difficulties in a case of unilateral neglect: A pilot study. *Neuropsychological Rehabilitation*, *1*, 175–183.

Robertson, I.H., Hogg, K. & McMillan, T.M. (1997). Rehabilitation of unilateral neglect: Improving function by contralesional limb activation. *Neuropsychological Rehabilitation*, *8*, 19–29.

Robertson, I.H. & North, N. (1992). Spatio-motor cueing in unilateral left neglect: The role of hemispace, hand and motor activation. *Neuropsychologia*, *30*, 553–563.

Robertson, I.H. & North, N. (1993). Active and passive activation of left limbs: Influence on visual and sensory neglect. *Neuropsychologia*, 31, 293–300.

Robertson, I.H., North, N. & Geggie, C. (1992). Spatio-motor cueing in unilateral neglect: Three single-case studies of its therapeutic effectiveness. *Journal of Neurology, Neurosurgery and Neuropsychiatry*, *55*, 799–805.

Rothi, L.J.G. & Heilman, K.M. (1997). *Apraxia: The neuropsychology of action*. Hove: Psychology Press.

Roy, E.A. & Square, P.A. (1985). Common considerations in the study of limb, verbal and oral apraxia. In E.A. Roy (Ed.) *Neuropsychological studies of apraxia and related disorders* (pp.111–161). Amsterdam: Elsevier Science Publishers B.V.

Schlageter, K., Gray, B., Hall, K., Shaw, R. & Sammet, R. (1993). Incidence and treatment of visual dysfunction in traumatic brain injury. *Brain Injury*, *7*, 439–448.

Schwartz, M., Reed, E.S., Montgomery, M.M., Palmer, C. & Mayer, N.H. (1991). The quantitative description of action disorganisation after brain damage: A case study. *Cognitive Neuropsychology*, *8*, 381–414.

Schwartz, M.F. & Buxbaum, L.J. (1997). Naturalistic action. In L.J.G. Rothi & K.M. Heilman (Eds.) Apraxia: The neuropsychology of action (pp.269–289). Hove: Psychology Press.

Schwartz, M.F., Montgomery, M.W., Buxbaum, L.J., Lee, S.S., Carew, T.G., Coslett, R.H., *et al.* (1998). Naturalistic action impairment in closed head injury. *Neuropsychology*, *12*, 13–27

Schwartz, M.F., Segal, M., Veramonti, T., Ferraro, M. & Buxbaum, L.J. (2002). The Naturalistic Action Test: A standardised assessment for everyday action impairment. *Neuropsychological Rehabilitation*, *12*, 311–339.

Seron, X., Deloche, G. & Coyette, F. (1989). A retrospective analysis of a single case neglect therapy: A point of theory. In X. Seron & G. Deloche (Eds.) *Cognitive approaches in neuropsychological rehabilitation* (pp.289–316). Hillsdale, NJ: Lawrence Erlbaum Associates.

Sheridan, J. & Humphreys, G.W. (1993). A verbal-semantic category-specific recognition impairment. *Cognitive Neuropsychology*, *10*, 143–184.

Sohlberg, M.M. & Mateer, C.A. (2001). *Cognitive rehabilitation. An integrative neuropsychological approach*. New York: The Guilford Press.

Spreen, O. & Strauss, E.A. (1998). *Compendium of neuropsychological tests* (2nd edn). New York: Oxford University Press.

Steinthal, P. (1871). *Abriss der sprach wissenschaft*. Berlin.

Stewart, F., Parkin, A.J. & Hunkin, H.N. (1992). Naming impairments following recovery from herpes simplex encephalitis. *Quarterly Journal of Experimental Psychology*, *44A*, 261–284.

Strano, C.M. (1989). Effects of visual deficits on ability to drive in traumatically brain-injured population. *Journal of Head Trauma and Rehabilitation*, *4*, 35–43.

Streff, J.W. (1996). Visual rehabilitation of hemianoptic head trauma patients emphasising ambient pathways. *Neurorehabilitation*, *6*, 173–181.

Tate, R.L. & McDonald, S. (1995). What is apraxia? The clinician's dilemma. *Neuropsychological Rehabilitation*, *5*, 273–297.

Tromp, E., Dinkla, A. & Mulder, T. (1995). Walking through doorways: An analysis of navigation skills in neglect patients. *Neuropsychological Rehabilitation*, *5*, 319–331.

Umiltà, C.A., Rizzolatti, G., Marzi, C., Zamboni, G., Franzini, C., Camarda, R., *et al.* (1974). Hemispheric differences in the perception of line orientation. *Neuropsychologia, 12*, 165–174.

Ungerleider, L.G. & Mishkin, M. (1982). Two cortical visual systems. In J. Ingle, M.A. Goodale & R.J.W. Mansfield (Eds.) *Analysis of visual behaviour* (pp.549–586). Cambridge, MA: MIT Press.

Valkenberg, C.T. (1908). Zur Kenntis der gestoerten Tiefenwahrnehmung. *Deutsche Zeitschrift fur Nervenheilkunde, 34*, 322–337.

Warrington, E.K. (1984). *Recognition Memory Test.* Windsor: NFER-Nelson.

Warrington, E.K. & James, M. (1986). Visual object recognition in patients with right hemisphere lesions: Axes or features? *Perception, 15*, 355–356.

Warrington, E.K. & James, M. (Eds.) (1991). VOSP: The visual object and space perception battery. Bury St. Edmunds: Thames Valley Test Company.

Warrington, E.K. & Taylor, A. (1973). The contribution of the right parietal lobe to object recognition. *Cortex*, 9, 152–164.

Wechsler, D. (1991). *Wechsler Adult Intelligence Scale-III.* New York: Psychological Corporation.

Wilson, B.A. (1999). *Case studies in neuropsychological rehabilitation.* New York: Oxford University Press, 384pp.

Wilson, B.A., Cockburn, J. & Halligan, P. (1987). *Behavioural Inattention Test.* Titchfield: Thames Valley Test Company.

Wilson, F.C. & Manly, T. (2003). Sustained attention training and errorless learning facilitates self-care functioning in chronic ipsilesional neglect following severe traumatic brain injury. *Neuropsychological Rehabilitation, 13*, 537–548.

Worthington, A. (1995a). Rehabilitation of acquired visuospatial disorders. *British Journal of Clinical Psychology, 34*, 314–318.

Worthington, A. & Beevers, L. (1996). Two arms, three hands – a supernumerary phantom phenomenon after right middle cerebral artery stroke. *Neurocase, 2*, 135–140.

Worthington, A. & Young, Y. (1996). Focal and global visual attention in left visuo-spatial neglect. *Neurocase, 2*, 441–447.

Worthington, A.D. (1995b). Single case design experimentation. *British Journal of Therapy and Rehabilitation, 2*, 536–538, 555–557.

Worthington, A.D. (1996). Cueing strategies in neglect dyslexia. *Neuropsychological Rehabilitation, 6*, 1–17.

Worthington, A.D. (2003). The natural recovery and treatment of executive disorders. In P.W. Halligan, U. Kischka & J.C. Wade (Eds.) *Handbook of clinical neuropsychology* (pp.322–339). New York: Oxford University Press.

Young, G.C., Collins, D. & Hen, M. (1983). Effect of pairing scanning training with block design training in the remediation of perceptual problems in left hemiplegics. *Journal of Clinical Neuropsychology, 5*, 201–212.

Zeki, S. (1993). *A vision of the brain.* Oxford: Blackwell Scientific Publications.

Zihl, J. (2000). *Rehabilitation of visual disorders after brain injury.* Hove: Psychology Press.

Zihl, J. & Von Cramon, D. (1979). Restitution of visual function in patients with cerebral blindness. *Journal of Neurology, Neurosurgery and Psychiatry, 42*, 312–322.

Zihl, J., Von Cramon, D. & Mai, N. (1983). Selective disturbance of movement vision after bilateral brain damage. *Brain, 106*, 313–340.

Zoccolotti, P. & Judica, A. (1991). Functional evaluation of hemineglect by means of a semistructured scale: Personal extrapersonal differentiation. *Neuropsychological Rehabilitation, 1*, 33–44.

9

Executive and Attentional Problems

Jonathan J. Evans

Introduction

Executive functioning is the term used to encompass a range of cognitive skills including problem solving, planning and organisation, self-monitoring, initiation, error correction and behavioural regulation. Attention refers to the ability to focus the mind's eye on something, and to sustain that attention in the face of competing distractions, be they external distractions such as other stimuli in the environment or internal distractions such as other thoughts. Executive and attention functions are considered together for several reasons. The executive system has been viewed by some as an attentional controller, and both functions are associated with the frontal lobes of the brain.

This review will begin with a description of the nature of executive and attentional skills and the types of problems that occur when the functioning of these systems is disrupted by brain injury. Within the frontal lobes, different regions are responsible for various different executive and attentional functions and these will be discussed. Techniques including standardised tests and practical task observation that can be used in the assessment of executive and attentional skills will then be described. The most important issue in the rehabilitation setting is how to help with such problems and various approaches to rehabilitation will be considered. Finally a case example will illustrate the rehabilitation process for one man with a combination of executive and attentional impairment after a head injury.

Executive Functioning and Attention: Theory

Executive functioning

Almost all of the theories of executive functioning have arisen from attempts to understand the role of the frontal lobes in cognition. Luria (1966) conceptualised the frontal lobes as being involved in problem solving, a process which includes the three phases of strategy selection, application of operations and evaluation of outcomes. Duncan (1993) described the role of the frontal lobes in terms of 'goal maintenance'. He argued that the frontal lobes are involved in identifying 'goals' or behavioural objectives and managing actions that will lead to the achievement of those goals. Duncan suggested that frontal lobe damage causes 'goal neglect', whereby the individual with a brain injury is able to identify what he or she needs to achieve and may be able to derive a plan, but during the course of the operation of the plan, the main goals may become neglected and actions no longer lead to achieving the goal. Whilst not completely random, behaviour is no longer goal-directed.

Baddeley and Wilson (1988) drew on the work of Rylander (1939) who described how individuals who suffer damage to the frontal lobes have impairments in attention (being easily distracted), have difficulties grasping the whole of a complicated state of affairs (an abstraction problem), and whilst they may be able to work along routine lines, they have difficulties in new situations. Baddeley (1986) coined the term dysexecutive syndrome as a replacement for the term 'frontal lobe syndrome'. He wanted to move away from an anatomically based description for a set of cognitive impairments, in favour of a common cognitive or functional link between the diverse set of problems that can occur after frontal lobe damage. He suggested that one of the functions of the frontal lobes is that of the 'central executive' component of the working memory model. Baddeley suggested that impairment in the central executive results in a 'dysexecutive' syndrome.

Baddeley (1986) equated the concept of the central executive with that of the 'supervisory attention system' (SAS), described by Norman and Shallice (see Shallice, 1988). They discussed the control of action in terms of two levels of control: an automatic schema-driven level (involving a non-conscious automatic control process referred to as contention scheduling) and the more conscious level referred to in terms of the SAS. This supervisory system was seen as responsible for dealing with novel situations through planning and problem solving. More specifically, the SAS was described as being required in situations that involve: (i) planning or decision making; (ii) error correction or troubleshooting; (iii) responses that are not well learned or where they contain novel sequences of actions; (iv) dangerous or technically difficult decisions; (v) situations that require the overcoming of a strong habitual response or resisting temptation.

Shallice and Burgess (1996) argued that the SAS can be fractionated into a set of basic sub-components, or sub-processes, and present evidence (based on neuropsychological dissociations and functional brain imaging) for the fractionation. They argued that responding appropriately to novelty requires three processes, each of which consists of a further set of sub-processes. Within their model (see Shallice & Burgess, 1996, p.1407) they posit the need for (1) a set of psychological operations that lead to the generation of a plan or solution for solving a novel problem, (2) a special-purpose working memory that is required for the implementation of the plan and (3) a system that monitors, evaluates and accepts or rejects actions depending upon their success in solving the novel problem. This model is illustrated in Figure 9.1.

A task clearly illustrating the distinction between automatic and conscious control of action is preparing a meal. When cooking a familiar meal, the whole process may

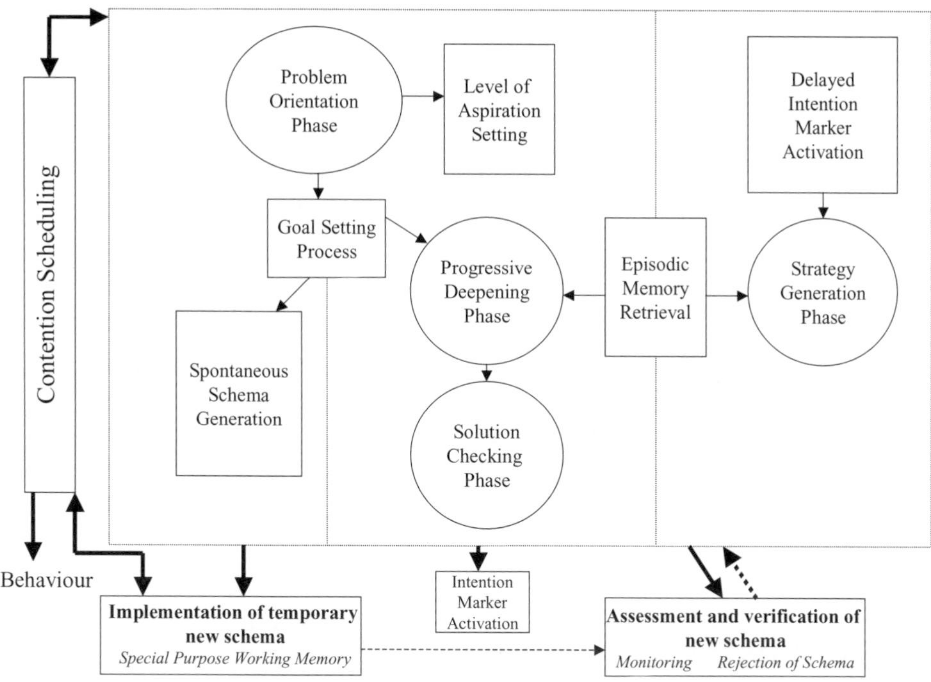

Figure 9.1 An adapted version of Shallice and Burgess's (1996) model of the fractionation of the supervisory attention system

be relatively automatic. The ingredients and where they can be bought are well known, and the various steps involved in preparation can be undertaken without a great deal of conscious attention. It is possible to hold a conversation, listen to the radio or watch television at the same time. However, if the task is to prepare an unfamiliar meal for a group of friends then much more conscious attention to actions is required. A recipe must be chosen and ingredients identified. A plan for obtaining ingredients may be needed. During the preparation, conscious attention to the steps involved, timings and undertaking new tasks may mean that it is not possible to dual-task; the chef may not be able to engage in conversation or listen to the radio. Problem solving in the kitchen may necessitate anti-social behaviour!

One source of evidence that the SAS can be fractionated is that the sub-processes of the SAS dissociate. Patients with brain injury may have difficulty with one or more of the processes, whilst others remain intact. For example, some patients appear to be aware that a problem exists, but may fail to identify more than one potential solution or make an adequate plan. Consequently, the patient may respond to a problem with impulsive actions. Impulsivity is a relatively common consequence of brain injury, particularly where the frontal lobes have been involved. The individual appears to 'act without thinking', doing the first thing that comes to mind, failing to think of alternative solutions to a problem and failing to anticipate the consequences of the chosen action. In contrast, some patients are able to generate a plan, but plans are never translated into action. In each case the end result will

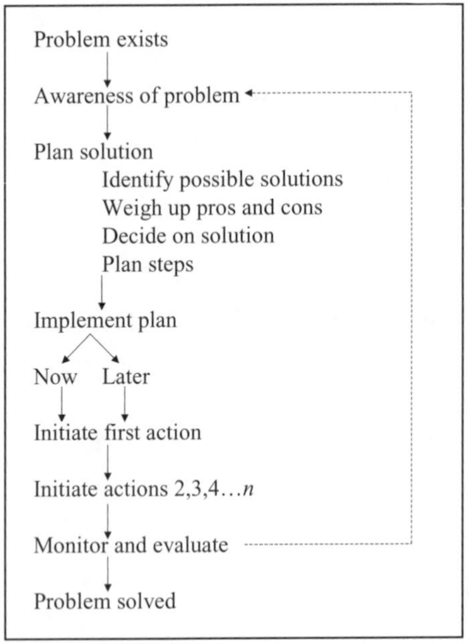

Figure 9.2 A simplified problem-solving framework

be essentially the same in that the problem is not dealt with adequately, but for different reasons. Those reasons become important when considering the assessment and rehabilitation of these problems, which are discussed later. The stages of the Shallice and Burgess (1996) model can be summarised in a simplified form, similar to the description of the problem-solving process described by d'Zurilla and Goldfried (1971; see also Evans, 2003), and this is illustrated in Figure 9.2.

Attention

As Manly and Mattingly (2004) note, 'although attention has a compelling subjective reality, it is notoriously difficult to define and still harder to measure' (p.243). One thing about attention that is now fairly well agreed is that attention, like memory, is not just one cognitive process, but rather there are several forms of attention. One of the most influential cognitive-anatomical models of attention has been that of Posner and Peterson (1990). They suggested that there are three separate circuits in the brain responsible for sustained attention (or vigilance), selective attention and spatial orientation. The latter circuit is concerned with the ability to attend to stimuli in the visual field. Deficits in this circuit (especially when combined with deficits in the sustained attention system which modulates the functioning) lead to the phenomenon of unilateral neglect (see Robertson *et al.*, 1995; Robertson, 1999). Spatial attention and unilateral neglect are addressed in another chapter and so will not be discussed in detail here. Sustained attention has been defined as 'the ability to self-sustain mindful, conscious processing of stimuli whose repetitive, non-arousing qualities would otherwise lead to habituation and distraction to other stimuli' (Robertson *et al.*, 1997a, p.747). In other words, the sustained attention system enables you to keep your mind on something from which you would otherwise 'switch off'. Attending to a boring lecture being delivered in a monotone, reading an uninteresting book and watching a radar screen are all examples of situations requiring the sustained attention system, if the stimulus (the lecture, the book or the radar screen) is to remain in conscious attention. Selective attention refers to the ability to attend to, pick out, or focus on a particular stimulus in the context of a complex background of other, distracting stimuli. The ability to pick out the particular brand of toothpaste from all of the other brands on the supermarket shelf, the ability to focus on one person's voice in amongst all the others at a party, the ability to notice danger ahead on a busy motorway are all examples of the selective attention system at work. The ability to divide attention is assumed to be subsumed within this selective attention system.

Van Zomeren and Spikman (2005) discuss a slightly simpler framework for thinking about assessment and remediation of attention, drawing the distinction between speed of processing and control of attention. Under the heading of control of attention they include control of focused and divided attention and control of sustained attention.

Pathology of Executive and Attention Deficits

Executive and attention functions depend upon the frontal lobes. Indeed our understanding of these cognitive skills has largely arisen from attempts to understand just what the frontal lobes do. What has emerged over many years of study of patients with lesions in the frontal lobes, and more recent studies of the functioning of intact frontal lobes using brain imaging techniques, is that different regions of the frontal lobes seem to have markedly different roles and thus damage causes different problems. Eslinger *et al.* (1995) summarised the neurobehavioural impairments associated with damage to specific frontal lobe regions and these are shown in Table 9.1.

Table 9.1 Neurobehavioural impairments associated with damage to specific frontal lobe regions (adapted from Eslinger *et al.*, 1995)

Superior mesial	Inferior mesial	Dorsolateral	Orbital
Akinesia	Amnesia	Poor integration and synthesis	Personality change
Mutism	Confabulations	Disorganised thinking and behaviour	Impulsive actions
Apathy	Disinhibition Lack of motivation Inattention	Perseveration Cognitive rigidity Poor planning	Poor social judgement Reduced empathy Lack of goal-directed behaviour
	Utilisation behaviour	Impulsive responding Stimulus boundedness Lack of empathy Impaired self-regulation	

One of the problems with this classification of impairments is that there is considerable overlap, or even duplication in the nature of impairments between regions. For example, impulsivity is attributed to both dorso-lateral and orbital regions. Lack of goal-directed behaviour, akinesia and disorganised behaviour feature in three regions, and yet there is considerable similarity between these concepts. Nevertheless, the point is made that there is probably regional specificity in functioning within the frontal lobes and that any attempt to identify a particular cognitive process as the one and only function of the frontal lobe is unlikely to succeed. Robbins (1996) notes that the fact that the prefrontal cortex is not a homogenous structure, having several different cytoarchitectronic regions, also supports a notion that there might be several functionally specialised areas within the prefrontal cortex.

The table suggests that the cognitive processes associated with planning and organisational skills appear to be dependent upon the dorso-lateral frontal lobes and evidence for this comes from a variety of other sources. Morris *et al.* (1993) demonstrated that this region was important for the planning element of performance on a computerised version of the Tower of London test (Shallice, 1988), an archetypal problem-solving task based on the Tower of Hanoi problem using a SPECT imaging technique. Robbins (1996) also reported on the use of a computerised version of the Tower of London test using positron emission tomography imaging, which highlighted the function of a combination of parietal lobe, premotor area, dorso-lateral prefrontal cortex bilaterally and fronto-polar cortex on the right. The extent to which the various sub-processes highlighted in the Shallice and Burgess (1996) model described above can be ascribed to separate regions of the frontal lobes is not yet clear, though the fact that there is evidence that the various processes do dissociate suggests that it will be possible to identify process-specific regions of the frontal lobes.

The three attention circuits described by Posner and Peterson (1990) are also located in different regions of the brain, though interact together. The sustained attention system is considered to be a function of the right hemisphere and in particular the right frontal lobe. Evidence for the involvement of the right frontal lobe in sustaining attention has come from several sources, including a study by Wilkins *et al.* (1987). In this study, patients were required to count auditory or tactile stimuli (2–11 stimuli per group of stimuli). Stimuli were presented at various different rates. It was found that for a presentation rate of one per second, patients with right frontal lesions were poorer at counting the stimuli. This task has been adapted and incorporated into the Test of Everyday Attention (Robertson *et al.*, 1994), which is described later.

The selective attention system described by Posner and Peterson (1990) is said to depend upon the anterior cingulate gyrus, whilst the orientation system is dependent upon posterior parietal regions.

The Consequences of Executive and Attentional Problems after Brain Injury

Impairments in executive functioning can cause devastating social handicaps, even in the context of well-preserved memory, perceptual and general intellectual skills.

This was dramatically illustrated in the most famous of all 'dysexecutive' patients, Phineus Gage. He was an American railway worker, who in 1848 suffered the trauma of losing part of his frontal lobes as a consequence of a tamping iron (an iron rod used to tamp down dynamite in a hole ready for detonation) being accidentally blasted through his skull. The remarkable thing about Phineus Gage was that he survived the injuries and in many ways made a good recovery. Nevertheless, he had a tendency to be disinhibited and had an inability to follow through with intended plans. The consequences of his impairments were described by the physician John Harlow, who had treated him, as resulting in the conclusion that he was 'No longer Gage'. Phineus Gage failed to keep his job, a clear indication of the handicap associated with suffering a dysexecutive syndrome. Similarly, patient EVR described by Eslinger and Damasio (1985), who had a large orbito-frontal meningioma removed, was described as having an IQ of over 130 and the ability to perform well on a wide variety of cognitive tasks, but appeared to be suffering with an impairment in his executive and problem-solving difficulties. As a consequence his life became disastrously disorganised. He had previously been a successful professional and a respected member of the community. However, he ended up losing his job, going bankrupt, being divorced, subsequently marrying a prostitute and divorcing again. He was described as having immense difficulties in making simple decisions, such as where to go out to dinner or what toothpaste to buy. The three patients described by Shallice and Burgess (1991) were all similar to EVR in that they appeared to have a combination of adequate general intellectual ability, impaired executive ability and disastrously organised lives. Patient RP (Evans *et al.*, 1998) similarly showed adequate general intellectual and memory functioning but impaired attention and executive skills. As a consequence, RP was unable to translate intention into action, to plan ahead, and sustain attention whilst carrying out tasks. She was unable to work or effectively manage the household and required constant support and supervision from her husband who had to give up his job to care for her. Crepeau and Scherzer (1993) provide further evidence of the social handicap caused by dysexecutive syndrome. They describe the results of a meta-analytic study of factors that predict return to work following traumatic brain injury which showed that the presence of impairments in executive functioning was a significant factor predicting whether or not individuals will return to work.

Problems with attention and concentration can also be severely disabling in both work and domestic settings. People with attention difficulties, particularly after head injury, frequently complain that they are unable to tolerate noise or any other distractions. For example, trying to hold a conversation with someone in the presence of young children is often an impossibility, as is speaking on the phone whilst the television is on. In these contexts, attention problems combined with reduced frustration tolerance can lead to irritability and anger. Another very problematic situation is coping with conversations in group settings. Here, problems with keeping up with conversations and in particular switching from one topic to another can be so difficult that individuals simply avoid such situations. The ability to sustain attention is often a major limiting factor in determining whether an individual returns to work or education. Robertson (1999) has also highlighted the importance of attention in the whole process of recovery and rehabilitation after brain injury, with evidence that sustained attention capacity predicts recovery of function over time following stroke (Robertson *et al.*, 1997b). Evans *et al.* (2003) also found that attentional functioning was a key factor in predicting which memory-impaired people will learn to make good use of memory aids.

Assessment of Executive Functions and Attention

Executive functioning

Wherever the process of problem solving breaks down, the consequence is essentially the same in that the individual fails to deal effectively with novel situations. Returning to Shallice and Burgess's (1996) model, a failure at any stage in any of the processes will lead to the same outcome – a failure to solve the problem. However, if we are to use our understanding of a person's difficulties to guide our interventions we need to establish the nature of the impairment in terms of the stages in the process of problem solving. This issue was highlighted by Crepeau *et al.* (1997) who showed dissociations between impairments at different stages of the problem-solving process amongst a group of brain-injured individuals. They used a four-stage model of problem solving: (1) analysis of the problem, (2) formulation of a general solution, (3) planning of the specific stages and (4) monitoring during execution. For assessing each of these stages they used a particular neuropsychological test, with another control test to measure more basic underlying cognitive processes (such as perceptual, visuo-spatial and memory functions) which, if impaired, could contribute to poor performance. Thus, for example, to assess the analysis of a problem they used the Picture Completion Test (a test involving the identification of key missing components from drawings of objects) from the Wechsler Adult Intelligence Scale–Revised as the target test, with the Boston Naming Test (which involves naming 60 line drawings of objects) used to control for visual and verbal functions. To assess formulation of a general solution, they used a form of the Tinkertoy Test (which involves making 'a free construction without the constraints of a model to copy or pre-determined solution', Lezak, 1995, p.659), with a second version of the test (in which subjects simply have to reproduce a model) acting as the control test. To assess planning they used the Self-ordered Pointing Test (requires the subject to organise a sequence of pointing responses to series of 6, 8, 10, and 12 representational pictures of living and artificial objects), with a second administration, in which the examiner determines the order, being used as the control. Finally, to assess monitoring they used the Wisconsin Card Sorting Test (a test of category formation which is sensitive to perseveration), with the control test being a Category Identification Test. Crepeau *et al.* attempted to validate this assessment structure by examining how performance on these tests related to performance on a series of photocopying tasks, designed as 'real-life' tests of each of their four components in their model of problem solving. The study revealed heterogeneity in performance amongst a brain-injured group, on both the neuropsychological tests and the photocopying tests (which they interpret as demonstrating dissociations and double dissociations amongst stages in the problem-solving process), but in fact there was little in the way of correlation between performance on the neuropsychological tests of a purported stage in problem solving and the corresponding 'real-life' test. However, Crepeau *et al.* noted that 'The results thus strongly suggest that more attention should be directed to the assessment of the components of executive functions rather than relying on a global score . . . [since] . . . use of a single score may lead to the conclusion that the patient has little or no residual executive capacities when in fact only one of the components is disrupting the capacity. This is particularly important for rehabilitation as the identification of an individual's strength constitutes the first step towards the remediation of deficits in problem-solving' (p.160).

Several other neuropsychological tests have traditionally been used for the assessment of executive functioning. The Controlled Oral Word Association (Verbal Fluency) task is often used as a test of executive functioning, though it could be argued that whilst it may be sensitive to frontal lobe damage, it is not clear how useful it is for assessing aspects of executive functioning. The test involves producing, in 60 seconds, as many words as possible beginning with particular letters of the alphabet. One way in which this test does make demands on executive functioning is that performance is improved by the application of strategies (e.g. producing words with similar stems). The test can also be sensitive to perseveration, or the tendency to become 'stuck in set', which is also seen as a characteristic frontal lobe executive deficit. However, the test is also vulnerable to word-finding problems, in the domain of language rather than executive functions. Maze tasks, such as Porteus Mazes, are also used as tests of planning (see Lezak, 1995). There is little evidence of the relationship between performance on the Mazes and practical planning tasks, though there is evidence that performance on the Mazes predicts performance on a driving task (see Lezak, p.657). A number of the traditional tests of executive function have now been brought together, along with some new ones, in the Delis–Kaplan Executive Function System (D-KEFS; Delis *et al.*, 2001), which consists of nine tests selected on the basis of demonstrated sensitivity to frontal lobe dysfunction. This battery has very extensive norms and therefore provides a very useful battery of tests which can be used selectively or as a complete set. The battery includes the Tower Test, a version of the Tower of Hanoi/Tower of London tasks which are useful in the assessment of problem solving and have been demonstrated to rely on dorsolateral frontal lobe functioning (Morris *et al.*, 1993; Robbins, 1996). Two other tests that are useful and have been shown to be sensitive to frontal lobe damage are the Hayling and Brixton Tests (Burgess and Shallice, 1997). The Hayling Test involves completing a spoken sentence with, in part I, a word that makes sense in the context of the sentence and, in part II, a word that does not make sense in the context of the sentence. The test can be said to be sensitive to impulsivity/inhibition and also to strategy application (as those who perform normally often adopt a strategy such as using items from the room) in part II. The Brixton Spatial Anticipation Test measures the ability to detect rules and to respond to changes in those rules (similar in nature to the Wisconsin Card Sorting Test).

One of the criticisms of many of the traditional tests of frontal lobe function has been that there is a lack of evidence of a clear relationship between test performance and functioning in day-to-day life. This issue was highlighted by Shallice and Burgess (1991), who noted that the problem with many of these tests is that 'the patient typically has a single explicit problem to tackle at any one time, the trials tend to be short . . . , task initiation is strongly prompted by the examiner and what constitutes successful trial completion is clearly characterised' (pp.727–728). By contrast, most of life's everyday problems are relatively unpredictable, have more than one possible 'correct' solution, and may require actions to be carried out over a long period of time. A further difficulty in assessing an individual's ability to solve a novel problem is that what is novel to one individual may be entirely routine for another.

This particular problem led Shallice and Burgess (1991) to develop two tasks, the Multiple Errands Test and the Six Elements Test. The Multiple Errands Test required individuals to carry out various tasks in a shopping centre (e.g. buying various things, meeting at a particular place), without breaking certain task rules (such as not going into a shop more than once, or not going into a shop unless to buy something). Shallice and Burgess showed that three patients who all had well-preserved IQs, and performed well on traditional frontal lobe tests, performed poorly on this task. These patients also performed poorly on the Six Elements Test. On this test, three tasks, each with two sub-tasks, must be undertaken over the course of a 10-minute period without breaking various task rules. The test was structured so that more points were awarded for earlier items, which meant that the optimum performance involved moving on to a new task before completing any one task. A modified and simplified version of this test was incorporated into the Behavioural Assessment of the Dysexecutive Syndrome Battery (BADS; Wilson *et al.*, 1996). This is a battery of six tests designed (or adapted from existing tests) to capture many of the aspects of the dysexecutive syndrome, including the ability to solve problems in novel situations. The problem with presenting patients with more complex tests is that they may fail, but the reasons for that failure are harder to discern. The tests are ecologically valid, but not process specific. However, this issue is relevant to most cognitive tests – there are no pure tests of cognitive processes. It is therefore the task of the therapist or clinician to develop a formulation of an individual's difficulties from the pattern of performance across a range of tests, and by careful observation of the apparent nature of problems on particular tests. For example, on the Modified Six Elements Test in the BADS, the patient may indicate that he or she has a plan, but then not stick to that plan, perhaps getting 'stuck' on just one of the tasks. In this case there may be a failure of monitoring. Alternatively, on the Zoo Map Test from the BADS, the patients may fail to take time to plan a solution, and so make errors. Included with the BADS is a 20-item questionnaire, the Dysexecutive Questionnaire. This has two forms, a self-rating and relative-rating form, and covers a range of problem areas. Burgess *et al.* (1998) showed that the DEX Other score and the DEX Other–DEX Self score (viewed as a measure of insight) correlated with scores of tests of executive function, whilst the DEX Self score did not (reflecting poor insight as a component of the dysexecutive syndrome). More recently, Bennett *et al.* (2005) showed that the DEX Questionnaire was sensitive to executive dysfunction (as defined by performance on the BADS battery), particularly when completed by rehabilitation team members (occupational therapists and neuropsychologists).

For some clients it appears that a particular difficulty is translating intentions to act into action. Thus a problem might have been noticed and a plan developed, but the client fails to translate that plan into action. For some people this problem is likely to be related to mood and motivational factors. However, for others (such as patient RP described above), an explanation simply in terms of mood or motivation does not seem to capture the nature of the deficit. Luria (1973) perhaps best described this type of problem in his description of patients with frontal lobe lesions. He noted that 'in these patients the verbal command remained in their memory, but it no longer initiated action and lost its regulating influence' (p.200). Assessment of this area of functioning is probably best undertaken through observation in informal settings as formal test situations often exert a strong prompt to action, so that the difficulty is not observed. However, it is important to be careful in interpreting apparent 'initiation' deficits in terms of a failure to translate intention into action, since some patients have initiation problems because they fail to notice a problem or fail to generate a plan in the first place, rather than failing to translate a plan into action. Once again discussion with the client, consideration of other test results and careful observation are the key to identifying the specific nature of an initiation problem.

Important information on the ability to solve problems is obtained through the use of observation of the client in functional situations. The processes of noticing problems and translating intention into action are perhaps best assessed in such functional settings. Most standard tests present problems rather directly to the patient and prompt task completion, so there is little demand on the ability to 'notice' or define the problem, nor to self-initiate task completion. The individual may not be aware that there is a gap between an intended goal (either self- or externally generated) and the individual's ability to achieve that goal (i.e. not notice there is still a problem to be solved). In the Oliver Zangwill Centre, the task of planning and preparing an unfamiliar meal is used as an example of a complex task which requires at least some, and often a lot, of problem solving, as is an in-house version of Shallice and Burgess's (1991) Multiple Errands Test (MET), in which clients are required to carry out various tasks around the hospital. Alderman *et al.* (2003) also developed a simplified version of the MET, which has subsequently been adapted for use in a hospital setting (Knight *et al.*, 2002).The need for this form of qualitative assessment, in addition to standardised assessment, also highlights the value of the interdisciplinary team working closely together in planning an individual's assessment and in formulating problems identified during assessment. In the Oliver Zangwill Centre, the team plans the client's assessment together. Typically, the psychologists carry out the neuropsychological tests of executive functioning (as part of a broader neuropsychological assessment) along with informal assessment on the in-house hospital version of the multiple-errands test. The occupational therapists also undertake some standardised assessment (e.g. Chessington Occupational Therapy Neurological Assessment Battery) and carry out the functional assessment using tasks such as planning and preparing an unfamiliar meal and sometimes a work-related project task. At the summary of assessment meeting information from the standardised tests, the functional assessment as well as qualitative observation information from other team members who have carried out other assessments (e.g. speech and language therapist, physiotherapist, neuropsychiatrist) is brought together in a formulation of the client's current problems, which is then documented in an interdisciplinary report.

Attention

Posner and Peterson's (1990) theoretical model of the attention systems in the brain provides a useful framework for considering the assessment of attention. Tests of visuo-spatial orienting (tests for unilateral neglect) are not, however, considered here as they are covered in a separate chapter. Ponsford (2000) provides a useful summary of tests of attention from the perspective of the Posner and Peterson model. There are very few widely available tests specifically designed to assess sustained attention. The one exception is the Test of Everyday Attention (Robertson *et al.*, 1994), which is a battery of eight sub-tests. A factor analytic study concluded that three tests (Elevator Counting, Telephone Search while Counting and Lottery) loaded on to a vigilance or sustained attention factor. The Elevator Counting Task requires the subject to count strings of tones presented at a variable rate. The Telephone Search while Counting is a dual-tasking test, but loads on a sustained attention factor rather than a selective attention factor. It involves searching a telephone directory for symbols while counting tones at the same time. The Lottery task requires the subject to listen to a tape of winning lottery ticket numbers/letters (e.g. HL855) and when tickets ending with 55 occur, the first two letters (i.e. HL) must be written down.

The Test of Everyday Attention also has several tests of selective attention. The Map Search (which requires subjects to search a map and locate symbols) and Telephone Search (searching a Yellow Pages for symbols) both make demands on visual selective attention and speed of information processing. The Elevator Counting with Distraction task requires the subject to count particular tones, while ignoring others. The Visual Elevator and Elevator Counting with Reversal tasks make demands on the ability to change attentional set flexibly and rapidly.

Speed of information processing is often assessed in the context of attention, and in fact it has been argued that deficits in speed of processing may underlie all impairments on tests of attention (van Zomeren & Brouwer, 1994). Many different tests make demands on speed of information processing, though it is often necessary to be cautious in interpreting a slow speed on tests with a motor component, where the slowness may be in motor, rather than cognitive processing. One test of selective attention that makes demands on the ability to focus on one stimulus and ignore another, which is also sensitive to speed of processing deficits, is the Stroop Test (see Ponsford, 2000, p.373 for a detailed discussion of this test). There are two forms of this test. The first involves reading out the colour words printed (in various colours) in columns across a page. The second form involves saying the name of the colour of the ink used to print a colour word, when the ink colour conflicts with the word (i.e. the word blue is written in red ink and the correct response is red). Ponsford (2000, p.364) also describes in some detail use of the Paced Auditory Serial Addition Task (PASAT). This is described as a measure of 'information processing capacity and rate'. It involves adding together a series of pairs of numbers presented as a continuous string (i.e. 4, 2, 6, 3, 5 should produce the response 6, 8, 9, 8). There are several versions of the test, which are varied in terms of the speed of presentation. It has been shown that this test is sensitive to head injury, including mild head injury. It is more sensitive to diffuse white-matter damage caused by acceleration/deceleration forces, rather than more static or focal injuries such as an assault. The Trail Making Test (see Lezak, 1995) is used as a measure of attention, and to some extent as a measure of executive functioning too. It has two parts; in Part A the subject must join a series of encircled numbers which are randomly spaced around a sheet of paper. This task therefore makes demands upon visual scanning skills, speed of information and motor processing. In Part B the subject must alternate between numbers and letters in ascending order (i.e. 1, A, 2, B, 3, C . . .). The subject must therefore inhibit the tendency to continue a sequence with either numbers or letters.

From the perspective of rehabilitation, the Test of Everyday Attention is probably the most useful attention test, though even here there are limitations on the ability of the tests to capture subtle changes in attentional skills and in particular the ability to sustain attention over time. As with the assessment of executive functioning, more qualitative, observational assessment is necessary. Collecting examples of apparent problems with attention and concentration while a client attends the rehabilitation programme is vital. Once again the task of preparing an unfamiliar meal provides ample opportunity to assess attention in a multi-tasking situation.

Rehabilitation of Executive and Attention Impairments

A key issue in rehabilitation is whether interventions should be aimed at treating the underlying impairment (i.e. restoring the lost function) or seek to provide clients with strategies that enable them to compensate for the impairment. As discussed below, the evidence that executive or attention problems can be restored is not wholly convincing, whilst there is more evidence that mental strategies or external aids can produce real benefits.

Retraining or restoring impaired executive and attention functioning

Executive functioning

Evidence that executive dysfunction can be returned to normal is limited, though a small number of studies do suggest that various forms of problem-solving training may be helpful. Beginning, however, with pharmacological approaches, placebo-controlled single-case studies of the drug Idazoxan (Sahakian *et al.*, 1994) in patients diagnosed with frontal lobe dementia are promising. However, it is not clear that frontal lobe dementia is a good model for non-progressive, single-event brain damage. Nevertheless, this work clearly needs expanding so that the potential benefit of pharmacological interventions is adequately assessed. Further work must also address the extent to which improvement of performance on specific tests of planning, such as those used in studies to date, generalises to everyday problem solving.

Retraining approaches to rehabilitation make the assumption that practising a particular cognitive function through tasks and exercises will enable that function to return, in a more or less normal fashion. von Cramon *et al.* (1991) and von Cramon and Matthes-von Cramon (1992) describe a group-based training programme described as 'problem-solving therapy', which is seen as a retraining approach. von Cramon and colleagues note that the broad aim of problem-solving therapy is to provide patients 'with techniques enabling them to reduce the complexity of a multi stage problem by breaking it down into more manageable portions. A slowed down, controlled and step-wise processing of a given problem, should replace the unsystematic and often rash approach these patients spontaneously prefer' (1991, p.46). The therapy approach adopts a problem-solving framework which draws on the work of d'Zurilla and Goldfried (1971). The specific aims of the therapy are to enhance the patients' ability to perform each of the separate stages of problem solving, through practice on tasks that are designed to exercise the skills required for each of the separate stages. These stages include (a) identifying and analysing problems; (b) separating information relevant to a problem solution from unimportant and irrelevant data; (c) recognising the relationship between different relevant items of information and if appropriate combining them; (d) producing ideas/solutions; (e) using different mental representations (e.g. verbal, visual, abstract patterns such as flow charts) in order to solve a problem; and (f) monitoring solution implementation and evaluate solutions.

von Cramon *et al.* (1991) compared a group of patients who received problem-solving therapy ($n = 20$), with a group of patients who received a control 'Memory Therapy' Group ($n = 17$). The control group allowed for the possibility that clients might benefit from general advice and group activity, rather than specifically from the tasks aimed at exercising executive skills. They showed that patients who underwent problem-solving therapy showed some improvement in tests of general intelligence and problem solving (Tower of Hanoi) compared with controls. von Cramon and colleagues demonstrated some generalisation of problem-solving skills to untrained test tasks but there was no evidence of generalisation to everyday situations. Evidence for the latter is hard to obtain because of measurement difficulties but it is clearly important that some evidence is obtained of generalisation to situations outside of formal test sessions.

Rath *et al.* (2003) also described an evaluation of a problem-solving training group. They compared outcome for 27 patients who undertook the problem-solving training with a control group of 19 patients who underwent what they described as 'conventional' treatment. The conventional treatment combined general cognitive remediation training and psychosocial work and involved 24 sessions, with 2–3 hours per week contact. The problem-solving group also involved 24 sessions, with one two-hour group per week. The impact of the group was measured with a range of neuropsychological tests, questionnaires and also a role-play of a problem-solving scenario that was rated by independent raters. Rath *et al.* found that the problem-solving training group improved (and the conventional group did not) on Wisconsin Card Sorting Test performance, on self-assessed ratings of problem-solving skills, clear thinking and emotional regulation, and perhaps most importantly on the observer ratings on the role-played scenario. Improvement was also maintained at a six-month follow-up. The major limitation of the study is, of course, the lack of evidence of generalisation to everyday life, but as noted already, this is a major difficulty for studies of this kind.

Attention

Robertson (1999) provides an overview of a number of studies that have looked at the impact of retraining approaches to attention. Most of these studies have used computerised presentation of tasks that make demands on the ability to concentrate over the course of a series of training sessions. The results have been rather mixed. Furthermore, many of the studies are subject to significant methodological problems and have been limited in scope, offering no evidence of generalisation to everyday situations. Several studies have found change over time, but those changes were not demonstrated to be a direct result of training.

One of the most methodologically rigorous studies is that of Ponsford and Kinsella (1988). They studied 10 patients who had suffered head injury. There were four conditions; no training, computerised attentional training, computerised attention training with additional therapist feedback and return to baseline (no training). They used a single-case experimental design, a multiple baseline across subjects with baseline lengths of three and six weeks. The computerised training included various tasks such as reaction time training, vigilance training (spot the letter on the screen), and visual search tasks. The measures used to assess the impact of training on attention were a four-choice reaction time task, a letter cancellation task and a symbol-digit test. A rating scale was also completed by occupational therapists relating to the patient's day-to-day attention and performance on a practical clerical task that made demands on attention. The study found improvements over time of the measures used, but it was noted that the improvement did not appear to link directly to the training. Whilst there was improvement over time, it was not possible to attribute this directly to the training.

Probably the most impressive results of computerised training approaches have come from Sturm and colleagues. Sturm *et al.* (1983; see Robertson, 1999, p.305) compared the performance of two groups of mixed head-injured and stroke patients using a crossover design (training followed by no training for one group and vice versa for the other group). Two groups of matched non-brain-injured subjects underwent the same procedure in order to control for practice effects. The training was on a range of attention tasks contained within the Vienna Test System. Sturm and colleagues found improvements on a range of neuropsychological tests of attention (and some other more general tests of cognitive function) following training. Similar results were found on another study by Sturm *et al.* (1997). They trained a group of 38 stroke patients on a series of attention tasks, but what was different about this intervention was that there was an attempt to train specific attention deficits (e.g. sustained attention or selective attention) using process-specific tasks. Sturm *et al.* found improvement in the type of attention targeted, with no comparable change on untargeted measures. Positive results from attention training were also found in studies by Gray and Robertson (1989) and Gray *et al.* (1992), though again there was no demonstration of generalisation to everyday life.

For the clinician who wants to use evidence to guide practice, the attention-training studies described above leave the clinician in somewhat of a dilemma. Whilst some have demonstrated change, few can confidently attribute any change to training and few have demonstrated that any change that occurs generalises to everyday life for the patient. Fortunately studies of internal and external strategies for managing attention are somewhat more convincing in their efficacy and relevance to everyday life.

Internal strategies

A number of interventions aimed at helping clients with attention and executive difficulties might be considered as 'internal' strategies. Typically this means that the individual is using a mental routine or self-instructional technique of some sort.

Executive functioning

Self-instruction in the management of impulsivity

Cicerone and Wood (1987) provide a good example of the use of the self-instructional technique in a 20-year-old man with a severe head injury. He was described as functioning relatively independently, but impulsively interrupted conversations and generally appeared not to think before he did something. They used the Tower of London Test as a training task, asking the client to state each move he was about to make while attempting to solve the problem and then to state the move while he performed it. In stage two the patient was asked to repeat the first stage except to whisper rather than speak aloud. Finally in the third stage he was asked to 'talk to himself' (i.e. to think through what he was doing). This approach was successful in improving performance on the trained task, but more importantly, there was generalisation to two other untrained tasks. In addition, with some generalisation training, there were improvements in general social behaviour, rated by independent raters. The main change brought about by this simple self-instructional technique was that it helped the patient to slow his approach to the task in hand and, in effect, develop a habit of thinking through his actions rather than responding impulsively.

Internalisation of an external checklist

von Cramon and Matthes-von Cramon (1995) provide an example of an internalised checklist routinely applied to compensate for executive deficits. They describe GL, a 33-year-old physician who had a traumatic brain injury at the age of 24, resulting in bilateral frontal lobe damage. Despite the injury, GL passed his medical exams post-injury (though after several failures). He was described as having 'drifted' through several jobs in neurosurgery, pathology and the pharmaceutical industry. His problems were characterised as involving a lack of overview and being dependent upon meticulous instructions. He was unable to benefit from feedback, spending too much time on routine activities and being unable to adapt himself to the requirements of novel or changing situations. In the study, a protected work trial was established in a hospital pathology laboratory and he was provided with prototypical reports on autopsy. It was noted that he tended to jump to conclusions about diagnosis and he was therefore taught a set of rules/guidelines for the systematic process of diagnosis. These rules were initially provided in the form of a written checklist, which, over time, GL learned and was able to apply without the need to refer to the checklist. GL improved his ability to diagnose correctly and to write reports. However, there was no generalisation to a novel planning task.

Using a problem-solving framework

Another approach is to teach a more general strategy that can be applied in a variety of situations. Evans (2003) describes a group approach, adapted from the von Cramon group described above and from the Goal Management Training of Robertson (1996; see also Levine *et al.*, 2000) described in more detail below. The Attention and Problem Solving Group is one component of a holistic rehabilitation programme. The first few sessions of the group (which runs twice a week for 8–10 weeks) primarily address attentional difficulties, and the later sessions are used to introduce a problem-solving framework to the clients. This framework is presented as a paper-based checklist of the stages of problem solving. An accompanying template is also provided that can be used to proceed through the stages using a written format, but clients are encouraged, through practice at using the framework with the template, to internalise the framework so that in time the use of the framework becomes more automatic. Miotto and Evans (2005) have undertaken a formal evaluation of this group format and demonstrated improved outcome on both neuropsychological tests of executive functioning and everyday functioning as measured by the DEX Questionnaire. The successful use of this framework by one client, Steven, is described later.

Goal management training

Levine *et al.* (2000) describe the use of a goal management training (GMT) technique in two studies. Study 1 evaluated the technique with a group of head-injured patients on paper-and-pencil tasks. The second study described the use of this technique with one post-encephalitic patient seeking to improve her meal preparation abilities. The GMT technique was derived from Duncan's (1986) concept of 'goal neglect'. The principle is that patients with frontal lobe damage fail to generate goal (or sub-goal) lists of how to solve problems (and achieve goals), and/or may fail to monitor progress towards achieving sub- or main goals. The training has five stages, which are first defined for the patient: (1) Stop and think what I am doing, (2) Define the main task, (3) List the steps required, (4) Learn the steps, (5) Whilst implementing the steps, check that I am on track, or doing what I intended to do. After each stage is introduced, illustrative examples from the patient's own life are used as well as mock examples. In the first study, the GMT was applied in a single one-hour session, with testing on several target tasks undertaken afterwards. Levine *et al.* showed improved performance on three paper-and-pencil tasks, but no generalisation to everyday life was demonstrated. However, Study 2 addressed the question of application of GMT in a more practical task, preparing a meal, with patient KF who suffered from a meningo-encephalitic illness, which resulted in some general intellectual decline, attentional, memory and executive functioning deficits. A particular problem for KF was meal preparation, with four particular areas of difficulty: failure to assemble the necessary ingredients, misinterpretation of written instructions, repeated checking of instructions and sequencing/omission errors. Using the number of problem behaviours evident during meal preparation tasks (as well as performance on the paper-and-pencil tasks used in Study 1), GMT was shown to be helpful, though the specific contribution of the specific components of the intervention package could not be determined.

Autobiographical memory cueing as a means of improving problem solving

Shallice and Burgess's (1996) model of the problem-solving processes associated with the functioning of the supervisory attentional system highlights the importance of the retrieval from memory of past experience. When faced with a novel situation or perhaps an infrequently encountered situation, the strategy of recalling incidents of tackling similar problems in the past may help in the present situation. However, Dritschel *et al.* (1998) demonstrated that people with head injury often fail to refer to previous experiences in solving practical planning tasks, such as describing how they would book a holiday, get a new job or find a new place to live. Hewitt *et al.*

(2000) hypothesised that if patients were given a brief training relating to the retrieval of autobiographical memories, they would improve in their ability to plan practical tasks. The training took the form of an illustration of the value of recalling specific autobiographical experiences from the past in practical problem solving, a cue-card to prompt specific memory retrieval and practice at doing this in order to plan how to tackle a particular task. The performance of two groups of subjects was compared, one receiving the training and the other not. The results showed that the training group improved significantly more than the no-training group, suggesting that incorporating some form of training relating to retrieval of specific incidents may be helpful in a problem-solving training programme.

Attention

Self-instructional techniques have also been used in the rehabilitation of attention, particularly in the domain of sustained attention. Robertson *et al.* (1995) describe a self-instructional training method for sustained attention *and* unilateral neglect. Their rationale was that the sustained attention system has an important modulating effect on the posterior spatial orienting system. In cases of persisting unilateral neglect it is hypothesised that there is a combination of deficits in both of these systems. Therefore, if it is possible to improve sustained attention, this may benefit the orienting system and neglect may be reduced. The intervention was essentially a self-alerting technique to enhance sustained attention. Patients were assessed on tests of neglect, sustained attention, and control tasks (i.e. tests where performance was not expected to improve as a result of training). During the training procedure, individuals practised tasks that required sustained attention skills for successful completion. The rationale for the training was explained and whilst the patient carried out the task the trainer would rap sharply on the desk at unpredictable intervals (between 20 and 40 seconds) and say 'attend' in a loud voice. After several repetitions, the patient was asked to say 'attend' (or some other alerting statement) when the trainer rapped on the table. In the next step, patients were cued to rap the desk themselves and say 'attend'; then the patient rapped the desk and said 'attend' sub-vocally, and finally the patients were required simply to signal whenever they were mentally knocking the desk and saying 'attend' to themselves. They were also given instructions about the usefulness of trying to apply this self-alerting strategy habitually in everyday life situations. Significant improvements were found on both neglect and vigilance tasks, with (as predicted) no changes on the control tests. It seems likely that this method works both by increasing the client's level of alertness or arousal and also by ensuring that the client frequently reviews what they are doing and keeps on task. The idea of patients developing a 'checking routine' is an important aspect of the development of internal strategies for coping with problem-solving situations.

As part of the Oliver Zangwill Centre Attention and Problem-Solving Group (Evans, 2003; Miotto & Evans, 2005), clients are often encouraged to develop a 'mental checking' routine. This is in effect the same as Stage 5 of Robertson's (1996) GMT. Patients are encouraged to regularly check that they are on track in a particular task, using a personal catchphrase (e.g. STOP: THINK; am I doing what I should be? am I on track?). This might be facilitated through the use of an alarm (such as a watch alarm) sounding at intervals and might be combined with a cue card containing the client's own self-monitoring statement. This is also illustrated with patient Steven discussed below.

External strategies

Executive functioning

The most common strategy in the rehabilitation of memory problems is to teach the use of external aids, such as checklists, diaries or electronic organisers. Such aids are also useful for people who have planning and organisational problems. It was noted earlier that a problem-solving framework in the form of a template can be used to support a systematic approach to dealing with some novel situations. For some individuals, the process of writing things down seems to be the critical step in that it prevents a more impulsive style of responding to situations. For others, the process of writing things down makes the process of generating possible solutions and weighing up the pros and cons of those solutions more manageable. For individuals with significant working memory or speed of information-processing deficits, it may be difficult to use the framework 'in mind', and an external written approach may be more helpful.

Poor sequencing of tasks is a possible consequence of executive disorder and in some cases checklists prove to be useful. The case of GL, the doctor who improved his performance in writing pathology reports, was described above. He used a checklist approach, but was able to internalise the checklist so that the task, even though complex, became essentially routine. Burke *et al.* (1991) describe six case studies where checklists were used in order to help clients develop and carry out plans.

For some people, particularly those with very severe executive impairments or with a combination of executive and other difficulties, the provision of external aids might not be effective and it is necessary to consider changing some aspect of their physical or social environment. Work with family, friends and colleagues is one form of environmental modification approach. Helping relatives and carers to understand the nature of executive difficulties can help to minimise negative responses to problems arising from a dysexecutive syndrome. For example, one of the most difficult things for families to appreciate is that an initiation difficulty is not laziness. Another is that the person may remember some things and not others owing to attentional problems rather than not bothering to remember. Education can have an important role in helping families both to understand, and to modify their own behaviour in relation to clients (for a case example, see O'Brien *et al.*, 1988). A combination of difficulties can sometimes result in problem behaviour such as aggressive or stereotyped behaviour, each of which may prevent the client from participating in other rehabilitation activities and cause significant disruption for family, friends and carers. In this situation, it is often necessary to provide a highly structured environment with the opportunity for very frequent feedback in order to help clients to shape and modify their behaviour. The work of Alderman and colleagues (Alderman & Burgess, 1990, 1994; Alderman & Ward, 1991) illustrates the use of behaviour modification techniques, originally developed in the context of work with people with complex patterns of neuro-behavioural disability, which are relevant in the context of the combination of memory and executive impairments in this client group.

Attention

'SUDDEN LOUD NOISES!!' grab attention very easily. This orienting response is automatic, biologically pre-programmed and, from an evolutionary perspective, vital to survival. In this situation, basic arousal is maximal and attention to task (identifying the source of potential threat) is facilitated. For people with significant difficulty sustaining attention, the presence of a naturally occurring orienting response opens the possibility that this phenomenon can be harnessed to good use. The study of Robertson *et al.* (1995) used this to help individuals develop an internal self-alerting technique, though starting out with an external alerting stimulus (someone banging a table). However, rather than try to train an internal strategy, another option is to rely on the alerting impact of a repeated external stimulus.

Such an approach was used with Patient RP (Evans *et al.*, 1998), who suffered a cerebro-vascular accident as a result of a ruptured aneurysm. Her main problem was that she had difficulty translating intention into action. She was also highly distractible and had difficulty completing tasks. Despite adequate memory and intelligence, RP's combination of executive and attentional deficits had a significant impact on her day-to-day life. Although she could accurately say what she had to do, she had to be prompted to do many things, such as take her medication, or water her plants. When she did manage to set off to do a task, she was frequently distracted by something else along the way and failed to return to the original task. She therefore took a huge amount of time to get things done. She also found it difficult to be organised and planful enough to cook a family meal. The intervention used with RP was a paging-based reminder system known as Neuro-Page®. This system was developed by Hersh and Treadgold (1994) and it was evaluated with a group of people with memory problems by Wilson *et al.* (1997). The system utilises radio paging technology and involves the patient wearing an alphanumeric pager. Reminders of things to do are entered onto a central computer using NeuroPage® software. This automatically sends out the message via a modem to a paging company, which then sends out the message to the patient's pager, which bleeps and delivers a text message. A study of RP's performance in carrying out a range of day-to-day tasks, using an ABAB single-case experimental design, showed that the system was highly effective in helping RP to complete tasks she needed to do on time. This significantly reduced the stress on her husband. Evans *et al.* noted that there appeared to be two important aspects to the success of the paging system. The first was the presentation of an external text message that appeared to be important for RP and prompted behaviour in a way that an internal intention to act failed to do. The second aspect was the bleeping of the pager, which provided an arousal boost to facilitate RP's initiation of tasks and help her sustain attention during the course of task completion. One issue in the use of alerting devices is the possibility that the individual will habituate to the sound and it will lose its alerting effect. This is a danger if alerts are being used very frequently and so highlights the importance of managing the frequency so that it retains its alerting capacity.

Manly *et al.* (2002) also examined the impact of external alerting. Performance of patients who had suffered traumatic brain injury on a multi-element task was tested under two conditions. The task used, the Hotel Test, is similar in format to the Six Elements Test. It involves the patient completing six different tasks, including a prospective remembering task, that are presented as tasks that might be given to an assistant hotel manager (e.g. making up bills, arranging conference delegate cards, looking up phone numbers, sorting charity box coins, proof-reading a leaflet and pushing a button to open a door). Like the Six Elements, not everything from all of the tasks can be completed in the 15 minutes allocated. Two parallel versions were used in the two experimental conditions. In one condition an external alert (a tone on an audio tape) was presented at random, relatively infrequent intervals. In the other condition no tone was presented. The study used a counterbalanced, crossover design. The results showed that participants performed more effectively during the bleeped condition than during the control condition. It was argued that the alerting tones improved the link between a well-represented goal and current behaviour. The tones did not specifically prompt task switching, but rather seemed to improve the ability to switch task at other, more appropriate, times.

Case 9.1

This example illustrates how some of the strategies described above were used with one man who had experienced a traumatic head injury.

Case details

Prior to his head injury, Steven was a successful businessman. He had no history of neurological or psychiatric problems. At the age of 35, Steven was driving a car when he was involved in a road traffic accident. On arrival at hospital his Glasgow Coma Scale score was 6. CT brain scans showed the presence of diffuse axonal injury and right frontal lobe contusions. The length of coma was difficult to be certain of as records were not available, though he had a period of post-traumatic amnesia which lasted several weeks. Initially he had a right hemiparesis and significant dysarthria. He was discharged from acute hospital care after three months. He had been living independently prior to his injury, but went to live with a family member after leaving hospital. He then had outpatient speech therapy, physiotherapy and cognitive rehabilitation for a period of nine months. It was noted that he had a degree of general intellectual deterioration, with specific problems in attention, mental control, reasoning, executive functioning, including impulse control, sequencing, planning, problem solving and abstract thinking skills. He made progress during this time, but it was felt that he would benefit from an intensive neuropsychological rehabilitation programme and so he was referred to a post-acute neuropsychological

Continued

rehabilitation programme (at the Oliver Zangwill Centre – see Wilson *et al.*, 2000), with the aim of helping him return to work and independent living. The programme has an interdisciplinary team of psychologists, occupational therapists, a speech therapist, a physiotherapist and rehabilitation assistants. He was seen for a preliminary (one-day) assessment one year after his accident, followed shortly afterwards by a two-week detailed assessment period. The presenting problems that Steven identified were difficulties with concentration, difficulty problem solving, being slower than he used to be, poor articulation, poor motor skills (being wobbly on his feet) and frustration at his situation. His main aim was to return to work. He also wanted to live independently, to understand the nature of his problems better and to be able to sit and read a novel.

Assessment

Recent cognitive assessment of Steven had shown evidence of mixed performance on the Wechlser Adult Intelligence Scale–Revised, with the poorest performance being on tests of Arithmetic, Block Design, Object Assembly and Digit Span. He showed some evidence of impaired verbal and visual memory on the Wechsler Memory Scale–Revised and on the recall items from the Doors and People Test. He was better on the Doors and People tests of recognition memory, and the Warrington Recognition Memory Test. There was some evidence of a mild reduction in working memory skills. He showed no major object or space perception deficits, though there was some evidence of a difficulty performing mental rotation tasks. Steven had problems on tests of language, including the Test for the Reception of Grammar (difficulty in the interpretation of reversible passive sentences, and embedded sentences). There was some difficulty on reading comprehension tasks, but these were affected by memory and attentional problems. There were also some mild reading and spelling problems. He showed significant impairment on a range of attention tests from the Test of Everyday Attention, including tests of selective attention (Map Search) and sustained attention (Lottery). He performed normally on the Modified Wisconsin Card Sorting Test, but executive dysfunction was evident from difficulties on several tasks from the Behavioural Assessment of the Dysexecutive Syndrome, including the Key Search and Zoo Map Tests. He was, however, able to complete the Modified Six Elements Test successfully.

Several sub-tests from the Chessington Occupational Therapy Neurological Assessment Battery were administered. On the 'following written instructions' task, he was borderline in his ability and below average for the time taken. He was observed to begin the task before the task instructions had been completed, but then interrupted his performance to ask questions. He had difficulty following the instructions as they became more complex so that he eventually improvised in his attempt to complete the task, which involves making a coat hanger. His performance on following visual instructions was better. He had some problems following spoken instructions, failing to select and sequence cards as per the instructions.

The assessment process included several more practical tasks, used for qualitative assessment of Steven's functioning. During a communication group he took part in a debate and whilst he showed he could put across a point forcefully, he tended to dominate the session. Monitoring by staff highlighted that he was excessively excitable at times and there was some evidence of socially inappropriate laughter. He was able to plan and prepare a meal satisfactorily. He undertook a budgeting task, but had difficulties with balancing an account effectively. As part of an assessment of his previous work role he was asked to complete a written account of his job. Initially it was difficult to obtain a clear account from his written work, which had spelling errors and lacked appropriate grammar, punctuation and sentence structure. He was better when given more structure to follow.

In an assessment of mood, Steven indicated that he had some difficulty in managing relationships since his injury. He was aware that he had difficulty expressing himself and tended to be impulsive. At times he was abrupt with people, particularly his family. While he did not report significant depression, he did admit to feeling sad and tearful on occasion. He was anxious at times in crowds. He had some difficulty falling off to sleep and waking early. He had been prescribed antidepressants and sleeping pills, but had discontinued them several months previously.

Rehabilitation programme

Steven undertook a 20-week rehabilitation programme, the first 10 weeks of which involved attendance at the centre 5 days per week. The second half of the programme involved part-time attendance initially 2–3 days per week, reducing to 1 day per week towards the

Continued

end. Eight specific rehabilitation programme goals were identified. Some of these were related to functional activities (e.g. identifying work roles and being engaged in them with support, or to be engaged in a physical leisure activity on at least a weekly basis), some were related to specific physical goals (e.g. be able to walk for one hour without having to rest), some were related to the development of strategies aimed at compensating for cognitive deficits (e.g. Steven will rate himself and be rated by the team as using strategies effectively for planning and organising activities, for managing attentional problems in functional settings, for managing impulsivity, for managing spelling difficulties), and one related to increasing writing speed. He also worked to increase his understanding of his difficulties.

The first half of Steven's programme, the intensive phase, included group work, individual sessions with members of the interdisciplinary team. Steven learned to manage his tendency to be impulsive with a range of techniques. He was able to identify that one factor causing him to act impulsively, particularly in conversations, was a concern that he would forget things if he did not say them straight away. He therefore learned to make notes during conversations, particularly in his work setting. He developed his use of an electronic organiser in order to improve his general management of his schedule. He also learned 'active listening' (basic counselling) skills, in order to improve his attention to conversations and to encourage him to listen properly in conversations as a means of reducing his tendency to jump in and interrupt. Through attendance at an Attention and Problem-Solving Group (see Evans, 2003 for details of this group) Steven also learned to use a problem-solving framework, which he used 'in mind', and this seemed to help him to slow down his approach to problems. The group involves learning about the steps involved in problems solving (recognising a problem, identifying a goal, generating potential solutions, deciding on solution and plan, implementing plan, monitoring success), practising steps with exercises and learning to use the framework initially in the form of an external cue and then as a mental checklist. A cue-sticker, initially placed on his electronic organiser and later entered on to his organiser for him to see every day in the morning, reminded him to 'Stop! Slow Down!' Steven became less impulsive, though it was noted that while this improved considerably in situations with more structure, in free-flowing interactions in which he was very engaged, it was more difficult for him to manage his impulsivity. Steven's difficulties with attention and concentration were helped through the use of the strategies for managing impulsivity. However, he also identified that in some situations it was necessary for him to try to manage his environment to reduce distractions. He was able to do this at work through organising his work setting. To improve spelling Steven had to develop his awareness of letter–sound relationships (consonants then vowels) and then work on a strategy of splitting words into syllables so that he could apply a phonetic approach to spelling. Further assessment of writing suggested that this was affected by a number of problems, including impaired fine motor control and coordination, difficulty forming some letters, difficulty spelling and working-memory problems (only being able to hold one word in mind when copying something). An adapted pen had little effect on speed. He practised pre-writing skills and then writing tasks and it was found that he could increase his speed (by 15 per cent, but not 20 per cent), but in that case quality of writing was poorer, or he could increase quality, but with no increase in speed. It was decided that as he was not required to write that often, the latter improvement was the more beneficial. Walking tolerance was improved through practice and Steven developed a good routine of attending the gym and swimming.

With regard to work, Steven identified with work colleagues a potential work role, which involved training and helping to manage a sales team. He attended work on a part-time basis during the integration phase of his programme. As part of the programme, Steven was asked to identify the situations or tasks at work that his difficulties could affect and how he could use strategies he had been learning to try to minimise the impact of his difficulties. For example, he was able to identify how impulsivity problems could impact on his ability to run meetings, to listen properly to staff and to give good, considered, advice. Table 9.2 shows a list of problem areas, situations at work where those problems might have an impact and the strategies he uses to compensate. Initial feedback from colleagues identified that he did have an aggressive and impulsive style in some situations at work, but over time this improved considerably.

Outcome

At the end of the programme Steven was working three days a week, which he then increased to four days. It was reported that he was able to take on the training of new and existing staff in sales techniques. He was referred to his local service for ongoing monitoring, which settled into a pattern of monthly sessions, which Steven reported he valued as a means of helping him to maintain use of strategies.

Table 9.2 Steven's list of problem areas, situations that could be affected and strategies to overcome difficulties

Problem area	Situations that might be affected	Strategies to compensate for problem
Working memory	Conversations, meetings, advising staff	Notes Dictaphone
Attention and impulsivity	Meetings, listening to staff; advising staff; reading	Stop! Slow down Active listening Manage the environment to reduce distractions
Memory	Reading work (e.g. sales technique texts) Conversations (incidental requests)	Use notes and aids Use associations Use PQRST Active listening – attend carefully to information
Communication (speaking and writing)	Meetings; giving advice; writing notes and reports.	Manage impulsivity as above Manage fatigue as below Use spelling strategies Use others (e.g. secretary) to check work Use joined writing
Fatigue	All aspects of work	Build up gradually at work Manage time Pacing! Keep up with fitness work

Summary and Conclusions

The areas of attention and executive functioning are still developing in terms of theory, assessment and rehabilitation. The concept of executive functioning, and the notion of a dysexecutive syndrome, has proved a useful step away from the anatomically based idea of a frontal lobe syndrome. However, theoretical developments are moving towards a fractionation of these global concepts in an attempt to identify a number of separate cognitive processes that work together to enable us to plan and problem solve. As these changes in theory take place, assessment tools will need to be adapted and developed to reflect changes in thinking. A prime function of assessment tools should also be to enable the clinician to predict the nature of the problems the individual is likely to experience in day-to-day life. In recent years there have been assessment batteries developed for the assessment of attention and executive functions, which have considerably more face and ecological validity. There have also been developments in the rehabilitation of attention and executive functioning. As with much of cognitive rehabilitation, many of the interventions might be considered to be compensatory strategies (some internal or mental, whilst others are external, utilising aids). Evidence that attention and executive functions can be restored through training programmes is equivocal, but needs to continue to be explored. For most individuals in rehabilitation a range of interventions will need to be used in a systematic way, and this was illustrated in the case of Steven, who managed to return to work as a senior manager. A key factor in Steven's rehabilitation was the coordinated interventions applied by an interdisciplinary neuropsychological rehabilitation team in liaison with Steven, his work colleagues and ongoing support services. Such interdisciplinary working is likely to be the key to more effective treatment of attention and executive dysfunction.

Recommended Reading

Alderman, N. & Ward, A. (1991). Behavioural treatment of the dysexecutive syndrome: Reduction of repetitive speech using response cost and cognitive overlearning. *Neuropsychological Rehabilitation*, *1*, 65–80.
A good example of the use of behaviour modification techniques in the context of severe dysexecutive syndrome and challenging behaviour. Interesting discussion of why certain techniques are not helpful and others are helpful in the context of executive dysfunction.

Baddeley, A.D. & Wilson, B.A. (1988). Frontal amnesia and the dysexecutive syndrome. *Brain and Cognition*, *7*, 212–230.
One of the first accounts of the notion of a dysexecutive syndrome and how it is manifested in day-to-day problems.

von Cramon, D., Matthes-von Cramon, G. & Mai, N. (1991). Problem-solving deficits in brain injured patients: A therapeutic approach. *Neuropsychological Rehabilitation*, *1*, 45–64.
Description and evaluation of a treatment group for problem-solving difficulties, which involves practice on exercises designed to make demands characteristic of the various stages of the problem-solving process.

Goldstein, L.H. & McNeil, J. (Eds.) (2004). *Clinical neuropsychology: A practical guide to assessment and management*. Chichester: Wiley.
A textbook which has chapters that provide very useful overviews of approaches to management of attention and executive disorders.

Halligan, P. & Wade, D. (Eds.) (2005). *The effectiveness of rehabilitation for cognitive deficits*. Oxford: Oxford University Press.
A text which covers theory, assessment and approaches to rehabilitation of a range of cognitive disorders, including chapters on attention and executive functioning.

Shallice, T. & Burgess, P. (1991). Deficits in strategy application following frontal lobe damage in man. *Brain*, *144*, 727–741.
Key paper that discusses the concept of executive function after frontal lobe injury, and the limitations of traditional tests of frontal lobe functioning. Also introduces the Six Elements and Multiple Errands Tests.

References

Alderman, N. & Burgess, P.W. (1990). Integrating cognition and behaviour: A pragmatic approach to brain injury rehabilitation. In R.Ll. Wood & I. Fussey (Eds.) *Cognitive rehabilitation in perspective* (pp.204–228). Basingstoke: Taylor and Francis.

Alderman, N. & Burgess, P. (1994). A comparison of treatment methods for behaviour disorder following herpes simplex encephalitis. *Neuropsychological Rehabilitation*, *4*, 31–48.

Alderman, N., Burgess, P.W., Knight, C. & Henman, C. (2003). Ecological validity of a simplified version of the multiple errands shopping test. *Journal of the International Neuropsychological Society*, *9*, 31–44.

Alderman, N. & Ward, A. (1991). Behavioural treatment of the dysexecutive syndrome: Reduction of repetitive speech using response cost and cognitive overlearning. *Neuropsychological Rehabilitation*, *1*, 65–80.

Baddeley, A.D. (1986). *Working memory*. Oxford: Oxford University Press.

Baddeley, A.D. & Wilson, B.A. (1988). Frontal amnesia and the dysexecutive syndrome. *Brain and Cognition*, *7*, 212–230.

Bennett, P.C., Ong, B. & Ponsford, J. (2005). Measuring executive dysfunction in an acute rehabilitation setting: Using the dysexecutive questionnaire (DEX). *Journal of the International Neuropsychological Society*, *11*, 376–385.

Burgess, P.W., Alderman, N., Evans, J.J., Emslie, H. & Wilson, B.A. (1998). The ecological validity of tests of executive function. *Journal of the International Neuropsychological Society*, *4*, 547–558.

Burgess, P.W. & Shallice, T. (1997). *Hayling and Brixton Tests*. London: Harcourt.

Burke, W.H., Zencius, A.H., Wesolowski, M.D. & Doubleday, F. (1991). Improving executive function disorders in brain injured clients. *Brain Injury*, *5*, 241–252.

Cicerone, K.D. & Wood, J.C. (1987). Planning disorder after closed head injury: A case study. *Archives of Physical Medicine and Rehabilitation*, *68*, 111–115.

von Cramon, D. & Matthes-von Cramon, G. (1992). Reflections on the treatment of brain injured patients suffering from problem-solving disorders. *Neuropsychological Rehabilitation*, *2*, 207–230.

von Cramon, D. & Matthes-von Cramon, G. (1995). Back to work with a chronic dysexecutive syndrome. *Neuropsychological Rehabilitation*, *4*, 399–417.

von Cramon, D., Matthes-von Cramon, G. & Mai, N. (1991). Problem-solving deficits in brain injured patients: A therapeutic approach. *Neuropsychological Rehabilitation*, *1*, 45–64.

Crepeau, F. & Scherzer, P. (1993). Predictors and indicators of work status after traumatic brain injury: A meta analysis. *Neuropsychological Rehabilitation*, *3*(1), 5–35.

Crepeau, F., Scherzer, P., Belleville, S. & Desmarais, G. (1997). A qualitative analysis of central executive disorders in a real-life work situation. *Neuropsycholgical Rehabilitation*, *7*, 147–165.

Delis, D.C., Kaplan, E. & Kramer, J.H. (2001). *Delis–Kaplan executive function system*. San Antonio, TX: Harcourt.

Dritschel, B.H., Kogan, L., Burton, A., Burton, E. & Goddard, L. (1998). Everyday planning difficulties following brain injury: A role for autobiographical memory. *Brain Injury*, *12*, 875–886.

Duncan, J. (1986). Disorganisation of behaviour after frontal lobe damage. *Cognitive Neuropsychology*, *3*, 271–290.

Duncan, J. (1993). Selection of input and goal in the control of behaviour. In A.D. Baddeley & L. Weiskrantz (Eds.) *Attention: Selection, awareness and control: A tribute to Donald Broadbent* (pp.53–71). Oxford: OUP.

Eslinger, P.J. & Damasio, A.R. (1985). Severe disturbance of higher cognition after bilateral frontal lobe ablation: Patient EVR. *Neurology, Cleveland*, *35*, 1731–1741.

Eslinger, P.J., Grattan, L.M. & Geder, L. (1995). Impact of frontal lobes on rehabilitation and recovery from acute brain injury. *NeuroRehabilitation*, *5*, 161–182.

Evans, J.J. (2003). Rehabilitation of executive deficits. In B.A. Wilson (Ed.) *Neuropsychological rehabilitation: Theory and Practice* (pp.53–70). Lisse: Swets and Zeitlinger.

Evans, J.J., Emslie, H. & Wilson, B.A. (1998). External cueing systems in the rehabilitation of executive impairments of action. *Journal of the International Neuropsychological Society*, *4*, 399–408.

Evans, J.J., Needham, P., Wilson, B.A. & Brentnall, S. (2003). Which memory impaired people make good use of memory aids? Results of a survey of people with acquired brain injury. *Journal of the International Neuropsychological Society*, *9*, 925–935.

Gray, J. & Robertson, I.H. (1989). Remediation of attentional difficulties following brain injury: Three experimental case studies. *Brain Injury*, *3*, 163–170.

Gray, J., Robertson, I.H., Pentland, B. & Anderson, S.I. (1992). Microcomputer based cognitive rehabilitation for brain damage: A randomised group controlled trial. *Neuropsychological Rehabilitation*, *2*, 97–116.

Hersh, N. & Treadgold, L. (1994). *Prosthetic memory and cueing for survivors of traumatic brain injury*. Unpublished report obtainable from Interactive Proactive Mnemonic Systems, 6657 Camelia Drive, San Jose, California.

Hewitt, J., Evans, J.J. & Dritchel, B. (2000). *Improving planning skills in people with traumatic brain injury through the use of an autobiographical episodic memory cueing procedure*. Paper presented at the Autumn Meeting of the British Neuropsychological Society, 23 November, Nottingham, UK.

Knight, C., Alderman, N. & Burgess, P.W. (2002). Development of a simplified version of the multiple errands test for use in hospital settings. *Neuropsychological Rehabilitation*, *12*(3), 231–255.

Levine, B., Robertson, I.H., Clare, L., Carter, G., Hong, J., Wilson, B.A., *et al.* (2000). Rehabilitation of executive functioning: An experimental-clinical validation of Goal Management Training. *Journal of the International Neuropsychological Society*, *6*, 299–312.

Lezak, M.D. (1995). *Neuropsychological rehabilitation* (2nd edn). Oxford: OUP.

Luria, A.R. (1966). *Higher cortical functions in man*. New York: Basic Books.

Luria, A.R. (1973). *The working brain: An introduction to neuropsychology*. New York: Basic Books.

Manly, T., Hawkins, K., Evans, J.J., Woldt, K. & Robertson, I.H. (2002). Rehabilitation of executive function: Facilitation of effective goal management on tasks using periodic auditory alerts. *Neuropsychologia*, *40*, 271–281.

Manly, T. & Mattingly, J. (2004). Visuospatial and attentional disorders. In L.H. Goldstein & J. McNeil (Eds.) *Clinical neuropsychology: A practical guide to assessment and management* (pp.229–252). Chichester: Wiley.

Miotto, E. & Evans, J.J. (2005). *Rehabilitation of executive functioning: A controlled cross-over study of an attention and problem-solving group intervention*. Paper presented at Neuropsychological Rehabilitation, University of Galway, Ireland, 11–12 July.

Morris, R.G., Ahmed, S., Syed, G.M. & Toone, B.K. (1993). Neural correlates of planning ability: Frontal lobe activation during the Tower of London test. *Neuropsychologia*, *31*, 1367–1378.

O'Brien, K.P., Prigatano, G.P. & Pittman, H.W. (1988). Neurobehavioural education of a patient and spouse following right frontal oligodendroglioma excision. *Neuropsychology*, 2, 145–159.

Ponsford, J. (2000). Attention. In G. Groth-Marnet (Ed.) *Neuropsychological assessment in clinical practice* (pp.355–400). New York: Wiley.

Ponsford, J. & Kinsella, G. (1988). Evaluation of a remedial programme for attentional deficits following closed head injury. *Journal of Clinical and Experimental Neuropsychology, 10*, 693–708.

Posner, M. & Peterson, S.E. (1990). The attention system of the human brain. *Annual Review of Neuroscience, 13*, 25–42.

Rath, J.F., Simon D., Langenbahn, D.M., Sherr, L. & Diller, L. (2003). Group treatment of problem solving deficits in outpatients with traumatic brain injury: A randomized outcome study. *Neuropsychological Rehabilitation, 13*, 461–488.

Robbins, T.W. (1996). Dissociating executive functions of the prefrontal cortex. *Philosophical Transactions: Biological Sciences, 351*, 1463–1471.

Robertson, I.H. (1996). *Goal Management Training: A clinical manual.* Cambridge: PsyConsult.

Robertson, I.H. (1999). The rehabilitation of attention. In D.T. Stuss, G. Winocur & I.H. Robertson (Eds.) *Cognitive rehabilitation* (pp.302–313). Cambridge: CUP.

Robertson, I.H., Manly, T., Andrade, J., Baddeley, B. & Yiend, J. (1997a). Oops! Performance correlates of everyday attentional failures: The Sustained Attention to Response Task. *Neuropsychologia, 35*, 747–58

Robertson, I.H., Ridgeway, V., Greenfield, E. & Parr, A. (1997b). Motor recovery after stroke depends on intact sustained attention: A two-year follow up study. *Neuropsychology, 11*, 290–295.

Robertson, I.H., Tegner, R., Tham, K., Lo, A. & Nimmo-Smith, I. (1995). Sustained attention training for unilateral neglect: Theoretical and rehabilitation implications. *Journal of Clinical and Experimental Neuropsychology, 17*, 416–430.

Robertson, I.H., Ward, T., Ridgeway, V. & Nimmo-Smith, I. (1994). *The Test of Everyday Attention.* Flempton: Thames Valley Test Company.

Rylander, G. (1939). *Personality changes after operations on the frontal lobes. Acta Psychiatrica et Neurologica* Supplementum XX. Copenhagen: Ejnar Munksgaard.

Sahakian, B.J., Coull, J.J. & Hodges, J.R. (1994). Selective enhancement of executive function in a patient with dementia of the frontal lobe type. *Journal of Neurology, Neurosurgery and Psychiatry, 57*, 120–121.

Shallice, T. (1988). *From neuropsychology to mental structure.* Cambridge: Cambridge University Press.

Shallice, T. & Burgess, P. (1991). Deficits in strategy application following frontal lobe damage in man. *Brain, 144*, 727–741.

Shallice, T. & Burgess, P. (1996). The domain of the supervisory process and temporal organisation of behaviour. *Philosophical Transactions: Biological Sciences, 351*, 1405–1412.

Sturm, W., Dahman, W., Hartje, W. & Willmes, K (1983). Ergebnisse eines Trainginsprogramms zur Verbesserung der visuellen Auffassungsshnelligkeit und Konzentrationsfahigkeit bei Hirngeschaditgen. *Archiv für Psychiatrie und Nervenkrankheiten, 233*, 9–22.

Sturm, W., Willmes, K., Orgass, B. & Hartje, W. (1997). Do specific attention deficits need specific training? *Neuropsychological Rehabilitation, 7*, 81–176.

Wilkins, A.J., Shallice, T. & McCarthy, R. (1987). Frontal lesions and sustained attention. *Neuropsychologia, 25*, 359–365.

Wilson, B.A., Alderman, N., Burgess, P. Emslie, H. & Evans, J.J. (1996). *The Behavioural Assessment of the Dysexecutive Syndrome.* Flempton: Thames Valley Test Company.

Wilson, B.A., Evans, J.J., Brentnall, S., Bremner, S., Keohane, C. & Williams, W.H. (2000). The Oliver Zangwill Centre for Neuropsychological Rehabilitation: A partnership between health care and rehabilitation research. In A-L. Christensen & B.P. Uzzell (Eds.) *International handbook of neuropsychological rehabilitation* (pp.231–246). New York: Kluwer Academic/Plenum Publishers.

Wilson, B.A., Evans, J.J., Emslie, H. & Malinek, V. (1997). Evaluation of NeuroPage: A new memory aid. *Journal of Neurology, Neurosurgery and Psychiatry*, *63*, 113–115.

Van Zomeren, A.H. & Brouwer, W.H. (1994). *Clinical neuropsychological assessment of attention*. New York: Oxford University Press.

Van Zomeren, A.H. & Spikman, J. (2005). Assessment of attention. In P. Halligan & D. Wade (Eds.) *The effectiveness of rehabilitation for cognitive deficits* (pp.71–80). Oxford: Oxford University Press.

d'Zurilla, T.J. & Goldfried, M.R. (1971). Problem-solving and behaviour modification. *Journal of Abnormal Psychology*, *78*, 107–126.

Part III

Behavioural and Emotional Interventions

10

Behaviour Problems

Andrew D. Worthington and Rodger Ll. Wood

Introduction

Traumatic brain injury (TBI) is a major cause of long-term disability in industrialised and developing countries across the world. The World Health Organisation has predicted that road accidents alone, which account for many instances of TBI, will constitute the third largest contributor to the global burden of disease and disability (after heart disease and depression) by 2015 (Murray & Lopez, 1997). In terms of long-term outcome and recovery, it has been recognised for some time that disturbances of mood and behaviour constitute the most debilitating aspects of brain injury (Brooks *et al.*, 1983; MacLean *et al.*, 1983; Oddy *et al.*, 1985; Tate, 1987). In contrast to impairments of specific cognitive abilities such as reading or memory, disturbances of emotion and behaviour (often accompanied by executive dysfunction) are more likely to result in wholesale changes in a person's character or personality. The term neurobehavioural disability (Wood, 2001) has been adopted to encompass the diverse range of disabilities associated with these underlying executive, emotional and behavioural disorders. The key feature of neurobehavioural disability is that there is a recognised cerebral basis to a clinical presentation, even if it is not sufficient to account for all the apparent disability (Wood & Worthington, 2001a). The resulting changes in personality are often reported by family members as constituting the greatest source of stress and burden (Brooks & McKinlay, 1983; Lezak, 1978). Successful treatment of behaviour disorders is therefore fundamental to reducing the barriers to community integration and achieving optimal psychosocial outcomes (Eames & Wood, 1985; NIH, 1999; Ponsford *et al.*, 1995; Rappaport *et al.*, 1989). The purpose of this chapter is to outline the nature of behaviour and personality disorders after TBI (linking these to different forms of brain damage or dysfunction where possible) in order to provide a rational basis for selecting and evaluating treatment.

Understanding Behaviour Disorder after TBI

Rehabilitation, as many readers will be fully aware, is a complex undertaking. The primary concern is with physical, cognitive, emotional and behavioural changes secondary to neurological insult. However, brain injury often occurs in the context of existing health problems, including concurrent mental health difficulties, which may compromise recovery. We know, for instance, that outcomes are poorer for people with a history of alcohol or substance abuse (Bogner *et al.*, 2001; Bombardier *et al.*, 2002) and poor academic achievement (Haas *et al.*, 1987). Medical conditions which were previously well controlled, such as diabetes or epilepsy, can become life-threatening after brain injury. Behavioural disturbance after TBI may exacerbate existing medical vulnerabilities and anti-social traits. Socially too, the onset of brain injury can threaten just about every aspect of a person's life: their work and home-life, the ability to drive, play sport, and manage their finances. These diverse aspects of everyday living are all legitimate concerns for a rehabilitative process that seeks to reduce handicap associated with disability and increase participation in social roles.

In this context it can be appreciated that the management of behaviour disorders poses particular problems for rehabilitation practitioners. Behaviour disorder can be exacerbated by, and contribute to, other deficits in a variety of ways, summarised by Wood and Worthington (2001a), as follows:

- Attention and information processing deficits can contribute to poor comprehension and judgment, as well as fatigue, irritability and poor learning.
- Executive dysfunction can impede execution of adaptive behaviour, and can lead to defective appraisal of situations resulting in inappropriate behaviour.
- Ability to cooperate with therapy can be undermined by disinhibition, lability of mood, intolerance and impulsive tendencies resulting from damage to regulatory mechanisms.
- Personality change following brain injury may be associated with a degree of denial, reduced self-awareness or *anosognosia*[1] with the result that a person does not demonstrate appreciation of the significance of their disabilities.

The constraints imposed by brain injury on social independence are considerable, but the nature of neurobehavioural disability and its relationship to brain dysfunction are not fully appreciated by many clinicians. One reason for this is that many individuals who are seriously handicapped by disorders of behaviour and personality after TBI often have no physical disability and may not be significantly impaired in respect of cognitive function (Lezak, 1995; Newcombe, 1987). Often clinicians have to rely on information obtained from relatives to elucidate the full impact of cognitive and personality changes on personal relationships and social functioning (see Powell & Wood, 2001). Where possible, one should seek to obtain information from structured observations undertaken over many days and weeks. This should constitute the initial basis of any admission to a specialist centre for treatment (and is far more fruitful than brief formal clinical assessment) but some form of structured record-keeping can also be instigated at home with relatives (Powell & Wood, 2001; Wood & Worthington, 2001b).

Behaviour problems and personality changes after brain injury are the product of complex interactions involving neurological disabilities, social demands, previously established behaviour patterns, and personal reactions to a combination of these factors. However, as Lezak (1995) points out, patients with similar lesions can also show different patterns of impairment and behaviour change. She concludes that the notion of 'brain damage' is useful as an organising concept for a broad range of behaviour disorders but when dealing with individual patients it only becomes meaningful to talk in terms of specific behavioural dysfunction. Although this is generally accepted (and hence the unhelpful term 'frontal lobe syndrome' is now rarely used), there is no formal taxonomy of behaviour disorders to help clinicians distinguish organic consequences of TBI from a person's psychological reactions to injury. Indeed, some authorities suggest that such distinctions are meaningless (Ben-Yishay & Gold, 1990) and it is important to recognise that 'behavioural, cognitive and emotional sequelae of even minor head injuries may be organically based' (p.195). Certainly, inappropriate use of psychiatric constructs leads to questionable diagnoses (such as psychosis) during post-traumatic amnesia (PTA) and an over-diagnosis of depression in patients with reduced drive or motivation (see below). The influence of psychiatric terminology is apparent in describing such organically induced losses as a 'pseudo-depression' (Stuss & Benson, 1986). One still encounters terms like 'pseudo-psychopathy' (Stuss & Benson, 1986) and 'acquired sociopathy' (Blair & Cipolotti, 2000) in relation to disturbances of social conduct resulting from frontal brain damage. Moreover, the distinction between positive and negative symptoms in psychiatry resonates in the differentiation between negative and positive disorders of behaviour (Wood & Eames 1981). Positive disorders are those that actively interfere with rehabilitation and social reintegration. Positive signs include aggression, disinhibition, intolerance and emotional lability. Negative signs represent problems because of a patient's passivity, and essential lack of behaviour. Negative signs reflect the relative absence of productive, effortful, interested or motivated behaviour. Such behaviours act as an obstacle to the amount or quality of cooperation patients can give in rehabilitation and therefore, reduce a patient's potential for recovery. Apathy, lethargy and a lack of motivation to cooperate in therapy are just as serious an obstacle to the achievement of rehabilitation goals as are the more intrusive and purposeful disorders of behaviour. The remainder of this chapter will address the identification and treatment of different forms of behaviour disorder from a psychological perspective.

The Organic Basis of Behaviour and Personality Problems after TBI

Neuropsychology is primarily concerned with the relationships between brain and behaviour, and contemporary neuropsychological theory is heavily influenced by the notion of modularity as an organising principle (Shallice, 1988). This means that damage to certain areas or circuits within the brain will produce certain forms of impairment while leaving other functions relatively unimpaired. Likewise, the severity of neurobehavioural disability reflects the severity of damage to particular brain regions rather than simply being proportionate to the overall amount of brain damage (the latter amounting to a theory of 'mass action', now largely discredited). Think about your computer and you have an idea how it is feasible for one software package to have a glitch without it necessarily affecting the operation of another. This theoretical position dominates neuropsychology because it is widely supported by research indicating that certain types of brain dysfunction can be linked to particular disorders of cognition and behaviour. If this relationship can be established it may be easier to predict patterns of recovery, or to understand variations of behaviour in different situations, or in response to different treatment methods. There is now general acceptance in the clinical neurosciences that the majority of behaviour and personality disorders after TBI are linked, to some degree at least, with damage to the frontal systems of the brain. The prefrontal cortex in particular is believed to be a critical region with many specialised areas operating discrete cognitive processes (Braver *et al.*, 2002). The matter is more complicated if one accepts that brain circuits or systems are maintained in balance, such that damage to system A may cause system B (the intact system) to take precedence in a way that would not occur if both were left intact or damaged to an equal extent (LeVere, 1988). This has important implications for understanding behaviour disorder because intelligent adaptive behaviour is dependent on effective mechanisms of cognitive control. When it is the control itself that is lacking, behaviour may reflect inappropriate use of intact cognitive functions, rather than operation of an appropriate but defective skill. Consider the contrast between the disinhibited use of a colourful vocabulary and the inability to produce the right words. Both convey a level of disability in social situations, but in the former case the problem is one of the application of language, not in language *per se*.

As a guide to such possibilities, clinicians should pay close attention to the mechanism of injury in a case of TBI, as it is an important factor determining the type of brain injury sustained. In turn, this helps clinicians predict future patterns of behaviour and personality. Professionals should make it part of their assessment routine to find out as much as possible about the circumstances and nature of a person's brain injury. Most TBIs are closed head injuries (i.e. do not involve penetration of the cranium), the majority of which are caused by road accidents. Where there is evidence that speed has been involved in the injury (such as a road accident or a fall from height) one should remember that the frontal systems of the brain are particularly vulnerable to decelerative mechanisms of closed head injury (Adams *et al.*, 1982; Pang, 1989). The resulting damage is found predominantly around the orbital, medial and dorso-lateral areas of the prefrontal cortex, as well as the anterior temporal regions (Tronsco & Gordon, 1996). Following TBI the location and extent of frontal brain injury are largely responsible for the behavioural presentation. In many cases, especially where neuronal damage is diffuse, the clinical picture is one of mixed cognitive, emotional and behavioural consequences.

Behavioural Syndromes

Formal clinical nomenclatures, in the form of ICD-10 and DSM-IV codes, are not particularly helpful when trying to understand the nature and character of behaviour and personality disorders after TBI. DSM-IV (APA, 2000) contains an Axis I reference to 'personality disorder due to a general medical condition' (310.1) which is subdivided according to the predominant features (e.g. disinhibition, aggression, lability, apathy). ICD-10 (WHO, 1992) has the category 'organic personality disorder' (F07.0), comprising such characteristics as: disinhibited, tactless and over-familiar behaviour; being over-talkative, making inappropriate jokes that reflect errors of judgement and sexual indiscretion; a fatuous, euphoric mood associated with a lack of regard for the feelings of others; poor attention and diminished insight. The ICD classification essentially describes one cluster of behaviour characteristics, usually seen in association with orbito-frontal injury, whereas at least three syndromal clusters have been outlined which can have a serious impact on social behaviour (Cummings, 1985; Stuss & Benson, 1986). Each syndrome has distinct features that can be associated with different anatomical systems within the fronto-temporal complex. However, the syndromes are not mutually exclusive and clinically one finds that a mixture of behavioural characteristics is more common than the expression of a single 'frontal syndrome'.

Orbital-frontal syndrome

The orbito-frontal cortex is strongly implicated in social and emotional judgements (Moll *et al.*, 2005) and the formation of stimulus-reinforcement associations (Rolls, 1999, 2002). Damage to this area is therefore commonly associated with anti-social conduct. The presentation largely corresponds to the diagnosis of organic personality disorder referred to in ICD-10. It incorporates such features as disinhibition; acting impulsively without thought of consequences; shallow affect; a lack of concern for social values or correct performance; distractibility, poor self-awareness and social judgement. Mood is often euphoric, sometimes accompanied by inappropriate jocularity (*witzlsuch*); an over-active, erratic, behaviour pattern, with a low tolerance of frustration; emotional lability, unstable, easily irritated, egocentric, with short-lived enthusiasm for ill-judged projects. Such patients often experience weaknesses of attention and information processing that interfere with day-to-day memory and general problem solving but few other neurological or neuropsychological abnormalities (Varney & Menefee, 1993). Nies (1999), for example, reported a 47-year-old woman with a right inferior orbito-frontal lesion who showed minimal problems on neuropsychological testing. Yet she exhibited signs of poor social judgement and emotional insensitivity resulting in an inability to manager her own business and social relationships.

Orbital-frontal patients demonstrate impairment of high-level judgement that involves anticipation of consequences, empathy and decision making but typically do not exhibit marked cognitive impairment of the kind associated with dorso-lateral frontal damage (see below). Orbito-frontal dysfunction may be quite subtle but it is often pervasive and may have a devastating effect in real-life situations because of the role of the orbital-frontal system in social behaviour. In cases of mild head injury the absence of confirmed neuropsychological deficit does not exclude the possibility of genuine psycho-social problems arising from orbito-frontal damage. In more severe cases behaviour disorder is thought to arise either as a result of poor inhibition of aggressive impulses in response to threat (the basis for the somatic marker hypothesis of Damasio *et al.* (1999)), or from poor perception of social cues

– the so-called social response reversal model (Blair, 2001). Impulsive, reactive aggression is particularly associated with damage to orbito-frontal regions (Brower & Price, 2001). Clinicians should be aware of the diversity of psycho-social sequelae incorporating self-awareness, sensitivity to the impact of one's behaviour on others and self-regulation.

Medial-frontal syndrome

This syndrome is characterised by low arousal, absence of drive and poor motivation. It has been variously identified with the mesial or medial and ventral aspects of the frontal lobes, and therefore is known by a variety of terms. Furthermore, due to anatomical proximity to the orbito-frontal cortex, patients with medial frontal damage often present with a combination of signs and symptoms, hence use of hybrid terms like 'orbito-medial frontal syndrome' (Malloy *et al.*, 1993). Likewise the notion of a ventro-medial area (incorporating some orbital cortex) has been proposed as a key region for assimilating emotion and behaviour (Tranel, 2002). Notwithstanding these nuances of terminology, it is important for the clinician to understand the distinct features of damage to the ventral and medial aspects of the frontal lobes.

Typically patients appear lethargic and apathetic, and are sometimes referred to as showing *adynamia*, a state often misinterpreted as depression or dementia though the patient usually denies low mood. In acute serious conditions the patient appears *akinetic* (i.e. mute, lacking spontaneous movement, and failing to respond to command). Frontal lobe lesions are among the localised disorders producing catatonia with lesions particularly located in the inferior and medial regions (Cummings, 1985). Equally important, however, is the notion that ventral and basal frontal regions are intimately connected to subcortical structures – not least the basal ganglia – which form numerous fronto-subcortical circuits (also implicating areas such as the cingulate gyrus, and cerebellum). Injury that spares white matter connections to other regions have a better prognosis (Eslinger & Geder, 2000). Unfortunately, TBI usually produces diffuse damage. This means that disruption to any part of these neural pathways can lead to significant frontal lobe dysfunction (i.e. both the apathetic ventro-medial picture and the dysexective dorsolateral presentation) without any clear evidence of frontal lobe damage (see Passingham, 1993).

In chronic states *bradykinesia* (poverty of movement) and lack of expressiveness has been described (Eames, 1990). These features are often seen in association with a lack of spontaneity and a low level of activity, from which many patients can be temporarily roused by novel stimuli or a very stimulating environment. The most frequent characteristic is *abulia* (inability to carry out voluntary actions due to loss of volition) associated with loss of dopamingeric neurons in the meso-cingulate circuit (Fisher, 1983). Patients can be briefly energised into action with sufficient environmental stimulation or a contextually relevant trigger (e.g. the telephone ringing). In milder cases, patients appear placid and less active. Disorders of mobility associated with medial frontal injury may respond to structured behavioural intervention (Worthington *et al.*, 1997). Clinical experience also suggests that at least some patients with prefrontal injury may benefit from treatment with bromocriptine, a dopamine agonist (Barrett, 1991; McDowell *et al.*, 1998; Powell *et al.*, 1996).

Bromocriptine is effective in response to so-called *extrapyramidal signs* – involuntary movements such as tremor and restlessness (Lieberman *et al.*, 1989). Hence when the behavioural features of abulia are seen in combination with extrapyramidal signs, suggesting subcortical involvement, this treatment should be explored (Ross & Stewart, 1981), though it can have adverse effects (Zasler, 1995).

Dorso-lateral frontal syndrome

Sometimes referred to as the frontal convexity syndrome, this behavioural type can share features of impaired social perception, inability to sustain affection and shallow affect that typify the orbito-frontal syndrome (Mah *et al.*, 2004). The most predominant features of dorsolateral damage, however, are those associated with executive dysfunction, such as poor initiative, an inability to plan, sequence, organise or sustain goal-directed behaviour, all of which lead to a loss of response capability. Functional imaging studies reveal that dorsolateral prefontal cortex is involved in working memory tasks (Bunge *et al.*, 2001; Petrides *et al.*, 1993) and verbal self-monitoring (McGuire *et al.*, 1996). Experimental studies also suggest that the region is important for multi-tasking (Burgess *et al.*, 2000). Consequently, dorsolateral damage produces widespread executive dysfunction which can undermine key cognitive skills underpinning social behaviour. Distractibility and an inability to maintain a way of thinking mean that patients lose track of ideas or activities in which they are engaged. Thinking is often quite concrete, they fail to abstract or categorise ideas and actions, or display difficulty interpreting idioms or metaphors which is a major reason for their failure to recognise or interpret social cues or to learn from normal social experience. Consequently, persons with dorsolateral damage are more likely to reveal signs of frontal dysfunction on neuropsychological assessment than are those with damage to other prefrontal regions.

Behavioural legacies of dorsolateral damage can be more apparent than cognitive deficits revealed by traditional psychometric evaluation. Many display a stereotyped, rigid, ritualistic behaviour pattern, often including 'organic orderliness' and compulsive hoarding. Patients frequently describe how a particular activity or task should be carried out yet fail to apply their knowledge when engaged in the activity. In cognitive terms, this suggests a distinction between the ability to articulate how something is done and the capacity to carry out the activity spontaneously. The first author can vividly recall a patient, asked to raise and lower her arms repeatedly, continuing to do so despite assuring her examiner that she had obeyed his subsequent instruction to place her arms by her side. This striking dissociation was recognised by Luria (1973), who noted 'lesions of the frontal lobes disturb only the most complex forms of regulation of conscious activity and in particular activity which is controlled by motives formulated with the aid of speech' (p.199).

Mechanisms Underlying Behaviour Disorders

The neurological tradition of describing behaviour in terms of syndromes has its limitations, although, as far as the frontal lobes are concerned, there is a robustness to the broad distinctions between different 'frontal presentations' described above. In response to the weakness of gross anatomical approaches (such as 'frontal lobe syndrome') psychologists have been instrumental in devising models of brain function which cut across and elaborate the functions of particular brain regions. The term dysexecutive syndrome is now in widespread use (Baddeley & Wilson, 1988) to describe a diverse range of cognitive, emotional and behavioural sequelae of brain dysfunction. It should be borne in mind however, that executive deficits can be observed without evident frontal lobe damage, for example after cerebellar lesions (Levisohn *et al.*, 2000; Schmahmann & Sherman, 1998; Silveri *et al.*, 1998). Conversely, frontal lobe injury can occur without manifest executive dysfunction. Thus the clinician must become familiar with both anatomical and functional descriptions of behaviour, as both have their place in understanding and ultimately rehabilitating behaviour disorders.

Models of executive control

Whilst executive disorders, are the subject of another chapter, the role of executive dysfunction in the production of behaviour and personality disorders should not be overlooked or under-emphasised. There are many theories of executive function. Some focus on single objectives like maintaining goals (Duncan *et al.*, 1996) or manipulating information in working memory (Kimberg & Farah, 1993; Petrides, 1998). Others emphasise a core set of control functions that operate in integrated fashion (Fuster, 2002; Norman & Shallice, 1986). Norman and Shallice's (1986) theory of how attention is used to regulate behaviour via a *supervisory attentional system* (SAS) is part of a frontal organising system performing the *programming*, *regulation* and *verification* operations on behaviour which formed an integral part of Luria's influential interpretation of frontal functioning (Luria, 1973).

An alternative approach is to consider the temporal sequence or stages involved in controlling everyday actions, as emphasised in a recent scheme proposed by Worthington (2002). This model distinguished three stages in behavioural control based on the concept of action units or *schemata*. A distinction is made between the preparatory assembling of actions relevant to a task, the initiation of a behaviour, and its subsequent regulation. Such a model, based on an understanding of normal behaviour (Jeannerod, 1997), provides clinicians with a useful heuristic framework for understanding many acquired disorders of behaviour in terms of a breakdown at one of the three key stages of behavioural control (see Table 10.1). Choice of intervention will depend on the stage at which the problem has arisen (Worthington, 2002).

In contrast, the Norman and Shallice SAS is hypothesised to operate across all stages of behavioural organisation but only in certain situations, characterised by:

- planning and decision making;
- error correction and troubleshooting;
- mediating actions in novel activities or situations where responses are not well learned;

Table 10.1 A three-stage cognitive model of the executive basis of behaviour disorders

I	**Schema assembly** Assembling the components for action *Executive deficits at this level cause disorders of goal articulation and planning*
II	**Schema activation** Activation of the required actions *Executive deficits at this level cause disorders of initiation and sequencing*
III	**Schema regulation** Coordination and modification of behaviour once initiated *Executive deficits cause cognitive disorders of monitoring and evaluation and behavioural disorders of inhibition and control*

- mediating actions in activities judged to be dangerous or technically difficult; and
- situations in which one needs to resist a strong habitual response or temptation.

This model has proved useful in thinking about rehabilitation of behaviour disorders that are underpinned by executive dysfunction (Burgess & Alderman, 1990; Burgess & Wood, 1990). Burgess and Wood (1990), for example, argue that in the absence of a fully working SAS there will be a loss of flexibility of thought and reduced ability to solve novel problems. The fact that the control mechanism operates at many levels means that malfunctioning can affect high-level cognitive processes mediating insight and social awareness. In terms of the Norman and Shallice model of information processing, social behaviour can be viewed as a set of 'routines' that are adapted and changed to fit changing social situations. This means that the mannerisms and language adopted will be different when we are socialising with our friends or attending a job interview. How one sits, the tone of one's voice, gestures and affectations will (or should) vary according to the social demands of a situation. These aspects of social interaction are all behavioural schemata which consist of many action units. We move from one action unit or schemata to another, often without conscious awareness, as a result of a *contention-scheduling* process which automatically selects appropriate behavioural schemata (see also Shallice, 1988). However, in conditions where the contention-scheduling process initiates schemata involving anger, for example, considerable conscious supervisory control may be necessary to inhibit a largely reflexive emotional response. Rehabilitation involves retraining self-regulatory skills so that self-restraint can be exercised when it is socially appropriate to do so. The problem for practitioners is that the very processes on which one usually depends for learning (e.g. motivation, concentration and memory) are often deficient after frontal injury. Attempts have been made to advance understanding of behaviour disorders by linking the type of executive deficit to the area of brain injury. For example, damage to frontal-subcortical circuits causes impairments of activation whereas dorsolateral lesions are responsible for subsequent derailing of activity once initiated. Recent evidence, including data from functional imaging studies, suggests that different component processes of the SAS may also have different anatomical substrates (Shallice, 2002).

Thus functional models of behaviour, being based on cognitive processes, offer fresh means of understanding the organic bases of behaviour disorders. However, not all behaviour disturbances after TBI are directly caused by the injury; some seem to be associated with a reaction to the injury or its consequences. Clinicians should become familiar with behaviour disorders of organic origin in order to identify and intervene appropriately. While many behaviour disorders can be characterised as dysfunctions within a cognitive framework (e.g. Worthington, 2002), there is no single scheme that can accommodate all forms of behaviour disturbance. Behaviour disturbance often arises from damage to subcortical structures and the (medial) temporal lobes. It is helpful to consider these in some detail too, because rehabilitation planning and management requires an ability to distinguish neurobehavioural from psychiatric disorders, and to discern in disorders such as aggression and motivation the relative contribution of frontal and non-frontal pathology.

Drive and motivation disorders

Drive has been described as a property of the organism (Wood & Eames, 1981) and a force that activates human impulses (Stuss & Benson, 1986). In an attempt to provide a basis for discriminating the role of drive and motivation in rehabilitation, Wood & Eames (1981) defined motivation as 'the amount of *effort* a person with a given level of *drive* is prepared and *able* to exert in order to achieve a certain *goal*'. Reduction in motivation as a primary organic disorder should be distinguished from reduced motivation as a symptom of depression. It is also important to distinguish deficiencies in drive and motivation from higher-level executive deficits in action planning and initiation. The latter are likely to be associated with other signs of executive dysfunction, whereas the former may occur in the absence of clear frontal damage e.g. after subcortical or brainstem lesions (Habib, 2000).

More recently, Wood (2001) has commented on the relationship between motivation and hedonic responsiveness. He referred to two disorders of motivation, (a) motivational deficit and (b) abnormal motivation. Motivational deficit is characterised by apathy, lethargy, loss of enthusiasm, often mistakenly diagnosed as depression. This has been discussed earlier in the context of medial frontal injury. Abnormal motivation is a more complex problem, involving both conscious and 'unconscious' motivation, making awareness a central issue. Psychodynamically oriented psychologists have considered motivation in terms of denial and other ego-defence mechanisms (Lewis, 1991). Cognitive approaches tend to focus on the modulation of mood upon information processing (e.g. Teasdale, 1993), but cognitive-behavioural constructs such as learned helplessness can also be helpful. The more neurologically inclined have formulated explanations in terms of damage to particular brain regions (Eames, 1992) whereas neuropsychological models have tried to bridge psychological and biological paradigms (Prigatano & Johnson, 2003; Schacter, 1989).

In extreme cases of abnormal motivation, patients may demonstrate curious behaviour reminiscent of game-playing. Experienced observers may note inconsistencies between behaviour under examination and naturalistic settings. The first author recalls a patient providing a detailed drawing of a bicycle when asked to reproduce the Rey complex figure, despite adequate functional memory ability. Responses to questions may be approximate but highly suggestive of the patient 'knowing' at some level the correct answer (the Ganser syndrome). This is akin to the pathological demand avoidance seen in disturbed children (Newson, 1989, cited in Eames, 2001). Alternatively, everyday behaviour may reveal discrepancies between behaviour and apparent disability. Contrasting examples are the so-called 'blind' man who skilfully negotiates his way unaided through the dining area without tripping over any obstacles, and the equally 'blind' lady who managed to bump into every passing tree while walking in the hospital grounds (Wood, 1987). Such instances can be perplexing to the uninitiated and may lead to misdiagnosis. Yet although such phenomena do occur, this remains a controversial and poorly understood aspect of brain injury. Eames (1992) has likened such behaviour to hysteria, because there appears to be a dissociation between forms of awareness, and proposed that structures mediating reward associated with the basal ganglia represent a plausible neurological basis to this condition.

Disorders of inhibitory and regulatory control

Lack of self-control is one of the most common complaints being made by families and carers of brain-injured people (Anderson *et al.*, 2002; Knight *et al.*, 1998; Wood *et al.*, 2005). This incorporates such traits as social and sexual disinhibition, comprising tactless and facetious remarks that cause offence and embarrassment, or more serious and intrusive behaviours that may involve inappropriate touching, lewd comments, public masturbation or sexual assault. Other self-control problems involve poor impulse control, low tolerance, disproportionate emotional reactions which escalate out of control, and a loss of social awareness or the ability to interpret social cues that normally inhibit or redirect behaviour. The cerebral basis for these kinds of behaviour problems is frequently damage to the orbito-frontal cortex. However, the tendency of such problems to increase over time if left untreated suggests that learning plays a part in the development of such problems.

Labile mood and volatile temperament are possibly the most frequent and pervasive behavioural legacies of closed head injury. Shifts of mood are often sudden and occur with an alarming frequency, even though there may be no obvious pattern or cycle. The unpredictable, episodic nature of these moods imposes enormous stress on relatives and has been identified as a significant factor underlying the breakdown of relationships after head injury (Wood & Yuidakul, 1997). Typical mood disorders after head injury include episodes of tense, agitated behaviour, often associated with feelings of fatigue, social withdrawal and headaches (usually referred to as 'a pressure' in the head). The majority of patients experience a depressive phase and this may lead to a misdiagnosis because clinicians may focus on the depressive features without recognising their episodic character in association with other symptoms which are not typical of depressive disorders *per se*. These episodic syndromes are variously referred to as temporo-limbic affective disorders (Eames, 1990) or, in more serious cases, episodic dyscontrol (Elliott, 1982). This is not a recognised 'diagnosis' though it shares features with the DSM-IV category of intermittent explosive disorder or IED (see Table 10.2 – italics added).

Intermittent explosive disorders have been reported in clinical literature for over 100 years. Kaplan (1899) used the term 'explosive diasthesis'. He referred to 'a rage which follows the most trivial cause . . . grotesque gesticulation, excessive movement of the face, . . . explosiveness of speech, cursing and outbreaks of violence, often directed at things; there may or may not be amnesia afterwards. The outburst may terminate in an epileptic fit.' Hooper *et al.* (1945) also describe explosive rage

Table 10.2 Intermittent explosive disorder (DSM-IV)

Failure to resist aggressive impulses resulting in several discrete episodes of serious assaultive acts or damage to property
The degree of aggression is out of proportion to any precipitating psychosocial stressors
The aggressive episodes are *not* better accounted for by another mental disorder, substance or general medical condition *such as head trauma*

following head injury. They point out that rage reactions are different from irritability because they have an explosive element which lifts the behaviour out of a background of normal mood and depression. Elliott (1982), reporting on 262 cases of patients with recurring attacks of uncontrolled rage, described an irregular and unpredictable pattern of angry behaviour with intervals of days, weeks or months. The onset was often sudden with little or no warning, although some cases experienced increasing moodiness for several hours or days (including a feeling of pressure in the head). The outburst itself usually lasts a few minutes but there may be several hours during which the patient is irrational and unreachable. The personality changes for the worse (patient's family usually deploy descriptions such as 'Jekyll and Hyde'). Whilst control is usually absent in respect of the outburst itself, there is some indication of control being present in the *direction* of aggression (the patient will attack furniture, not people). The explosive rage can involve either verbal or physical aggression. When physical there is often a primitive response, comprising biting, spitting, gouging, clawing and stabbing. The episodes are out of character with the patient's usual pattern of behaviour and personality.

Despite head injury being a contra-indication to the diagnosis of IED, the term is used to describe outbursts of aggression associated with epilepsy. Distinct from aggression and irritability following frontal lobe injury, there is a range of episodic disorders of mood which are probably related to dysfunction within the limbic system. One hypothesis links these disorders with epileptiform activity, possibly involving kindling activity which affects dopamine transmission and therefore produces an alteration in mood and behaviour rather than a motor seizure (see Eames & Wood, 2003). A recent study of patients with and without such 'affective aggression' who have temporal lobe epilepsy suggested that there may be a dual pathology. Van Elst (2002) proposed that damage to the amygdala or related structures predisposed patients to hyperarousal (i.e. becoming angry in the context of trivial events), while frontal pathology left patients unable to suppress the resulting behavioural impulses. The first-line treatment should be anti-convulsants – with the best evidence pointing to carbamazepine (Trimble, 1988; Yatham & McHale, 1988) – as this may alleviate symptoms and significantly improve everyday functioning (Roberts *et al.*, 1996). Woody (1988) described associated nursing and behavioural interventions alongside pharmacological treatment in a case of episodic dyscontrol following head injury.

Disorders of insight and social awareness

Severe and circumscribed problems of denial and anosognosia are less frequently seen after TBI than after stroke, but some degree of diminished self-awareness is

Table 10.3 Characteristics of impaired awareness following frontal lobe dysfunction (after Stuss, 1991)

Impaired awareness is related to changes in the Self (i.e. it affects 'self-awareness') and may influence all aspects of behaviour, rather than specific domains of cognition.
Impaired self-awareness is compatible with normal memory and intellectual abilities (including reasoning).
Disorders of self-awareness may fractionate (i.e. may affect some aspects of a person's functioning and not others).
Knowledge is distinct from awareness. Inability to reflect on the implications for oneself of one's knowledge and understanding is often a feature of disturbed self-awareness.
Disturbed self-awareness involves a loss of the sense of immediacy and warmth associated with direct experience, so experience becomes detached from personal meaning.
Disordered self-awareness may incorporate inability to appreciate implications of past experience for the future.

common following TBI. This may take various forms but typically includes a lack of awareness of one's own behaviour or the impact it has on others (Eames & Wood, 1984). In contrast to anosognosia, the person is often very aware of their physical disabilities and may have insight into practical problems of everyday living, but shows no real appreciation of their emotional or behavioural changes (Prigatano, 1996).

Unawareness of deficits depends not only on how severely the brain is damaged, but which regions are damaged, with research suggesting that this may lead to different forms of unawareness (see Prigatano, 1999). Impaired awareness associated with frontal lobe damage has characteristics features (see Table 10.3).

Problems of insight and social awareness following frontal injury are often associated with attentional deficits. The comment made by William James (1890) – 'my experience is what I agree to attend to, only those items I notice shape my mind', is particularly apt. Social awareness depends upon the ability to process and comprehend information in the shape of social cues and then monitor one's response to such cues in order to evaluate its social impact. This allows a person to decide if a response is appropriate or inappropriate, which is a prerequisite for social judgement.

Van Zomeren and Brouwer (1994) interpret impaired social awareness as a problem of social attentiveness. They comment on how relatives of head-injured patients complain that the patient is insensitive or uninterested. They fail to respond to subtle jokes, hearing the words but not perceiving the irony in the voice of the speaker. They argue that such problems can be explained on the basis that social cues are not recognised, or on the basis of slow or otherwise poor information processing. Kreutzer (1993) has also commented on the failure of brain-injured people to recognise social cues, pointing out the implications of this in a work environment. The attentional demands of any social situation are complex, often involving multiple sources of information, numerous distractions, figure–ground distinctions (processing words in conversation from background noise – which may be of greater volume than the conversation), and the ability to sustain conversation to keep track of the conversational content. Social behaviour during such interactions also relies heavily on attentional mechanisms to perceive subtle cues in facial expression, verbal intonation, emotional content of remarks, or the impact of one's own contribution on others (are you being boring, offensive, etc?).

In some cases insight is preserved, in the sense that a person is aware that a behaviour problem exists and that other people suffer as a consequence, but they are not able to judge the impact in order to evaluate the degree to which other people suffer. This is most frequently seen in adolescents who lack maturity and the capacity for empathy. Thomsen (1989) noted that the combination of immaturity and the lack of insight is a poor prognostic indicator as far as social outcome from head trauma is concerned. Problems of awareness can impose major constraints on rehabilitation and the reintegration of head-injured people into the community (Brooks & McKinlay, 1983). Prigatano (1999) argues that the key to improving psycho-social outcome is to promote a person's capacity for self-awareness because this can improve emotional control, acceptance of psychological problems and a willingness to adopt compensatory techniques, as well as better psychological adjustment, and greater ability to interact successfully with others.

Treatment of Behaviour Disorders

Behaviour management in context

The treatment of behaviour problems in brain-injured people presents a major challenge because of the complex diversity of factors that need to be addressed as part of a rehabilitation plan. In addition to premorbid experiences which shape our thinking and personality, clinicians have to consider the emotional impact of: the injury, the change of lifestyle and status, personal adjustment to disability, family attitudes, and the environment in which behaviour problems are displayed. To all these factors one must add the impact of the brain injury itself and how it directly alters awareness, judgement, empathy, emotional expression, and a host of other functions implicit to human relationships and behavioural self-regulation. Ben-Yishay and Gold (1990) expressed the view that brain injury rehabilitation must try to simultaneously address various combinations of cognitive, behavioural and interpersonal problems displayed by patients. They argue that remedial interventions should not be artificially partitioned into purely physical treatments, such as occupational or physiotherapy, nor into narrowly defined and isolated cognitive remedial training. Nor should treatment focus exclusively on insight-producing psychotherapies to improve self-awareness or disability adjustment.

If we consider rehabilitation as a process of optimising a person's social participation and psychological well-being, then alleviation of behaviour disorder is obviously a crucial goal of a person's treatment. Clinicians should be aware not simply of what intervention techniques are available, but of how and why they are effective. Yet many rehabilitation outcome reports do not address the efficacy of behavioural management techniques *per se*, separately from other aspects of rehabilitation (Cope *et al.*, 1991; Corrigan *et al.*, 1998; Malec *et al.*, 1993; Schalen *et al.*, 1994). It is therefore difficult to assess the overall contribution of behavioural techniques to the kinds of global outcome reported from integrated rehabilitation programmes.

Fortunately, there is also an established literature testifying to the specific effectiveness of behavioural modification techniques with traumatic brain injury. This includes treatment manuals (Ashley *et al.*, 1995; Carnevale & DeGrauw, 1995; Jacobs, 1993), detailed single cases of treatment efficacy (Alderman & Burgess, 1994; Godbout, 1997; Persel *et al.*, 1997; Wood, 1987, 1989b), reviews of practical techniques (McGlynn, 1990; Worthington, 2005; Yody *et al.*, 2000) and outcome studies from neurobehavioural-based services (Eames *et al.*, 1995; Wood *et al.*, 1999; Worthington, 2001, 2006). Wood *et al.* (1999) showed that a minimum period of six months' residential rehabilitation can significantly reduce long-term supervision and support, and improve individuals' integration into their communities. The cost-benefits are most evident within the first one to two years of injury but have been established for persons receiving treatment after many years (Wood *et al.*, 1999; Worthington *et al.*, 2006). The benefits of treatment for behaviour disorders which otherwise prevent social adaptation become clear when one considers the reduction in lifetime care costs, making it an extremely cost-effective form of intervention. This is also reflected in recent suggestions that behaviour modification is no longer viewed as a dehumanising form of intervention, and is increasingly being recognised as an important approach to intervention (Katz *et al.*, 2000).

Recent interest has focused upon whether cognitive neuropsychological characterisations of behaviour disorder can inform treatment approaches. This approach appears promising. For example, Alderman and Ward (1991) suggested that severe attentional deficits are likely to undermine treatment programmes based exclusively upon positive reinforcement. Deficits in working memory capability have been associated with poor response to traditional conditioning methods (Alderman, 1996). Finally, it has been shown that even routine behaviours can be disrupted after brain injury, and formerly automatic skills may require hitherto a degree of self-regulation (Humphreys & Forde, 1998).

However, there are a number of caveats, of which the clinician should be aware. In large studies the nature of behavioural disorders is often unclear. Aetiology is particularly important in diagnosis, and it is difficult to appreciate the effectiveness of a programme without knowing something about the difficulties that people present. For example, some rehabilitation programmes specifically exclude people who are unmotivated towards rehabilitation, while others require the prospective client to show some insight into their deficits. People with behaviour disorders are unlikely to benefit from such programmes. Therefore, reports of good treatment outcomes need to be judged critically against admission criteria.

Secondly, the nature of intervention techniques is often under-specified, making it difficult to compare results across centres. Yet anecdotal evidence of clinical effectiveness is often accumulated in this way. Reports that a given technique works well, on the basis that one or two different centres have reported success, must be considered cautiously, if details of its application in each case have not been specified. Finally, attention must be paid to the design of the intervention in question. In particular, one needs to consider first the baseline period, during which the natural frequency of the behaviour is supposedly established. Too short a measurement period, instability in the baseline or inadequate functional analysis can all produce misleading information about the target behaviour to be modified. Similarly, a good intervention will show signs of lasting behaviour change, and in this respect there should be a reasonable period of post-intervention or follow-up observation. Evidence of rapid behaviour change does not imply that such change is consolidated, and one should always look for signs of sustained improvements in behaviour over at least six months. If these basic guidelines are followed, clinicians will have an empirical basis to select therapeutically sound, conceptually well-grounded methods to incorporate into their professional practice. Examples of several forms of therapy will be illustrated with reference to patient RB with whom the first author worked closely. Relevant clinical information concerning RB is summarised below (some details have been altered to preserve anonymity).

Case 10.1: RB

RB was a 29-year-old clerical worker who sustained a severe TBI in a road accident, requiring surgical intervention via a right frontal lobectomy. RB made a good physical recovery and was discharged home after four months. His intellectual functions were weak (Verbal IQ: 74, Performance IQ: 69) and memory was severely impaired. Residual behaviour problems consisted of:

- labile mood;
- dysexecutive disorder;
- poor social communication skills;
- disinibited social behaviour;
- persistent spitting; and
- elaborate ritualistic behaviours associated with toilet use.

After unsuccessful out-patient treatment, he was admitted for specialist neurobehavioural rehabilitation.

Psychotherapy

The complex nature of brain-injury-related problems of behaviour means that many psychotherapists have been reluctant to work with this group of individuals because of the seemingly immutable nature of the problems (Manchester & Wood, 2001). Developing a therapeutic relationship and treatment goals with a person who might have premorbid personality problems, family pathology, and defects in basic cognitive processes is a daunting prospect, even for a skilled clinician. Access to psychotherapy is probably as important a factor determining treatment choice as the attitude and competence of individual clinicians. For this reason it is understandable why the application of insight therapies to brain-injured people has been much more prevalent in America than in Britain (Ben-Yishay *et al.*, 1985; Geva & Stern, 1985; Prigatano 1986; Stern & Stern, 1985; Tadir & Stern, 1985).

A recent survey of practitioners in the UK offering psychotherapy to brain-injured persons identified lack of insight, inflexible thinking and impaired memory as the main challenges to forming a working alliance in therapy (Judd & Wilson, 2005). However, this is a selective sample relating to recipients of psychotherapy and one may assume that many persons with behaviour disorder would not have been considered appropriate for such treatment. Yet for many people success in rehabilitation is dependent on people with brain injury becoming aware of their difficulties and learning to compensate for them. This involves recognising the need for, and value of, some kind of therapeutic activity. Prigatano has advocated the use of psychotherapy within a general rehabilitation programme to facilitate awareness and acceptance of disability. He has employed individual and family counselling within a social milieu treatment programme and reported improvement of insight and psychosocial problems (see Prigatano, 1999). He also acknowledges that psychotherapy, while advocated for patients showing denial, is unlikely to be fruitful in cases of neurologically induced loss of self-awareness (Prigatano, 2005).Other successful outcomes using insight psychotherapy have also been reported (Geva & Stern, 1985; Stern & Stern, 1985; Tadir & Stern, 1985). Successful outcomes of group psychotherapy have been reported, used in both in-patient and out-patient centres (Carberry & Burd, 1983; Corrigan *et al.*, 1985; Jackson & Gouvier, 1992; Leer, 1986; Leer & Sonday, 1986). Power and Dell Orto (1980) have also described successful family therapy in the treatment of psychosocial problems following brain injury.

However, not all people with acquired brain injury will respond to these methods. Lewis and Rosenberg (1991) argue that the brain-injured client needs adequate attentional and language skills in order to participate effectively in dialogue over the course of a therapeutic session. Equally, lack of awareness, poor judgement and insight, inaccuracy in verbal self-report, and motivational problems can act as barriers to psychotherapy (Alderman, 2001; Burgess & Wood, 1990). Successful participation in group psychotherapy, for example, is usually dependent on the brain-injured person having already made a 'moderately good cognitive and behavioural recovery' (Jackson & Gouvier, 1992, p.322).

Continued

Outcome from psychotherapy programmes needs to take into account admission criteria. For Prigatano (1986) this meant WAIS and WMS scores of not less than 75; digit symbol score not less than 5; absence of psychotic disorder or severe disturbance of personality; the ability to talk about painful issues; ability to keep appointments; motivation to engage in cognitive retraining and psychotherapeutic tasks. The latter criteria, which disqualify admission to Prigatano's programme, are precisely those required for admission into a neurobehavioural programme (see below). Unless this type of information is made clear, inaccurate estimates of the utilitarian value of different rehabilitation procedures will ensue. RB would not have met Prigatano's criteria for inclusion into a neuropsychological rehabilitation programme. Although he remained articulate and intelligent, psychotherapy was contra-indicated by his labile mood, impaired self-awareness, dysexecutive disorder (poor abstract reasoning, judgement and concentration) and social disinhibition, including persistent interrupting and verbal perseveration.

Behaviour management approaches

Behavioural techniques have a long history in neurorehabilitation. Goodkin (1966, 1969) reported the use of behaviour modification methods with people who suffered traumatic brain injury and other neurological disorders. Behaviour modification approaches have also been incorporated into interventions concerned with the rehabilitation of cognitive deficits (for example: Diller & Weinberg, 1977; Lincoln, 1979; Weinberg *et al.*, 1979). However, the predominant use of behaviour modification has been in the management of psychosocial, emotional and behavioural problems (Alderman & Burgess, 1990; Alderman & Ward 1991; Booream & Seacat, 1972; Ince, 1976; Taylor & Persons, 1970; Wood 1984, 1987, 1989b). Space does not permit an extensive consideration of behavioural techniques but there are several excellent reviews of behaviour management approaches in the recent literature on brain-injury rehabilitation (Alderman, 2001; Carnevale & DeGrauw, 1995; Giles, 1999; Goldstein, 2003; Ponsford *et al.*, 1995). Alderman (2001) pointed to the advantages of behaviour modification in the treatment of behaviour problems after brain injury. These include:

- the variety of treatment techniques available to both decrease and increase behaviour;

- human behaviour modification can draw upon theoretical principles found in learning theory, developmental psychology, information processing, and social learning theory;
- assessment of behaviour problems lead directly to the choice of subsequent treatment approaches;
- specific targets and goals of treatment are designated prior to commencement of treatment;
- it provides a clear set of procedures to follow when implementing a treatment programme, to ensure that a consistent and objective approach is adopted by all who are involved in treatment;
- treatment is continuously evaluated through objective observation and recording processes, which Powell (1981) states are essential features of any applied science; and
- behaviour modification programmes are individualised and take into account variables such as the neurological and neuropsychological condition of the person, antecedent causes, consequences, plus social and environmental factors.

Behavioural interventions were introduced for RB's spitting and toilet rituals. Rehabilitation staff were asked to record all aspects of RB's behaviour (including duration) whenever he asked to use the toilet, for one week. From this information, a more structured recording form was established incorporating RB's principal inappropriate behaviours associated with use of the toilet. These were: tearing up tissue paper and blocking the sink; turning taps full on and leaving them running; persistent spitting; and engaging in repetitive chanting. This structured recording form was used to provide baseline data prior to treatment. The data also suggested a relationship between staff presence, the likelihood of engaging in maladaptive behaviour and the length of time spent in the toilet.

Given these relationships, treatment was based upon manipulating access to the trigger to the behaviour. In this case, this meant that RB was to be supervised by a support worker who would accompany RB to the toilet. The team member would remind him of the inappropriate (target) behaviours and set a time limit of five minutes, after which RB would have to exit, unless he asked for more time and had not engaged in any (or some acceptable level) of the target behaviours. RB would also be informed when two minutes were left, and then would be 'counted down'. This last step was not in the original programme but experience showed it to be helpful in breaking the repetitive chanting and focusing RB on the task at

Continued

hand. Compared with a baseline period of six weeks, when RB spent an average of 20 minutes in the toilet, this was reduced to an average of just five minutes. There was a corresponding reduction in incidents of maladaptive behaviour during the toileting procedure.

Spitting was an ever-present problem. It was assessed in two ways. A semi-structured interview undertaken by a clinical psychologist sought to ascertain the triggers and maintaining factors underlying the behaviour. A time-sampling approach was also employed, whereby staff recorded the frequency of spitting for 15-minute periods every hour. In this way it was possible to record a full 12 hours of spitting (9:00am. to 9:00pm) over a 10-day period (see Wood & Worthington, 1999). This method also allowed staff to explore any relationship between spitting and situational or interpersonal factors. Assessment had shown that RB's spitting occurred throughout the day, especially around structured activities when demands were being made of him, for example in the early morning. At other times, however, this behaviour could be held in abeyance for up to 30 minutes if he was engrossed in an activity. Rehabilitation staff were given guidelines in the general management of such behaviour, prior to any specific intervention being employed. Within these guidelines staff were instructed to initiate social interaction with RB whenever he was noted to be refraining from spitting (thus positively reinforcing such inhibitory control). They were also trained to briefly disengage from interaction whenever RB started to spit, and then to re-engage after approximately 30 seconds if the spitting had ceased. By using this method of time-out-on-the-spot, RB was being positively reinforced for non-spitting. It was planned to develop this approach into a more formal programme of DRI (differential reinforcement of incompatible behaviour), but RB continued to show generalisable behavioural changes under the general procedure. When the time-sampling recordings were repeated after some 12 weeks, there had been an overall reduction in instances of spitting of almost 70 per cent. This is both clinically very important and also satisfies statistical tests of significance ($F = 21.9$, $p < .001$).

Cognitive-behavioural therapy

The constraints upon learning and understanding imposed by neurobehavioural disorder are capable of being addressed by adapting cognitive–behavioural techniques in brain injury rehabilitation. Traditional behaviour management has its limitations, both in respect of the range of behaviours that can be effectively changed and the circumstances in which behavioural methods can be administered (Alderman & Burgess, 1990). Some brain-injured people do not respond to reinforcement contingencies because of drive or hedonistic weaknesses. Other individuals with different forms of brain injury, such as predominantly frontal dysfunction, often learn social or functional skills in a behaviourally oriented environment but fail to generalise those skills into the wider community (Corrigan *et al.*, 1998; McGlynn, 1990). Another criticism made by many psychologists is that behaviour management's early emphasis on reinforcement contingencies and purely observable behaviour exposed it to the criticism of it being unable to explain complex, emotionally driven behaviour (Allen, 1998).

The principal difference between cognitive behaviour therapy (CBT) and behaviour modification is the role assigned to cognition and emotion. In CBT, cognitions and emotions are assumed to reflect self-regulatory processes that allow a person to plan, execute and evaluate his or her own behaviour (Schefft *et al.*, 1997). Manchester and Wood (2001) emphasise the role of CBT in promoting awareness and motivation to achieve successful rehabilitation and social outcome. They give examples of how the structure implicit in CBT interview techniques helps shape a client's thinking and improve their awareness of socially acceptable ways to express their emotional problems, reducing or removing potential barriers to cooperation and motivation in rehabilitation. They describe the role of verbal mediation strategies to assist goal-directed behaviour and impulse control, emphasising that the aim of the CBT approach is to help brain-injured people improve their capacity for self-regulation and thereby gain greater control over their social environment. Recipients are trained in techniques of accurate self-monitoring, realistic goal setting, and time management to improve a range of social and functional skills. They are also trained in coping skills to help prepare for, and deal appropriately with, various stressful situations they may encounter. There is greater emphasis on engagement and motivation for change to tackle resistances that may otherwise undermine progress (see Miller & Rollnick, 2002). Feedback from staff, peers and family is an important element of CBT (Ben-Yishay & Lakin, 1989) because it helps to raise awareness, often in highly pertinent situations, of social signals exhibited by others and the need to inhibit, or alter the style of, one's behaviour.

RB's behaviour during his early morning washing and dressing routine was treated using a verbal mediation technique (Wood &

Continued

Worthington, 2001a; Worthington, 2002). A support worker, accompanying the supervising occupational therapist, recorded the different behaviours that RB engaged in during this activity. After one week these initial recordings were used as the basis for a structured recording form which contained the key components of the task and the target maladaptive behaviours. These were: spitting, repetitive questioning, and attending to task-irrelevant objects in the vicinity.

A prompt sheet was devised consisting of specific verbal instructions which the therapist delivered and which RB repeated immediately prior to performance of the action to which the prompts referred. This has two advantages: it focuses the client's attention on the task at hand and prevents them engaging in time-consuming irrelevancies, and it also helps to establish a link between the prompt and its action, which the client learns to internalise with repeated practice. After just two weeks of the intervention RB was able to get up, wash and dress in about half the time (i.e. approximately 30 minutes), showing a 43 per cent reduction in the amount of prompting required. RB required less assistance because the intervention was successful both in improving his attention to task and in increasing his initiation of components of his morning routine.

Pharmacological management

Medication can have an important role in management of behaviour disturbance, especially in the early acute and sub-acute phase. Some examples of effective drug treatment have been mentioned elsewhere in the chapter. The reader should be aware of a positive publication bias in the literature on drug treatment after brain injury, and most drugs are prescribed on an empirical basis. The best evidence for effectiveness in relation to agitation and aggression comes from carbamazepine and propranolol, but there are several reviews of potentially beneficial drugs for behaviour disorder (Cassidy, 1999; Deb & Crownshaw, 2004; Griffin *et al.*, 2003; Whyte, 1994; Wroblewski & Glenn, 1994) and their possible adverse consequences (Boyeson & Harmon, 1994; Goldstein, 1995; Stanislav, 1997). One promising approach is the use of serotonin re-uptake inhibitors (SSRIs) in the management of affective disorders after TBI, including anxiety and ritualistic behaviour (Zafonte *et al.*, 2002). In RB's case it was decided to embark on a trial of paroxetine, an SSRI with anxiety-reducing potency. In an integrated effort by the psychiatrist and clinical psychologist on the team the effects of behavioural interventions were compared with a stepwise introduction of paroxetine. This systematic evaluation revealed that the behavioural interventions alone were effective; the addition of an SSRI had no demonstrable effect.

The treatment environment

The final aspect of behaviour management to be considered is the treatment environment. Ben-Yishay and Gold (1990) argued that a patient's potential for recovery could be optimised using a therapeutic milieu that has the structure and organisation to systematically integrate and time the introduction of various treatment interventions. A similar approach was adopted by Prigatano (1986) in his neuropsychological rehabilitation programme. Neuropsychological factors also need to be considered as a preliminary to any behavioural rehabilitation approach because the ability of brain-injured people to learn is constrained in various ways by cognitive deficits (Alderman, 1991, 2001). To this end, Wood and others have advocated that the principles of behaviour modification and those of neuropsychology should be combined to form what is now called a *neurobehavioural paradigm* (see Wood 1987, 1990; Wood & Worthington, 2001a). Clinicians need to assimilate an understanding of the nature of brain injury, the neuropsychological impairments and the behavioural disorders, for which one must ascertain antecedents and consequences to behaviour, the state of the environment and other relevant variables.

Specialised neurobehavioural units have grown from this early paradigm. They attempt to organise the service they provide to minimise the effect of cognitive impairment whilst maximising opportunities for new learning, using structure, repetition and routine (see Wood & Worthington, 2001b). In a neurobehavioural rehabilitation unit, structure is sustained through the physical environment, the format of the day, strong interdisciplinary teamwork, appropriate levels of expectation regarding participation within rehabilitation, and the use of behaviour modification strategies. The emphasis is on promoting adaptive behaviours, often as habit patterns which act as a platform for all activities of daily living upon which the client will rely to promote independence (McNeny, 1990). This entails application of behaviour management, and functional skills training using behavioural techniques, in real-life settings. Unless the process of *acquiring* a skill is associated with its *application*, what is learned may never be spontaneously implemented. Failure to appreciate this important aspect of learning has been a criticism levelled at cognitive approaches to brain injury rehabilitation (Baddeley, 1993). Neurobehavioural rehabilitation addresses this dilemma by employing a procedural approach to learning (see Wood & Worthington, 2001b), in which the practice of a skill in real-life situations forms the basis of how the skill is acquired.

When services are organised in this way, the net effect is the provision of a daily routine within which skills that aim to maximise independence and quality of life are practised repeatedly and acquired through procedural learning in the form of new habits. Good communication within the interdisciplinary team, together with a programme that is grounded in behavioural methods, helps ensure rehabilitation is established at the appropriate level for each individual, that goals are shared, and that management, including contingencies to behaviour, is consistent. The success of specialised neurobehavioural programmes has been well documented (for example, see: Alderman & Knight, 1997; Alderman *et al.*, 1995; Burgess & Alderman, 1990; Wood, 1987; Youngson & Alderman, 1994).

Conclusion

There is now an established literature of individual treatment techniques and service-related programmes which provide with a strong evidence-base for clinical practice. Given the potential impact of mood and behavioural changes after brain injury, and the range of treatment approaches available, behavioural management skills should be at the core of any rehabilitation service. The ability to identify, formulate, and intervene effectively can open up new opportunities for rehabilitation previously inaccessible to individuals and their families. If this chapter tempts the reader unfamiliar with behaviour disorders to explore the topic a little further, the benefits may exceed their expectations. The novice practitioner used to the slow processes of cognitive recovery or emotional adjustment may be surprised how quickly lasting and meaningful change can take place.

Note

1 This term was introduced by Babinski in 1914 to describe apparent unawareness of hemiplegia and the phenomenon was well known in the nineteenth century. The term remains in use to refer to a partial or complete unawareness of an impairment or denial of disability.

Recommended Reading

Ponsford, J. (2004). *Cognitive and behavioral rehabilitation.* New York: Guilford Press.
A very readable overview of cognitive rehabilitation methods for use with behavioural problems, with good chapters on challenging behaviour, executive dysfunction and self-awareness, and TBI.

Sheldon, B. (1995). *Cognitive behavioural therapy.* London: Routledge.
An excellent text bridging the gap between cognitive psychology and behavioural therapy. It contains much useful theoretical background material and practical examples that can be applied to TBI.

Wood, R.Ll. (1990). *Neurobehavioural sequelae of traumatic brain injury.* London: Taylor & Francis.
An accessible introduction to behavioural problems after TBI and the relationships between underlying cognitive (especially executive) dysfunction and behaviour disorder. Somewhat dated but many chapters contain good working case examples.

Wood, R.Ll. & McMillan, T.M. (2001). *Neurobehavioural disability and social handicap following traumatic brain injury.* Hove: Psychology Press.
An updated summary of neurobehavioural problems at a conceptual and practical level, written with practitioners in mind. It also contains good chapters for professionals on service provision and capacity issues.

References

Adams, J.H., Graham, D.I., Murray, L.S. & Scott, G. (1982). Diffuse axonal injury due to nonmissile head injury in humans: An analysis of 45 cases. *Annals of Neurology*, *12*, 557–63.

Alderman, N. (1991). The treatment of avoidance behaviour following severe brain injury by satiation through negative practice. *Brain Injury*, *5*(1), 77–86.

Alderman, N. (1996). Central executive deficit and response to operant conditioning methods. *Neuropsychological Rehabilitation*, 6, 161–186.

Alderman, N. (2001). Managing challenging behaviour. In R.Ll. Wood & T.M. McMillan (Eds.) *Neurobehavioural disability and social handicap following traumatic brain injury* (pp.175–207). London: Taylor and Francis.

Alderman, N. & Burgess, P.W. (1990). Integrating cognition and behaviour: A pragmatic approach to brain injury rehabilitation. In R.Ll. Wood & I. Fussey (Eds.) *Cognitive rehabilitation in perspective* (pp.204–228). London: Taylor and Francis.

Alderman, N. & Burgess, P. (1994). A comparison of treatment methods for behaviour disorder following herpes simplex encephalitis. *Neuropsychological Rehabilitation*, *4*, 31–48.

Alderman, N., Fry, R.K. & Youngson, H.A. (1995). Improvement of self-monitoring skills, reduction of behaviour disturbance and the dysexecutive syndrome. *Neuropsychological Rehabilitation*, *5*, 193–222.

Alderman, N. & Knight, C. (1997). The effectiveness of DRL in the management and treatment of severe behaviour disorders following brain injury. *Brain Injury*, *11*, 79–101.

Alderman, N. & Ward, A. (1991). Behavioural treatment of the dysexecutive syndrome: Reduction of repetitive speech using response cost and cognitive overlearning. *Neuropsychological Rehabilitation*, *1*, 65–80.

Allen, N.B. (1998). Cognitive psychotherapy. In S. Bloch (Ed.) *An introduction to the psychotherapies*. Oxford: Oxford Medical Publications.

Anderson, M.I., Parmenter, T.R. & Mok, M. (2002). The relationship between neurobehavioural problems of severe traumatic brain injury (TBI) and family functioning and the psychological well-being of the spouse/caregiver: Path model analysis. *Brain Injury*, *16*, 743–757.

American Psychiatric Association (2000). *Diagnostic and statistical manual of mental disorders, 4th edition* (Text Rev.) [DSM-IV-TR]. Washington: APA.

Ashley, M.J., Krych, D.K., Persel, C.S. & Persel, C.H. (1995). *Working with behavior disorders*. San Antonio: Psychological Corporation.

Baddeley, A.D. (1993). A theory of rehabilitation without a model of learning is a vehicle without an engine: A comment on Caramazza and Hillis. *Neuropsychological Rehabilitation*, *3*, 217–296.

Baddeley, A.D. & Wilson, B. (1988). Frontal amnesia and the dysexecutive syndrome. *Brain and Cognition*, *7*, 212–230.

Barrett, K. (1991). Treating organic abulia with bromocriptine and lisuride: Four case studies. *Journal of Neurology, Neurosurgery and Psychiatry*, *54*, 718–721.

Ben-Yishay, Y. & Gold, J. (1990). A therapeutic milieu approach to neuropsychological rehabilitation. In R.Ll. Wood (Ed.) *Neurobehavioural sequelae of traumatic brain injury* (pp.194–215). London: Taylor Francis.

Ben-Yishay, Y. & Lakin, P. (1989). Structured group treatment for brain-injury survivors. In D. Ellis and A.L. Christensen (Eds.) *Neuropsychological treatment of head injury* (pp.271–295). Boston: Martinus Nijhoff.

Ben-Yishay, Y., Rattock, J., Lakin, P., Piasetsky, E.B., Ross, B., Silver, S., *et al.* (1985). Neuropsychologic rehabilitation: Quest for a holistic approach. *Seminars in Neurology*, *5*, 252–258.

Blair, R.J.R. (2001). Neurocognitive models of aggression: The antisocial personality disorders, and psychopathy. *Journal of Neurology, Neurosurgery and Psychiatry*, *71*, 727–731.

Blair, R.J.R. & Cipolotti, L. (2000). Impaired social response reversal. A case of 'acquired sociopathy'. *Brain*, *123*, 1122–1141.

Bogner, J.A., Corrigan, J.D., Mysiw, W.J. & Clinchot, D. (2001). A comparison of substance abuse and violence in the prediction of long-term rehabilitation outcomes after traumatic brain injury. *Archives of Physical Medicine and Rehabilitation*, *82*, 571–577.

Bombardier, C.H., Rimmele, C.T. & Zintel, H. (2002). The magnitude and correlates of alcohol and drug use before traumatic brain injury. *Archives of Physical Medicine and Rehabilitation*, *83*, 1765–1773.

Booream, C.D. & Seacat, G.F. (1972). Effects of increased incentive in corrective therapy. *Perceptual and Motor Skills*, *34*, 125–126.

Boyeson, M.G. & Harmon, R.L. (1994). Acute and postacute drug-induced effects on rate of behavioral recovery after brain injury. *Journal of Head Trauma Rehabilitation*, *9*, 78–90.

Braver, T.S., Cohen, J.D. & Barch, D.M. (2002). The role of prefrontal cortex in normal and disordered cognitive control: A cognitive neuroscience perspective. In D.T Stuss & R.T. Knight (Eds.) *Principles of frontal lobe function* (pp.428–447). New York: Oxford University Press.

Brooks, D.N. & McKinlay, W.W. (1983). Personality and behavioural change after severe blunt head injury: A relative's view. *Journal of Neurology, Neurosurgery and Psychiatry*, *46*, 336–344

Brower, M.C. & Price, B.H. (2001). Neuropsychiatry of frontal lobe dysfunction in violent and criminal behaviour: A critical review. *Journal of Neurology, Neurosurgery and Psychiatry*, *71*, 720–726.

Bunge, S.A., Oschsner, K.N., Desmond, J.E., Glover, G.H. & Gabrieli, J.D.E. (2001). Prefrontal regions involved in keeping information in and out of mind. *Brain*, *124*, 2074–2086.

Burgess, P.W. & Alderman, N. (1990). Rehabilitation of dyscontrol syndromes following frontal lobe damage: A cognitive neuropsychological approach. In R.Ll. Wood & I. Fussey (Eds.) *Cognitive rehabilitation in perspective* (pp.183–203). London: Taylor & Francis.

Burgess, P.W. & Wood, R.Ll. (1990). Neuropsychology of behaviour disorders following brain injury. In R.Ll. Wood (Ed.) *Neurobehavioural sequelae of traumatic brain injury* (pp.110–133). London: Taylor & Francis.

Burgess, P.W., Veitch, E., de Lacy Costello, A. & Shallice, T. (2000). The cognitive and neuroanatomical correlates of multi-tasking. *Neuropsychologia*, *38*, 848–863.

Carberry, H. & Burd, B. (1983). Social aspects of cognitive retraining in an outpatient group setting for head trauma patients. *Cognitive Rehabilitation*, *1*, 5–7.

Carnevale, G.J. & DeGrauw, W.P. (1995). *Natural setting behavioural management. Traumatic brain injury and behavior management: Applied programming in the home, work and school environment. A manual for therapists.* East Orange, NJ: Kesler Institute for Rehabilitation.

Cassidy, J.W. (1999). Neuropharmacological contributions to the rehabilitation of patients with traumatic brain injury. In D.T. Stuss, G. Winocur & I.H. Robertson (Eds.) *Cognitive neurorehabilitation* (pp.136–152). Cambridge: Cambridge University Press.

Cope, N.D., Cole, J.R., Hall, K.M. & Barkans, H. (1991). Brain injury: Analysis of outcome in a post-acute rehabilitation system. Part1: General analysis. *Brain Injury*, *5*, 111–125.

Corrigan, J.D., Arnett, J.A., Houck, L.J. & Jackson, R.D. (1985). Reality orientation for brain injured patients: Group treatment and monitoring of recovery. *Archives of Physical Medicine and Rehabilitation*, 66, 626–630.

Corrigan, J.D., Smith-Knapp, K. & Granger, C.V. (1998). Outcomes in the first 5 years after traumatic brain injury. *Archives of Physical Medicine and Rehabilitation*, *79*, 298–305.

Cummings, J.L. (1985). *Clinical neuropsychiatry*. London: Grune and Stratton.

Damasio, A.R., Tranel, D. & Damasio, H. (1999). Somatic markers and the guidance of behavior: Theory and preliminary testing. In H.S. Levin, H.M. Eisenberg & A.L. Benton (Eds.) *Frontal lobe function and dysfunction* (pp.217–229). New York: Oxford University Press.

Deb, S. & Crownshaw, T. (2004). The role of pharmacotherapy in the management of behaviour disorders in traumatic brain injury patients. *Brain Injury*, *18*, 1–31.

Diller, L. & Weinberg, J. (1977). Hemi-inattention in rehabilitation: The evolution of a rational remediation program. In E.A. Weinstein & R.P. Friedland (Eds.) *Advances in neurology*, *18*. New York: Raven Press.

Duncan, J., Emslie, H., Williams, P., Johnson, R. & Freer, C. (1996). Intelligence and the frontal lobe: The organisation of goal-directed behaviour. *Cognitive Neuropsychology*, *30*, 257–303.

Eames, P., Cotterill, G., Kneale, T.A., & Storrar, A. (1995). Outcome of intensive rehabilitation after severe brain injury: A long-term follow-up study. *Brain Injury*, *10*, 631–650.

Eames, P. & Wood, R.Ll. (1985). Rehabilitation after severe brain injury: A follow-up study of a behaviour modification approach. *Journal of Neurology, Neurosurgery and Psychiatry*, *48*, 613–619.

Eames, P. & Wood, R.Ll. (2003). Episodic disorders of behaviour and affect after acquired brain injury. *Neuropsychological Rehabilitation*, *13*, 241–258.

Eames, P.G. (1990). Organic bases of behaviour disorders after traumatic brain injury. In R.Ll. Wood (Ed.) *Neurobehavioural sequelae of traumatic brain injury* (pp.134–150). London: Taylor & Francis.

Eames, P.G. (1992). Hysteria following brain injury. *Journal of Neurology, Neurosurgery and Psychiatry*, *55*, 1046–1053.

Eames, P.G (2001). Distinguishing the neuropsychiatric, psychiatric, and psychological consequences of acquired brain injury. In R.Ll. Wood & T.M. McMillan (Eds.) *Neurobehavioural disability and social handicap following traumatic brain injury* (pp.29–45). Hove, UK: Psychology Press.

Eames, P.G. & Wood, R.Ll. (1984). Consciousness in the brain-damaged adult. In M. Stevens (Ed.) *Aspects of consciousness, Vol. 4: Clinical issues*. New York: Academic Press.

Elliott, F.A. (1982). Neurological findings in adult minimal brain dysfunction and the dyscontrol syndrome. *Journal of Nervous and Mental Disease*, *170*, 680–687.

Eslinger, P.J. & Geder, L. (2000). Behavioral and emotional changes after focal frontal damage. In J. Bogousslavsky & J.L. Cummings (Eds.) *Behavior and mood disorders in focal brain lesions* (pp.217–260). Cambridge: Cambridge University Press.

Fisher, C.M. (1983). Abulia minor vs. agitated behaviour. *Clinical Neurosurgery*, 31, 9–31.

Fuster, J.M. (2002). Physiology of executive functions; the perception-action cycle. In D.T. Stuss & R.T. Knight (Eds.) *Principles of frontal lobe function* (pp.96–108). New York: Oxford University Press.

Geva, N. & Stern, J.M. (1985). The mourning process with brain injured patients. *Scandinavian Journal of Rehabilitation Medicine, Supplement 12*, 50–52.

Giles, G.M. (1999). Management of behaviour dysregulation and non-compliance in the post-acute severely brain injured adult. In G.M. Giles & J. Clark-Wilson (Eds.) *Rehabilitation of the severely brain injured adult*. Cheltenham, UK: Stanley Thornes Ltd.

Godbout, A. (1997). Structured habituation training for movement provoked vertigo after severe traumatic brain injury: A single case experiment. *Brain Injury*, *11*, 629–641.

Goldstein, L.B. (1995). Prescribing potential harmful drugs to patients admitted to hospital after head injury. *Journal of Neurology, Neurosurgery and Psychiatry*, *58*, 753–755.

Goldstein, L.H. (2003). Behaviour problems. In R.J. Greenwood, M.P. Barnes, T.M. McMillan & C.D. Ward (Eds.) *Handbook of neurological rehabilitation* (pp.419–432). Hove: Psychology Press.

Goodkin, R. (1966). Case studies in behavioural research in rehabilitation. *Perceptual and Motor Skills*, *23*, 171–182.

Goodkin, R. (1969). Changes in word production, sentence production and relevance in an aphasic through verbal conditioning. *Behaviour Research and Therapy*, *7*, 93–99.

Griffin, S.L., van Reekum, R. & Masanic, C. (2003). A review of cholinergic agents in the treatment of neurobehavioral deficits following traumatic brain injury. *Journal of Neuropsychiatry and Clinical Neurosciences*, *15*, 17–26.

Haas, J.F., Cope, D.N. & Hall, K. (1987). Premorbid prevalence of poor academic performance in severe head injury. *Journal of Neurology, Neurosurgery and Psychiatry*, *50*, 52–56.

Habib, M. (2000). Disorders of motivation. In J. Bogousslavsky & J.L. Cummings (Eds.) *Behavior and mood disorders in focal brain lesions* (pp.261–284). Cambridge: Cambridge University Press.

Hooper, R.S., McGregor, J.M. & Nathan, P.W. (1945). Explosive rage following head injury. *Proceedings of the Royal Society of Medicine*, *2*, 458–471.

Humphreys, G.W. & Forde, E.M.E. (1998). Disordered action schema and action disorganisation syndrome. *Cognitive Neuropsychology*, *15*, 771–811.

Ince, L.P. (1976). *Behaviour modification in rehabilitation medicine*. London: Williams and Wilkins.

Jackson, W.T. & Gouvier, W.D. (1992). Group psychotherapy with brain-damaged adults and their families. In C.J. Lang & L.K. Ross (Eds.) *Handbook of head trauma: Acute care to recovery*. New York: Plenum Press.

Jacobs, H.E. (1993). *Behavior analysis guidelines and brain injury rehabilitation*. Gaithersburg, MD: Aspen Publishers Inc.

James, W. (1890). *The principles of psychology*. New York: Holt.

Jeannerod, M. (1997). *The cognitive neuroscience of action*. Oxford: Blackwell.

Judd, D. & Wilson, S.J. (2005). Psychotherapy with brain injury survivors: An investigation of the challenges encountered by clinicians and their modifications to therapeutic practice. *Brain Injury*, *19*, 437–449.

Kaplan, K. (1899). Cited by Hooper, R.S., McGregor, J.M. & Nathan, P.W. (1945). Explosive rage following head injury. *Proceedings of the Royal Society of Medicine*, 2, 458–471.

Katz, R.C., Cacciapaglia, H. & Cabral, K. (2000). Labelling bias and attitudes toward behavior modification revisited. *Journal of Behavior Therapy*, *31*, 67–72.

Kimberg, D.Y. & Farah, M.J. (1993). A unified account of cognitive impairments following frontal lobe damage: The role of working memory in complex organized behavior. *Journal of Experimental Psychology: General*, *122*, 411–428.

Knight, R.G., Devereux, R. & Godfrey, H.P.D. (1998). Caring for a family member with a traumatic brain injury. *Brain Injury*, *12*, 467–481.

Kreutzer, J.S. (1993). Improving the prognosis for return to work after brain injury. In P. Frommelt & K.D. Wiedman (Eds.) *Neurorehabilitation: A perspective for the future*, Deggendorf Conference Proceedings.

Leer, W.B. (1986). Brain injured activity group for cognitive retraining in a rehabilitation setting. Abstract, Proceedings of the 5th Annual Meeting of the National Academy of Neuropsychology. *Archives of Clinical Neuropsychology*, *1*, 55.

Leer, W.B. & Sonday, W.E. (1986). Brain injured client coping skills group in a rehabilitation setting. Abstract, Proceedings of the 6th Annual Meeting of the National Academy of Neuropsychology. *Archives of Clinical Neuropsychology, 1*, 277.

LeVere, T. E. (1988). Neural system imbalances and the consequences of large brain injuries. In S. Finger, T.E. LeVere, C.R. Almli & D.G. Stein (Eds.) *Brain injury and recovery: Theoretical and controversial issues* (pp.15–28). New York: Plenum Press.

Levisohn, L., Cronin-Golomb, A. & Schmahmann, J.D. (2000). Neuropsychological consequences of cerebellar tumour resection in children. *Brain, 123*, 1041–1050

Lewis, L. (1991). Role of psychological factors in disordered awareness. In G.P. Prigatano & D.L. Schacter (Eds.) *Awareness of deficit after brain injury* (pp.223–239). New York, Oxford University Press.

Lewis, L. & Rosenberg, S.J. (1991). Psychoanalytic psychotherapy with adult brain injured patients. *Journal of Nervous and Mental Diseases, 178*, 69–77.

Lezak, M.D. (1978). Living with the characterologically altered brain injured patient. *Journal of Clinical Psychiatry, 39*, 592–593.

Lezak, M.D. (1995). *Neuropsychological assessment* (3rd edn). Oxford: Oxford University Press.

Lieberman, J.A., Alvir, J., Mukherjee, S. & Kane, J.M. (1989). Treatment of tardive dyskinesia with bromocriptine. *Archives of General Psychiatry, 46*, 908–913.

Lincoln, N.B. (1979). *An investigation of the effect of the effectiveness on language retraining methods with aphasic stroke patients.* Unpublished doctoral dissertation, University of London.

Luria, A.R. (1973). *The working brain.* Harmondsworth: Penguin.

MacLean, A., Temkin, N.R., Dikmens, S. & Wyler, A.R. (1983). The behavioural sequelae of head injury. *Journal of Clinical Psychology, 5*, 361–376.

Mah, L.M., Arnold, M.C. & Grafman, J. (2004). Impairment of social perception associated with lesions of the prefrontal cortex. *American Journal of Psychiatry, 161*, 1247–1255.

Malec, J.F., Smigielski, J.S., DePompolo, R.W. & Thompson, J.M. (1993). Outcome evaluation and prediction in a comprehensive-integrated post-acute brain injury rehabilitation programme. *Brain Injury, 7*, 15–29.

Malloy, P., Bihrle, A., Duffy, J. & Cimino, C. (1993). The orbitomedial frontal syndrome. *Archives of Clinical Neuropsychology, 8*, 185–201.

Manchester, D. & Wood, R.Ll. (2001). Applying cognitive therapy in neurobehavioural rehabilitation. In R.Ll. Wood & T.M. McMillan (Eds.) *Neurobehavioural disability and social handicap following traumatic brain injury* (pp.157–174). Hove, UK: Psychology Press.

McDowell, S., Whyte, J. & D'Esposito, M. (1998). Differential effect of a dopaminergic agonist on prefrontal function in traumatic brain injury. *Brain, 121*, 1155–1164.

McGlynn, S.M. (1990). Behavioral approaches to neuropsychological rehabilitation. *Psychological Bulletin, 108*, 420–441.

McGuire, P.K., Siulbersweig, D.A. & Frith, C.D. (1996). Functional neuroanatomy of verbal self-monitoring. *Brain, 19*, 907–917.

McNeny, R. (1990). Daily living skills: The foundation of community living. In J.S. Kreutzer & P. Wehman (Eds.) *Community integration following traumatic brain injury* (pp.105–113). York, PA: Paul H. Brookes.

Miller, W.R. & Rollnick, S. (2002). *Motivational interviewing.* New York: Guilford Press.

Moll, J., de Oliveira-Souza, R., Bramati, I.E. & Grafman, J. (2005). Functional networks in emotional moral and nonmoral social judgments. In J.T. Cacioppo & G.G. Berntson (Eds.) *Social Neuroscience.* New York: Psychology Press.

Murray, C.J.L. & Lopez, A.D. (1997). Alternative projections of mortality and disability by cause 1990–2020: Global Burden of Disease Study. *The Lancet, 349*, 1498–1504.

Newcombe, F. (1987). Psychometric and behavioural evidence: Scope, limitations, and ecological validity. In H.S. Levin, J. Grafman & H.M. Eisenberg (Eds.) *Neurobehavioral recovery from head injury*. New York: Oxford University Press.

Nies, K.J. (1999). Cognitive and social-emotional changes associated with mesial orbitofrontal damage: Assessment and implications for treatment. *Neurocase*, *5*, 313–324.

NIH Consensus development panel on rehabilitation of persons with traumatic brain injury (1999). *Journal of the American Medical Association*, *282*, 974–983.

Norman, D. & Shallice, T. (1986). Attention to action. In R.J. Davidson, G.E. Schwartz & D. Shapiro (Eds.) *Consciousness and self-regulation* (pp.1–18). New York: Plenum Press.

Oddy, M., Coughlan, T., Tyerman, A. & Jenkins, D. (1985). Social adjustment after closed head injury: A further follow-up seven years after injury. *Journal of Neurology, Neurosurgery and Psychiatry*, *48*, 564–568.

Pang, D. (1989). Physics and pathophysiology of closed head injury. In M. Lezak (Ed.) *Assessment of the behavioural consequences of head trauma* (pp.1–17). New York: Alan Liss.

Passingham, R. (1993). *The frontal lobes and voluntary action*. New York: Oxford University Press.

Persel, C.S., Persel, C.H., Ashley, M.J. & Krych, D.K. (1997). The use of noncontingent reinforcement and contingent restraint to reduce physical aggression and self-injurious behaviour in a traumatically brain injured adult. *Brain Injury*, *11*, 751–760.

Petrides, M. (1998). Specialised systems for the processing of mnemonic information within the primate frontal cortex. In A.C. Roberts, T.W. Robbins & L. Weiskrantz (Eds.) *The prefrontal cortex: Executive and cognitive functions* (pp.103–116). Oxford: Oxford University Press.

Petrides, M., Alivisatos, B., Meyer, E. & Evans, A.C. (1993). Functional activation of the human frontal cortex during the performance of verbal working memory tasks. *Proceedings of the National Academy of Sciences*, *90*, 878–882.

Ponsford, J., Olver, J.H. & Curran, C. (1995). A profile of outcome: 2 years after traumatic brain injury. *Brain Injury*, *9*, 1–10.

Powell, G.E. (1981). *Brain function therapy*. Aldershot, UK: Gower Press.

Powell, G.E. & Wood, R.Ll. (2001). Assessing the nature and extent of neurobehavioural disability. In R.Ll. Wood & T.M. McMillan (Eds.) *Neurobehavioural disability and social handicap following traumatic brain injury* (pp.65–90). London: Taylor & Francis.

Powell, J.H., Al-Adawi, S., Morgan, J. & Greenwood, R. (1996). Motivational deficits after brain injury: Effects of bromocriptine in 11 patients. *Journal of Neurology, Neurosurgery and Psychiatry*, *60*, 416–421.

Power, P.W. & Dell Orto, A.E. (1980). Approaches to family intervention. In P.W. Power & A.E. Dell Orto (Eds.) *Role of the family in the rehabilitation of the physically disabled*. Baltimore: University Park Press.

Prigatano, G.P. (1986). *Neuropsychological rehabilitation after brain injury*. Baltimore, MD: John Hopkins University press.

Prigatano, G.P. (1996). Behavioral limitations TBI patients tend to underestimate: A replication and extension to patients with unilateralised cerebral dysfunction. *Clinical Neuropsychologist*, *10*, 191–201.

Prigatano, G.P. (1999). Disorders of self-awareness after brain injury. In G.P. Prigatano, *Principles of neuropsychological rehabilitation* (pp.265–293). New York: Oxford University Press.

Prigatano, G.P. (2005). Disturbances of self-awareness and rehabilitation of patients with traumatic brain injury. A 20-year perspective. *Journal of Head Trauma Rehabilitation*, *20*, 19–29.

Prigatano, G.P. & Johnson, S.C. (2003). The three vectors of consciousness and their disturbances after brain injury. *Neuropsychological Rehabilitation*, *13*, 13–29.

Rappaport, M., Herrero-Backe, C., Rappaport, M.H. & Winterfield, K. (1989). Head injury outcome up to ten years later. *Archives of Physical Medicine and Rehabilitation*, *70*, 885–892.

Roberts, M.A., Verduyn, W.H., Manshadi, F.F. & Hines, M.E. (1996). Episodic symptoms in dysfunctioning children and adolescents following mild and severe traumatic brain injury. *Brain Injury*, *10*, 739–747.

Rolls, E.T. (1999). The functions of the orbitofrontal cortex. *Neurocase*, *5*, 301–312.

Rolls, E.T. (2002). The functions of the orbito-frontal cortex. In D.T. Stuss & R.T. Knight (Eds.) *Principles of frontal lobe function* (pp.354–375). New York: Oxford University Press.

Ross, E.D. & Stewart, R.M. (1981). Akinetic mutism from hypothalamic damage: Successful treatment with dopamine agonists. *Neurology*, *31*, 1435–1439.

Schacter, D.L. (1989). On the relation between memory and consciousness: Dissociable interactions and conscious experience. In H.L. Roediger & F.I.M. Craik (Eds.) *Varieties of memory and consciousness* (pp.355–389). Hillsdale, NJ: Lawrence Erlbaum.

Schalen, W., Hansson, L., Nordstrom, G. & Nordstrom, C-H. (1994). Psychosocial outcome 5–8 years after severe traumatic brain lesions and the impact of rehabilitation services. *Brain Injury*, *8*, 49–64.

Schefft, B.K., Malec, J.F., Lehr, B.K. & Kanfer, F.H. (1997). The role of self-regulation therapy with the brain injured patient. In M.E. Maruish & J.E. Moses (Eds.) *Clinical neuropsychology* (pp.237–283). Hillsdale, NJ: Lawrence Erlbaum Associates.

Schmahmann, J.D. & Sherman, J. (1998). The cerebellar cognitive affective syndrome. *Brain*, *121*, 561–579.

Shallice, T. (1988). *From neuropsychology to mental structure.* Cambridge: Cambridge University Press.

Shallice, T. (2002). Fractionation of the supervisory system. In D.T. Stuss & R.T. Knight (Eds.) *Principles of frontal lobe function* (pp.261–277). New York: Oxford University Press.

Silveri, M.C., Di Betta, A.M., Filippini, V., Leggio, M.G. & Molinari, M. (1998). Verbal short-term store-rehearsal system and the cerebellum. *Brain*, *121*, 2175–2187.

Stanislav, S.W. (1997). Cognitive effects of antipsychotic agents in persons with traumatic brain injury. *Brain Injury*, *11*, 335–341.

Stern, B. & Stern, J.M. (1985). On the use of dreams as a means of diagnosis of brain-injured patients. *Scandinavian Journal of Rehabilitation Medicine, Supplement 12*, 44–46.

Stuss, D.T. (1991). Disturbances of self-awareness after frontal system damage. In G.P. Prigatano & D.L. Schacter (Eds.) *Awareness of deficit after brain injury. Clinical and theoretical issues* (pp.63–83). New York: Oxford University Press.

Stuss, D.T. & Benson, D.F. (1986). *The frontal lobes.* New York: Raven Press.

Tadir, M. & Stern, J.M. (1985). The mourning process with brain injured patients. *Scandinavian Journal of Rehabilitation Medicine, Supplement No 12*, 50–52.

Tate, R.L. (1987). Issues in the management of behaviour disturbance as a consequence of severe head injury. *Scandinavian Journal of Rehabilitation Medicine*, *19*, 13–18.

Taylor, G.P. & Persons, R.W. (1970). Behaviour modification techniques in a physical medicine and rehabilitation centre. *Journal of Psychology*, *74*, 117–124.

Teasdale, J.D. (1993). Selective effects of emotion on information-processing. In A. Baddeley & L. Weiskrantz (Eds.) *Attention: Selection, awareness and control* (pp.374–389). New York, Oxford University Press.

Thomsen, I.V. (1989). Do young patients have worse outcomes after severe blunt head trauma? *Brain Injury*, *3*, 157–62.

Tranel, D. (2002). Emotion, decision making, and the ventromedial prefrontal cortex. In D.T. Stuss & R.T. Knight (Eds.) *Principles of frontal lobe function* (pp.338–353). New York: Oxford University Press.

Trimble, M.R. (1988). Carbamazepine and mood: Evidence from patients with seizure disorders. *Journal of Clinical Psychiatry*, *49*(4, Suppl.), 7–11.

Tronsco, J.C. & Gordon, B. (1996). Neuropathology of closed head injury. In M. Rizzo & D. Tranel (Eds.) *Head injury and post-concussive syndrome* (pp.47–56). New York: Churchill Livingstone.

Van Elst, L.T. (2002). Aggression and epilepsy. In M. Trimble & B. Schmitz (Eds.) *The neuropsychiatry of epilepsy* (pp.81–106). Cambridge: Cambridge University Press.

Van Zomeren, A.H. & Brouwer, W.H. (1994). *Clinical neuropsychology of attention*. New York: Oxford University Press.

Varney, N.R. & Menefee, L. (1993). Psychosocial and executive deficits following closed head injury: Implications for orbital frontal cortex. *Journal of Head Trauma Rehabilitation*, *8*, 32–44.

Weinberg, J., Diller, L., Gordon, W.A., Gerstman, L.J., Lieberman, A., Lakin, P., *et al.* (1979). Training sensory awareness and spatial organisation in people with right brain damage. *Archives of Physical Medicine and Rehabilitation*, *60*, 491–496.

World Health Organisation (WHO) (1992) International Classification of Diseases, 10th edn. Geneva: WHO.

Whyte, J. (1994). Toward rational psychopharmacological treatment: Integrating research and clinical practice. *Journal of Head Trauma Rehabilitation*, *9*, 91–103.

Wood, R.Ll. (1984). Behaviour disorders following severe head injury: Their presentation and psychological management. In N. Brooks (Ed.) *Closed head injury, psychological, social and family consequences* (pp.195–200). New York: Oxford University Press.

Wood, R.Ll. (1987). Brain injury rehabilitation: A neurobehavioural approach. London: Croom Helm.

Wood, R.Ll. (1989a). Management of behaviour disorders in a day hospital setting. *Journal of Head Trauma Rehabilitation*, *3*, 53–62.

Wood, R.Ll. (1989b). Behaviour problems and treatment after head injury. *Physical Medicine and Rehabilitation State of the Art Reviews*, *3*, 123–43.

Wood, R.Ll. (1990). Neurobehavioural paradigm for brain injury rehabilitation. In R.Ll. Wood (Ed.) *Neurobehavioural sequelae of traumatic brain injury* (pp.153–174). London: Taylor & Francis.

Wood, R.Ll. (2001). Understanding neurobehavioural disability. In R.Ll. Wood & T.M. McMillan (Eds.) *Neurobehavioural disability and social handicap following traumatic brain injury* (pp.1–28). Hove, UK: Psychology Press.

Wood, R.Ll. & Eames, P. (1981). Applications of behaviour modification in the rehabilitation of traumatically brain injured patients. In G. Davey (Ed.) *Applications of conditioning theory*. London: Croom Helm.

Wood, R.Ll., Liossi, C. & Wood, L. (2005). The impact of head injury neurobehavioral sequelae on personal relationships: Preliminary findings. *Brain Injury*, *19*, 845–851.

Wood, R.Ll., McCrea, J.D., Wood, L.M. & Merriman, R.N. (1999). Clinical and cost-effectiveness of post-acute neurobehavioural rehabilitation. *Brain Injury*, *13*, 69–88.

Wood, R.Ll. & Worthington, A.D. (1999). Outcome in community rehabilitation: Measuring the social impact of disability. *Neuropsychological Rehabilitation*, *9*, 505–516.

Wood, R.Ll. & Worthington, A.D. (2001a). Neurobehavioural rehabilitation: A conceptual paradigm. In R.Ll. Wood & T.M. McMillan (Eds.) *Neurobehavioural disability and social handicap following traumatic brain injury* (pp.107–131). Hove: Psychology Press.

Wood, R.Ll. & Worthington, A.D. (2001b). Neurobehavioural rehabilitation in practice. In R.Ll. Wood & T.M. McMillan (Eds.) *Neurobehavioural disability and social handicap following traumatic brain injury* (pp.133–155). Hove: Psychology Press.

Wood, R.Ll. & Yuidakul, L.K. (1997). Change in relationship status following traumatic brain injury. *Brain Injury*, *11*, 491–502.

Woody, S. (1988). Episodic dyscontrol syndrome and head injury: A case presentation. *Journal of Neuroscience Nursing*, *20*, 180–184.

Worthington, A.D. (2001). Out on a limb? Developing an integrated rehabilitation service for adults with acquired brain injury. *Clinical Psychology*, *23*, 14–18.

Worthington, A.D. (2002). The natural recovery and treatment of executive disorders. In P.W. Halligan, U. Kischka & J. Marshall (Eds.) *Handbook of clinical neuropsychology* (pp.322–339). Oxford: Oxford University Press.

Worthington, A.D. (2005). Effective treatment of related disabilities. In P.W. Halligan & D.T. Wade. *The effectiveness of rehabilitation for cognitive deficits*. Oxford: Oxford University Press.

Worthington, A., Matthews, S., Melia, Y. & Oddy, M. (2006). Cost-benefits associated with social outcome from neurobehavioural rehabilitation. *Brain Injury*, *20*, 947–957.

Worthington, A.D., Wiliams, C., Young, K. & Pownall, J. (1997). Re-training gait components for walking in the context of abulia. *Physiotherapy and Practice*, *13*, 247–256.

Wroblewski, B.A. & Glenn, M.B. (1994). Pharmacological treatment of arousal and cognitive deficits. *Journal of Head Trauma and Rehabilitation*, *9*, 19–42.

Yatham, L.N. & McHale, P.A. (1988). Carbamazepine in the treatment of aggression: A case report and a review of the literature. *Acta Psychiatrica Scandinavica*, *78*, 188–190.

Yody, B.B., Schaub, C., Conway, J., Peters, S., Strauss, D. & Heslinger, S. (2000). Applied behaviour management and acquired brain injury: Approaches and assessment. *Journal of Head Trauma Rehabilitation*, *15*, 1041–1060.

Youngson, H.A. & Alderman, N. (1994). Fears of incontinence and its effects on a community based rehabilitation programme after severe head injury: Successful remediation of escape behaviour using behaviour modification. *Brain Injury*, *8*, 23–26.

Zafonte, R.D., Cullen, N. & Lexell, J. (2002). Serotonin agents in the treatment of acquired brain injury. *Journal of Head Trauma Rehabilitation*, *17*, 322–334.

Zasler, N.D. (1995). Bromocriptine: Neuropharmacology and clinical caveats. *Journal of Head Trauma Rehabilitation*, *10*, 101–104.

11

Fear, Anxiety and Depression

Joanna Collicutt McGrath

Introduction

Traumatic brain injury is an acute and dramatic life event with multiple and long-term ramifications. The immediate consequences are likely to include both cognitive and physical impairments such as amnesia, dysphasia, hemiparesis or ataxia. These will be evident as disabilities such as disorientation, inability to make one's wishes known to others, inability to walk or to reach for desired objects. Physical appearance may change beyond recognition. In addition, the brain-injured person's social situation changes dramatically. He or she becomes a 'patient', may be admitted to hospital, and may become a long-term resident in a rehabilitation facility. Thus, in a matter of hours dramatic, and often long-term, changes in physical and social status take place. The person will have experienced an event that may have brought him or her close to death and may pose a continuing threat to life. The prognosis is uncertain, in the early stages at least.

Over a period of time the person may come to realise that he or she may no longer be in a position to derive meaning and satisfaction from certain roles such as being a leading academic, skilled footballer or competent homemaker, and must search for satisfaction elsewhere. The ability to act freely may have been compromised by disability and changed social status, so that new limits to personal autonomy must be accepted. Lastly, and perhaps most importantly, personal identity is profoundly challenged by the general loss of cohesion to personal life brought about by disorganisation and fragmentation of cognitive and physical systems (Collicutt McGrath, 2007; Kay, 1986; Mohl & Burstein, 1982).

Each brain-injured person brings a personal and social history and a unique set of coping resources to this situation. Unfortunately, these very resources are likely to be diminished as a result of the brain injury. For instance, a person who previously was able calmly to think through problems in life may no longer be able to utilise such a strategy owing to cognitive impairment. At the very time that resources need to be effectively marshalled, they are unavailable (Lewis & Rosenberg, 1990; Miller, 1992).

It might therefore be expected that major psychological distress would be an inevitable consequence of traumatic brain injury. However, traumatic brain injury survivors show a wide range of emotional responses, including positive feelings such as relief at being alive, hope of further or full recovery or thankfulness at an opportunity to review a previously dysfunctional lifestyle (Collicultt McGrath & Linley, 2006; McGrath, 2004).

The more unpleasant emotions reported by people with acquired brain injury include frustration (almost ubiquitous), sadness, confused feelings, fear, worry and proneness to tears (McGrath & Adams, 1999).

This chapter is concerned with fear, anxiety and depression. These terms are widely, and often inconsistently, used. They will therefore now be defined, and their relationship with each other discussed.

Fear

Fear is an emotion characterised by behaviour that occurs in response to clear threat. The type of behaviour involved is generally divided into:

- passive avoidance, including freezing;
- active avoidance, including social submission or placatory behaviours;
- attachment behaviour (seeking close proximity to a familiar and trusted person);
- escape or attempts to escape; and
- defensive aggression.

This behaviour is usually accompanied by characteristic thoughts concerned with personal vulnerability, and signs and symptoms of physiological arousal such as changes in heart activity and muscle tension, increased perspiration, feeling too hot or too cold, shortness of breath, dizziness, stomach sensations, or desire to urinate or defecate.

Anxiety

Anxiety is closely related to fear, but is more often thought of as a response to unfocused or only partly conscious threat (Beck & Emery, 1979; Lazarus, 1994), often involving emotional conflict. For this reason, clinical states whose core emotion is extreme fear (Izard, 1972) are described as anxiety disorders. (The fear is out of proportion to the objective danger or is not focused on any identifiable threat.) The degree of physiological arousal may be so extreme that it culminates in a *panic attack*. Panic attacks can then themselves become the focus of fear and avoidance.

Beck and Emery (1992) argue that anxiety is characterised by thoughts that look towards the future, anticipating danger, in contrast to depression which is characterised by thoughts of regrets concerning the past. Anxious thoughts are said to be tentative and exploratory of the 'What if . . .?' variety, whereas depressive thoughts are more fixed, with clear negative expectations. Preoccupation with both these types of thoughts constitutes *worry*. Self-blame may occur in both conditions but in anxiety the blame is attached to specific actions, whereas in depression it reflects a general characterological evaluation.

Depression

Depression is a clinical state whose core emotion is extreme sadness or hopelessness but in which other emotions such as guilt, anxiety or anger occur. It is also characterised by biological features including sleep disturbance, fatigue, loss of appetite with consequent weight loss, and loss of sexual desire. There are often problems with cognition and ability to make decisions, and a loss of interest in normal pleasurable activities. Beck (1967) describes a key triad of beliefs in depression:

- The self is worthless.
- The future is hopeless.
- The world is meaningless.

These beliefs are thought to underpin the preoccupation with death and suicidal behaviour of seriously depressed people.

It can be seen that depression is a higher-order concept, which can incorporate anxiety. Psychiatric diagnostic systems are hierarchical in nature, and anxiety states are sometimes treated as symptoms of a more fundamental depressive disorder.

These definitions of fear, anxiety, and depression make it clear that it is possible to experience distressing levels of emotion without necessarily showing signs of clinical anxiety or depression. Even if the distress does take the form of clinically severe anxiety or depression, a person may not be considered to be suffering from a formal psychiatric disorder because the distress does not seem to be out of proportion to his or her life circumstances (for instance in bereavement). The emotional behaviour of people with traumatic brain injury can often be seen as a normal response to an abnormal situation. Who can say that a fear of developing hydrocephalus is unwarranted, if previous treatment attempts have had only short-lived success? or that fear of going out if there is significant risk of falling is out of proportion to the actual risk involved? or that suicidal thoughts are unreasonable on learning that one will never walk again?

For this reason the management of emotional distress in people with acquired brain injury must place at least as much emphasis on the modification of the person's situation (his or her physical environment, functional skill levels, and social support systems) as on the modification of internal psychological processes such as negative automatic thoughts. This is a difference in emphasis from that usually found in the psychological treatment of people with mental health problems (see, for instance, Greenberger & Padesky, 1995; Kinney, 2001; Whitehouse, 1994).

Other related states: (I) Emotionalism

Emotionalism following brain injury is a behavioural pattern that is characteristic of neurological patients and is not addressed by current psychiatric classification systems. It is distinct from depression but is sometimes mistaken for it. It is also sometimes referred to as 'emotional lability', 'inappropriate emotion', 'emotional incontinence', 'pathological crying or affect', 'pseudobulbar affect', and has been described in a wide range of neurological disorders, including traumatic brain injury (McGrath, 2001). Its main clinical feature is an increased readiness to cry or, more rarely, laugh (Allman, 1991).

Systematic descriptions of emotionalism are largely confined to studies of stroke patients. House and colleagues note that, while emotionalism is clearly distinct from depression, many of their sample showed signs of both conditions (House *et al.*, 1989). Crying tended to occur in 'emotional' contexts and was therefore not inappropriate but excessive. In other studies of stroke patients the crying occurred with some warning and was most usually provoked by thoughts of family or the illness, kind gestures, the arrival or departure of visitors, television or music, disagreements, and the inability to perform a task (Allman *et al.*, 1990; Allman 1991b). These findings have been confirmed for a mixed sample which included patients with traumatic brain injury (McGrath, 2001).

This problem may be confined to the post-acute period, resolving spontaneously over time. Low doses of antidepressants can be helpful in treatment (Allman, 1992; Sloan *et al.*, 1992).

Other related states: (II) Apathy

Apathy is a behavioural concept that incorporates lack of engagement in activities, reduced initiation, psychic fatigue and apparent emotional indifference. It is a feature of depression which is readily observable, but may also be particularly applicable to neurological patients who are not actually experiencing depressed mood (Kant *et al.*, 1998; Nyenhuis *et al.*, 1997; Riley, 2000). It is possible that apathy may be functional in some circumstances, for instance allowing the individual necessary time to rest and recuperate after action or trauma (Rothbaum *et al.*, 1982).

A study of apathy in a mixed sample of neurological patients, which included people with traumatic brain injury, showed that it was most characteristic of patients with right-sided or subcortical lesions, that it often appeared in combination with depressed mood, but also occurred independently (Andersson *et al.*, 1999).

When trying to help the heterogeneous group of people who experience apathy it is therefore necessary to be clear about the mechanism underlying it. Where problems with initiating action predominate, treatment with a dopamine agonist could be considered (Powell *et al.*, 1996).

Other related states: (III) 'Organic' alexithymia

This is an acquired difficulty in identifying or describing emotional feelings, which may or may not be underpinned by a loss or impoverishment of affective experience. It is associated with some types of mental health problems but is increasingly recognised as a complication of traumatic brain injury (Becerra *et al.*, 2002; Williams *et al.*, 2001). While most people with acquired brain injury report a rich and nuanced emotional experience (McGrath, 2002), some may deny unpleasant emotional experience, some may have a restricted range of experience because of depressed mood, and those with alexithymia may have lost the capacity to experience emotions. Careful questioning is often necessary to identify this sort of problem which, like the loss of the ability to feel pain, may not be unpleasant for the patient, but can have disastrous effects on intimate relationships.

Other related states: (IV) The role of medication

Apathetic behaviour is a phenomenon that straddles the domains of emotion and cognition. It is also an example of a common end point for a number of processes including physical fatigue and weakness, depression, and dysexecutive problems such as inertia or anhedonia. Medication-induced states or reactions to the withdrawal of medication can superficially resemble anxiety states. Patients with acquired brain injury can be very susceptible to the effects of psychotropic medication (which may have been prescribed in an attempt to sedate them in the acute phase), including unwanted side effects. For instance, one side effect of the major tranquillisers is *akathisia* expressed as marked motor and mental restlessness which can easily be mistaken for agitation (Trimble, 1996).

Incidence and prevalence of anxiety and depression following traumatic brain injury

While there is an association between traumatic brain injury and psychiatric disorder (Fann *et al.*, 2004; Silver *et al.*, 2001), specific incidence and prevalence rates are likely to vary in relation to severity of brain injury and time since injury. The assessment of incidence and prevalence also obviously depends on the chosen definitions of anxiety and depression. The number of people assessed as suffering formal anxiety or mood disorders is likely to be less than the number who show some signs and symptoms of anxiety and depression, which is in turn likely to be less than the number of people who experience private subjective fear, worry or sadness. There are also problems with both defining and measuring these phenomena in people with traumatic brain injury (see below). The literature in this area is quite small, much more attention having been paid to behavioural and cognitive sequelae of traumatic brain injury.

Anxiety is a very common problem following mild head injury (see King, 1997). Studies suggest that anxiety may also be a significant problem in people with severe head injury, with phobic and generalised anxiety and panic disorder reported (Deb *et al.*, 1999; Fann *et al.*, 1995; Lishman, 1973; Roberts, 1979). Post-traumatic stress disorder is also increasingly recognised (see chapter 12). Using the Leeds Scale for Anxiety (Snaith *et al.*, 1976) Tyerman and Humphrey (1984) found that 44 per cent of their sample of head-injured patients scored above the cut-off, indicating 'clinically severe' levels of anxiety. Sixty per cent of their sample showed evidence of depression. Kinsella and colleagues, also using this scale, found that 26 per cent of their sample scored at a level indicative of 'clinically severe' anxiety, and 33 per cent showed evidence of depression (Kinsella *et al.*, 1988). Both these studies involved patients who had suffered head injury within the past two years.

Van Zomeren and Van den Bing (1985) used a problem checklist with a sample of patients two years after the injury. Eighteen per cent of their sample reported being troubled by anxiety, 19 per cent were troubled by depression, and 21 per cent by emotionalism. Linn and colleagues also examined a sample of chronic subjects with a mean time since injury of six years (Linn *et al.*, 1994). Using the SCL 90-R (Derogatis, 1983) they found 50 per cent of their sample to be troubled by anxiety and 70 per cent by depression. However, the SCL 90-R is not an ideal assessment tool as it involves somatic and cognitive symptoms that may be directly caused by brain injury. The rates of anxiety and depression reported are therefore likely to be overestimates.

Reported incidence rates of formal depressive disorder have been as high as 42 per cent in the first year after traumatic brain injury (Fedoroff *et al.*, 1992; Jorge *et al.*, 1993a, 1993b, 1994). This group of investigators note a significant number of anxiety symptoms in their samples but effectively ignore them, describing them as 'clinical manifestations' of depression. They used a version of the Present State Examination (Wing *et al.*, 1978) to assess mental state. Like the SCL 90-R, this contains items that many of be attributed to the direct effects of brain injury, particularly apathy, and again many of these studies probably overestimate of the incidence of depression.

Clinical Description of Fear, Anxiety and Depression in Traumatic Brain Injury

Emotional behaviour

It is likely that the experience of and expression of emotional distress takes specific forms in people with traumatic brain injury. This is for at least two reasons: first, their ability to organise and control their own behaviour, including emotional behaviour, is reduced; secondly, there are specific sources of stress in their situation, so their worries, fears, and depressive preoccupations may have a similarly specific focus.

Emotional behaviour involves facial expression, prosodic aspects of speech, verbal self-report, crying and laughing, body posture and action. Yet the cognitive and motor systems involved in this may be compromised in brain injury. Facial expression may be limited by paralysis, weakness, or Parkinsonism, such that the person may look 'flat' or 'sad' no matter what emotion is actually being experienced. Speech may be slow, monotonic, lacking nuances, unintelligible, reduced in volume, or absent, lacking the urgency and rapidity usually associated with fear or anxiety. The person may not physically be able to say how he or she is feeling. Body movement and posture may be severely limited. Emotional behaviour may therefore be difficult for observers to detect and identify.

The emotional behaviour of people with acquired brain injury undergoing in-patient rehabilitation has been studied in some detail by the author (McGrath, 1998). This study used occupational therapists and physiotherapists who knew the participants well as observers, and found that *some* participants showed behaviour that could be recognised by these observers as signifying specific emotional states such as fear and sadness. Fearful behaviour included reluctance, resistance and avoidance of specific activities, attachment behaviour directed towards the therapist, clinging to stable objects in the environment, screaming, freezing and physiological signs such as sweating and hyperventilating. Sadness was identified mainly through facial expression and tearfulness. However, when directly questioned by an independent investigator, *many more* participants reported feeling these emotions to a very distressing degree, yet they had not disclosed it previously and it was not apparent in their behaviour to the therapist observers. In fact, when making judgements about participants' emotional state the therapist observers relied most heavily on what the participants spontaneously said, rather than on their non-verbal behaviour, perhaps because they could not always 'read' this behaviour easily.

These findings highlight the particular problems faced by people with traumatic brain injury who have speech and language impairment in communicating their emotions to others. The findings also suggest that even those people who have intact speech and language may experience significant emotional distress, which goes undetected by professionals unless they are questioned directly about it.

Emotional concerns

The study also examined the focus of specific fears and feelings of sadness in this group using both self-report and therapist observations. The results indicate that the things feared by this sample of brain-injured people (most of whom had at least mild problems with mobility) are rather different from those feared either by people with mental health problems or by the general population. Both observers and participants gave highly consistent reports in this respect. By far the most commonly feared event was falling (Collicutt McGrath, in press). Fear occurred in situations involving some degree of physical risk, usually personal mobility (for instance, standing, walking or transferring) or car travel. There was also considerable fear of novel situations or activities. When describing the experience of fear, these participants referred to their own vulnerability in a threatening environment. They thought themselves at risk of falling, and vulnerable to the effects of a fall:

> I just get panicky. I start to do things but then I panic. I can get up and stand straight for a while and then I just get panicky – I freeze. I know I'm standing but I feel I'm going to fall, I go to grab – I feel willing in my body but I can't understand why it isn't there.

The deeper fear underlying this was accessed through more detailed questioning concerning automatic thoughts, underlying assumptions and core fears. This was often a fear of sustaining further injury (either another head injury or a fractured limb), and the perceived cost in terms of the process of recovery. The participants expressed fears and worries concerning their prognosis. Their goal was to get better as quickly as possible and they did not want anything to get in the way of this:

> I might damage myself further and put back my return to a normal life.

Fear of falling is fairly common in elderly people (Delbaere *et al.*, 2004; Fletcher & Hirdes, 2004; Isaacs, 1978), and fear of moving about in open spaces, termed 'space phobia' (Marks & Bebbington, 1976), has been reported in people with a range of physical problems, including neck injury and cerebrovascular disease (Jeans & Orvell, 1991; Lishman, 1978; Marks, 1981; McCaffrey *et al.*, 1990; McNally, 1990). It may therefore be characteristic of patients with mobility problems following traumatic brain injury, but not unique to them.

The participants in this study were at a relatively early stage in their rehabilitation. They were concentrating on becoming physically well and spent much time in a protected hospital environment. This perhaps explains why they showed less fear than might be expected of social situations (such as meeting old friends or eating in public). It is likely that social fears emerge more consistently after discharge when physical status has stabilised and the demands made by community living and return to family life become more evident.

This move from hospital to the community is also a potentially significant factor in the emergence of depressed mood. Discharge from rehabilitation signals the end of major recovery and, sadly, often the loss of professional support networks. Patients can feel abandoned at the very time that the realities of their long-term situation are beginning to dawn on them (Tyerman, 1988).

In the early stages of recovery from traumatic brain injury, sadness appears to be focused on separation from home and family, and a loss of familiar routines (McGrath & Adams, 1999). These people often describe a particularly quality of sadness characterised by intense feelings of isolation and a longing for things to return to the way they were prior to the injury.

Depression can be difficult to diagnose in people with traumatic brain injury because the biological features may be attributable to their physical condition (for instance, sleep disturbance due to pain, weight loss due to dysphagia), it can be hard to distinguish from apathy or emotionalism, and cognitive or communication problems may prevent patients articulating their beliefs and feelings. However, the cognitive triad identified by Beck can be seen in the preoccupations of brain-injured people who can communicate, though it is focused on their specific situation. Thus, a person may see herself as worthless because she no longer looks conventionally attractive. She may see the future as hopeless because she has been told that she will never be able to return to her university studies, and she may see the world as meaningless because the injury happened to her apparently at random. This is clearly reflected in the three key questions dominating the thoughts of traumatic brain injury survivors identified by Prigatano (1991) as:

- Will I be normal?
- Is life worth living after this brain injury?
- Why did this happen to me?

These questions refer to the self, the future, and the world respectively. The struggle with such questions can be seen as part of a normal process of psychological adaptation to this major life event. However, where fixed themes of worthlessness, hopelessness or meaninglessness emerge it becomes appropriate to invoke the label of depression.

Links with Pathology

The role of particular brain structures in the experience and expression of emotion remains controversial. Neural models of fear are better developed than those of general anxiety and depression. The summary presented below is a simplification of an extremely complex and rapidly developing area of research.

The key structure implicated in both the experience of fear and the learning of fear associations is the amygdala (LeDoux, 1992, 1995; Scott *et al.*, 1997). A two-system model has been proposed involving, first, a rapid automatic but undifferentiated system mediated by subcortical pathways, and second, a slower more detailed and accurate system mediated via the cerebral cortex and hippocampus and accessible to consciousness. The subcortical system involves direct sensory input to thalamic nuclei which project to the lateral nucleus of the amygdala, and thence to the central nucleus which enables a motor and physiological response. The second system, acting in parallel, enables more detailed perceptual analysis to take place in the cortex, with the septo-hippocampal system being instrumental in appraisal of the significance and meaning of the stimulus. Output from the hippocampus to the amygdala enables the initial automatic response to be developed or inhibited as necessary. Thus, the second system acts as a check on and backup to the first system.

For instance, the rapid response system may underpin the initial withdrawal response from a spider-like object, and the conscious system may ascertain that the object is in fact only a tomato top and inhibit further fear.

Fearful responding to signals of danger is rapidly learnt and only unlearnt with some difficulty (Marks, 1987). The initial learning of fear can be abolished, at least in animals, by lesions to the amygdala, and the unlearning of fear associations can be abolished by lesions of orbito-frontal cortex (Jones & Mishkin, 1972; Morgan *et al.*, 1993; Rolls, 1986). Thus selective lesions to the amygdala (which occur very rarely under natural conditions) might render a person unable to learn that a particular place was associated with something unpleasant. In contrast, lesions to orbito-frontal cortex (common in traumatic brain injury) might make it very difficult for a person who had *already* learnt to fear a particular place to learn that it was in fact now safe (Freedman, 1990; King, 2002).

One implication of the two-system account of fear is that the learning of fear can still take place if one of the systems is disabled or destroyed. This has very important clinical significance for people with brain injury. The medial temporal lobe structures, including the hippocampus, are very vulnerable to surface shearing effects and pressure from oedema in traumatic brain injury (Brooks, 1989). Damage to these structures results in at least impairment of learning and memory and at most in dense amnesia. However, these people may still retain the rapid response subcortical fear system. They can learn unconsciously to be frightened of certain people, places, smells, but they cannot reflect on this or place a conscious check on it. There is plenty of clinical evidence that this actually occurs (e.g. Black *et al.*, 1977; Claparede, 1911), and this mechanism may have been operating in the rehabilitation case presented later in this chapter. Claparede's famous amnesic patient was completely unable to recall having met him the previous day, but was nevertheless unwilling to shake his hand because he had secreted a drawing pin in his palm on the previous occasion. It must never be assumed that because a person has very impaired explicit memory he or she cannot learn to be afraid.

Lesion models of depression have proved easier to construct. These have been based on experimental animal studies, studies of humans with stroke (Robinson *et al.*, 1983, 1984), and studies of humans with traumatic brain injury (Jorge *et al.*, 1993a, 1993b). This group of investigators claims a link between left hemisphere lesions located towards the frontal pole and clinical depressive disorder. They argue that it is mediated by depletion of noradrenaline in cortical pathways, arising from these left hemisphere lesions. However, the findings of this group remain controversial and not consistently replicated by other investigators. Changed activity in the caudate nuclei of the basal ganglia, which have projections to frontal cortex, has also been implicated in depressive disorder (Krishnan *et al.*, 1992).

While it is theoretically possible that depression following traumatic brain injury may arise as an exclusively biological 'complication' of damage to the brain, it is likely that the mechanisms at work involve a more complex interplay between premorbid personality, degree and site of brain lesions, and situational factors.

Psychological Theory

There are several cognitive behavioural theories of emotion. The model presented below is based on the work of Lazarus (1966) but its components are common to most theories:

- circumstances in the environment (stimuli);
- interpretation of the significance of these stimuli in terms of personally valued goals (primary appraisal);
- judgement of ability to cope with these stimuli using personal resources or other resources available in the environment (secondary appraisal);
- coping reaction patterns (response repertoire).

Primary appraisal

If environmental stimuli pose a significant threat to a person's valued goals, fear will be experienced. If the person appraises his or her ability to deal effectively with the source of threat as good, then this fear will be ameliorated. Fear will also be reduced if the person can identify helpful resources available from someone else through social support. However, if the person judges his or her own coping abilities as poor, and there is no one else on whom to rely, then fear will increase.

Some stimuli pose universal threats (for instance, a fire burning out of control). However, there is infinite variability in the way in which stimuli are interpreted by individuals in terms of their relation to personal history, culture or currently valued goals. For instance, the risk of sustaining a small injury through falling may be interpreted as extremely threatening if the person is already injured and on a fairly fragile road to recovery.

Secondary appraisal

Appraisal of ability to cope is influenced by objective features of the person's situation. For instance, an inability to move independently reduces the range of available coping reactions when faced with physical threat, presumably leading to an increase in experienced fear. However, personal beliefs about the self will also influence this process. These personal beliefs are based in part on past experience of attempts at coping.

The effectiveness of past coping reactions influences subsequent secondary appraisals of available psychological resources. That is the experience of success not only makes a person more likely to utilise a similar strategy when in a similar situation (positive reinforcement of the coping reaction), it also makes the same situation appear less threatening on subsequent occasions because self-efficacy is perceived to be high (Bandura, 1997). This principle has influenced cognitive behavioural approaches to phobic anxiety which emphasise behavioural experiments in which the patient is exposed to the feared situation and enabled to cope with it (Butler, 1989).

On the other hand, repeated perceived failures to cope are likely to result in a view of the self as unable to cope, and reduce the likelihood of attempting effective action (Abramson *et al.*, 1978). Negative beliefs about the self ('worthless') and lack of engagement with activities ('hopeless', 'meaningless') underpin discouragement and depressed mood. These negative beliefs help maintain the depressed state by influencing interpretation of attempts at coping (Beck, 1967), so that they are too readily dismissed as ineffectual. The environmental stimuli that began as threats signalling potential losses are realised as perceived actual losses.

This theory helps explain why fear appears to be fairly common in the early stages of acquired brain injury, but depression may take some time to emerge (Fleminger *et al.*, 2003; Harrick *et al.*, 1994; Jorge *et al.*, 1993a, 1993b). The environment of the brain-injured person is full of perceived threats, but these threats may be seen as time limited while the person is physically vulnerable, hence the acute desire to regain physical strength and abilities. The person may believe that he or she will be able to cope as effectively as before the injury once these abilities return (hence the enthusiasm that many patients show for physiotherapy). The vulnerable state is seen as an unpleasant temporary phase. Over time the hoped-for physical recovery may not be achieved, and insight into other problems such as persisting cognitive deficits and a loss of social support networks emerges. The person may then reappraise his or her long-term coping potential as poor, with consequent discouragement and depression.

Coping

The fear behaviours described in the first section can be thought of as coping responses that occur under conditions of threat. Avoidance occurs in response to fear signals with a view to pre-empting a potentially dangerous situation. Attachment behaviour reduces the perceived threat of such a situation. Escape or aggression occurs in response to an existing painful or escalating dangerous situation; in such cases avoidance may have been tried first and failed, or avoidance may not have been an available option. This point has important clinical implications. People with traumatic brain injury may be unable to avoid things that frighten them because of mobility problems, because they lack the cognitive or communication ability to express the need to avoid, or because their attempts at avoidance are thwarted owing to their reduced power as patients in a hospital environment. The threshold for defensive aggression is therefore reduced (McGrath & Davis, 1992). In brain-injured people aggression often signifies fear.

Coping responses are not limited to overt behaviour (Lazarus & Folkman, 1984). Active mental attempts to reappraise the significance of an event can reduce the degree of threat it poses. For instance, on not being successful at a job interview it would be possible to decide that one had never really wanted the job in the first place, so that self-concept is no longer threatened. Cognitive behavioural approaches to anxiety and depression actively encourage reappraisal of stimuli in terms of the threat they pose, and critical examination of habitual negative self-appraisals, reflected in automatic thoughts (Padesky & Greenberger, 1995). Dramatic improvements in mood can often be effected through the modification of these appraisal processes.

It might be thought that people with traumatic brain injury would be unable to utilise cognitive coping techniques. However, the McGrath (1998) study found that at least rudimentary 'positive thinking' was a strategy spontaneously used by many participants:

> Come on, you'll be able to do it soon if you persevere. Keep your patience. I went to the loo on my own the other night. I felt really chuffed with myself that I could do it.

These people often said that it helped to see that other people in the rehabilitation unit were worse off than themselves, presumably because this placed their own coping abilities and situation in a more favourable light:

> I try to think about some of the other patients. At least I can stand. Other people will take a lot longer to reach the stage I am at if they ever do. It puts it more in perspective.

This type of thinking apparently gave them the courage to engage in activities such as physiotherapy which caused them some fear, but which they knew would help them to become less vulnerable in the longer term.

People with traumatic brain injury have good reason to see threat or actual loss in their environment. They may be in a novel hospital environment. This may expose them to threatening degrees of space, height, noise or illumination. They may be touched and handled unexpectedly. They may be left alone or, more likely, separated from family and friends. Sudden loss of physical support on lifting may occur. (All these things are stimuli which have been shown to elicit innate fear responses across a wide range of species.) In addition, these patients may experience pain at the hands of health-care professionals, for instance through attempts to exercise contracted limbs or administer injections, and quickly learn to be afraid of them. This all occurs against a background of potential major losses, which include permanent disability, unemployment, homelessness, poverty, divorce or separation, and death.

People with traumatic brain injury also have good reason to believe that their coping abilities are poor. The brain injury renders them less competent to deal with threat situations because of physical or cognitive disability and social disempowerment. They may no longer be able to walk away from situations they find threatening, such as large social gatherings, or to think out solutions to problems in living effectively. Communication problems limit control over the actions of others, for instance in giving consent to unpleasant procedures. Incarceration in hospital may render them incapable of dealing with pressing situations at home or at work.

In many respects therefore, their appraisals of themselves as vulnerable and their situation as threatening are realistic. However, there are additional factors arising from brain injury which may distort appraisal processes, making people with traumatic brain injury even more susceptible to feelings of fear, anxiety or depression. The hospital environment is novel to most sick people, but it is rendered profoundly novel to many brain-injured patients because of cognitive problems such as amnesia or spatial perceptual impairment. In addition, the experience of normal activities of daily living such as moving or speaking may have become distorted, with the relation between intention and result being unpredictable. Where there is loss of sensation, feelings of being unsupported by one's limbs and unawareness of the safety signals provided by solid surfaces are likely to be evident.

Thus, for people with traumatic brain injury the environment poses a real threat, effective resources for coping with threat are depleted, and the environment is appraised as even more threatening owing to deficiencies in processing environmental stimuli.

Certain cognitive problems may exacerbate this situation. As discussed in an earlier section, damage to the frontal lobes may prevent the unlearning of initial fear responses that are no longer appropriate. Frontal lobe damage can also result in reduced flexibility of thinking (Eslinger *et al.*, 1995), so that the person gets stuck with certain ideas and beliefs such as 'I am a cripple.' This may mean that unhelpful reasoning patterns are held with rigid intensity. For instance, 'If I can't walk normally no attractive girl will ever want me, therefore I am worthless.'

Finally, other cognitive problems may protect the person with acquired brain injury from emotional distress, at least for a time. Unawareness of deficits, sometimes evident as an almost delusional denial of disability (anosognosia), is traditionally associated with large lesions to the non-dominant hemisphere (Prigatano, 1994). However, while these people may deny disability or attribute their problems to external factors, they can still become indignant and angry to a distressing degree at what they interpret as the unreasonable behaviour of those around them in placing constraints upon their freedom of action. It has also been argued that depression following right hemisphere lesions may be missed because it is masked by apparent unconcern (Finset, 1988).

Assessment Techniques

People with traumatic brain injury have short attention spans and fatigue easily, at least in the acute stages. They may not be able to write owing to acquired physical disability. Their vision may be too impaired to read, or they may have acquired dyslexia. They may not be able to speak owing to dysarthria. They may not comprehend or be able to produce expressive language. Thus the process of cognitive and emotional assessment is enormously challenging for the clinician.

Given the variety of needs and abilities in this population, access to a range of instruments designed to assess emotional distress is desirable. The objective of carrying out the assessment should always be kept clearly in mind. This is mainly to drive the selection of instruments, but a coherent explanation of the reason for going through the process can be very reassuring to the examinee.

It is tempting to rely on reports or ratings of observers (professionals or family members) in assessing the emotional status of brain-injured people, especially if they have significant communication problems. However, there are problems with this approach. Observers can only comment on overt behaviour, and these observations cannot be treated as equivalent or superior in validity to self-report. For instance, the behavioural aspects of fear may not be synchronised with the subjective aspects (Mathews, 1971). Behaviour is situation specific, and it is likely that brain-injured people behave differently with professionals and with family. Family members may themselves be suffering from mood disturbance or have their own personal agendas, and it therefore cannot be assumed that their ratings have a high degree of objectivity. Nevertheless, observer ratings provide useful information. Examples of such measures in clinical use are the Katz Social Adjustment Scale (Hogarty & Katz, 1971), the Neurobehavioral Rating Scale (Levin *et al.*, 1987), and the relative's form of the Neuropsychology Behaviour and Affect Profile (Nelson *et al.*, 1989). These scales have varying amounts of data concerning reliability and validity. The most promising scale of this sort, with good data on its validity with respect to assessing mood, is the Neurobehavioral Functioning Inventory (Kreutzer *et al.*, 1996).

Instruments relying on self-report should be relatively short, reliable, and contain items that are appropriate and relevant to this population. Scales that were designed as brief paper-and-pencil questionnaires for use with other groups may have to be treated more like structured interviews, with sufficient time allowed. Some patients will require instruments that do not rely on the written or spoken word.

Open-ended questions can be useful in this respect, allowing articulate people the opportunity to give an account of their emotional experience in their own words. However, they may also need to make use of structure in order to formulate their responses, and they may find non-directive interviews socially ambiguous and anxiety provoking. Open-ended questions can prove particularly difficult for people with traumatic brain injury who have impaired executive function, being analogous in some respects to a verbal fluency task.

A selection of the more useful scales is given below.

Profile of Mood States (POMS)

The POMS (McNair *et al.*, 1981) consists of 65 single words describing mood states. The use of single words means that it is applicable to patients who have impaired language function but are still capable of single word comprehension. It is able to give a total mood disturbance score, and scores on each of six derived factors; tension-anxiety, depression-dejection, anger-hostility, fatigue-inertia, vigour-activity, confusion-bewilderment. It has proven reliability and a stable factorial structure. However, it is long, and several shortened versions have been developed (Cella *et al.*, 1987; Schacham, 1983) which may be more appropriate for use with people with traumatic brain injury.

The Beck Depression Inventory (BDI)

The BDI (Beck *et al.*, 1961) is the instrument of choice to assess depression in non-brain-injured populations. However, its length, its linguistic complexity, and its inclusion of somatic items which might be direct effects of brain injury limit its usefulness in traumatic brain injury (Green *et al.*, 2001; Sliwinski *et al.*, 1998). Nevertheless, it remains a highly clinically useful tool for those patients who are able to complete it, if interpreted with caution.

The Hospital Anxiety and Depression Scale (HADS)

The HADS (Zigmond & Snaith, 1983) is a widely used scale whose main advantages are that it is short and that it gives separate anxiety and depression scores. It was developed for use with patients who are physically ill. Despite this, the depression scale contains several items that could relate to physical or cognitive symptoms of brain injury. The wording of some items is complex and cumbersome. There is no item in the depression scale relating to sadness or low mood. The anxiety scale is again quite physically based, with an emphasis on generic physiological arousal, useful in cases of generalised anxiety, tension or distress, but not useful for phobic anxiety. It is not sensitive or specific in identifying clinical anxiety or depression disorders in brain-injured populations (Johnson *et al.*, 1995; McGrath, 1998).

The Visual Analog Mood Scale (VAMS)

The VAMS (Nyenhuis *et al.*, 1997) is a seven-item scale using single words together with pictorial facial representations of the seven mood states represented. It is therefore short and applicable to patients with significant language impairment. The VAMS is unipolar, anchored on a neutral stimulus, and presented vertically rather than horizontally, so that the risk of error owing to perceptual impairment or inattention is minimised. There are norms available for stroke patients, and its reliability in this population is good (Arruda *et al.*, 1997).

All the above scales can be used as screens for the presence of anxiety or depressive disorders, but their predictive validity in this respect is ambiguous owing to the difficulty of making such diagnoses in this population. The instruments can also form the basis of psychological formulations and treatment, and are probably more useful if treated in this way.

The Rivermead Fear Questionnaire (Appendix 11.1)

This is an unpublished instrument used as a simple checklist of feared situations in patients attending the Oxford Centre for Enablement. It has proved clinically useful in identifying potential problem situations in patients who are newly admitted to the unit. The questionnaire consists of 20 items selected because they represented the most frequent responses given by a pool of 53 brain-injured participants who were interviewed about situations or activities that elicited fear. Each item is rated on a four-point scale with respect to the degree of subjective distress it causes and the degree to which it would be avoided. The questionnaire appears to have reasonable test–retest and reliability. Two administrations, separated by two weeks, on 10 people with long-standing acquired brain injury gave Kendall's correlation coefficients of 0.91 for total distress score and 0.80 for total avoidance score. There was also 86 per cent agreement across the two administrations on the identity of the feared items.

Rehabilitation

Some general points need to be borne in mind in the management of emotional distress in people with traumatic brain injury. First, the person has often been referred by someone else (a relative or professional) and may not see any need for treatment. Ethical considerations regarding consent to treatment procedures, which may involve distress getting worse before it gets better, therefore become very important. For instance, if a patient with traumatic brain injury refuses to participate in hydrotherapy because of a fear of water, it would only be acceptable to treat the fear using a graded exposure to water-based activities if the patient agrees. This can be frustrating for therapists, and the rights of the patient sometimes have to be balanced against a duty of care or against staff safety. Nevertheless, other things being equal, the patient must have the final say.

Second, assessment and one-to-one treatment of emotional distress should take place in a private setting, and confidentiality should be ensured as far as possible. Sensitive information should be shared on an 'as needed' basis, and this sharing should generally be restricted to the team directly involved in the patient's care.

Third, periods of distress in people in the post-acute stages of traumatic brain injury can settle fairly quickly without the necessity of major intervention (McGrath & Adams, 1999). Furthermore, there is evidence that moderate levels of anxiety or distress may actually be functional, indicating a degree of healthy psychological engagement with the reality of the situation (Collicutt McGrath & Linley, 2006).

Fourth, all interventions should have clear objectives that fit in with any team rehabilitation aims (McGrath & Davis, 1992; Wade, 1999), or with a wider sense of purpose in the patient's life. An example of such an objective would be 'for X to be able to attend his son's school sports day with a level of anxiety that he can manage', rather than 'for X to have 10 sessions of cognitive therapy' (which is merely an action plan).

Fifth, all interventions should be guided by a psychological theory. Treatment techniques can then be selected on a rational basis, rather than just being picked of the shelf at random. For instance, the theory presented earlier in this chapter lays down a number of processes that may be targeted in the management of emotional distress in people with traumatic injury.

Threats in the environment

These can be identified and minimised, for instance by positioning of the bed and adjacent furniture to give a sense of physical security; carrying out physiotherapy in a small room rather than in a large echoing gym; adjusting illumination and noise levels; providing clear safety signals at the end of unpleasant procedures.

Appraisal of threat

This may be based on a misunderstanding of something the person has been told, or on a partial understanding of the situation (for instance, beliefs about the healing of skull fracture). Therefore, one thrust of treatment is to ensure that the patient has an accurate understanding of the facts of his or her case. These may refer to the medical history, the medical prognosis or the therapy plan. If there are memory problems, then a simple written record easily accessible in a diary or on audiotape may be necessary. Excessive reassurance seeking (arising either from memory problems or anxiety) can be dealt with simply by writing answers to repeated questions in a diary, and referring the patient to the diary without further comment when these questions arise.

Where the simple facts of the situation are accurately understood, but perceived as threatening, then cognitive behavioural methods of reducing threat through reappraisal can be used (see e.g. Padesky & Greenberger, 1995). This involves looking at the actual losses that may follow from, for instance, being unable to walk or to resume work, which may not be as catastrophic as initially envisaged (McGrath & Adams, 1999).

Where visual perception or language comprehension problems contribute to threat appraisal, handling techniques may need to be modified. For instance, it may be helpful always to approach people with neglect or visual field loss from the 'good' side so that they are not startled. It may be helpful for the team to use an agreed consistent warning sign before hoisting a person with receptive dysphasia.

Self-appraisal

This can be supported by the provision of accurate feedback about rehabilitation progress and achievements. This may happen as part of the general rehabilitation system of goal planning, but some patients may require a more individualised approach. For instance, patients with memory loss can be given simple written records supplemented by photographs of their achievements (such as standing in a frame or paying a visit to town). If the person tends to dismiss such achievements as trivial, the valid feelings behind this response must be genuinely acknowledged. However, it is also the role of the clinician to provide challenges to this view, emphasising the link between apparently small steps and the final rehabilitation aims, which themselves *must* correspond to the patient's basic values if this argument is to be effective (McGrath *et al.*, 1995).

Coping reaction patterns

These may need little more than support from the clinician. Many people with traumatic brain injury are capable of thinking through the implications of this significant life event if they can be provided with ways around the problems with memory, writing or speech that might otherwise limit the process. Counselling sessions can give the opportunity and space to express emotion, and continuity between sessions can be established if the clinician or patient writes down summaries of the key points. Again, these can be usefully incorporated into diaries for private reflection between sessions, enabling emotion-focused coping.

Some coping reaction patterns are frankly dysfunctional, for instance defensive aggression. Where this occurs, offering the patient an alternative effective response that achieves the same communication function (La Vigna & Donnellan, 1986) can be helpful. For instance, teaching a patient who was previously biting to signal 'stop' during aversive procedures, and persuading the rehabilitation team not to ignore this less compelling response.

Denial of disability can be the expression of a specific form of cognitive impairment, as discussed in an earlier section. However, it can also reflect an emotional coping process aimed at self-protection. Dealing with the distress experienced by patients who have limited insight into their disabilities, of whatever origin, requires great tact and sensitivity on the part of the clinician. The objective in such cases is to achieve as accurate an awareness of the situation as is necessary for safety at least, but to maintain dignity and positive self-regard. It is preferable to set up a process of self-discovery rather than to confront the patient directly. This can be done by constructing a series of 'safe' failure experiences in a protected environment so that humiliation is avoided; for instance, asking a university lecturer to give a talk on some aspect of his work to a small staff group. General discussion about the problems following traumatic brain injury can also take place. Here it can be helpful to talk in the third person to reduce threat, for instance asking the patient what sort of problems he or she thinks a person with traumatic brain injury might have.

People with limited insight have a tendency to blame others for their own mistakes. They may complain about environmental signposting, accuse therapists of making mistakes about appointment times, or of changing offices. It is tempting to respond with outright correction when this occurs, but it is better practice to develop some tolerance of this behaviour, not colluding, but thinking carefully before actually challenging. Lack of insight may have a functional advantage of protecting the person from depression (Druss & Douglas, 1988; Fleminger *et al.*, 2003), at least in the first year of recovery.

Specific Approaches to Depression

Antidepressant medication (both traditional tricyclics and new generation serotonin specific re-uptake inhibitors (SSRIs)) can be of great use in the treatment of depression in traumatic brain injury survivors, particularly where biological symptoms predominate, or the person is incapable of engaging in psychological approaches. If depressed mood is contributing towards cognitive problems, the administration of antidepressants may result in an improvement in cognition. However, most antidepressants increase the risk of epileptic seizures (Trimble, 1978). This is an important consideration because any benefit achieved by the antidepressant may be completely cancelled out by the experience of a single seizure. This is a discouraging experience, particularly so because of its implications for return to driving.

As discussed above, conventional cognitive behavioural approaches to depressed mood can be used with traumatic brain injury survivors. The modifications required are (above all) therapist acknowledgement of the enormity of the experienced losses, a more directive and concrete style, briefer sessions but longer course of treatment, and the use of written records including flashcards for answers to negative automatic thoughts.

Suicidal thoughts and expressed intentions should always be taken seriously, but should be distinguished from the often-expressed wish to have died from the initial injury. When closely questioned about this the person may clarify, 'I sometimes wish I had died then, but I don't want to die now.'

Specific Approaches to Fear and Anxiety

Anxiolytic medication such as the benzodiazepines may be useful for limited short-term management of acute anxiety and distress but they also carry some risk of seizures and may impair cognition.

Relaxation techniques (e.g. Bernstein & Borkovec, 1973) may be useful in reducing arousal, and provide the patient with an additional coping strategy to deal with stress. Indeed, biofeedback-assisted relaxation has been used in single cases to ameliorate myoclonus and ataxia secondary to acquired brain injury (Duckett & Kramer, 1994; Guercio *et al.*, 1997). This type of physical problem can be worsened by anxiety, and its management can be a fruitful area for interdisciplinary cooperation.

Some care should be taken in the application of relaxation procedures to neurological patients. The use of active muscle tensing should be avoided where there are problems with increased muscle tone. Where there is paralysis or weakness in specific body parts, these parts may have to be omitted from the relaxation procedure or treated with especial care. Deep relaxation is sometimes frightening for people whose bodies already seem to be outwith their control, and may be a precipitant for some sorts of seizures. Especial care should be taken to avoid hyperventilation during deep breathing procedures. In addition, the patient may not have the attentional capacity to engage in a lengthy relaxation procedure and may benefit from frequent short sessions. If language comprehension is a problem then use of music or natural relaxing sounds can be investigated.

It is particularly helpful to question the patient on relaxation strategies that he or she used prior to the brain injury. Where possible, the resumption of their use should be encouraged and assisted inventively. This supports the person's own coping responses.

Where fear is focused on identified situations or activities the principles of graded exposure treatment for phobias (e.g. Butler, 1989) can be applied. The patient is exposed to the fear situation and learns to cope with it (rather than to master it). In general this is a highly effective procedure (taking place naturally in most rehabilitation programmes), and its success can be explained at the physiological, behavioural and cognitive levels. Again, some care should be taken in its application. Exposure to feared stimuli can sometimes result in an *increase* in fear, a phenomenon termed 'sensitisation'. This is most likely to occur if the patient is under particular stress from other sources (Ormel & Wohlfarth, 1991) or if the exposure procedure is carried out in a haphazard way. There is also some danger of this occurring in patients who are over-ambitious in setting goals for themselves. This is a phenomenon rarely seen in conventional mental health practice, but it is a feature of people with acquired brain injury who are desperate to return to normal and have limited understanding of their own limits. The clinician's job is to place a brake on this enthusiasm rather than to be swept along by it. For further details of graded exposure procedures, see the section on joint working.

People with traumatic brain injury may have significant health anxiety that is based in reality but nevertheless prevents them from taking 'reasonable' risks. For instance, they may avoid leaving the house for fear of suffering an epileptic seizure, or they may constantly monitor themselves for symptoms of hydrocephalus. The cognitive behavioural approach to health anxiety (e.g. Salkovskis, 1989) tends to be based on the assumption that all symptoms experienced are physically benign but misinterpreted by the patient as signifying illness. This assumption does not hold for this population, whose physical symptoms are likely to be multifactorial in nature. The focus of therapy in these cases is to carry out a cost–benefit analysis of the avoidance or self-monitoring behaviour with the patient, to agree on an acceptable risk levels, and to generate additional coping strategies so that they can get on with their lives. For instance, if the risk of having a seizure is one in twenty, and the person is given a strategy for dealing with a seizure if warning signs occur, and leaving the house gives access to valued social contacts, then leaving the house may become an acceptable (but not anxiety-free) option.

The use of diaries, audiotapes and written aids has been emphasised in this section. These can form a useful adjunct to face-to-face therapy, and are as least as useful in the management of anxiety and depression as they are in the management of cognitive problems. Indeed, the review by Carney *et al.* (1999) made the point that cognitive rehabilitation is an effective treatment of anxiety in acquired brain injury.

Joint Working

As indicated in previous sections, the ideal approach to the management of emotional distress in traumatic brain injury survivors involves an interdisciplinary rehabilitation team. Behavioural experiments are an integral part of most psychological approaches to anxiety and depression (McGrath & King, 2004). These experiments can be incorporated into occupational therapy programmes, especially those focusing on community skills such as use of public transport or shops. In these cases a graded hierarchy of situations can be agreed between the patient, occupational therapist and psychologist. It is important to remember that a hierarchy of feared situations may not correspond completely with the degree of functional difficulty presented by these situations. An apparently easy task may therefore have to

Case 11.1: Rehabilitation example

R, a 30-year-old steel presser, sustained a very severe head injury (post-traumatic amnesia 6 weeks) as the result of being knocked off his bicycle by a hit and run driver on the way to work early one autumn morning. It was still dark and the weather was wet at the time of the accident. A CT scan showed a small sub-dural haematoma, which was not treated surgically. In addition to the head injury, R suffered several orthopaedic injuries: a fractured left knee complicated by an effusion, a fractured pelvis and a fractured right metatarsal. There was also a hepatic haematoma.

R had a prior history of intermittent binge drinking which had resulted in severe marital stress. However, he had not drunk alcohol for several weeks prior to the accident. He was the father of two-year-old twins.

Three months after the accident R was transferred from his district general hospital to the rehabilitation unit, which he attended five days a week, returning to the family home at weekends. At this

Continued

time he was completely physically independent, but walked with a limp, was physically weak and had suffered some weight loss. Neuropsychological assessment indicated a retrograde amnesia of approximately six weeks (he therefore had no recollection of the accident or circumstances leading up to it), and continuing memory, executive and attentional impairment.

In the early stages of his time in the unit R was fearful of going outside after dark. In particular, he froze and reported feelings of overwhelming panic when he saw car headlights approaching him. He completely avoided going outside his front door at night. He was also fearful of going into busy environments where his physical vulnerability placed him in danger of being knocked over. The following extract describing his fears is taken from the transcript of an interview with R:

> . . . the car headlights would look as though they were coming directly at me, although they weren't coming at me they felt as though they were, and I felt a shudder of fear going down my spine. . . . It was a fear of the dark, and quite often kids ride mopeds round our estate because they use it as a short cut, and that was playing on the back of my mind, the thoughts of kids scooting round the corner on these mopeds – would they see me? . . . especially if it was dark and it was raining as well, the thought of a car coming towards me in the rain because it was raining when my accident happened. . . . In myself I didn't feel able to get out of the way quick enough. Once my wounds started to heal . . . the fear subsided . . . now I can jump out of the way if I see something coming.
>
> Before the accident I had this attitude that 'It'll never happen to me' . . . now I know how vulnerable we all are, how easily it can be wiped out just like that.

Treatment consisted of simple graded exposure, and a physical fitness programme jointly administered by his psychologist and physiotherapist. All avoidance behaviour was eliminated, and progress was maintained over a six-month follow-up period. However, during this time R began to experience extended periods of derealisation and depersonalisation, which seemed to occur when he was engaging in physically or cognitively demanding activity. (His lifestyle was very busy as he was actively involved in caring for his young children while he was at home.) These experiences caused both him and his wife a great deal of worry. He described them as follows:

> . . . it was an eerie feeling like everything was really happening around me and I felt almost invisible to it. It was a feeling of being separated and distanced from reality. It wasn't pleasant at all . . . I wouldn't wish it on my worst enemy – it was horrible . . . life is going on around you

> and you are behind a glass sheet seeing everything, hearing everything, but nobody can see or hear you – it's very strange.
>
> There was no evidence of epilepsy. The physiotherapist hypothesised that the experiences appeared to be linked to fatigue and excessive self-monitoring. R was therefore treated with a cognitive behavioural approach which included scheduling rest periods into his weekly routine. The experiences ceased immediately and did not recur during the follow-up period.

be left until a later stage in the process. Potential coping strategies should be discussed and practised in advance. These may include relaxation, or methods of coping with communication difficulties. The involvement of a speech and language therapist is obviously important in such cases.

In a similar way, behavioural experiments may be carried out in therapy situations which the patient finds difficult. This often involves the delivery of nursing care or physiotherapy, with their physical demands, potentially risky activities, and physical handling. Again, a hierarchy of feared activities may need to be generated. This may depart from the usual order of treatment or care plan, and negotiation, possibly involving written contracts, will be necessary. It is important for nurses and therapists to stick to an agreed routine, and not to exceed what has been agreed with the patient even if he or she appears to be doing well. (This reduces the chance of sensitisation.) Where periods of activity interspersed with rests have been agreed, the use of a kitchen timer kept in view of the patient, and which rings to alert patient and therapist alike, can be helpful. The patient may need to be helped to endure certain procedures by the use of relaxation tapes, counting, or distraction, for instance being helped to read magazines while in a standing frame. This may involve joint input from the whole team.

Where a patient is clearly not tolerating an activity or withdrawing consent the activity should be terminated, but if possible this should not happen until the patient has asked appropriately, in response to a direct question if necessary. (If unpleasant activities are terminated by the nurse or therapist in response to biting, screaming, etc., these behaviours are reinforced and are likely to occur more frequently.) Again, the role of the speech and language therapist is important here in teaching the patient to communicate his or her needs appropriately, and to teach the team to communicate appropriately with the patient. (Team members often overestimate the language comprehension abilities of their patients, and make excessive linguistic demands or over-stimulate them with questions and choices.)

Where the patient requires good information about his or her medical status, prognosis and rehabilitation progress, all members of the team have a role in presenting this information in a helpful and comprehensible way. The input of medical practitioners is particularly important in explaining the role of medication and the significance of continuing medical problems such as post-traumatic epilepsy. This information can be collated into one document for the patient, and this is also helpful for family and carers.

Where this information is unpalatable, for instance that the chances of attaining normal independent walking are low, then a considered team approach to the sharing of this information is desirable. If two members of the team take responsibility for sharing this news they can support both the patient and each other in what can be a distressing business for all concerned.

Where a patient is troubled by outbursts of emotionalism in response to certain topics of conversation, it is a good idea to designate one member of the team to talk to the patient about these things in private, and for the rest of the team to agree to avoid these topics. Completely avoiding these topics may rob the person of the chance to process emotionally what has happened, or to converse about deeply loved family, friends or pets.

Specialist help from a psychiatrist *experienced in traumatic brain injury* is often valuable, but should definitely be sought in cases where suicidal intent is expressed, or where the person's distress appears to be driven by internal processes such as hallucinations. Help from professionals experienced in the treatment of psychological trauma should also be sought when post-traumatic stress disorder is suspected.

Final Considerations

This chapter has dealt with the psychological treatment of emotional distress, particularly fear, anxiety and depression following traumatic brain injury. There is a paucity of outcome data based on controlled group studies, but clinical experience and an increasing number of single case reports indicate that this is an area where a psychological approach has much to offer (Williams *et al.*, 2003).

Psychological treatments are underpinned by psychological theory, and should ideally arise from a specialist assessment by a clinical psychologist, but are often delivered by the whole rehabilitation team, ideally with support and supervision from a psychologist (McGrath & King, 2004). Much of the clinical experience on which this chapter has been based has been with patients with relatively recent and severe head injuries. Thus the emphasis has been on in-patient and early out-patient treatment programmes. The principles are also applicable to people who have returned to living in the community. Nevertheless, there are significant differences in physical and psychosocial context, and patterns of health and social care delivery, between these two groups. Early rehabilitation is focused on physical recovery, and emotional distress arises within this ethos. Nursing care and physiotherapy tend to dominate at this stage, and members of these professions may need to incorporate psychological techniques into their work. As the person moves back into family life and begins to cope at home and to consider a return to work, occupational therapy becomes increasingly important. Occupational therapists are often the key health professionals involved in the psychological care of people at later stages of recovery, where close working with families, colleagues, friends and community agencies replaces the in-patient interdisciplinary team approach.

Recommended Reading

House, A. (1992). Management of mood disorder in adults with brain damage: Can we improve what psychiatry has to offer? In P.J. Cowen & K. Hawton (Eds.) *Practical problems in clinical psychiatry* (pp. 51–62). Oxford, Oxford University Press.

Overview and discussion of the range of psychiatric and psychological management options for patients with acquired brain injury and mood disorder.

King, N.S. (1997). Mild head injury: Neuropathology, sequelae, measurement, and recovery. *British Journal of Clinical Psychology*, *36*, 161–184.
Literature review of mild head injury and the post concussion syndrome including psychological treatment options when emotional factors are in operation.

Lazarus, R. & Folkman, S. (1984). *Stress, appraisal, and coping*. New York, Springer.
A classic text outlining psychological conceptualisations of stress and anxiety disorders with their associated treatment implications.

McGrath, J. & King, N. (2004) Acquired brain injury. In J. Bennett-Levy, G. Butler, M. Fennell, A. Hackmann, M. Mueller & D. Westbrook (Eds.) *The Oxford guide to behavioural experiments in cognitive therapy*. Oxford: Oxford University Press.
Practical overview of how a cognitive behavioural approach can be applied to the treatment of patients with acquired brain injury and emotional disorders. Case study material is used to demonstrate the use of behavioural experiments with this client group.

Ownsworth, T. & Oei, T. (1998). Depression after traumatic brain injury: Conceptualization and treatment considerations. *Brain Injury*, *12*, 735–751.
Theoretical and practical considerations when understanding and treating patients with depression and traumatic brain injury.

Useful Resources

Mind over mood (1995). Greenberger, D. & Padesky, C.A. Guilford, New York.
Managing anxiety: A training manual (1995). Kennerly, H. Oxford University Press, Oxford.
Manage your mind (1995). Butler, G. & Hope, T. Oxford University Press, Oxford.
Oxford Cognitive Therapy Centre Self Help Booklets: *Managing anxiety* (Butler, G.), *Controlling anxiety* (Fennell, M. & Butler, G.), *Managing depression* (Westbrook, D.), *Overcoming social anxiety* (Butler, G.), *Understanding health anxiety* (Küchemann, C. & Sanders, D.), *Understanding panic* (Westbrook, D. & Rouf, K.), *How to relax* (Norris, R. & Küchemann, C.), *Overcoming phobias* (Sanders, D.), *Managing anxiety: A user's manual* (Kennerly, H.), *Obsessive-compulsive disorder* (Westbrook, D.) www.octc.co.uk
Understanding your reactions to trauma; a guide for survivors of trauma and their families – revised version (2002). Herbert, C. Blue Stallion Publications, Witney, Oxon.

References

Abramson, L.Y., Seligman, M.E.P. & Teasdale, J.D. (1978). Learned helplessness in humans: Critique and reformulation. *Journal of Abnormal Psychology*, *87*, 49–74.
Allman, P. (1991a). Depressive disorders and emotionalism following stroke. *International Journal of Geriatric Psychiatry*, *6*, 377–383.
Allman, P. (1991b). Emotionalism following brain damage. *Behavioural Neurology*, *4*, 57–62.
Allman, P. (1992). Drug treatment of emotionalism following brain damage. *Journal of the Royal Society of Medicine*, *85*, 423–424.
Andersson, S., Krogstad, J.M. & Finset, A. (1999). Apathy and depressed mood in acquired brain damage: Relationship to lesion localization and psychophysiological reactivity. *Psychological Medicine*, *29*, 447–456.

Arruda, J.E., Stern, R.A., Somerville, J.A. & Bishop, D.S. (1997). Description and initial validity evidence for the Visual Analog Mood Scales in a neurologically impaired population. [Abstract]. *Journal of Neuropsychiatry and Clinical Neurosciences*, *9*, 152.

Bandura, A. (1997). *Self-efficacy: The exercise of control*. New York: Freeman.

Becerra, R., Amos, A. & Jongenelis, S. (2002). Organic alexithymia; a study of acquired emotional blindness. *Brain Injury*, *16*, 633–645.

Beck, A.T. (1967). *Depression: Clinical, experimental and theoretical aspects*. New York: Harper & Row.

Beck, A.T. & Emery, G. (1979). *Cognitive therapy of anxiety and phobic disorders*. Philadelphia: Center for Cognitive Therapy.

Beck, A.T., Ward, C.H., Mendelson, M., Mock, J. & Erbaugh, J. (1961). An inventory for measuring depression. *Archives of General Psychiatry*, *4*, 561–571.

Bernstein, D.A. & Borkovec, T.D. (1973). *Progressive relaxation training: A manual for the helping professions*. Champaign, IL: Research Press.

Black, A.H., Nadel, L. & O'Keefe, J. (1977). Hippocampal function in avoidance learning and punishment. *Psychological Bulletin*, *84*, 1107–1129.

Brooks, D.N. (1989). Closed head trauma: Assessing the common cognitive problems. In M.D. Lezak (Ed.) *Assessment of the behavioral consequences of head trauma* (pp. 61–85). New York: Alan Liss.

Butler, G. (1989). Phobic disorders. In K. Hawton, P. Salkovskis, J. Kirk & D. Clark (Eds.) *Cognitive behaviour therapy for psychiatric problems* (pp. 97–128). Oxford, Oxford University Press.

Carney, N., Chesnut, R.M., Maynard, H., Mann, N.C., Patterson, P. & Helfand, M. (1999). Effect of cognitive rehabilitation on outcomes for persons with traumatic brain injury: A systematic review. *Journal of Head Trauma Rehabilitation*, *14*, 277–307.

Cella, D.F., Jacobsen, P.B., Orav, E.J., Holland, J.C., Silberfarb, P.M. & Rafla, S. (1987). A brief POMS measure of distress for cancer patients. *Journal of Chronic Disease*, *40*, 939–942.

Claparede, E. (1911). Recognition et moiïté. *Archives de Psychologie Geneve*, *11*, 79–90.

Collicutt McGrath, J. (2007). *Ethical practice in brain injury rehabilitation*. Oxford: Oxford University Press.

Collicutt McGrath, J. (in press). Fear of falling after brain injury. *Clinical Rehabilitation*.

Collicutt McGrath, J. & Linley, P.A. (2006). Posttraumatic growth following acquired brain injury. *Brain Injury*, *20*, 767–773.

Deb, S., Lyons, I., Koutzoutkis, C., Ali, I. & McCarthy, G. (1999). Rate of psychiatric illness 1 year after traumatic brain injury. *American Journal of Psychiatry*, *156*, 374–378.

Delbaere, K., Crombez, G., Vanderstraeten, G., Willems, T., & Cambier, D. (2004). Fear related avoidance of activities, falls, and physical frailty. A prospective community centred cohort study. *Age and Aging*, *33*, 368–373.

Derogatis, L.R. (1983). *S.C.L.90-R. Administration, scoring, and procedures manual–II*. Tarson, MD: Clinical Psychometric Research.

Druss, R. & Douglas, C. (1988). Adaptive responses to illness and disability: Healthy denial. *General Hospital Psychiatry*, *10*, 163–188.

Duckett, S. & Kramer, T. (1994). Managing myoclonus secondary to anoxic encephalopathy through EMG biofeedback. *Brain Injury*, *8*, 185–188.

Eslinger, P.J., Grattan, L.M. & Geder, L. (1995). Impact of frontal lobe lesions on rehabilitation and recovery from acute brain injury. *Neurorehabilitation*, *5*, 161–182.

Fann, J., Burington, B., Leonetti, A., Jaffe, K., Katon, W. & Thompson, R. (2004). Psychiatric illness following traumatic brain injury in an adult mental health maintenance organization population. *Archives of General Psychiatry*, *61*, 53–61.

Fann, J., Katon, W., Uomoto, J. & Esselman, P. (1995). Psychiatric disorders and functional disability in outpatients with traumatic brain injuries. *American Journal of Psychiatry*, *152*, 1493–1499.

Fedoroff, J.P., Starkstein, S.E., Forrester, A.W., Geisler, F.H. *et al.* (1992). Depression in patients with acute traumatic brain injury. *American Journal of Psychiatry*, *149*, 918–923.

Finset, A. (1988). Depressed mood and reduced emotionality after right hemisphere brain damage. In M. Kinsbourne (Ed.) *Cerebral hemisphere function in depression* (pp. 49–64). Washington, American Psychiatric Press.

Fleminger, S., Oliver, D., Williams, W.H. & Evans, J. (2003). The neuropsychiatry of depression after brain injury. *Neuropsychological Rehabilitation*, *13*, 65–87.

Fletcher, P. & Hirdes, J. (2004). Restriction in activity associated with fear of falling among community-based seniors using home care services. *Age and Ageing*, *33*, 273–279.

Freedman, M. (1990). Object alternation and orbitofrontal system dysfunction in Alzheimer's and Parkinson's disease. *Brain & Cognition*, *14*, 134–143.

Green, A., Flemingham, K., Baguley, I.J., Slewa-Younan, S. & Simpson, S. (2001). The clinical utility of the Beck Depression Inventory after traumatic brain injury. *Brain Injury*, *15*, 1021–1028.

Greenberger, D. & Padesky, C.A. (1995). *Mind over mood.* New York: Guilford.

Guercio, J., Chittum, R. & McMorrow, M. (1997). Self-management in the treatment of ataxia: A case study in reducing ataxic tremor through relaxation and biofeedback. *Brain Injury*, *11*, 353–362.

Harrick, L., Krefting, L., Johnston, J., Carlson, P. & Minnes, P. (1994). Stability of functional outcomes following transitional living programme participation: Three year follow up. *Brain Injury*, *8*, 439–447.

Hogarty, G.E. & Katz, M.M. (1971). Norms of adjustment and social behaviour. *Archives of General Psychiatry*, *25*, 470–480.

House, A., Dennis, M., Molyneux, A., Warlow, C. & Hawton, K. (1989). Emotionalism after stroke. *British Medical Journal*, *298*, 991–994.

Isaacs, B. (1978). *Recent advances in geriatric medicine* (Vol. 1). Edinburgh: Churchill Livingstone.

Izard, C. (1972). *Patterns of emotions: A new analysis of anxiety and depression.* San Diego, CA: Academic Press.

Jeans, V. & Orvell, M.W. (1991). Behavioural therapy of space phobia: A case report. *Behavioural Psychotherapy*, *19*, 285–288.

Johnson, G., Burvill, P.W., Anderson, C.S., Jamrozik, K., Stewart-Wynne, E.G. & Chakera, T.M.H. (1995). Screening instruments for anxiety and depression following stroke: Experience in the Perth Community Stroke Study. *Acta Psychiatrica Scandinavica*, *91*, 252–257.

Jones, B. & Mishkin, M. (1972). Limbic lesions and the problem of stimulus reinforcement associations. *Experimental Neurology*, *36*, 362–377.

Jorge, R.E., Robinson, R.G. & Arndt, S. (1993). Are there symptoms that are specific for depressed mood in patients with traumatic brain injury? *Journal of Nervous and Mental Disease*, *181*, 91–99.

Jorge, R.E., Robinson, R.G., Arndt, S.V., Forrester, A.W., Geisler, F. & Starkstein, S.E. (1993a). A comparison between acute and delayed onset depression following traumatic brain injury. *Journal of Neuropsychiatry and Clinical Neurosciences*, *5*, 43–49.

Jorge, R.E., Robinson, R.G., Arndt, S.V., Starkstein, S.E., Forrester, A.W. & Geisler, F. (1993b). Anxiety and depression in traumatic brain injury. *Journal of Affective Disorders*, *27*, 233–243.

Jorge, R.E., Robinson, R.G., Starkstein, E. & Arndt, S.T. (1994). Influence of major depression on one year outcome in patients with traumatic brain injury. *Journal of Neurosurgery*, *81*, 726–733.

Kant, R., Duffy, J. & Pivovarnik, A. (1998). Prevalence of apathy following brain injury. *Brain Injury*, **12**, 87–92.

Kay, T. (1986). *Minor head injury: An introduction for professionals.* Framingham, MA: National Head Injury Foundation.

King, N.S. (1997). Mild head injury: Neuropathology, sequelae, measurement, and recovery. *British Journal of Clinical Psychology*, *36*, 161–184.

King, N.S. (2002). Perseveration of traumatic re-experiencing in P.T.S.D. *Brain Injury*, *16*, 65–74.

Kinney, A. (2001). Cognitive therapy and brain injury: Theoretical and clinical issues. *Journal of Contemporary Psychotherapy*, *31*, 89–102.

Kinsella, G., Moran, C., Ford, B. & Ponsford, J. (1988). Emotional disorder and its assessment within the severe head injured population. *Psychological Medicine*, *18*, 57–63.

Kreutzer, J., Marwitz, J., Seel, R. & Serio, C. (1996). Validation of a neurobehavioral functioning inventory for adults with traumatic brain injury. *Archives of Physical Medicine & Rehabilitation*, *77*, 116–124.

Krishnan, K.R.R., McDonald, W.M., Escalona, P.R. *et al.* (1992). MRI of the caudate nuclei in depression. *Archives of General Psychiatry*, *49*, 553–557.

La Vigna, G.W. & Donnellan (1986). *Alternatives to punishment: Solving behavior problems with non-aversive strategies.* New York: Irvington.

Lazarus, R. (1966). *Psychological stress and the coping response.* New York: McGraw Hill.

Lazarus, R. (1994). Universal antecedents of the emotions. In P. Ekman & R.J. Davidson (Eds.) *The nature of emotion: Fundamental questions* (pp. 163–171). Oxford: Oxford University Press.

Lazarus, R. & Folkman, S. (1984). *Stress, appraisal, and coping.* New York: Springer.

LeDoux, J.E. (1992). Brain mechanisms of emotion and emotional learning. *Current Opinion in Neurolobiology*, *2*, 191–197.

LeDoux, J.E. (1995). Emotion: clues from the brain. *Annual Review of Psychology*, *46*, 209–235.

Levin, H.S., High, W.M. Goethe, K.E., Sisson, R.A., Overall, J.E., Rhoades, H.M., *et al.* (1987). The Neurobehavioural Rating Scale: Assessment of the behavioural sequelae of head injury by the clinician. *Journal of Neurology, Neurosurgery, and Psychiatry*, *50*, 183–193.

Lewis, L. & Rosenberg, S.J. (1990). Psychoanalytic psychotherapy with brain injured adult psychiatric patients. *Journal of Nervous and Mental Disease*, *178*, 69–77.

Linn, R.T., Allen, K. & Willer, B. (1994). Affective symptoms in the chronic stage of traumatic brain injury: A study of married couples. *Brain Injury*, 2, 135–147.

Lishman, W.A. (1973). The psychiatric sequelae of head injury: A review. *Psychological Medicine*, *3*, 304–318.

Lishman, W.A. (1978). Psychiatric sequelae of head injuries: Problems in diagnosis. *Journal of the Irish Medical Association*, *71*, 306–314.

Marks, I.M. (1981). Space 'phobia': A pseudo-agoraphobic syndrome. *Journal of Neurology, Neurosurgery, and Psychiatry*, *44*, 387–391.

Marks, I. M. (1987). *Fears, phobias, and rituals*. Oxford: Oxford University Press.

Marks, I.M. & Bebbington, P. (1976). Space phobia: Syndrome or agoraphobic variant? *British Medical Journal*, *2*, 345–347.

Mathews, A.M. (1971). Psychophysiological approaches to the investigation of desensitization and related procedures. *Psychological Bulletin*, *76*, 73–91.

McCaffrey, R.J., Rapee, R.M., Gansler, D.A. & Barlow, D.H. (1990). Interaction of neuropsychological and psychological factors in two cases of 'space' phobia'. *Journal of Behaviour Therapy and Experimental Psychiatry*, *21*, 113–120.

McGrath, J. (1998). *Fear following brain injury*. Unpublished doctoral thesis, Oxford Brookes University, UK.

McGrath, J. (2001). A study of emotionalism in patients undergoing rehabilitation following severe acquired brain injury. *Behavioural Neurology, 12, 201–207.*

McGrath, J. (2002). The phenomenology of distressing emotion in patients with severe acquired brain injury. *Third World Congress in Neurological Rehabilitation*, Venice.

McGrath, J. (2004). Beyond restoration to transformation: Positive outcomes in the rehabilitation of acquired brain injury. *Clinical Rehabilitation*, *18*, 767–775.

McGrath, J. & Adams, L. (1999). Patient-centered goal planning: A systemic psychological therapy? *Topics in Stroke Rehabilitation*, *6*, 43–50.

McGrath, J. & Davis, A. (1992), Rehabilitation: Where are we going and how do we get there? *Clinical Rehabilitation*, *6*, 255–235.

McGrath, J. & King, N. (2004) Acquired brain injury. In J. Bennett-Levy, G. Butler, M. Fennell, A. Hackmann, M. Mueller & D. Westbrook (Eds.) *The Oxford guide to behavioural experiments in cognitive therapy* (pp. 331–348). Oxford: Oxford University Press.

McGrath, J., Marks, J. & Davis, A. (1995). Towards interdisciplinary rehabilitation. Further developments at Rivermead Rehabilitation Centre. *Clinical Rehabilitation*, *9*, 320–326.

McGrath, J., Wade, D. & Linley, P.A. (2004). Posttraumatic growth in acquired brain injury: A small scale study. *Second European Conference on Positive Psychology Proceedings* (pp.128–130). Milan: Arcipelago Edizioni. www.gallup-europe.be/PositivePsychology/presentations.htm.

McNair, D.M., Lorr, M. & Droppleman, L.F. (1981). *EDITS manual for the Profile of Mood States*. San Diego, CA: Educational and Industrial Service.

McNally, R.J. (1990). Another case of 'space phobia'? *Phobia Practice and Research*, *3*, 79–80.

Miller, L. (1992). Cognitive rehabilitation, cognitive therapy, and cognitive style: Toward an integrative model of personality and psychotherapy. *Cognitive Rehabilitation*, *10*, 18–29.

Morgan, M.A., Romanski, L.M. & LeDoux, J.E. (1993). Extinction of emotional learning: Contribution of medial prefrontal cortex. *Neuroscience Letters*, *163*, 109–113.

Mohl, P.C. & Burstein, A.G. (1982). The application of Kohutian self-psychology to consultation-liaison psychiatry. *General Hospital Psychiatry*, *4*, 113–119.

Nelson, L. Satz, P., Mitrushinna, M., van Gorp, W., Cichetti, D., Lewis, R. & Van Lancker, D. (1989). Development and validation of the Neuropsychology Behaviour and Affect Profile. *Psychological Assessment*, *1*, 266–272.

Nyenhuis, D.L., Stern, R.A., Yamamoto, C., Luchetta, T. & Arruda, J.E. (1997). Standardization and validation of the Visual Analog Mood Scales. *The Clinical Neuropsychologist*, *11*, 407–415.

Ormel, J. & Wohlfarth, T. (1991). How neuroticism, long term difficulties, and life situation change influence psychological distress: A longitudinal model. *Journal of Personality and Social Psychology*, *60*, 744–755.

Padesky, C.A. & Greenberger, D. (1995). *Clinician's guide to mind over mood*. New York: Guilford.

Powell, J.H., al-Adani, S., Morgan, J. & Greenwood, R.J. (1996). Motivational deficits after brain injury: Effect of bromocriptine in eleven patients. *Journal of Neurology, Neurosurgery and Psychiatry*, *60*, 416–421.

Prigatano, G.P. (1991). Disordered mind, wounded soul: The emerging role of psychotherapy in rehabilitation after brain injury. *Journal of Head Trauma Rehabilitation*, *6*, 1–10.

Prigatano, G.P. (1994). Individuality, lesion location, and psychotherapy after brain injury. In A-L. Christensen & B. Uzzell (Eds.) *Brain injury and neuropsychological rehabilitation: International perspective* (pp. 173–199). Hillsdale, NJ: Lawrence Erlbaum.

Riley, R. (2000). Geriatric depression and neuropsychological impairment: An exploration of frontal lobe functioning, hetereogeneity of depression, and global cognitive decline. *International Dissertation Abstracts*, *61*(1-B), 547.

Roberts, A.H. (1979). *Severe accidental head injury: An assessment of long term prognosis*. London: McMillan.

Robinson, R.G., Kubos, K.L. Starr, L.B., Rao, K. & Price, T.R. (1983). Mood changes in stroke patients: Relationship to lesion location. *Comprehensive Psychiatry*, *24*, 555–566.

Robinson, R.G., Kubos, K.L. Starr, L.B., Rao, K. & Price, T.R. (1984). Mood disorders in stroke patients: Importance of lesion location. *Brain*, *107*, 81–93.

Rolls, E.T. (1986). Neural systems involved in emotion in primates. In R. Plutchik & H. Kellerman (Eds.) *Emotion: Theory, research and experience* (Vol. III, pp. 125–148). New York: Academic Press.

Rothbaum, F., Weisz, J.R. & Snyder, S.S. (1982). Changing the world and changing the self. *Journal of Personality and Social Psychology*, *42*, 5–37.

Salkovskis, P.M. (1989). Somatic problems. In K. Hawton, P. Salkovskis, J. Kirk & D. Clark (Eds.) *Cognitive behaviour therapy for psychiatric problems* (pp. 235–276). Oxford: Oxford University Press.

Schacham, N. (1983). A shortened version of the profile of mood states. *Journal of Personality Assessment*, *47*, 305–306.

Scott, S.K., Young, A.W., Calder, A.J., Hellawell, D.J., Aggleton, J.P. & Johnson, M. (1997). Impaired auditory recognition of fear and anger following bilateral amygdala lesions [Letter to the editor]. *Nature*, *383*, 254.

Silver, J., Kramer, R., Greenwalds, S. & Weissman, M. (2001). The association between head injuries and psychiatric disorders: Findings from the New Haven NIMH Epidemiologic Catchment Area Study. *Brain Injury*, *15*, 935–945.

Sliwinski, M., Gordon, W.A. & Bogdany, J. (1998). The Beck Depression Inventory: Is it a suitable measure for individuals with traumatic brain injury? *Journal of Head Trauma Rehabilitation*, *13*, 40–46.

Sloan, R.L., Brown, W. & Pentland, B. (1992). Fluoxetine as a treatment for emotional lability after brain injury. *Brain Injury*, *6*, 315–319.

Snaith, R.P., Bridge, G.W. & Hamilton, M. (1976). *The Leeds scale for the self assessment of anxiety and depression*. London: Psychological Test Publishers.

Trimble, M.R. (1978). Non-MAOI antidepressants and epilepsy. *Epilepsia*, *19*, 241–250.

Trimble, M.R. (1996). *Biological psychiatry*. Chichester: Wiley.

Tyerman, A. (1988). Personal and social rehabilitation after head injury. In F. Watts (Ed.) *New developments in clinical psychology* (pp. 189–207). Leicester: Wiley/British Psychological Society.

Tyerman, A. & Humphrey, M. (1984). Changes in self concept following severe head injury. *International Journal of Rehabilitation Research*, *7*, 11–23.

Van Zomeren, A.H. & Van den Bing, W. (1985). Residual complaints of patients two years after severe head injury. *Journal of Neurology, Neurosurgery, and Psychiatry*, *48*, 21–28.

Wade, D. (1999). Goal planning in stroke rehabilitation: How? *Topics in Stroke Rehabilitation*, *6*, 16–36.

Whitehouse, A.M. (1994). Applications of cognitive therapy with survivors of head injury. *Journal of Cognitive Psychotherapy: An International Quarterly*, *8*, 141–60.

Williams, H.W., Evans, J. & Fleminger, S. (2003). Neurorehabilitation and cognitive-behaviour therapy of anxiety disorders after brain injury. *Neuropsychological Rehabilitation*, *13*, 133–148.

Williams, K., Galas, J., Light, D., Pepper, C., Ryan, C., Kleinmann, A., *et al.* (2001). Head injury and alexithymia: Implications for family practice care. *Brain Injury*, *15*, 349–356.

Wing, J., Cooper, J. & Sartorius, N. (1978). *The measurement and classification of psychiatric symptoms. W.H.O. 78 Mental disorders: Glossary and guide to their classification in accordance with I.C.D.-9*. Cambridge: Cambridge University Press.

Zigmond, A. & Snaith, P. (1983). The Hospital Anxiety and Depression Scale. *Acta Psychiatrica Scandinavica*, *67*, 361–370.

Rivermead Fear Questionnaire

Name . . . . .
Date . . . . .

Below is a list of situations that sometimes make people upset because of fear or other unpleasant emotions. Please underline the reply which comes closest to how you have been feeling about each situation in the past week. If any of the situations don't apply to you (for instance if you are a wheelchair user) then just tick the item and go on to the next one.

1. Walking

Not upset		Would not avoid it
A bit upset	and	Slightly avoid it
Very upset		Definitely avoid it
Extremely upset		Completely avoid it

2. Using the toilet

Not upset		Would not avoid it
A bit upset	and	Slightly avoid it
Very upset		Definitely avoid it
Extremely upset		Completely avoid it

3. Transferring e.g. from bed to chair

Not upset		Would not avoid it
A bit upset	and	Slightly avoid it
Very upset		Definitely avoid it
Extremely upset		Completely avoid it

4. Being touched

Not upset		Would not avoid it
A bit upset	and	Slightly avoid it
Very upset		Definitely avoid it
Extremely upset		Completely avoid it

5. Being a car passenger

Not upset		Would not avoid it
A bit upset	and	Slightly avoid it

Appendix 11.1 Rivermead Fear Questionnaire

Very upset		Definitely avoid it
Extremely upset		Completely avoid it

6. Large open spaces

Not upset		Would not avoid it
A bit upset	and	Slightly avoid it
Very upset		Definitely avoid it
Extremely upset		Completely avoid it

7. Being in hospital

Not upset		Would not avoid it
A bit upset	and	Slightly avoid it
Very upset		Definitely avoid it
Extremely upset		Completely avoid it

8. Being alone

Not upset		Would not avoid it
A bit upset	and	Slightly avoid it
Very upset		Definitely avoid it
Extremely upset		Completely avoid it

9. Doing something new or going somewhere new

Not upset		Would not avoid it
A bit upset	and	Slightly avoid it
Very upset		Definitely avoid it
Extremely upset		Completely avoid it

10. Being in busy places e.g. shops or pubs

Not upset		Would not avoid it
A bit upset	and	Slightly avoid it
Very upset		Definitely avoid it
Extremely upset		Completely avoid it

11. Going up or downstairs

Not upset		Would not avoid it
A bit upset	and	Slightly avoid it
Very upset		Definitely avoid it
Extremely upset		Completely avoid it

12. Meeting old friends

Not upset		Would not avoid it

Appendix 11.1 *Continued*

A bit upset Very upset Extremely upset	and	Slightly avoid it Definitely avoid it Completely avoid it

13. Being examined or tested by doctors or therapists

Not upset A bit upset Very upset Extremely upset	and	Would not avoid it Slightly avoid it Definitely avoid it Completely avoid it

14. Talking to other people - answering questions

Not upset A bit upset Very upset Extremely upset	and	Would not avoid it Slightly avoid it Definitely avoid it Completely avoid it

15. Thinking about what has happened to me (illness or injury)

Not upset A bit upset Very upset Extremely upset	and	Would not avoid it Slightly avoid it Definitely avoid it Completely avoid it

16. Eating in front of other people

Not upset A bit upset Very upset Extremely upset	and	Would not avoid it Slightly avoid it Definitely avoid it Completely avoid it

17. Thinking about the future

Not upset A bit upset Very upset Extremely upset	and	Would not avoid it Slightly avoid it Definitely avoid it Completely avoid it

18. Crossing the road

Not upset A bit upset Very upset Extremely upset	and	Would not avoid it Slightly avoid it Definitely avoid it Completely avoid it

19. Driving a car

Appendix 11.1 *Continued*

Not upset		Would not avoid it
A bit upset	and	Slightly avoid it
Very upset		Definitely avoid it
Extremely upset		Completely avoid it

20. Meeting new people

Not upset		Would not avoid it
A bit upset	and	Slightly avoid it
Very upset		Definitely avoid it
Extremely upset		Completely avoid it

Thank you for your help

Appendix 11.1 *Continued*

12

Post-traumatic Stress Disorder and Traumatic Brain Injury

Nigel S. King

Introduction

Post-traumatic stress disorder (PTSD) is a severe psychological reaction to a traumatic event. It involves the persistent re-experiencing of the trauma, avoidance of stimuli which remind the person of the event, increased physiological arousal and a numbing of emotional responses. It can be highly disabling and cause significant impairments in all areas of psychosocial functioning.

Traumatic brain injuries take place in circumstances where psychological trauma might also occur, and therefore where PTSD could be expected. Head injury may protect a person from developing PTSD, however, when it causes organic amnesia for the event in the form of unconsciousness, retrograde amnesia or post-traumatic amnesia (PTA). Nevertheless, this protection is probably not as common as investigators initially believed.

There are often specific challenges to assessing, intervening and providing rehabilitation for people with head injury and PTSD. This chapter aims to clarify what these challenges are and provide some guidance as to how they might be met. It will initially review the literature on PTSD in non-head-injured patients before addressing the literature on head injury and PTSD as the latter is relatively sparse. It will address (i) the definition of PTSD, (ii) psychological models, measures and interventions for PTSD, (iii) the means by which PTSD and head injury can co-occur and (iv) complications and challenges posed by the co-existence of PTSD and head injury and some of the ways these might be addressed. It will not address issues relating to the comorbid disorders which often accompany PTSD e.g. depression, as these are covered in a previous chapter.

PTSD

Definition

The symptoms of PTSD have been known about for a long time. They have been described by Shakespeare in *Henry IV*, by Pepys following the Great Fire of London, and more recently under headings such as 'shell shock' and 'battle fatigue' following combat experiences (Hacker Hughes & Thompson, 1994). PTSD, however, has been a formal psychiatric diagnosis only since 1980.

The *Diagnostic and Statistical Manual of Mental Disorders* (DSM-IV; APA, 1994) defines the disorder as occurring under the following circumstances:

1 The person is exposed to a traumatic event involving actual or threatened death or serious injury or a threat to the physical integrity of other people.
2 Their reaction to the event involved intense fear, helplessness or terror.
3 Following the event they persistently re-experience the trauma via: intrusive and distressing dreams of the event; intrusive and distressing images, thoughts, perceptions and recollections; acting or feeling as if the trauma was re-occurring; intense psychological distress or physiological reactivity to internal or external cues that symbolise or resemble aspects of the event.
4 They persistently avoid stimuli and situations which remind them of the event and/or experience a numbing of their emotional responses. This can occur in a number of ways: avoiding thoughts, feelings or conversations associated with the trauma; avoiding activities, places or people that arouse recollections of the trauma; an inability to remember important aspects of the event; greatly reduced interest or participation in significant activities; feelings of detachment from others; restricted range of feelings; sense of foreshortened future, e.g. not expecting to have a career, family or normal life span.
5 The person experiences increased physiological arousal. This can manifest as: difficulties falling or staying asleep; irritability or anger outbursts; concentration difficulties; hypervigilance; exaggerated startle response.
6 The symptoms cause significant distress and social impairment and last for more than one month.

Spontaneous improvement of PTSD symptoms

The lifetime prevalence for developing PTSD is around 8 per cent (Kessler *et al.*, 1995). It is approximately twice as prevalent in women as men and is associated with high levels of comorbidity, e.g. depression, substance misuse and other anxiety disorders. PTSD symptoms spontaneously improve and/or resolve within the first three to twelve months of the trauma for a significant proportion of sufferers. The likelihood of spontaneous improvement or recovery occurring after 9–12 months post-trauma, however, diminishes significantly, although a minority do improve up to six years post-trauma (Mayou & Bryant, 2002). Approximately a third of sufferers remain symptomatic beyond six years (Kessler *et al.*, 1995).

Psychological Models and Interventions for PTSD

There is only a very small literature on psychological models, measures or interventions for people with head injury and PTSD. Most clinicians therefore use models, measures and interventions from the substantial PTSD literature dealing with non-head-injured populations and adapt these to head-injured patients. There is emerging evidence that such adaptations are effective (Bryant *et al.*, 2003).

Models and interventions

The majority of psychological models and interventions for PTSD come broadly from cognitive–behavioural therapy (CBT) frameworks. Even psychodynamic and more specialist models share commonalities with CBT. These more specialist models would include eye movement desensitisation and reprocessing (EMDR) where rapid horizontal eye movements methods are combined with imaginal exposure, habituation and cognitive restructuring (Spector & Read, 1999). This chapter will therefore focus on CBT models and interventions.

There are two main conceptual strands in the CBT literature to explain PTSD. They frame the disorder primarily within a learning theory model or a social cognitive model (Fecteau & Nicki, 1999). Consequently, the interventions tend to have either a behavioural or a cognitive emphasis.

Learning theory model

Learning theory models view PTSD as arising when the perceptions, sensations, thoughts and impressions that occur during a traumatic event are conditioned with the intense feelings of fear, distress and helplessness that occur at the same time. The traumatic feelings therefore become inextricably associated with the perceptions and memories as an automatic, unconscious process. Consequently, following the event any stimulus which acts as a reminder of the trauma triggers the conditioned emotional responses and elicits extremely distressing feelings. Reminders can include symbols, internal states and any stimuli which resemble aspects of the trauma. A natural coping response is to attempt to avoid such cues as this results in a temporary reduction in distressing feelings. The reduction in distress, however, acts as a reinforcer for this coping behaviour, as it does in many anxiety disorders. The avoidance of talking, thinking or being reminded about the event then means that the unresolved feelings are never 'processed' or habituated to and emerge as intrusive flashbacks, dreams, images, etc.

The psychological intervention which follows from this model involves helping the patient to persistently re-expose themselves to the thoughts, feeling, images and memories of the trauma in such a way that habituation to these conditioned responses can occur. This often involves:

1 the patient giving very detailed narrations of the trauma;
2 imaginal exposure to memories and images of the event; and/or
3 real-life (*in-vivo*) exposure to avoided situations or stimuli.

The aim is for the conditioned association between the perceptions and memories and the distressing feelings to diminish over repeated exposures (Richards & Rose, 1991). This process can sometimes be accelerated by using a recorded narrative of the event which the patient listens to between sessions.

Social cognitive model

Social cognitive models view PTSD as arising when a traumatic event powerfully contradicts and puts into question fundamental beliefs which are necessary for everyday functioning. These beliefs are rarely consciously entertained but are vital for successful interaction with the world at large. They relate to the safety, benevolence, meaningfulness and predictability of the world and the stability, integrity and worthfulness of the person themselves. The traumatic event therefore powerfully undermines assumptions such as 'the world is generally a safe place for me', 'the environment is generally predictable for me and I have reasonable control over it' and 'I am generally a decent person with a stable and robust personality'. In addition to these assumptions being undermined, attributional factors that operated at the time of the trauma or soon afterwards may also play a significant role, e.g. the degree of control that the person perceived they had at the time or the amount of responsibility/blame they felt for the event. A more comprehensive cognitive model of PTSD (Ehlers & Clark, 2000) has also emphasised three further cognitive factors in the development of the disorder: (i) the appraisal that there is a serious, current and ongoing threat to the person even though the trauma is in the past, (ii) maladaptive beliefs about the PTSD symptoms themselves when they initially emerge, e.g. that the symptoms are permanent, harmful and/or will lead to insanity, and (iii) the lack of full access to explicit, conscious, chronological memory of the events surrounding the trauma, i.e. the person cannot piece together a personal 'narrative' of the event because the only memories they have access to are fleeting sensations, perceptions and conditioned responses. These cannot be elaborated on and integrated into a full memory of events because they evoke too much distress and are therefore avoided.

The conflict between these much-needed assumptions and the person's experiences during the traumatic event leads to intrusive thoughts and feelings as they struggle to make sense of the implications of the event. The distress caused by thinking about this conflict leads to an avoidance of any reflection or testing of changed assumptions and beliefs about the world and about themselves.

The main intervention approaches which derive from this type of model involve the cognitive restructuring of the beliefs and assumptions changed by the trauma. The ultimate aim is to re-establish an integrated system of assumptions which are viable in the face of the traumatic experience. This usually involves:

1 behavioural experiments to evaluate the evidence for any maladaptive cognitions;
2 rational discussions focusing on the meanings and potentially flawed logic underlying maladaptive assumptions (Socratic dialogue); and
3 generating a detailed chronological account of the events leading up to, during and after the trauma.

These two largely separate conceptualisations of PTSD may have some correlation with neurophysiological findings. These have demonstrated dissociations between the brain structures primarily associated with conscious, explicit recall (the temporocortical and hippocampal areas), and those primarily associated with implicit, conditioned memories (the amygdala and associated areas) (Bechara *et al.*, 1995). It is therefore possible that the features of PTSD best accounted for by learning theory models are mainly mediated by the amygdala and those best accounted for by the social cognitive models are mainly mediated by the hippocampal and corticotemporal areas.

Principal components of a CBT intervention for PTSD

The principal components of a CBT intervention which might be suitably adapted where head injury was also present would be those highlighted by Clark (1999). They might include:

1 establishing a safe context for therapy, an empathic relationship and an appropriate therapeutic alliance;
2 assessing the presenting PTSD problems and any premorbid factors which might affect therapy;
3 providing education about PTSD and rationale for treatment;
4 establishing techniques for dealing with intrusive thoughts;
5 helping the patient reclaim aspects of their lives lost as a result of the PTSD;
6 facilitating imaginal reliving and exposure to the memories of the traumatic event;
7 *in-vivo* exposure to avoided stimuli or situations;
8 cognitive restructuring.

Some discussion about how to cope with any resurgence of symptoms in the future and under what kinds of conditions they could occur might also be included.

Measures

There are no widely used measures of PTSD specifically designed for co-occurring head injury. Generic measures of PTSD are therefore commonly used and these are of two main types:

1 *Impact of Event Scale (Horowitz* et al., *1979).* This lists eight common avoidance symptoms and seven intrusion symptoms and asks the patient to rate how frequently they have experienced them over the previous week. It is a self-report measure and is the single most used instrument for assessing distress following traumatic events (Keane, 1995). It 'has demonstrated excellent discriminant validity in distinguishing patients with PTSD symptoms from traumatised asymptomatic control subjects in military and non-military populations' (McFall *et al.*, 1990). When used with head-injured patients its major strengths are its brevity, ease of use and the fact there are only one or two items which might

be endorsed solely due to head injury sequelae rather than PTSD symptoms. Its main weakness is that it is unsatisfactory as a PTSD diagnostic measure (Joseph, 2000). A revised version of the measure (Weiss & Marmar, 1997) may, however, prove to be a more satisfactory diagnostic tool.

2 *PTSD symptom scales based on DSM diagnostic criteria.* There are a large number of very similar measures based around the 17 key DSM PTSD diagnostic symptoms. They tend to use either a structured interview format administered by a clinician or a self-report format to generate ratings according to the frequency and/or intensity and/or the degree of stress associated with the 17 PTSD symptoms as experienced by the patient during the previous week or month. Some of the most commonly used are the Post-traumatic Stress Symptoms Scale (PSS; Foa *et al.*, 1993), Clinician Administered PTSD Scale (CAPS; Blake *et al.*, 1990), Post-trauma Diagnosis Scale (PDS; Foa *et al.*, 1997) and Structured Clinical Interview for DSM (SCID; Spitzer *et al.*, 1990). These are all well-validated, reliable measures which differentiate effectively between traumatised patients with and without PTSD and are reasonably sensitive to changes in PTSD symptoms. They are generally quite easy to use and some provide scoring norms to aid diagnostic questions. Their main weaknesses when used with patients with head injuries is the fact that almost half of the 17 items could be positively endorsed because of head injury symptoms alone and some can be quite lengthy to administer. Significant caution therefore has to be exercised when interpreting such measures with a head-injured population (Sumpter & McMillan, 2005).

Outcomes

There is a large and ever-growing body of evidence demonstrating that psychological interventions for PTSD are clinically effective in reducing symptoms (National Institute for Clinical Excellence Clinical Guidelines, 2005). The effect size tends to be greater than for pharmacological interventions and with lower dropout rates (e.g. 34 per cent and 14 per cent respectively) (Van Etten & Taylor, 1998). CBT interventions incorporating exposure and/or cognitive restructuring appear to be significantly more effective than anxiety management, supportive counselling, psychodynamic interventions, hypnotherapy and placebo (Hacker Hughes & Thompson, 1994; Spector & Read, 1999; Tarrier *et al.*, 1999; Van Etten & Taylor, 1998). Gains made via CBT interventions are generally well maintained at long-term follow-up (Tarrier *et al.*, 1999) and there is little evidence to suggest that specialist interventions like EMDR provide any increased efficacy beyond that attributable to their exposure elements (Spector & Read, 1999).

The most effective pharmacological interventions appear to be the serotonin specific re-uptake inhibitor (SSRI) antidepressants. More specifically, sertraline in 2001 became the first pharmacological treatment for PTSD endorsed by the US Food and Drug Administration (Bryant & Friedman, 2001). Similarly, in 2005 paroxetine became the first drug to secure a UK product licence for PTSD despite it demonstrating statistically but not clinically significant benefits for the disorder (National Institute for Clinical Excellence Clinical Guidelines, 2005). When SSRIs are maximally effective their effect size begins to approach the magnitude of some of the CBT psychotherapies (Van Etten & Taylor, 1998). Many antidepressants, however, (including SSRIs) increase the risk of epilepsy which may already be raised as the result of certain types of head injury. This in tandem with the proven efficacy of CBT means that psychological interventions focusing on exposure and/or cognitive restructuring will typically be the treatment of choice for people with head injury and PTSD to an even greater extent than for those with PTSD alone where such treatments are already the treatment of choice (National Institute of Clinical Excellence Clinical Guidelines, 2005). It should be noted, however, that when severe executive impairment arises as the result of a brain injury the cognitive elements of CBT may be very difficult to implement and in these circumstances behavioural approaches alone may be the treatments of choice.

Neuropsychological aspects of PTSD

A small number of group studies have investigated to what extent PTSD affects neuropsychological test performance and whether there are specific cognitive impairments associated with the disorder. Results from these are variable. Two large-scale group studies reported that PTSD was associated with mild or no cognitive impairment and that impairments which were present were most attributable to comorbid disorders (Barrett *et al.*, 1996; Zalewski & Thompsen, 1994). These studies, however, used non-treatment-seeking patients or those with only a lifetime diagnosis of PTSD. They may therefore have studied patients without current PTSD or those with relatively mild presentations. Smaller group studies of treatment-seeking patients and subjects with current PTSD have reported impairments in verbal short-term memory functioning and some also have found impairments in visuo-spatial short-term memory, verbal long-term memory, sustained attention and speed of information processing (Bremner *et al.*, 1993; Sutker *et al.*, 1991; Dalton *et al.*, 1989; Everly & Horton, 1989). It should also be noted that one small-scale group study which investigated treatment-seeking patients found severe and global impairments in this group over a wide range of neuropsychological functions, including verbal and visuo-spatial intellectual functioning, verbal and visuo-spatial short-term and long-term memory, remote memory, sustained attention, speed of information processing and executive functioning in the area of verbal fluency (Gil *et al.*, 1990).

Group studies therefore suggest that:

1 cognitive impairment should not automatically be expected with PTSD;
2 some, at least mild, impairments are quite probable with the disorder. Deficits in verbal short-term memory are most likely, although they may also occur in visuo-spatial short-term memory, verbal long-term memory, speed of information processing and sustained attention; and
3 severe and global impairments may be possible in some PTSD patients.

PTSD and Traumatic Brain Injury

The literature addressing the co-occurrence of PTSD and traumatic brain injury is relatively small and case studies often predominate. This is somewhat surprising as the circumstances where head injuries often occur are precisely those where 'actual or threatened death or serious injury' (DSM-IV) may be present and therefore where PTSD might be expected, e.g. road traffic accidents (RTA), assaults, industrial accidents, falls etc. (King, 1997a). The organic amnesia that often occurs as the result of a head injury, however, has long been considered to offer considerable protection against the development of PTSD and it is this assumption that may account for the lack of literature in this area.

Organic amnesia as protection against PTSD

Following head injury unconsciousness is common. Indeed, the depth of unconsciousness and length of unconsciousness are both useful measures of the severity of the injury. Similarly, there can be retrograde amnesia as the result of the brain injury, i.e. no conscious recall of a period of time immediately prior to the injury. Post-traumatic amnesia (PTA) is very common too – the period of time between receiving a head injury and regaining continuous, moment-by-moment memory for events. This includes both periods of time with no conscious recall of events and times where there are only isolated memories outside continuous memory ('islands' of memory). The length of PTA is also a useful measure of head injury severity. Traumatic brain injury may therefore lead to little or no conscious recall of the events surrounding a trauma and protect the person from developing PTSD (Bryant & Harvey, 1995; King, 1997a).

The following case example elegantly illustrates how head injury can protect a person from developing the disorder.

Case Example 12.1

CM, a 45-year-old man, and PG, his 46-year-old wife, were sitting on a bus, returning home from work together. At a bus stop two masked men with baseball bats suddenly jumped on the bus and proceeded to assault CM, hitting him over the head repeatedly. After rendering him unconsciousness they made their escape. CM suffered a severe head injury with 90 minutes retrograde amnesia, 15 minutes loss of consciousness and PTA of two days. His first memory after the assault was of being in a hospital ward approximately 18 hours later. When seen at six months post-injury for a routine head injury follow-up he reported having suffered no emotional consequences following the assault. PG, however, who had witnessed the assault but was not head-injured had developed significant PTSD sufficient to warrant clinical intervention.

This protective feature of at least some forms of TBI against PTSD directly contrasts with almost all other psychological and psychiatric disorders where TBI generally increases the likelihood of developing such problems (including suicidality) by a factor of between 2 and 4 (Fann *et al.*, 2004; Silver *et al.*, 2001; Simpson & Tate, 2002).

Mechanisms for developing PTSD with traumatic brain injury

In spite of the evidence demonstrating that head injury can protect against PTSD there are at least four different ways in which the two do co-occur:

1 Where the head injury is of mild severity and it leads to little or no PTA or retrograde amnesia. PTSD may then occur because the person has conscious memories for a part or parts of the traumatic event either immediately before the head injury or soon after it (Horton, 1993).
2 Where there are one or more 'islands' of memory during PTA and PTSD develops because there is conscious memory of a part of the traumatic event (King, 1997a).
3 Where there is no conscious, explicit memory for any of the events but the trauma is re-experienced by implicit, conditioned fear responses when the person is exposed to stimuli which are reminiscent of the event. Reminders of the event therefore trigger physiological and psychological fear responses which are presumed to have been present at the time of the trauma (Layton & Wardi-Zonna, 1995; McMillan, 1991; McNeil & Greenwood, 1996).
4 Where there is little or no memory for the event but where imagined or reconstructed memories are generated based on what the patient believes or has been told. These 'pseudomemories' consequently become the material for intrusive PTSD symptoms (Bryant, 1996; Harvey & Bryant, 2001; McMillan, 1996).

   PTSD may also develop because of traumatic experiences some time after the event, e.g. invasive or painful medical procedures, first experiences of physical/cognitive disability and/or confused perceptions while emerging from PTA.

Figure 12.1 illustrates the major subdivisions of memory which helps clarify how both explicit and implicit memories can play a part in the development of PTSD with traumatic brain injury.

Incidence rates

There are only a small number of group studies on PTSD and head injury and these have focused on incidence rates of the dual diagnosis and the types of PTSD symptoms most associated with such.

Small- and medium-scale prospective studies have found that 13–14 per cent of patients with mild head injury following events like road traffic accidents also fulfil PTSD diagnostic criteria at one month post-injury, 11–24 per cent at six months and 22 per cent at two years (Bryant & Harvey, 1998; Gil *et al.*, 2005; Harvey & Bryant, 1998, 2000). These figures compare with similar incidence rates of PTSD

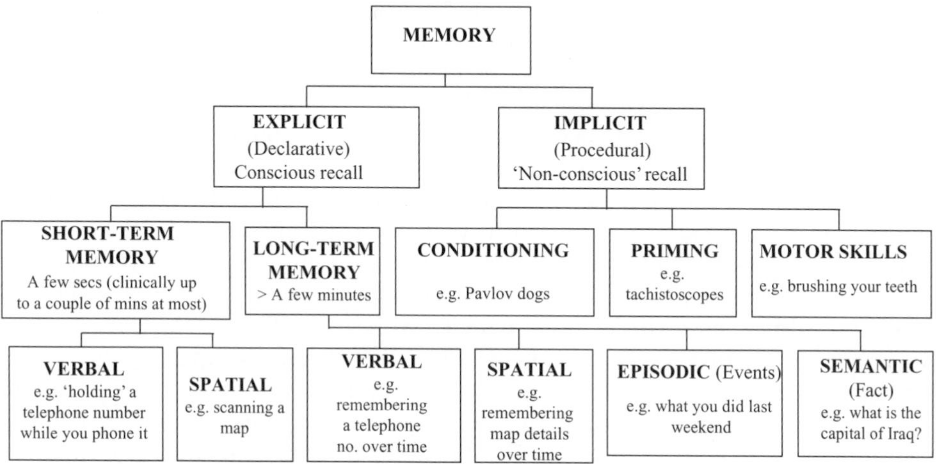

Figure 12.1 Major subdivisions of memory. *Source*: adapted from Hodges (1994)

following road traffic accidents where the large majority are without head injury (23 per cent at three months and 17 per cent at one year) (Ehlers *et al.*, 1998). Such studies suggest that mild head injury may be only minimally protective against PTSD at best.

A well-conducted large-scale study of 1441 consecutive attenders at a hospital emergency department following RTA has provided further, high quality incidence data (Mayou *et al.*, 2000). This study actually found higher rates of PTSD for those with concurrent mild head injury than for those with no head injury. They defined mild head injury as those resulting in unconsciousness of less than 15 minutes. Twenty-one per cent of their cohort fulfilled this criterion. At three months post-injury those with definite loss of unconsciousness had significantly higher rates of PTSD (48 per cent) than those without head injury (23 per cent) and those with only probable loss of consciousness (23 per cent). At one year post-injury the former group still had higher rates although not significantly so. They hypothesised that the increased incidence in those with definite unconsciousness might be due to disruptions in the information processing of the trauma. They concluded that PTSD 'was at least as common in those who suffer unconsciousness as those who were not unconscious' (Mayou *et al.*, 2000). Mild head injury therefore appears to offer little or no protection to the development of PTSD, and if anything, possibly increases the chances of the disorder occurring.

There are only a few incidence studies investigating severe head injury and concurrent PTSD. Some have found zero rates of PTSD in small cohorts of adults and children with severe head injury at six months and two years post-injury (Warden *et al.*, 1997; Max *et al.*, 1998). Similar results were also found in the large cohort of Mayou *et al.* (2000), of whom 1.5 per cent had a severe head injury. While these were excluded from formal PTSD follow-up none appeared to have developed the disorder from a review of their case notes. At least one unrepresentative sample of severely head-injured patients, however, has reported significant rates of PTSD (27 per cent) at six months post-injury (Bryant *et al.*, 2000). A more representative community sample has also found a high incidence rate (18 per cent) for those experiencing levels of post-traumatic stress symptoms high enough to be consistent with a PTSD diagnosis (Williams *et al.*, 2002). A similar incidence rate (11–16 per cent) was found in a mixed-severity sample (Greenspan *et al.*, 2006). Unfortunately, the former study was unable to provide an incidence figure due to the sampling procedures used (Bryant 2001a) and the latter two studies used measures that were insufficient to provide a firm PTSD diagnosis. A further study has demonstrated that severe head injury with no conscious memory for a traumatic event might have the same incidence of PTSD as no injury and full memory for a traumatic event (Turnbull *et al.*, 2001). A very low response rate of 15 per cent however severely limits this finding. There is evidence, none the less, that patients with severe TBI experience less intrusion symptoms than non-injured patients and that avoidance symptoms tend to predominate in this group (Bryant *et al.*, 2000; Powell & Chorlton, 1999; Turnbull *et al.*, 2001). It has also been hypothesised that when brain injury includes damage to the limbic system an increased probability of developing PTSD might be expected owing to the possibility of impairments in the regulation of emotions and memory, and in the extinction of conditioned fear (Harvey *et al.*, 2003).

Some of these anomalies are explained by the finding that self-report questionnaires often dramatically 'overdiagnose' PTSD in people with severe head injuries. Sumpter and McMillan (2005) found a 44–59 per cent incidence rate in their severe head injury sample when using self-report questionnaires but only a 3 per cent rate when a structured interview was used (Clinician-Administered PTSD Scale).

The overall picture is therefore that severe TBI does provide significant protection against PTSD but by no means complete protection.

Special issues for traumatic brain injury and PTSD

There are a number of special issues and challenges unique to working with people with head injury and PTSD. The following highlights some of the most important ones with reflections on how the challenges might be met.

Overlap of PTSD and head injury symptoms

Symptoms arising as the result of PTSD can be identical to those arising as the result of traumatic brain injury (O'Donnell *et al.*, 2003). It is often impossible therefore to accurately assess the proportion of presenting problems which should be attributed to either of them. This is particularly true after mild and moderate head injuries where post-concussion symptoms (PCS) are common. These are a series of symptoms caused by both organic and psychological processes which fully resolve within three to six months of the injury in the majority of cases. PCS overlap considerably with possible PTSD symptoms (Bryant & Harvey, 1999; King, 1997b). This can be powerfully illustrated by studying the list of common symptoms below and trying to ascertain whether they are taken from the PCS or PTSD literature:

sleep disturbance;
irritability;
poor concentration;
headaches;

fatigue;
nausea;
depression;
restlessness;
forgetfulness;
slowed thinking.

They are in fact taken from the PCS literature, although the vast majority could equally have been gleaned from the PTSD literature.

Neuropsychological impairments may also be difficult to interpret. Deficits which commonly follow severe head injury can be identical to those which follow PTSD (McGrath, 1997) – deficits in short-term memory, sustained attention and speed of information processing can be caused by both disorders while intellectual decline, executive dysfunction and long-term memory impairments which often follow head injury may also sometimes be caused by PTSD (Gil *et al.*, 1990).

Such diagnostic difficulties are not merely an academic question. They have important implications for the potential prognosis of presenting problems. This in turn affects the kind of information and advice that is provided and the kinds of realistic rehabilitative goals that might be worked towards. They can also have important implications in medico-legal contexts. In criminal law, for example, the diagnosis may affect whether or not someone is charged with actual bodily harm. In civil law it might inform whether or not a person will ever be able to return to work and therefore the amount of compensation to which they are entitled.

Some guide to the respective causes of impairments may be inferred from the severity and type of the cognitive deficits. When there is evidence of specific areas of damage to the brain, e.g. from neuroimaging scans, this will provide relatively obvious guidance for the types of impairment which are most attributable to the head injury. Also, severe neuropsychological impairments and those not attributable to short-term memory, sustained attention or speed of information processing are more likely to be due to severe head injury than PTSD. In addition, where the head injury is very mild it may be possible to assume that symptoms are unlikely to be due to PCS after three to six months post-injury as they would normally have recovered within this time. Such assumptions, however, are complicated by the fact that 7–8 per cent of mild head-injured patients continue to suffer PCS up to and beyond one year post-injury (Binder, 1997; King, 1997b). An accurate interpretation in many cases may be only possible when PTSD has been maximally treated and it can be assumed that its contribution has significantly diminished, i.e. that the majority of any remaining symptoms are most likely to be due to head injury sequelae. In a significant number of cases, however, an accurate judgement may remain impossible.

Interpretation of amnesia surrounding the event

Where there is a lack of memory surrounding events that have led to a head injury and PTSD it can be important to ascertain the extent to which this is due to psychological or organic factors. A lack of memory could be a PTSD symptom indicative of a form of psychological avoidance of distressing parts of the trauma. It could equally be a head injury symptom due to retrograde or post-traumatic amnesia (King, 1997b).

The judgement regarding the extent to which amnesia is psychogenic or organic amnesia is important as the treatment implications may be diametrically opposed depending on the conclusions reached. If amnesia is organic, intervention may well focus on:

1 providing education about organic amnesia and the impossibility of regaining memory lost as part of PTA and the very low probability of regaining memory lost as part retrograde amnesia;
2 facilitating the acceptance of the amnesia and addressing any frustration arising from a lack of memory for the events;
3 facilitating the reconstruction of events using witness statements, police statements, CCTV footage, etc. in appropriate cases (see section on 'real' and 'imagined' memories for further details); and
4 using generic stimuli in exposure work to facilitate habituation (e.g. videos of traffic) rather than relying on specific but patchy memories which might not be robust enough for the process to occur (Bryant, 2001b).

If, on the other hand, amnesia is psychogenic then it is likely that the patient will at some point be encouraged to recall the amnesic periods as part of the exposure therapy of intervention.

The judgement can be helped by the knowledge that organic amnesia is most common for events immediately following a head injury and that during PTA it may be the more distressing aspects of an event which are later recalled as 'islands' of memory rather than the less distressing aspects (King, 1997a). This is because 'islands' often occur 'when a stimulating event coincides with a peak arousal, providing enough external activation to push the peak above the threshold level for memory' (Gronwall & Wrightson, 1980). Therefore it is more likely that the amnesia is organic in circumstances where it is the *more* distressing aspects of the event that are remembered and the less distressing aspects are not (King, 1997a). Conversely, if psychogenic amnesia is conceptualised as a form of psychological avoidance of traumatic memories then it is likely that the more distressing aspects will not be remembered and the *less* distressing aspects will be. In these circumstances the amnesia is more likely to be psychogenic in nature.

Vicious circle of PTSD symptoms exacerbating head injury symptoms and vice versa

Neuropsychological impairments and PCS following traumatic brain injury are exacerbated by anxiety states, stress and fatigue. PTSD by definition causes significant anxiety and stress and often leads to sleep disturbance and fatigue. The interaction between head injury and PTSD sequelae can, therefore, easily become mutually exacerbating (Bryant & Harvey, 1999; King, 2003; McGrath, 1997). This vicious circle can be particularly pernicious as the patient is robbed of coping resources at precisely the time when they are most needed. They are less able to cope with PCS and/or neuropsychological impairments because of their PTSD and they are less able to cope with their PTSD symptoms owing to PCS and/or neuropsychological impairments. In addition, the ever-increasing stress and anxiety mean that the patient experiences more and more internal reminders of the trauma leading to potentially ever more disabling PTSD symptoms. The vicious circle can be summarised:

PTSD ⇄ ↑ anxiety & stress + ↓ sleep ⟶ ↑ PCS and/or cognitive impairment

Reduced coping

The types of intervention which might help minimise this vicious circle include the following:

1 Early education about the nature of the vicious circle and reassurance that deterioration in problems attributable to this are not physically harmful and will improve as head injury or PTSD disabilities diminish (King *et al.*, 1997). Such education will at times also be appropriate for those close to the patient. Some early cognitive restructuring may also be necessary if the sequelae are initially attributed by the patient to threatening factors (see Ehlers & Clark, 2000). Such attributions may be more likely with a dual diagnosis than with PTSD alone because the overall severity of symptoms is likely to be higher. Also, suffering a brain injury, in and of itself, can become the focus of anxiety inducing attributions.
2 The early provision of anxiety management training to facilitate some control over anxiety symptoms.
3 Close liaison with an appropriate medical doctor to assess whether PTSD symptoms or reduced sleep might be improved with antidepressant or other medication.
4 The provision of advice about behaviours which might maximise sleep – 'sleep hygiene advice'.
5 Provision of neuropsychological rehabilitation intervention and advice concurrently with PTSD intervention (King *et al.*, 1997) and/or the integration of psychotherapeutic and neuropsychological rehabilitation techniques (King & Tyerman, 2003; Tyerman & King, 2004; Williams *et al.*, 2003). This may lead to significant benefits in helping the patient reclaim back aspects of their lives lost as a result of their dual diagnosis which may, in and of itself, help facilitate PTSD improvement (see Clark, 1999). Under these circumstances close liaison and joint working between clinical psychologists, occupational therapists and work placement officers is likely to be essential.

Psychoeducation complications

The provision of accessible, accurate and appropriately paced information is often a key aspect of intervention in both traumatic brain injury and PTSD. The importance of this is magnified when both disorders occur together. There can, however, be a number of complications. First, it can be very difficult to convey to a patient how PTSD can develop when there is no memory of the traumatic event as this appears contradictory. Second, it may be very difficult to give information about prognosis as it may be unclear to what extent symptoms and disabilities are due to head injury or PTSD. Providing information and advice about the timing of attempts to return to work can be especially problematic in these circumstances. If the majority of disabilities are due to PTSD, they may be ameliorated by intervention or spontaneous remission and full recovery may be complete and relatively quick. If, however, they are mainly due to severe brain injury, full recovery is unlikely and the acceptance of this and significant changes in work practices may be necessary. Third, cognitive impairments may lead to the forgetting of information, a lack of understanding of information or an inability to act on information provided or on decisions made.

Some of the ways of meeting these challenges might include the following:

1 Using a 'scientific' hypothesis testing emphasis when providing information. A range of options regarding the causes of the patient's problems might be discussed and the potential prognostic implications associated with each option addressed. The information is thus framed within a dynamic context which is revisited as time and interventions proceed and is presented in terms of possibilities and probabilities to be reassessed periodically rather than as a single categorical statement.
2 Using concrete language, analogy and high frequency words to simplify and clarify concepts.
3 Using diagrams and concrete examples to illustrate difficult ideas, e.g. a model of a brain alongside Figure 12.1 could be used to help explain different types of memory and their neurophysiological correlates.
4 Close liaison between the patient's employer, clinical psychologist, occupational therapist and work placement officer may ensure that plans to return to work and working arrangements can be modified smoothly in line with changes in the patient's functioning.
5 Providing short written summaries to help remind the patient of information provided.
6 Using the first few minutes of each therapy session as a 'mini review' to remind the patient of information covered and intervention approaches agreed upon.

Real versus 'imagined' memories of the event

Patients with traumatic brain injury and PTSD are often frustrated by having only partial or no memories for the events surrounding their injuries. They can also be frustrated by being unsure whether their memories are real or reconstructions. This can pose a dilemma to the treating clinician. On one hand, helping the patient to develop an understanding of the event and a chronological narrative of it may help make sense of the event and be an important part of intervention (Clark, 1999). On the other hand, reconstructions might develop into traumatic images and 'pseudomemories' which become part of the intrusive symptomatology (Bryant, 1996; Harvey & Bryant, 2001; McMillan, 1996). In addition, pre-injury stressors and traumatic memories may be emotionally 'reawakened' as a result of a head injury because the patient's ability to manage distressing premorbid memories is compromised by cognitive impairments (McMillan *et al.*, 2003).

The decision about whether to pursue reconstructing the event will invariably be a collaborative one between clinician and patient. It will probably be dependent on: (i) the extent to which the patient believes pursuing this approach will be beneficial and (ii) an evaluation of (a) the extent to which the patient is prone to developing vivid images and (b) the extent to which the patient is able to control these images without them automatically being elaborated on. An assessment of how vivid a patient's imagination is and how much control they have over non-distressing images is therefore sensible, and may include behavioural experiments to test this.

The following case study highlights some of the complications addressed so far.

Case Examples 12.2 (for a fuller account see King, 2001)

DF, a 32-year-old male clerical officer, suffered a severe head injury and PTSD as the result of being a pedestrian in a road traffic accident involving a large lorry. The driver lost control of the lorry and it travelled at speed towards DF. It was only prevented from hitting him by it colliding with a lamppost a few feet in front of him. It was the buckling lamppost that caused DF's head injury. He had three minutes retrograde amnesia, unconsciousness for some minutes and post-traumatic amnesia for 24 to 48 hours. His first memory was of being in hospital approximately two hours after the accident.

He was referred to a specialist head injury service at 15 months post-injury following a breakdown in his ability to cope at work and being signed off sick by his GP for six months. Neuropsychological assessment revealed mild impairments in verbal short-term memory, speed of information processing and executive functions in the areas of verbal fluency and category alternation and moderate impairments in visuo-spatial intellectual functions and visuo-constructional abilities. Also, DF reported PTSD symptoms sufficient to fulfil the DSM-IV diagnostic criteria. These included: acute distress and physiological reactivity when seeing the head-on view of large lorries similar to the one involved in the accident, hearing air brakes or standing near large lorries; avoidance of driving situations where large white lorries were believed to be prevalent; a sense of foreshortened career; poor concentration; depression; sleep disturbance; headaches; irritability; generalised anxiety.

Intervention initially focused on providing information about head injury, PTSD, the interaction between their respective sequelae and the rationale for the intervention that might be attempted. This was backed up with written handouts. Particular attention was paid to providing information on implicit, conditioned memory as a mechanism for his PTSD as DF was confused as to how his PTSD

Continued

symptoms could have developed without any conscious memory for the accident. The main focus of intervention then turned to *in-vivo* graduated exposure to the specific views of lorries which elicited the physiological re-experiencing symptoms of fear and distress. Four sessions of anxiety management training were concurrently provided by an assistant psychologist. The *in-vivo* exposure began with DF sitting in his car on a busy industrial estate and him looking in his rear-view mirror as large lorries passed him. This approach proved to be only limitedly successful and after further discussion it was decided that DF would carry out exposure more naturalistically by not avoiding the driving situations he previously evaded. With his permission his employer was contacted and they were provided with information about head injury and PTSD and the potential prognostic implications. A graduated return to work was negotiated with them which included reduced hours, decreased workload and regular short breaks. This was reinforced with written information to the employer. Cognitive rehabilitation advice was given to help minimise DF's cognitive disabilities and their impact on his work and social life.

Following successful naturalistic exposure, reduction in PTSD symptoms and a successful return to work (part-time), DF became increasingly concerned about not knowing what had happened during and after the accident. He felt that seeing the CCTV coverage of the accident might be beneficial. This was obtained from the police and the clinical psychologist watched it to gauge how traumatic it was. It was felt to be sufficiently devoid of traumatic material to be useful and as there was no evidence of DF being prone to either vivid imagery or elaboration it was left that he would decide if he wished to watch the film or not. Following discussions with his wife DF decided not to watch the film but used witness statements instead to gain an understanding of the accident. Some time later DF's employer became unable to maintain the modifications to his work and it once again became unsustainable. Joint intervention with a specialist work placement officer was therefore commenced so that an alternative job could be pursued which would be sustainable in the long term.

Dissociative fugue states and post-traumatic epilepsy

The development of dissociative fugue type states, although uncommon following PTSD, do sometimes occur. During fugue states a patient has amnesia for a circumscribed period, often travels away from their home situation with no memory of their travels and in some cases has disturbances of identity during this time (where they are unable to remember who they are or assume a different identity). Psychogenic fugues are often viewed as a form of emotional avoidance where the patient escapes from overwhelming feelings of fear, distress, anger, etc. Sufferers of fugue states can be very distressed as they struggle to make sense of gaps in their episodic memory and can be very confused and worried about how they come to be in places with no recollection of travelling there. There may also be anxieties about how they might have behaved during the fugue. When they occur in the context of PTSD and traumatic brain injury it is particularly important to ascertain whether they are psychogenic in nature or due to complex partial epileptic activity as both can cause the phenomenon (Reither & Stoudemire, 1988) and the probability of developing epilepsy is significantly increased following certain types of head injury.

Where fugue-like symptoms are reported by someone with PTSD and head injury, close liaison with a neurologist or similarly qualified medical practitioner is essential so that a full assessment of epilepsy can be made. The judgement is made easier where fugue states last for days or a number of hours rather than for minutes as it is unlikely that epileptic activity would lead to fugues over protracted lengths of time. Where the fugues are shorter, however, the judgement may be more difficult and hence there is a requirement for a full assessment for the presence of epilepsy.

If epilepsy is excluded it should normally be clearly conveyed to the patient so that a psychological explanation can be given with the maximum of confidence. Psychogenic fugues are rare, not well understood and can be difficult to explain and the patient is likely to require clear information about how they arise. It is unlikely that this can be given when an epileptic diagnosis has not been excluded. Following an explanation of fugue as a form of unconscious psychological avoidance of overwhelming feelings, psychological intervention might include the following:

1 Detailed examination of events leading to the fugue states to find potential triggers, e.g. increases in anxiety, anger or feelings of helplessness. If triggers can be found some control over the fugues may be possible by exploring 'emergency' behaviours which reduce the intensity of the feelings experienced in the situations where these are prone to occur, e.g. for a person whose fugues emerge when anger levels become high in specific driving conditions, an 'emergency behaviour' might be to pull over at a safe location as soon as anger levels begin to rise. Relaxation exercises might then be undertaken to reduce overall arousal levels.
2 Reassurance about the unlikelihood of the person behaving irresponsibly during fugue states based on their previous behaviours in everyday life and their previous fugue behaviours, e.g. reassuring that past behaviour is often the best predictor of future behaviour and the fact that the person has behaved responsibly both in everyday life and during previous fugue states means that they are likely to continue to behave responsibly in any future fugue states.
3 Where fugues occur for days and the person regularly travels away from their home environment, electronic tagging devices can be helpful in relocating the person. They can then be brought back to a place of psychological safety which may be beneficial in reducing the length and frequency of fugue episodes (Macleod, 1999).

Perseveration of traumatic re-experiencing

Perseveration is a neuropsychological impairment in executive functioning which causes the patient difficulty in changing their actions, ideas or sensations when these responses are no longer required (Hotz & Helm-estabrooks, 1995). If a traumatic brain injury has led to perseveration and PTSD is also suffered, it is possible that under rare circumstances the person can become 'stuck' while re-experiencing their traumatic event due to it becoming a perseverated response. The re-experiencing of the trauma may consequently become unavoidable and inescapable. In the single-case study which highlights this potential problem the perseveration of traumatic re-experiencing meant that it lasted for a number of days with extremely high levels of distress for the patient which eventually required psychiatric in-patient treatment to manage (King, 2002). While this may occur only in very rare circumstances (e.g. where there is co-occurring specific types of brain injury, PTSD and chronic pain) (King, 2002), the resultant extremes of prolonged distress that may arise mean that precautions should be entertained where perseveration and PTSD are present.

Although caution must be taken in making generalisations from a single case and particularly one which might describe a rare phenomenon, the treatment recommendations drawn from the above case include the following:

1 Close liaison with a psychiatrist prior to the commencement of interventions involving exposure work. This would enable the introduction of medications for PTSD and pain which might help prevent 'traumatic perseveration' developing. It would also allow for smoother and quicker access to in-patient services should these be necessary.
2 Psychological intervention should focus on all non-exposure aspects of therapy before exposure is attempted. This might allow the therapeutic relationship to be maximally robust should 'traumatic perseveration' develop and might help facilitate patient compliance with any emergency management procedures that might be necessary.
3 Techniques which help 'ground' and orientate a person when experiencing dissociative symptoms should be taught prior to exposure work (Kennerly, 1996). These might help refocus the person's thoughts and feelings on the present rather than on the trauma should 'traumatic perseveration' develop. These might include distraction techniques and tape recordings of the person reminding themselves where they are, that the trauma is over, etc.
4 Clear guidelines should be made regarding under what conditions exposure work should be conducted outside therapy sessions. This might reduce the possibility of poorly controlled exposure exercises acting as a trigger for 'traumatic perseveration'.

Other complications

There are at least two further complications which commonly arise when PTSD and head injury co-exist but which are not exclusive to this group.

Concurrent pain acting as a constant reminder of the trauma

When an event has led to head injury and PTSD it may also have led to chronic pain (particularly headache pain). This can act as a constant reminder of the traumatic event and therefore may exacerbate PTSD symptoms (Sharp & Harvey, 2001; Taylor *et al.*, 2001). It may also act as an unavoidable source of stress and anxiety leading to increased internal reminders of the trauma and therefore further exacerbate PTSD symptoms. A vicious circle may be set up where this additional source of stress leads to increased PTSD symptoms and/or cognitive impairment which in turn exacerbates the stress leading to more pain and so on. It can be summarised:

Pain ←——→ Stress ←——→ PTSD and/or cognitive impairment

Physical and cognitive impairments resulting from the trauma may also, in and of themselves, elicit feelings of helplessness, anger or anxiety which may act as further internal cues for the trauma and as such increase the likelihood of PTSD developing, being maintained or being exacerbated (Hembree *et al.*, 2004; Mellman *et al.*, 2001; O'Donnell *et al.*, 2004).

Where pain is present, early liaison with an appropriate medical practitioner to address its pharmacological treatment and early anxiety management may be beneficial in reducing the impact of the vicious circle outlined above. Psychological intervention for the PTSD should in most circumstances proceed at the same time as active pain management as PTSD intervention is believed to be a useful part of pain management in these circumstances (Eisendrath, 1995; Geisser *et al.*, 1996).

Legal proceedings which act as a constant reminder of the trauma

Criminal and civil legal proceedings often arise following events that have led to head injury and PTSD, e.g. criminal proceedings following an assault or civil compensation claims following a road traffic accident. This process is often very stressful and can also act as an ongoing reminder of the trauma. Both of these factors may set up a vicious circle similar to the one above relating to pain. The additional stress and constant reminders of the trauma exacerbate PTSD and head injury sequelae and this leads to increased stress and so on. There may be additional complications if the legal result is unsatisfactory and the patient perceives that justice has not been done. Clark (1999) recommends that the potential consequences of a negative legal result are openly discussed with the patient prior to them going to court so that coping strategies may be explored in advance. It may also be useful to help the patient develop a degree of cognitive and emotional distance between 'legal realities' and actual realities where the legal framework for accessing truth and justice is perceived as useful but not perfect. This may also help minimise the psychological impact of detrimental material which may emerge as part of the legal process.

Conclusions

PTSD is a highly distressing emotional response to a traumatic event and can be an extremely disabling disorder. The circumstances where traumatic brain injury occurs are often precisely those where PTSD might also occur. Organic amnesia following brain injury can protect against PTSD but this occurs less frequently than investigators previously thought. The dual diagnosis can develop where there are conscious memories of the trauma, where implicit conditioned 'memories' of the event have occurred or where reconstructed 'memories' occur. CBT interventions appear to be the treatment of choice for PTSD and these are the ones that have most commonly been adapted for patients with the dual diagnosis of head injury and PTSD. Little is known about the nature of the interaction between head injury and PTSD sequelae but it is highly likely that they are mutually exacerbating. Other potential complications with the dual diagnosis include: difficulties interpreting sequelae common to both PTSD and head injury; problems in interpreting periods of amnesia; challenges in delivering appropriate psycho-education; difficulties in interpreting fugue-type states; perseveration of traumatic re-experiencing; concurrent pain and concurrent legal proceedings. If PTSD is suspected by a member of a multidisciplinary team it is important that the patient is assessed by a clinical psychologist. In addition, close inter-professional and joint working may be imperative when PTSD and traumatic brain injury co-exist because of the potential complications highlighted in this chapter.

Recommended Reading

Ehlers, A. & Clark, D.A. (2000). A cognitive model of posttraumatic stress disorder. *Behaviour Research and Therapy*, *38*, 319–345.
A comprehensive cognitive behavioural model of PTSD which includes useful and practical intervention methods.

Hacker Hughes, J.G.H. & Thompson, J. (1994). Post traumatic stress disorder: An evaluation of behavioural and cognitive behavioural interventions. *Clinical Psychology and Psychotherapy*, *1*(3), 125–142.
A review of 16 case studies, 8 uncontrolled treatment trials and 8 controlled treatment trials which have assessed the efficacy of cognitive behavioural interventions for PTSD. It includes useful descriptions of the range of intervention methods used.

Kessler, R.C., Sonnega, A., Bromet, E., Hughes, M. & Nelson, C. (1995). Posttraumatic stress disorder in the national co-morbidity study. *Archives of General Psychiatry*, *52*, 1048–1060.
An impressive national study on the prevalence rates of PTSD in a representative sample of 5877 US citizens aged 15 to 54.

McGrath, J. (1997). Cognitive impairment associated with post-traumatic stress disorder and minor head injury: A case report. *Neuropsychological Rehabilitation*, *7*(3), 231–239.
One of the few papers which describes its treatment approach for a patient with PTSD and traumatic brain injury.

McMillan, T.M. (1991). Post traumatic stress disorder and severe head injury. *British Journal of Psychiatry*, *159*, 431–433.
Another of the few papers which describes its treatment approach for a patient with PTSD and traumatic brain injury.

McMillan, T.M., Williams, W.H. & Bryant, R.A. (2003). Post-traumatic stress disorder after traumatic brain injury: A review of causal mechanisms, assessment and treatment. *Neuropsychological Rehabilitation – Special Issue*, *1*, 149–164.
An excellent review of the literature on TBI and PTSD.

Van Etten, M.L. & Taylor, S. (1998). Comparative efficacy of treatments for post-traumatic stress disorder; a meta-analysis. *Clinical Psychology and Psychotherapy*, *5*, 126–144.

A meta-analytic review of 61 outcome trials assessing the efficacy of psychological and pharmacological treatments for PTSD. It has more of an emphasis on the effect sizes of differing treatments than on describing the intervention methods themselves.

Useful Resources

Herbert, C. (2002). Understanding your reactions to trauma: A guide for survivors of trauma and their families. Revised version. *Blue Stallion Publications*. ISBN-1904127029.

A comprehensive self-help booklet for managing PTSD.

King, N.S. (1997). Coping with post traumatic stress leaflet. In N.S. King, S. Crawford, F.J. Wenden, N.E.G. Moss & D.T. Wade (1997). Interventions and service need following mild and moderate head injury: The Oxford Head Injury Service. *Clinical Rehabilitation*, *11*, 13–27.

A single-page leaflet on managing post-traumatic stress symptoms.

References

American Psychiatric Association (1994). *Diagnostic and statistical manual of mental disorders, 4th edition (DSM IV)*. Washington, DC: APA.

Barrett, D.H., Green, M.C., Morris, R., Giles, W. & Croft, J. (1996). Cognitive functioning and posttraumatic stress disorder. *American Journal of Psychiatry*, *153*, 1492–1494.

Bechara, A., Trandel, D., Damasio, H., Adelphs, R., Rectland, C. & Damasio, A.R. (1995). Double dissociation of conditioning and declarative knowledge relative to amygdalae and hippocampus in humans. *Science*, *269*, 1115–1118.

Binder, L.M. (1997). A review of mild head trauma. Part II: Clinical implications. *Journal of Clinical and Experimental Neuropsychology*, *19*(3), 432–457.

Blake, D.D., Weathers, F.W., Nagy, L.M., Kaloupek, D.G., Klauminzer, G., Charney, D.S., *et al.* (1990). A clinician rating scale for assessing current and lifetime PTSD: The CAPS-I. *Behaviour Therapist*, *September*, 187–188.

Bremner, J.D., Scott, T.M., Delaney, R.C., Southwick, S.M., Mason, J.W., Johnson, D.R., *et al.* (1993). Deficits in short term memory in posttraumatic stress disorder. *American Journal of Psychiatry*, *150*(7), 1015–1019.

Bryant, R.A. (1996). Posttraumatic stress disorder, flashbacks and pseudomemories in closed head injury. *Journal of Traumatic Stress*, *9*(3), 621–629.

Bryant, R.A. (2001a). Posttramatic stress disorder and traumatic brain injury: Can they co-exist? *Clinical Psychology Review*, *21*(6), 931–948.

Bryant, R.A. (2001b). Posttraumatic stress disorder and mild brain injury; controversies, causes and consequences. *Journal of Clinical and Experimental Neuropsychology*, *23*(6), 718–728.

Bryant, R.A. & Friedman, M. (2001). Medication and non-medication treatments of post-traumatic stress disorder. *Current Opinion in Psychiatry*, *14*, 119–123.

Bryant, R.A. & Harvey, A.G. (1995). Acute stress response: A comparison of head injured and non-head injured patients. *Psychological Medicine*, *25*, 869–873.

Bryant, R.A. & Harvey, A.G. (1998). Relationship between acute stress disorder and posttraumatic stress disorder following mild traumatic brain injury. *American Journal of Psychiatry*, *155*, 625–629.

Bryant, R.A. & Harvey, A.G. (1999). Postconcussive symptoms and posttraumatic stress disorder after mild traumatic brain injury. *Journal of Nervous and Mental Disease, 187*, 302–305.

Bryant, R.A., Marosszeky, J.E., Crooks, J. & Gurka, J.A. (2000). Posttraumatic stress disorder after severe traumatic brain injury. *American Journal of Psychiatry, 157*(4), 629–631.

Bryant, R.A., Moulds, M., Guthrie, R. & Nixon, R.D. (2003). Treating acute stress disorder following mild traumatic brain injury. *American Journal of Psychiatry, 160*(3), 585–587.

Clark, D.M. (1999). Cognitive-behavioural treatment of PTSD. *Oxford Cognitive Therapy for Anxiety Disorders Group*. © D.M. Clark, 1999.

Dalton, J.E., Pederson, S.L. & Ryan, J.J. (1989). Effects of post-traumatic stress disorder on neuropsychological test performance. *International Journal of Clinical Neuropsychology, 11*, 121–124.

Ehlers, A. & Clark, D.A. (2000). A cognitive model of posttraumatic stress disorder. *Behaviour Research and Therapy, 38*, 319–345.

Ehlers, A., Mayou, R.A. & Bryant, B. (1998). Psychological predictors of chronic posttraumatic stress disorder after motor vehicle accidents. *Journal of Abnormal Psychology, 107*(3), 508–519.

Eisendrath, S.J. (1995). Psychiatric aspects of chronic pain. *Neurology, 45*(Suppl. 9), 526–534.

Everly, F.S. & Horton, A.M. (1989). Neuropsychology of posttraumatic stress disorder: A pilot study. *Perceptual and Motor Skills, 68*, 807–810.

Fann, J.R., Bart, M.P.H., Burington, M.S., Leonetti, M.S., Jaffe, K., Katon, W.J., *et al.* (2004). Psychiatric illness following traumatic brain injury in an adult health maintenance organisation population. *Archives of General Psychiatry, 61*, 53–61.

Fecteau, G. & Nicki, R. (1999). Cognitive behavioural treatment of post traumatic stress disorder after motor vehicle accidents. *Behavioural and Cognitive Psychotherapy, 37*, 201–214.

Foa, E.B., Cashman, L., Jaycox, L. & Perry, K. (1997). The validation of a self report measure of posttraumatic stress disorder: The posttraumatic diagnostic scale. *Psychological Assessment, 9*, 445–451.

Foa, E.B., Riggs, D.S., Dancu, C.U. & Rothbaum, B.O. (1993). Reliability and validity of a brief instrument for assessing post-traumatic stress disorder. *Journal of Traumatic Stress*, 6, 459–473.

Geisser, M.E., Roth, R.S., Bachman, J.E. & Eckert, T.A. (1996). The relationship between symptoms of post-traumatic stress disorder and pain, affective disturbance and disability among patients with accident and non-accident pain. *Pain, 66*, 207–214.

Gil, T., Avraham, C., Greenburg, D., Kugelmass, S. & Lerer, B. (1990). Cognitive functioning in post-traumatic stress disorder. *Journal of Traumatic Stress, 3*(1), 29–45.

Gil, G., Caspi, Y., Ben-Ari, I.Z., Koren, D. & Klein, E. (2005). Does memory of a traumatic event increase the risk of posttraumatic stress disorder in patients with traumatic brain injury? A prospective study. *American Journal of Psychiatry, 162*, 963–969.

Greenspan, A.I., Stringer, A.Y., Phillips, V.L., Hammond, F.M. & Goldstein, F.C. (2006). Symptoms of post-traumatic stress: Intrusion and avoidance 6 and 12 months after TBI. *Brain Injury, 20*(7), 733–742.

Gronwall, D. & Wrightson, P. (1980). Duration of post traumatic amnesia after mild head injury. *Journal of Clinical Neuropsychology*, 2, 51–60.

Hacker Hughes, J.G.H. & Thompson, J. (1994). Post traumatic stress disorder: An evaluation of behavioural and cognitive behavioural interventions. *Clinical Psychology and Psychotherapy, 1*(3), 125–142.

Harvey, A.G., Brewin, C.R., Jones, C. & Kopelman, M.D. (2003). Coexistence of posttraumatic stress disorder and traumatic brain injury: Towards resolution of the paradox. *Journal of the International Neuropsychological Society*, *9*, 663–676.

Harvey, A.G. & Bryant, R.A. (1998). Acute stress disorder after mild traumatic brain injury. *Journal of Nervous and Mental Disease*, *186*, 333–337.

Harvey, A.G. & Bryant, R.A. (2000). Two year prospective evaluation of the relationship between acute stress disorder and posttraumatic stress disorder following mild traumatic brain injury. *American Journal of Psychiatry*, *157*, 626–628.

Harvey, A.G. & Bryant, R.A. (2001). Reconstructing trauma memories; a prospective study of 'amnesic' trauma sufferers. *Journal of Traumatic Stress*, *14*(2), 277–282.

Hembree, E.A., Street, G.P., Riggs, D.S. & Foa, E.B. (2004). Do assault-related variables predict response to cognitive behavioural treatment for PTSD? *Journal of Consulting and Clinical Psychology*, *72*(3), 531–534.

Hodges, J.R. (1994). *Cognitive assessment for clinicians*. Oxford Medical Publications. Oxford: Oxford University Press.

Horowitz, M., Wilner, N. & Alvarez, W. (1979). Impact of event scale: A measure of subjective stress. *Psychological Medicine*, *41*, 209–218.

Horton, A.M. (1993). Posttraumatic stress disorder and mild head trauma: Follow up case study. *Perceptual and Motor Skills*, *76*, 243–246.

Hotz, G. & Helm-estabrooks, N. (1995). Perseveration. Part 1: A review. *Brain Injury*, *9*(2), 151–159.

Joseph, S. (2000). Psychometric evaluation of Horowitz's Impact of Event Scale: A review. *Journal of Traumatic Stress*, *13*(1), 101–113.

Keane, T.M. (1995). Guidelines for the forensic psychological assessment of posttraumatic stress disorder claimants. In R.I. Simon (Ed.) *Posttraumatic stress disorder in litigation: Guidelines for forensic assessment* (pp.99–115). Washington, DC: American Psychiatric Press.

Kennerly, H. (1996). Cognitive therapy of dissociative symptoms associated with trauma. *British Journal of Clinical Psychology*, *35*(3), 325–340.

Kessler, R.C., Sonnega, A., Bromet, E., Hughes, M. & Nelson, C. (1995). Posttraumatic stress disorder in the national co-morbidity study. *Archives of General Psychiatry*, *52*, 1048–1060.

King, N.S. (1997a). Post-traumatic stress disorder and head injury as a dual diagnosis; 'islands' of memory as a mechanism. *Journal of Neurology, Neurosurgery and Psychiatry*, *62*(1), 82–84.

King, N.S. (1997b). Literature Review; Mild head injury: Neuropathology, sequelae, measurement and recovery. *British Journal of Clinical Psychology*, *36*, 161–184.

King, N.S. (2001). 'Affect without recollection' in post-traumatic stress disorder where head injury causes organic amnesia for the event. *Behavioural and Cognitive Psychotherapy*, *29*, 501–504.

King, N.S. (2002). Perseveration of traumatic re-experiencing in PTSD; a cautionary note regarding exposure based psychological treatments for PTSD when head injury and perseveration are also present. *Brain Injury*, *16*(1), 65–74.

King, N.S. (2003). The post concussion syndrome: Clarity amid the controversy? *British Journal of Psychiatry*, *183*, 276–278.

King, N.S., Crawford, S., Wenden, F.J., Moss, N.E.G. & Wade, D.T. (1997). Interventions and service need following mild and moderate head injury: The Oxford Head Injury Service. *Clinical Rehabilitation*, *11*, 13–27.

King, N.S. & Tyerman, A. (2003). Neuropsychological presentation and treatment of head injury and traumatic brain damage. In P.W. Halligan, U. Kischau & J. Marshall Eds.) *Handbook of clinical neuropsychology* (pp.487–505). Oxford: Oxford University Press.

Layton, B.S. & Wardi-Zonna, K. (1995). Post-traumatic stress disorder with neurogenesis amnesia for the traumatic event. *The Clinical Neuropsychologist*, 9, 2–10.

Max, J.E., Castillo, C.S., Robin, D., Lindgren, S.D., Smith, W.L., Satoy, Y., *et al.* (1998). Posttraumatic stress symptomatology after childhood traumatic brain injury. *Journal of Mental and Nervous Disease*, *186*(10), 589–596.

Mayou, R.A., Black, J. & Bryant, B. (2000). Unconsciousness, amnesia and psychiatric symptoms following road traffic accident injury. *British Journal of Psychiatry*, *177*, 540–545.

Mayou, R. & Bryant, B. (2002). Outcome 3 years after a road traffic accident. *Psychological Medicine*, *32*, 671–675.

Macleod, A.D. (1999). Posttraumatic stress disorder, dissociative fugue and a locator beacon. *Australian and New Zealand Journal of Psychiatry*, *33*, 102–104.

McFall, M.E., Smith, D.E., Roszell, D.K., Tarver, D.J. & Malas, K.L. (1990). Convergent validity of measures of PTSD in Vietnam combat veterans. *American Journal of Psychiatry*, *147*, 645–648.

McGrath, J. (1997). Cognitive impairment associated with post-traumatic stress disorder and minor head injury: A case report. *Neuropsychological Rehabilitation*, 7(3), 231–239.

McMillan, T.M. (1991). Post traumatic stress disorder and severe head injury. *British Journal of Psychiatry*, *159*, 431–433.

McMillan, T.M. (1996). Post-traumatic stress disorder following minor and severe closed head injury: 10 single cases. *Brain Injury*, *10*(10), 749–758.

McMillan, T.M., Williams, W.H. & Bryant, R. (2003). Post-traumatic stress disorder after traumatic brain injury: A review of causal mechanisms, assessment and treatment. *Neuropsychological Rehabilitation – Special Issue*, *1*, 149–164.

McNeil, J.E. & Greenwood, R. (1996). Can PTSD occur with amnesia for the precipitating event? *Cognitive Neuropsychiatry*, *1*, 239–246.

Mellman, T.A., David, D., Bustamante, V., Fins, A.I. & Esposito, K. (2001). Predictors of post-traumatic stress disorder following severe injury. *Depression and Anxiety*, *14*, 226–231.

National Institute for Clinical Excellence (2005). *Clinical Guidelines: Post-traumatic stress disorder (PTSD): The management of PTSD in adults and children in primary and secondary care*. London: NHS National Institute for Clinical Excellence.

O'Donnell, M.L., Creamer, M., Bryant, R.A., Schnyder, U. & Shalev, A. (2003). Posttraumatic disorders following injury: An empirical and methodological review. *Clinical Psychology Review*, *23*, 587–603.

O'Donnell, M.L., Creamer, M., Pattison, P. & Atkin, C. (2004). Psychiatric morbidity following injury. *American Journal of Psychiatry*, *161*, 507–514.

Powell, G.E. & Chorlton, L. (1999). *Does head injury protect people from PTSD?* Paper Presented to the Annual Conference of the British Psychological Society, Belfast, April, 1999.

Reither, A.M. & Stoudemire, A. (1988). Psychogenic fugue state: A review. *Southern Medical Journal*, *81*(5), 568–571.

Richards, D.A. & Rose, J.R. (1991). Exposure therapy for posttraumatic stress disorder. *British Journal of Psychiatry*, *158*, 836–840.

Sharp, T.J. & Harvey, A.G. (2001). Chronic pain and posttraumatic stress disorder: Mutual maintenance? *Clinical Psychology Review*, *21*(6), 857–877.

Silver, J.M., Kramer, R., Greenwald, S. & Weissman, M. (2001). The association between head injuries and psychiatric disorders: Findings from the New Haven NIMH epidemiologic catchment area study. *Brain Injury*, *15*, 935–945.

Simpson, G. & Tate, R. (2002). Suicidality after traumatic brain injury: Demographic, injury and clinical correlates. *Psychological Medicine*, *32*, 687–697.

Spector, J. & Read, J. (1999). The current status of eye movement desensitisation and reprocessing (EMDR). *Clinical Psychology and Psychotherapy*, *6*, 165–174.

Spitzer, R.L., Williams, J.B.W., Gibbon, M. & First, M.B. (1990). *Structured interview for DSM III-R*. Washington, DC: American Psychiatric Press.

Sumpter, R.E. & McMillan, T.M. (2005). Misdiagnosis of post-traumatic stress disorder following severe traumatic brain injury. *British Journal of Psychiatry*, *186*, 423–426.

Sutker, P.B., Winstead, D.K., Galina, Z.H. & Allain, A.N. (1991). Cognitive deficits and psychopathology among former prisoners of war and combat veterans of the Korean conflict. *American Journal of Psychiatry*, *148*, 67–72.

Tarrier, N., Sommerfield, C., Pilgrim, H. & Humphreys, L. (1999). Cognitive therapy or imaginal exposure in the treatment of post-traumatic stress disorder. *British Journal of Psychiatry*, *175*, 571–575.

Taylor, S.T., Fedoroff, I.C., Koch, W.J., Thordarson, D.S., Fecteau, G. & Nicki, R. (2001). Posttraumatic stress disorder arising after road traffic collisions; patterns of response to cognitive-behavioural therapy. *Journal of Consulting and Clinical Psychology*, *67*, 13–18.

Turnbull, S.J., Campbell, E.A. & Swann, I.J. (2001). Post-traumatic stress disorder symptoms following a head injury; does amnesia for the event influence the development of symptoms? *Brain Injury*, *15*(9), 775–785.

Tyerman, A. & King, N.S. (2004). Interventions for psychological problems after brain injury. In L.H. Goldstein & J.E. McNeil (Eds.) *Clinical neuropsychology: A practical guide to assessment and management for clinicians* (pp.385–404). Chichester: Wiley.

Van Etten, M.L. & Taylor, S. (1998). Comparative efficacy of treatments for post-traumatic stress disorder; a meta-analysis. *Clinical Psychology and Psychotherapy*, *5*, 126–144.

Warden, D.L., Labdate, L.A., Salazar, A.M., Nelson, R., Sheley, E., Staudenmeier, J., *et al.* (1997). Posttraumatic stress disorder in patients with traumatic brain injury and amnesia for the event? *Journal of Neuropsychiatry and Clinical Neuroscience*, *9*(1), 18–22.

Weiss, D.S. & Marmar, C.R. (1997). The Impact of Event Scale–Revised. In J.P. Wilson & T.M. Keane (Eds.) *Assessing psychological trauma and PTSD* (pp.399–411). New York: Guilford Press.

Williams, W.H., Evans, J.J. & Wilson, B.A. (2002). Prevalence of posttraumatic stress disorder after severe traumatic brain injury in a representative community sample. *Brain Injury*, *16*(8), 673–679.

Williams, W.H., Evans, J.J. & Wilson, B.A. (2003). Neurorehabilitation for two cases of post-traumatic stress disorder following traumatic brain injury. *Cognitive Neuropsychiatry*, *8*(1), 1–18.

Zalewski, C. & Thompsen, W. (1994). Comparison of neuropsychological test performance in PTSD, generalised anxiety disorder and control Vietnam veterans. *Assessment*, *1*(2), 133–142.

13

Facilitating Psychological Adjustment

Andy Tyerman

Introduction

People with traumatic brain injury (TBI) often have difficulty in adjusting to the complex physical, sensory, cognitive, behavioural and emotional changes resulting from TBI and their wide-ranging personal, family, vocational and social effects. As Linge (1990), a clinical psychologist who sustained a serious TBI, comments, 'The far ranging effects of head injury on the survivor's life and that of his or her family cannot be overemphasised. In my own case I realize that it was for me the most significant event of my lifetime. The catastrophic effect of my injury was such that I was shattered and then remoulded by the experience, and I emerged from it a profoundly different person with a different set of convictions, values and priorities.'

This chapter focuses on how people may be guided and supported in making psychological adjustments following TBI. (Psychological interventions for specific emotional difficulties – fear, anxiety and depression – are discussed in chapter 11.) The need for psychological interventions to include a psychotherapeutic approach to facilitate adjustment (alongside cognitive rehabilitation, behavioural management and social skills training) has long been stressed (e.g. Prigatano, 1986; Tyerman & Humphrey, 1988). As Ponsford (1995) notes, 'The importance of addressing the myriad of psychological and adjustment problems faced by TBI individuals cannot be overemphasised. At an appropriate time after injury, all those who have sustained TBI should have access to counselling and/or group therapy to enhance the development of self-awareness, whilst maximising self-esteem and providing an opportunity to rebuild a new sense of self.'

The need to support people with neurological conditions in achieving a sense of well-being and in making long-term psychological adjustments to altered personal, family and social circumstances is recognised in the 'markers of good practice' for Quality Requirement 6 on 'Community Rehabilitation and Support' in the *National*

Service Framework for Long-term Conditions (Department of Health, 2005). The *National Clinical Guidelines on Rehabilitation following Acquired Brain Injury* (RCP/BSRM, 2003) include specific guidelines on provision of psychotherapeutic support:

127 Patients should be given information, advice and the opportunity to talk about the impact of brain injury on their lives with someone experienced in managing the emotional impact of acquired brain injury.

128 Patients should be provided with access to individual and/or group psychological interventions for their emotional difficulties, adapted to take into account individual neuropsychological deficits.

131 Patients should have access to specialist individual or group-based neuro-psychotherapeutic interventions to facilitate long-term psychological, family and social adjustment, including sexual relationships.

The chapter will consider the adjustment needs of people with TBI and approaches to facilitating psychological adjustment. The focus is on practical interventions based on clinical experience within the Community Head Injury Service in Aylesbury, illustrated by two case examples – one early and one late post-injury. (For an overview of adjustment see Yates (2003); for an evaluation of theories and research on psychosocial adjustment, on coping patterns and self-beliefs and on the role of pre-injury factors after TBI see Kendall and Terry (1996), Moore and Stambrook (1995) and Tate (2003), respectively.)

The Psychological Impact of TBI

The psychological impact of TBI is variable, depending upon specific disabilities, level of awareness, coping style and personal circumstances. Early after onset there may be a profound sense of confusion, reflecting an interaction of trauma, cognitive impairment and the bewildering array of symptoms of which the person may be only partially aware. Thereafter a wide range of emotional reactions may be experienced (e.g. irritability, anger, frustration, fear, anxiety, depression, mood swings, loss of confidence, etc.) (e.g. Brooks *et al.*, 1986; Hoofien *et al.*, 2001; Kersel *et al.*, 2001; Oddy *et al.*, 1985; Ponsford *et al.*, 1995; Tyerman & Humphrey, 1984). Some view the situation as unreal, others view themselves as no longer a 'real' or 'whole' person.

Whilst for some the psychological impact is experienced from early post-injury, others may be less concerned during early rehabilitation, confident of a full recovery. This may reflect reduced awareness of the extent of disabilities arising directly from TBI, but there may also be an element of psychological denial. As such, the psychological impact may surface later when the person has developed greater awareness and/or been confronted by their difficulties on attempting to resume former family, work and social roles (Tyerman, 1987, 1991). This may arise, for example, after return to work, on losing a previous job, on relationship breakdown or after repeated episodes of loss of behavioural control in social situations. When the full impact of TBI is realised many people are no longer receiving any professional support. People with TBI often behave in ways which are inconsistent with the person that they thought they were, an experience which Bannister (1974) described, in general, as 'perhaps the most disturbing and disorganising experience that man can undergo'.

Prigatano (1995) highlights existential questions about the meaning of life that often arise in post-acute rehabilitation (e.g. Will I be normal? Is this life worth living after brain injury?). Miller (1993) observes that many problems experienced after brain injury concern fundamental issues of life and meaning (i.e. death, isolation, meaninglessness and freedom). With increased awareness there may be questions about 'Why me?', sometimes tinged with resentment and anger, especially when someone else is held responsible. Stripped of their everyday skills, some people experience generalised anxiety, others specific fears (see chapter 11). Loss of control over one's skills, behaviour and emotions, combined with an inability to progress as expected, may provoke a profound sense of helplessness, particularly in view of the effort usually invested in rehabilitation. This may be compounded by difficulties in evaluating progress owing to lack of insight and/or memory impairment. There may also be enormous frustration with the slow rate and protracted course of recovery. Over time there may be increasing doubt about the extent of recovery and anxieties about the future (e.g. Will I ever walk again? Will I be able to drive? Will I be able to return to work? How will I care for the children?) (Tyerman & King, 2004).

TBI may result in a wide range of psychological disorders. The prevalence of any psychiatric disorder in the first year post-injury is reported to be 49 per cent for moderate to severe TBI and 34 per cent for mild TBI (Fann *et al.*, 2004). In a large community study, 32 per cent of people with a head injury reported at least one psychiatric disorder, with a higher incidence than the general population for alcohol abuse/dependence, phobic disorder, major depression, drug abuse/dependence, dysthymia, obsessive-compulsive disorder and panic disorder (Silver *et al.*, 2001). Reviewing the literature on depression Fleminger *et al.* (2003) estimate a prevalence rate of 20–40 per cent in the first year, with 50 per cent experiencing depression at some time. A three- to fourfold increased risk of suicide was also estimated, with about 1 per cent committing suicide over a 15-year period. Clinically significant levels of hopelessness (35 per cent), suicidal ideation (23 per cent) and suicide attempts (18 per cent) have also been reported (Simpson & Tate, 2002). Anxiety is also common after TBI (Williams *et al.*, 2003). There is often a major impact upon self-concept (Mann *et al.*, 2003), with people with very severe TBI rating their present selves markedly less positively than the past (e.g. more bored, unhappy, helpless, worried, dissatisfied, unattractive, irritable, dependent and inactive) (Tyerman, 1987).

The complex array of disability after TBI often has far-reaching personal, vocational, family and social effects. Many people with TBI lose full capacity for independent living, contribute less to family life (in terms of practical, social, parental and marital roles), experience a limited leisure and social life, have few friends and no boy- or girlfriend (e.g. Brooks *et al.*, 1986; Engberg & Teasdale, 2004; Finset *et al.*, 1995; Hoofien *et al.*, 2001; Klonoff *et al.*, 1986; Morton & Wehman, 1995; Oddy *et al.*, 1985; Ponsford *et al.*, 1995; Tate *et al.*, 1989; Tyerman *et al.*, 1994). Many will be unsuccessful in returning to employment (see chapter 14) and experience difficulties in marital, family and sexual relationships (see chapter 17). Life satisfaction has been found to be low relative to healthy controls, both overall and across all domains except financial (i.e. in activities of daily living, leisure, vocational situation, sexual life, partnership relations, family life and contact with friends) (Johansson & Bernspang, 2003).

The long-term consequences of TBI can be quite devastating and it is no surprise that many struggle to adjust to their new situation. Those no longer able to function independently and those unable to resume their former work, family and social roles face major challenges. Even those with more subtle disability may have to re-evaluate personal aspirations and goals. Others may recognise the need for change but make decisions (e.g. change of job) which do not take full account of their restrictions, leading to repeated failure and loss of confidence/self-belief. The process of adjustment to TBI may be compounded by executive difficulties (especially lack of awareness and reduced capacity for self-appraisal and problem solving), as well as by lack of emotional and behavioural control.

As noted previously (Carpenter & Tyerman, 2006), commonly observed difficulties in long-term adjustment include the following:

- preoccupation with lost skills/roles (with a failure to recognise remaining skills and potential);
- continued striving for an unattainable degree of recovery (thereby delaying or limiting positive adjustments);
- repeated failure and loss of confidence/self-belief (often arising from lack of insight and/or clinging to pre-injury expectations that can no longer be met);
- social withdrawal due to fear of loss of emotional and/or behavioural control;
- strained family relationships and social isolation.

Without specialist help people with TBI may flounder, unable to determine and/or implement positive psychological adjustments. Approaches to facilitate psychological adjustment after TBI will now be considered.

Approaches to Intervention

Interventions to promote psychological adjustment to a neurological condition are sometimes referred to as 'neuropsychotherapy' (i.e. the interface between neurological rehabilitation and psychotherapy). Neuropsychotherapy has been defined as 'the use of neuropsychological knowledge in the psychotherapy of persons with brain disorders' (Judd, 1999) or the use of psychotherapeutic approaches in the process of neurological rehabilitation (Tyerman & King, 2004).

Fundamental elements of neuropsychotherapy after TBI include: a holistic assessment of the effects of TBI; a framework within which the person and therapist can together make sense of the effects of TBI and their personal, family and social consequences; coping strategies to enable the person to participate effectively in the therapeutic process; and an effective therapeutic relationship. An early account of psychotherapy after brain injury was provided by Prigatano (1986), who suggested that psychotherapy should attempt to:

1 provide a model or models that help the patient understand what has happened to him or her;
2 help the patient deal with the meaning of the brain injury in his or her own life;
3 help the patient achieve a sense of self-acceptance and forgiveness for himself or herself and others who have caused the accident;
4 help the patient make realistic commitments to work and interpersonal relations;
5 teach the patient how to behave in different social situations (to improve competence);
6 provide specific behavioural strategies for compensating for neuropsychological deficits; and
7 foster a sense of realistic hope.

Approaches to psychological adjustment to TBI have drawn on various therapeutic perspectives, including cognitive–behavioural, neuropsychological and psycho-dynamic. Cognitive–behavioural therapy (CBT) has been advocated as particularly useful as it is structured, educational, focused and collaborative and involves problem solving, behavioural training/rehearsal, stress awareness/management, concrete goal setting, combating maladaptive thoughts and improving self-awareness (Whitehouse, 1994). CBT has been used for a range of difficulties after TBI, including anxiety, depression, irritability and aggression, pain and substance abuse (see Williams & Evans, 2003). Moore and Stambrook (1995) advocate a combination of cognitive–behavioural interventions with neuropsychologically based cognitive rehabilitation. Kendall and Terry (1996) stress the importance of increasing perceived control over the environment and of addressing inappropriate coping responses and appraisals. However, applying CBT with people with cognitive difficulties poses many challenges. The adaptation of psychological therapies for people with brain injury are discussed by many authors (e.g. Butler & Satz, 1988; Carberry & Burd, 1986; Cicerone, 1989; Judd, 1999; Laatsch, 1999; Miller, 1991; Tyerman & King, 2004; Whitehouse, 1994).

A core need is for education about TBI and its effects. Such provision should be appropriate (i.e. meeting the needs of the recipient), accessible (i.e. in terms of complexity, pace and style) and acceptable (i.e. sensitive to how the information is likely to be received) (Judd, 1999). After TBI, education needs to be delivered in a way that both takes into account cognitive constraints and is sensitive to reduced awareness and psychological denial.

Awareness of the effects of TBI is a major factor in psychological adjustment. Reduced awareness may prevent the person from experiencing their difficulties, from benefiting from educational material and from making positive adjustments (e.g. implementing and evaluating compensatory strategies and informed decision-making). Understanding self-perceptions is considered to be essential to the rehabilitation process and attempts to increase the capacity for self-observation often a specific goal of psychotherapy (Cicerone, 1989). The nature, assessment and management of reduced self-awareness after brain injury are addressed by several authors (e.g. Bach & David, 2006; Fleming & Ownsworth, 2006; Judd, 1999; Langer 1999; Langer and Padrone, 1992; Ownsworth *et al.*, 2000; Prigatano, 2005; Sherer *et al.*, 2005).

Judd (1999) stresses that brain injury is like few other experiences, because people may be fundamentally changed in their personalities, emotions and abilities. As such, there is often a need to reconstruct meaning through interpreting experiences and integrating them into a new self-image. In a model derived from dynamic psychotherapy, as well as TBI and trauma, Ellis (1989) suggests that the inability to observe and monitor behaviour is a prime reason for the disruption of the individual's narrative (i.e. the story one tells oneself and others about one's life and experiences). It is suggested that the high level of abstraction needed to observe oneself is 'shattered' and the person is caught up in the ongoing experience of day-to-day life, losing touch with reality because of an inability to grasp the unique differences between events. An understanding of the difference between what a person feels and what he or she observes is considered to be critical for self-monitoring. A person's observational level of awareness of his or her own narrative reflects the level of functioning; that is, the more aware of 'self' the person is, the better he or she is functioning.

For Ellis (1989) the primary goal of neuropsychotherapy is 'to help the brain-injured person form an integrated sense of identity, based in part on post-trauma elements of personality, as well as the person's personality before the trauma'. His model has three phases: (i) contract setting, building the therapeutic relationship and introducing techniques for communication; (ii) developing and communicating an in-depth understanding of the new identity and self-narrative; and (iii) helping the 'survivor' to use information-processing aids, support personnel, and community services to better enjoy his or her life. Through therapy 'the idealized pretrauma self' of the brain-injured individual has been allowed to 'die' and the 'survivor' has come to accept some, if not most, of the deficits and the many profound changes that have resulted from the trauma. Part of the primary goal of the treatment has been to help the 'survivor' integrate this acceptance of reality into his or her life in a meaningful way.

Group interventions can make a major contribution to facilitating adjustment and are a core element of holistic neuropsychological rehabilitation programmes (see chapter 4). Whilst some groups have an educational, skills or behavioural management focus (e.g. Whitehouse, 1994; Wilson *et al.*, 2000), others serve a broader psychotherapeutic function (e.g. Ben-Yishay & Lakin, 1989; Prigatano, 1986). Alongside their practical value, a major benefit of groups is the realisation for the person that they are not alone in experiencing and striving to manage complex difficulties after TBI. A core purpose of psychotherapeutically oriented groups is to assist the person in understanding and addressing the effects of the TBI on social interaction and relationships. A working example of integrated group programmes, including psychosocial, self-regulation and anger management groups, is described by Langerbahn *et al.* (1999).

Research on the efficacy of psychotherapeutic interventions is extremely limited. In reviewing the cost-effectiveness of psychotherapy, Pepping and Prigatano (2003) conclude that five benefits are frequently seen for people with TBI:

1 the reduction in anxiety and depression in the face of altered abilities;
2 a sense of hope that comes from not feeling 'alone' with their disturbances in higher cerebral functioning;
3 a meaningful reduction of confusion as to what is 'wrong' with their functioning and, therefore, a more reasonable approach to compensating for their disabilities;

4 the appropriate use of guidance regarding issues of productivity and interpersonal relationships; and
5 an experience that is truly 'emotionally corrective' in so far as it helps patients understand the fabric of their lives and thereby, either re-establish (or, for the first time, establish) meaning in the face of frustration and suffering.

A practical approach to facilitating psychological adjustment within a community brain injury service will be outlined.

Facilitating Psychological Adjustment

Within the Community Head Injury Service (CHIS) (described in detail in chapter 4) we have sought to facilitate psychological adjustment through the core assessment and feedback process, followed by group and/or individual interventions.

General management

In parallel with interdisciplinary team assessments to clarify the effects of TBI, it is important to understand the subjective experience of the person and family. This is addressed within a structured interview covering relevant social and clinical history, rehabilitation, current situation and problems, but also changes in self-concept, expectations of recovery and personal priorities and goals. Whilst self-reports/ratings may be affected by lack of awareness and/or denial, an understanding of the subjective experience is fundamental. It allows assessment feedback and rehabilitation goals to take account of self-perceptions, expectations and priorities, as well as cognitive constraints and emotional state. As such, the person is more likely both to feel understood (rather than just evaluated) and to engage positively in rehabilitation. (An example of a person-centred TBI initial assessment process is described in chapter 4.)

A carefully crafted feedback of assessment results not only increases understanding of specific TBI difficulties but establishes a framework which can be of both immediate and ongoing therapeutic benefit. A systematic approach to feedback and goal setting is required. Neurorehabilitation counselling can then assist the person to develop their understanding and enhance their coping, both practically and emotionally. This is likely to include some of the following: general information; detailed explanation about specific impairments; reinforcement of treatment rationale; joint monitoring of treatment goals; reinforcement of coping strategies; joint progress review/resettlement planning; and general advice and support (Tyerman & King, 2004).

Given the cognitive constraints of TBI, it is usually helpful to provide visual illustrations (e.g. charts, videotape recordings, etc.) of difficulties and progress alongside verbal information. It is important to help the person to develop a balanced view of strengths and weaknesses – it is easy for all concerned to become focused on the difficulties and lose sight of the skills and resources that remain. Ongoing monitoring and re-assessments/reviews can help to promote insight, accurate self-appraisal and more realistic expectations of recovery, thereby facilitating resettlement and laying the foundations for long-term adjustment. This role may be undertaken by identified members of the rehabilitation team (e.g. primary nurse or key worker), drawing on psychological expertise as appropriate. However, for those with complex cognitive, behavioural and emotional needs, this will often require the specialist skills of the clinical neuropsychologist.

Within CHIS education about TBI and its effects is provided in part through a Brain Injury Educational Programme (see chapter 4), currently comprising 12 (90-minute) sessions covering the nature and effects of TBI. Within a group setting it is not possible to address in detail individual educational needs and clients are encouraged to raise further questions with their key worker or other relevant staff member. Education and coping strategies are core components in other CHIS groups (cognitive rehabilitation, communication, leisure and lifestyle and personal issues groups – see chapter 4). Whilst most groups are tightly structured, the personal issues group is generally run as a more open group, focusing on emotional and behavioural changes. This allows clients the opportunity to raise any pressing concerns.

Assessment feedback, goal planning and neurorehabilitation counselling, combined with educational and other group programmes and individual psychological therapy for specific difficulties, can help to guide and support many people with TBI through the process of rehabilitation and resettlement, as illustrated in Case 13.1 below. However, some people with TBI require greater assistance in making long-term psychological adjustments to the effects of TBI. How can this be facilitated?

Exploring difficulties in long-term adjustment

In addressing difficulties in adjustment it is vital to anchor interventions in a full understanding of the impact of TBI on the person in their family and social context. A number of assessment techniques have been found helpful:

1 It is often helpful to revisit the personal meaning and impact of TBI through in-depth interviewing of the person (and relatives, as appropriate) about the person's life history, aspirations and plans prior to injury. It is important to understand not just where the person was but where they were headed. Experience suggests that this not only assists understanding of the impact of TBI but increases the client's confidence in that understanding and, as such, facilitates engagement in therapy.
2 It is equally important to track the course of recovery, both as experienced subjectively by the person and as reported by professionals. It is particularly important to reach an informed judgement about whether rehabilitation input was sufficient (taking into account the extent of cognitive difficulties) for the person to understand (as fully as possible) their own difficulties and implement effective coping strategies. If the person and/or family do not consider that appropriate and/or sufficient rehabilitation input has been provided, then hopes of further rehabilitation and recovery may be impeding psychological adjustment.
3 It is essential to establish the full range of long-term term effects of the TBI through a holistic assessment (see, for example, chapter 4). For clients who have

received early TBI assessment and rehabilitation, it may not be necessary to repeat neuropsychological and other assessments to clarify the extent of disability. However, it is important to consider whether such re-assessments may be helpful to the client when feedback of previous assessments may not have been provided in detail or was provided early and not retained over time. When the person is seeking to understand their own difficulties there is often much to be gained by repeating formal assessments, even where change is not expected. This provides an opportunity for shared experience, detailed feedback and the development of a joint in-depth understanding of the effects of the TBI. As noted, it may also be helpful to evaluate systematically self-perceptions and expectations of further recovery.

4 It is often helpful to evaluate in detail changes in life circumstances post-injury through some form of a life review, charting changes in personal and social circumstances from pre- to post-injury. Many people with TBI have difficulty in establishing a balanced view of the impact of their injury – some focusing unduly on what they have lost and losing sight of the skills, positive attributes and roles that remain, others playing down or denying their restrictions and resultant changes. Systematic evaluation, charting and feedback of changes in both skills and life circumstances often help to clarify the position.

5 Changes in self-concept may be evaluated through scales such as the Head Injury Semantic Differential scale (HISD), which is sensitive to change in rehabilitation (Tyerman & Humphrey, 1984; Tyerman, 1987). In its current form the HISD III comprises 18 adjective pairs (see Figure 13.1). (There is a parallel 18-item relatives' version, in which the items 'Attractive–Unattractive' and 'Of Value–Worthless' are replaced by 'Sensitive–Insensitive' and 'Cooperative–Uncooperative'.) The person and relative are asked to rate the 'Past' and 'Present' on initial assessment, with ratings of the 'Present' repeated on review and follow-up, as illustrated in Case 13.1 below. When using the scale in facilitating adjustment it may be helpful to include ratings of 'Future Self', as well as Past and Present.

6 For selected clients who are able to cope with a cognitive approach, it has on occasions been helpful to complete a repertory grid (see Fransella *et al.*, 2003), a technique drawn from personal construct psychotherapy. In essence, this involves eliciting bi-polar constructs and asking the client to rate self and significant others (elements) on these constructs. (This has similarities to the HISD but extracts the person's own constructs and values rather than using pre-determined ones.) The constructs are commonly elicited through the 'triad' method – asking the client a series of questions about how two of the elements differ from a third. The grid elements have typically included past self, current self, future self, ideal self, parents, sibling, partner, old friend (pre-injury), new friend (post-injury), 'typical person' (own sex/age), 'typical head-injured person', plus additional elements (e.g. 'a person you respect'), relevant to the individual. In an example of a repertory grid at three years post-injury the constructs which emerged were clearly influenced by TBI (e.g. 'brain injured'; 'non-driver'; 'non-head-injury expert'). The results of a simple principal components analysis is illustrated in Figure 13.2, with the vertical factor identified as 'head injured – not head injured' and the horizontal factor as 'not special – special'. The person with TBI viewed himself currently as 'head injured' but still 'special', distant

Name:.. **Dob:**.................... **Date:**.............. **Past/Present/Future**

Bored								Interested
Unhappy								Happy
In Control								Helpless
Worried								Relaxed
Satisfied								Dissatisfied
Despondent								Hopeful
Self Confident								Lacks Confidence
Unstable[1]								Stable
Attractive[2]								Unattractive *
Of Value								Worthless *
Aggressive								Unaggressive
Calm								Irritable
Capable								Incapable
Dependent								Independent
Inactive								Active
Withdrawn								Talkative
Friendly								Unfriendly
Patient								Impatient

[1] Emotionally [2] As a Person

(* Items Attractive–Unattractive & Of Value–Worthless are replaced in relatives' version – see text).

(Andy Tyerman, 08/03/02)

Figure 13.1 The Head Injury Semantic Differential

from his family and others. This illustrated well the isolated position he occupied post-injury.

7 For the more cognitively able person with TBI, self-descriptions pre- and post-injury may be informative – it may help to suggest people construct this as if

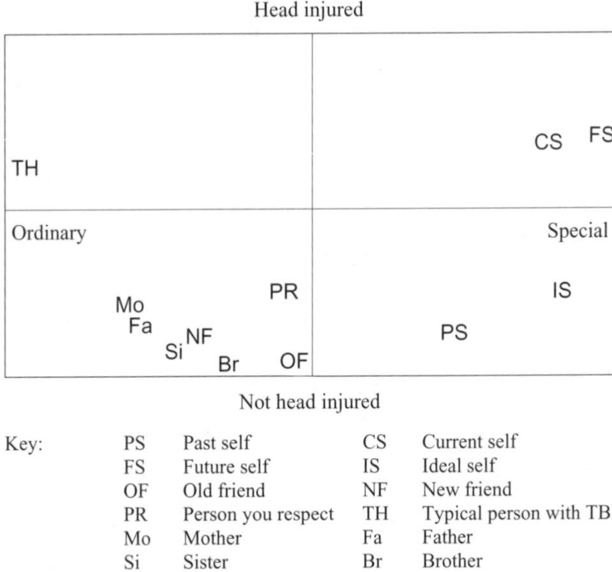

Figure 13.2 Repertory Grid Example: Principal Components Analysis

from the perspective of a close friend. This can also produce helpful insights into key issues in adjustment. An example of such self-descriptions is provided for B at nine years post-injury (see Case 13.2 and Table 13.1). B's description of his current self illustrates well his predominantly negative view of himself.

Facilitating psychological adjustment

Key aims of interventions to assist psychological adjustment include the following:

1 To help people to develop a clear understanding of the effects of TBI and its impact on their personal, family, vocational, leisure and social roles.
2 To identify and address (or refer on to other services) specific TBI difficulties requiring specific further treatment or management advice.
3 To model a positive, neuropsychologically informed, problem-solving approach, both in managing the effects of TBI and in exploring and rebuilding lives.
4 To assist people in adjusting and/or identifying and pursuing alternative personal, family, vocational, leisure and/or social roles.

A core requirement is to assist people with TBI in understanding and compensating for the effects of their cognitive, behavioural and/or emotional difficulties to enable them to function effectively in their daily lives. Whilst some people require assistance in addressing specific problem situations, others have much broader difficulties with adjustment to feeling a 'new' or 'different' person. A number of interventions have been found to be useful in facilitating psychological adjustment:

1 Reviewing the nature of brain injury and its effects to establish (or reinforce) an appropriate framework of understanding, through revisiting medical records, neuropsychological and other assessments and subjective/family accounts. A review of current difficulties and management may identify the need for new or 'refresher' sessions of therapy to address specific issues (e.g. anger management) and often highlights the need for refinement of existing coping strategies and/or the introduction of new strategies to reflect changes in current circumstances.
2 Providing explanations about the course of TBI recovery and adjustment can help to place current difficulties and progress in context. This may be facilitated through charting of progress and recovery curves to illustrate different scenarios (e.g. 'expected', 'high risk', 'optimal', 'managed' recovery). A common scenario is of a person striving unsuccessfully to make further progress late post-injury in order to return to pre-injury responsibilities with which they cannot now cope. It may be tempting here to seek to convince a person that they will not achieve a specific goal, in effect asking them to 'settle' for a life that they may view as unacceptable. If the person is putting themselves or others at risk, explicit advice may be required (e.g. fitness to drive). However, it is often effective to encourage the person to recognise that they are not currently able to cope with greater demands, whilst at the same time modelling how to test out the capacity to take gradual steps forward in the future. This may include setting up time-limited trials to evaluate readiness and to plan how advances might be implemented safely with the minimum of risk.
3 A key issue is to assist the person in reviewing what they can reasonably expect of themselves post-injury, so that they do not continue to judge themselves against pre-injury standards that they can no longer meet. Whilst some people will be reluctant to let go of long-standing expectations/standards, they may be prepared to suspend them and agree a new temporary baseline from which they can hopefully progress and give themselves credit and encouragement. It is important to be alert to outside pressure from family, friends, work colleagues or supervisors to resume former responsibilities, particularly by those with limited understanding of TBI and its effects. It may be necessary to assist the person in explaining their restrictions to others or to intervene directly through direct communication. Sometimes the person may need 'permission' to stop striving to regain their former self and life.
4 Most people with TBI are in unfamiliar territory with few (if any) friends or family with relevant experience to draw on. Aware that they cannot resume life as before, some lose their sense of direction and/or a belief in their capacity to move forward. Use of analogies with meaning for the individual (e.g. a car journey, mountain walk, sailing trip) may assist understanding and provide a positive way of viewing the situation. The analogy may serve to illustrate alternative ways of reaching a chosen goal or destination with reduced risk (e.g. through choice of route, speed, timing, number of stops or other support) which can be likened to the management of TBI restrictions. Understanding the process of adjustment through analogy may also help the person to 'normalise' the experience to some extent.
5 It is usually productive to promote a positive image of an informed person seeking to cope constructively with the effects of their injury and rebuild their

lives. If a person feels controlled by the effects of TBI, it may help to encourage them to see themselves not as 'a head-injured person', but rather as a 'person with specific restrictions after a head injury', who is seeking actively to understand and manage the changes. This may be facilitated by reviewing strengths alongside weaknesses, taking opportunities to emphasise remaining positive characteristics and skills, and identifying/addressing difficulties likely to be responsive to new coping strategies. The latter provides an opportunity to model positive problem solving and restore confidence that at least some difficulties after TBI can be managed.

6 Many people with TBI struggle to cope with the late effects of TBI due to their cognitive constraints. Executive difficulties are likely to impede coping if they are themselves compromised. Others may feel overwhelmed by the effects of TBI and not know how to start to address them. A wide range of situations may require assisted problem solving, including coping with and making decisions about work adjustments, financial management, alternative leisure pursuits, changes in family roles and relationships, sexual relations and performance, establishing new boy- or girlfriends, managing alcohol intolerance, communicating in groups, coping with large family and social gatherings etc. Compensating for cognitive and emotional difficulties and assisting the person in taking stock of their situation, in identifying priorities, and in formulating, appraising and implementing appropriate action plans may release compromised problem-solving skills. However, it is important to recognise that where problem solving and coping skills are affected by executive difficulties, the person is likely to need ongoing access to specialist help in dealing with future difficulties and life changes. Lack of resources to provide ongoing support needs to be considered to reduce the risk of encouraging progress but inadvertently setting someone up to fail. It is also sensible to encourage people to establish their limits at any given time but then to fall back slightly below this level in order to keep some resources in reserve.

7 No longer feeling the same person and unable to fulfil previous roles, people with TBI may need help in identifying, finding and evaluating new experiences in order to explore and redefine themselves and their life goals. Some may require guidance about suitable activities, taking into account the constraints of the TBI. Others may also require highly structured exercises and explicit instructions in order to explore and evaluate new experiences, for example using fixed role therapy from personal construct psychotherapy, as illustrated for Case 13.2 below. People with severe and/or multiple disability are likely to require guidance on potential activities and practical support in implementation. They may also be susceptible to suggestion. As such, great care is required to ensure that, as far as possible, suggestions are anchored by a full understanding of individual needs and preferences and made in close consultation with both relatives and other professionals involved (e.g. occupational therapists, social service care managers, independent case managers).

Drawing upon the above, it has proved possible to facilitate positive adjustments within the constraints imposed by TBI. When the person has received the benefit of specialist rehabilitation early in recovery, this is likely to represent one or more small steps forward rather than a transformation in psychological or social adjustment. However, even a small step forward in one sphere of life will often give a boost to self-confidence and sense of control and restore hope for the future. For those who have not received the benefit of specialist assessment or rehabilitation, transformation in understanding, coping and adjustment can sometimes be facilitated. In providing such interventions it has proved helpful on occasions for core neuropsychological assessment and rehabilitation to be undertaken by another clinical neuropsychologist within the service to avoid any potential confusion for the person with TBI or any disruption to the neuropsychotherapeutic process.

As noted previously (Tyerman & King, 2004), it often proved helpful to liken the process of adjustment to a journey of personal discovery. The aim of this journey is to move from a position of denying, feeling controlled by, or battling with the effects of TBI, to a position of understanding and coping, which enables the person to deal constructively with their altered circumstances and move forward in their lives. In facilitating adjustment it is vital to take into account the individual's capacity to maintain and build on the benefits of therapy. For those with executive difficulties and/or lack of self-belief, it is usually necessary to build in strategies and/or external support to help the person to maintain progress. Therapy will often need to be faded out gradually with provision for follow-up to respond to any emergent difficulties. For some clients ongoing but infrequent therapy will be required to maintain progress, as in Case 13.2 below.

Case 13.1: Example P

P was living with her teenage daughter and son at the time of injury, working as a critic and freelance writer, when she incurred a severe TBI (PTA six days) in a road traffic accident. A CT scan revealed a right occipital skull fracture, fluid in the sphenoid sinus and left frontal contusion. She was in intensive care for eight hours, in and out of consciousness the first day and conscious but confused the next day. She was desperate to return home and was discharged on day 12, still very confused and unwell. 'I just felt that I was on another planet, very weak and very emotionally fragile.' After a brief re-admission to a local hospital she was discharged home and referred to the Community Head Injury Service.

Assessment

P was seen for initial assessment with her boyfriend at one month post-injury. She had been very confused, sleeping a lot, intolerant of noise and experiencing panic attacks. She felt she was making progress but 'still getting into a terrible mess' and 'worried about

Continued

everything'. The major effects of her TBI were reported to be: fatigue, neck pain, headaches, loss of taste/smell, lack of confidence, poor memory, emotional lability and reduced sexual drive. On the Head Injury Semantic Differential (HISD) (see Figure 13.1) she rated herself pre-injury positively overall although not happy, in control, stable or calm and also fairly worried. (The latter ratings were considered to reflect at least in part the emotional consequences of the breakdown in her first marriage and her second husband leaving unexpectedly four years earlier.) Currently she rated herself lower on 15 of 20 dimensions, most notably so in being unhappy, helpless, lacking in confidence, emotionally unstable, aggressive, irritable, dependent, inactive and impatient (see Figure 13.3). On the Hospital Anxiety and Depression Scale (HADS) she reported marked anxiety but no significant depression.

A neuropsychological assessment indicated modest difficulties with speed of information processing, memory and attention, exacerbated by fatigue and anxiety. Occupational therapy assessment identified difficulties in 3-D construction and coordination with slow speed of function and limited problem solving. Speech and language assessment identified mild difficulties with auditory comprehension and associative naming, exacerbated by time pressure and anxiety. On discussing the test results it was agreed to provide psychological therapy to guide and support recovery.

Psychological therapy

P was seen initially on a fortnightly basis. The early focus was on: increasing understanding of the effects of TBI; establishing a sustainable daily routine; containing her anxiety; promoting recovery

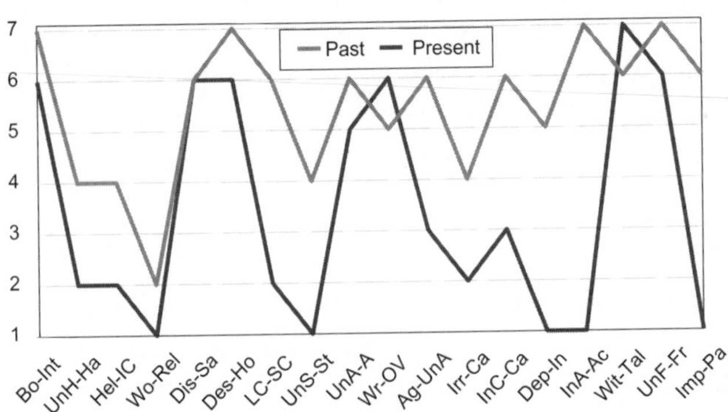

Figure 13.3 Head Injury Semantic Differential – P (at 1 mon.)

of cognitive function; and coping with the stresses of daily life. As P commented, 'My confidence was rock bottom . . . I was extremely needy, needing constant reassurance.' With progress P was encouraged to complete a graded series of exercises to explore her cognitive skills and prepare for a return to work (e.g. reviewing TV programmes, undertaking/writing up interviews, writing articles and attending media events). A central theme was the need to pace herself and plan her week carefully. She started to do some freelance interviewing and writing – whilst coping well technically she was initially very fatigued by any activity requiring sustained concentration and needed to stagger the work. She was also struggling to cope with the demands of her children. She continued to describe marked fluctuations in mood accompanied by emotional lability and volatility.

On review at eight months P reported good progress in stamina, cognitive function and emotional state. She had resumed a limited amount of writing, built up her leisure and social life and also become engaged. She reported a much more positive self-concept, now comparable with retrospective pre-injury ratings except for being more impatient. However, there remained marked anxiety. As such, she required support to prevent her anxiety from spiralling out of control, as well as ongoing help to manage a return to work, mood swings, lack of confidence, emotional vulnerability and impulsivity.

P continued to be seen fortnightly. She became increasingly anxious about her finances and decided to move house but was not coping with this and was advised to delay. Her difficulties were exacerbated by her unsettled relationship with her fiancé, with whom she broke up one year post-injury after two previous break-ups, described as 'an emotional roller-coaster'. After the final break-up she very distressed and required a great deal of support. 'I was just devastated and I thought I couldn't cope, I remember just feeling desperate, suicidal, all sorts of things and it was just like I had no reserve left to cope with. It was the most awful time – if it had not been for the head injury it would not have been like that, it threw it into a different dimension.' At this time P tape-recorded sessions both to help her memory of discussions but also to support her emotionally when feeling particularly low in-between sessions.

By 14 months post-injury P was coping better – she had completed about 20 interviews with several pieces published but struggled to sustain the workload. She had started a new relationship but was uncertain about this and continued to find coping with the children a major strain. She also experienced 'all encompassing' depressions

Continued

every 2–3 weeks lasting 1–2 days, during which everything was too much for her and she felt 'like giving up'. A low self-concept, severe anxiety and moderate depression were thought to reflect the break-up with her fiancé, combined with the strain of coping with work and financial pressures. P continued to be seen monthly to guide and support her adjustment. She was advised against full-time work – whilst stamina, recovery time and confidence had improved, mild difficulties with memory, concentration and word finding continued to slow her down and required additional effort which exacerbated her fatigue. She still needed help in managing fatigue, mood swings and emotional volatility and their impact on close relationships.

On review at two years post-injury her fatigue had improved but she still required regular rests. Her cognitive skills were considered to have reached a plateau. She now had a contract as an interviewer/writer and was using a number of coping strategies in her work: reading cuttings the night before and preparing her questions systematically; writing out her questions in detail rather than relying on a skeleton structure; avoiding driving long distances and using train journeys to refresh her memory of background and questions; creating a 'mind-map' of the interview from the tape-recording to structure and prompt her memory. These strategies were effective but time consuming. Outside work she was pursuing her interest in alternative therapies as well as an active leisure and social life. Her relationship with a new boyfriend helped her to relax but she expressed concern about her inconsistent feelings and emotional engagement, feeling 'drained by intense emotion'. She described herself as being 'quite changeable – very 'up' one minute, 'gloomy' the next, but 'much more optimistic and much happier' in herself. On the HISD she was more positive than when last reviewed after the break-up with her fiancé, close to her pre-injury ratings. The HADS indicated a moderate degree of anxiety but no significant depression, notably improved over her last review, now similar to initial assessment.

Therapy continued bi-monthly for a further 18 months. Sessions focused on managing her mood swings and their impact on close relationships. Her boyfriend reportedly commented that 'it was like living with two different people'. When feeling low in mood she was vulnerable and emotionally dependent and receptive to his wish to get married; when feeling positive she was 'strong independent woman', wanting to develop her own career. Whilst the relationship with her boyfriend was also causing conflict with her daughter, she doubted her ability to cope without the 'security blanket' that this provided – she continued to have bouts of depression with suicidal thoughts. At this stage her 'deep-seated need to be looked after', which she attributed to previous family and relationship experiences, was explored to promote understanding and coping. When the relationship eventually broke down, she required support but coped with this and other life events much more independently.

Follow-up

At follow-up at 44 months post-injury P was continuing to work as a freelance journalist/interviewer for magazines and newspapers. She was very involved in alternative therapies and had an active leisure/social life. She was very positive about life, commenting, 'I feel stronger today than I have been since the accident, maybe even stronger, I don't know, I feel the best now that I have felt for as long as I can remember.' At the time of writing, five years post-injury, P has recently completed an MA in Screenwriting. She is settled in a relationship with a new boyfriend and her children have both moved on positively.

Psychological therapy played a critical role in guiding and supporting P in her early, stormy recovery – in assisting her in understanding, monitoring and managing her fatigue, cognitive difficulties, mood swings, emotional/behavioural volatility, anxiety, depression and lack of confidence. She required ongoing assistance in managing her return to work and her close relationships, particularly following the break-up with her fiancé. Whilst she made encouraging progress in the first year it was critical that therapy continued to safeguard progress and assist her in managing her emotional difficulties and in coping with the pressures of work, home and close relationships.

Whilst P had some emotional vulnerabilities prior to her injury, she was positive and resourceful, drawing on alternative therapies. However, she required specialist help to guide her in recognising, understanding and managing the effects of her TBI and in making the necessary adjustments. As she commented later in a magazine article, 'Unlike external injuries to an arm or a leg, a head injury is different – your brain injury is the very essence of the person you are. And I really didn't know who that was anymore.' Reflecting on psychological therapy P commented, 'I couldn't have done it without it, I really couldn't. To me it feels like it has been the spine that supported me when I was fragile and confused and I needed support. It was always there, that knowledge gave me the confidence to know that I could work through it all . . . it helped me to put my life back together.'

Case 13.2: Example B

B was a highly qualified and experienced teacher in his late forties, living with his wife and teenage daughter. He was employed as a supply teacher when he incurred a severe TBI (PTA two weeks) including basal and occipital skull fractures and frontal lobe contusion/swelling in a road traffic accident. He was in intensive care for five days and in hospital for six weeks before transfer to a rehabilitation unit where he was an in-patient for five weeks and an out-patient for two months. His main complaints related to memory, word finding and feeling 'detached from reality' – he was noted to be 'extremely garrulous', irritable and anxious. As this early stage B expected to make a good recovery: 'I was in cloud-cuckoo land, in that I was under the impression that, like a broken leg it would take a bit of time to get back to normal but eventually my head, my mind, would be almost as before, so I expected to have a few difficulties at first and I would then be OK.'

B returned to work at 6 months but struggled with memory and word finding, returning home exhausted, extremely irritable and increasingly anxious and depressed. He stopped supply teaching and looked for a permanent position. He continued to receive psychological and psychiatric input over the next year. At one year post-injury he accepted a part-time post but did not cope well and was made redundant after six months. He subsequently started a Foundation Course with the Open University but 'could not face' the examinations. He later started to help out twice a week as a volunteer with a hospital library service. At four years a neuropsychiatrist noted difficulties with depression, control of behaviour/mood, paranoia and obsessionality. In-patient assessment in a specialist unit for people with behavioural difficulties after brain injury and case management input was recommended but not implemented. At seven years in-patient assessment was again recommended but not funded. B and his wife were seen by a psychiatrist for a few sessions of psychotherapeutic support and then referred by his GP to the Community Head Injury Service at eight years post-injury.

Assessment

When seen with his wife for initial assessment B reported mild residual physical difficulties (coordination, balance, fatigue), substantial cognitive difficulties (of a generalised nature) and marked behavioural/emotional difficulties (irritability, frustration, aggression, disinhibition, mood swings, lability, depression, anxiety and lack of confidence). The latter difficulties were noted to 'build up to explosion', placing a major strain on the family. (He was taking antidepressant medication and an anti-convulsant, tegratol, to assist behavioural control.) B presented as low in mood with limited insight, understanding and adjustment to the effects of his TBI. On the Head Injury Semantic Differential (HISD) he rated his current self very negatively, most notably in being bored, unhappy, worried, despondent, low in confidence, emotionally unstable, worthless, incapable, dependent, inactive and impatient. His wife rated him positively pre-injury but very negatively currently. On the Hospital Anxiety and Depression Scale (HADS) he reported moderate anxiety and mild depression.

A neuropsychological assessment indicated marked improvement over an assessment at six months post-injury, with a high level of intellectual skills but significant reductions in speed of information processing, memory and learning, psychomotor speed and executive function (e.g. poor self-monitoring) with evidence of impulsivity and disinhibition. The results of the assessments were discussed in detail with B and his wife. Subsequent family assessment confirmed B's reduced contribution to family roles, very low levels of marital intimacy and a very high level of marital discord. B's wife had taken over responsibility for the family since the TBI and provided a great deal of support. She was exhausted by years of coping and clearly could not continue to do so without support. The home situation was at breaking point.

Interventions

B was seen monthly to explore his difficulties in adjusting to the long-term effects of his TBI (his wife was seen in parallel by the family specialist). The following issues were identified: lack of insight/awareness; poor executive skills; preoccupation with himself and his problems; unrealistic expectations/goals; depression; behavioural volatility/aggressive outbursts; being stuck in the past; avoidance of sensitive issues; intolerant/critical of others; social isolation; egocentricity/insensitivity; and marital discord/dependence. B was deeply troubled by the person he had become – the loss of cognitive skills and 'worthlessness' about not teaching. He commented, 'It's very hard to constantly make allowances for what has happened to me, my head injury . . . living from hour to hour, one forgets, one behaves as it used to be before my head injury

Continued

and that causes problems . . . things I do wrong I castigate myself . . . egocentricity, self-vilification, self, around myself, around my ego all the time. I do make efforts, especially when people point it out to me, to try and counteract that, sometimes successfully, but basically that is me, that is how I have become, that is how I am now . . . I was more normal before.'

Early input focused on helping B to develop a framework for understanding his difficulties in the context of his TBI and also on challenging his negative beliefs, particularly self-blame. B found this very helpful, commenting 'You managed to elucidate the effects of my head injury and give me understanding and therefore feel better about it – that was a great relief to me.' On review a year later B rated himself much more positively on the HISD (notably so in being more interested, happy, relaxed, hopeful, confidant, stable, of value, caring, capable, independent and active) and also reported fewer symptoms of anxiety and depression. Intervention then switched to joint sessions with his wife, focusing on the effects of B's difficulties on family relationships. This highlighted his difficulty in coping with daily life without his wife's constant prompting. This appeared to reflect his lack of insight and other executive difficulties (e.g. preoccupation with self, poor self-monitoring, etc.), combined with a tendency to negative interpretation of events, leading to self-blame.

B believed that he could not control his thoughts or behaviour and lacked ideas about how else he might handle situations. As such, B's view of how he had changed as a result of his injury and how he might move forward were explored in depth. His self-descriptions of the past (pre-injury), present (last month) and future (one year ahead) – see Table 13.1 – formed the background to a series of exercises designed to provide B with experiences of behaving more positively. A variation of the 'fixed role profile' from personal construct psychotherapy (Bannister, 1974) was developed as follows:

1. Has some awareness of strengths and weaknesses.
2. Is realistic about what he can achieve.
3. Sustains input to achieve objectives.
4. Seeks a balanced view of events.
5. Shows interest in partner's feelings and needs.
6. Shares feelings with sensitivity.
7. Shares good moods, as well as bad.
8. Is willing to entertain social contact.
9. Makes an effort to understand others' views.
10. Lives for the present and the future.

Table 13.1 Self-descriptions: B at 9 years post-injury

Past self (one year pre-injury)
- Good natured, soft and sensitive
- Keeps self to self
- Never vilifies others
- Tries his best to meet needs of job
- Appreciates interest/sympathy
- Does not mind being told when wrong
- Prejudiced and thin-skinned
- Likes music
- Escapes to own intellectual world
- Not so good with people
- Very conscientious and trustworthy

Current self (9 years post-injury)
- Isolated, introverted and egocentric
- Regressed to childhood
- Forgets his weaknesses
- Self-critical – frustrated/depressed by failings
- Not normal – others find him strange
- Pre-occupied with self/pursues own interests
- Tries to do things well – reliable/conscientious
- Foul tempered and inappropriate in behaviour
- Reacts excessively and causes consternation
- Behaviour painful and tragic in outcome
- Relies on conditioned reflexes from the past

Future self (one year ahead)
- Wishes to:
  - Be less selfish
  - Be clear sighted, balanced and plan ahead
  - Be more systematic
  - Exploit selfish part to achieve results
  - Be more aware of limitations
  - Be more conscientious
  - Grasp things by the nettle, not put them off
  - Write things down and exploit what learnt
  - Learn selflessness
  - Utilise good moods

Over the next 18 months B was guided through a series of exercises to explore the above behaviours. B kept a diary of his attempts to implement the behaviours and their effects. A recurrent theme was the need to build in prompts to increase awareness and consideration of his wife's perspective and needs. These exercises were set and monitored individually as part of joint appointments with his wife and family specialist. The joint sessions were vital both in eliciting his wife's feedback and in responding to other issues (e.g.

Continued

B's relationship with his daughter; unrealistic expectations of voluntary work, etc.). Whilst a challenge the exercises demonstrated that it was possible for B to change his behaviour in spite of the constraints imposed by his TBI. Whilst B struggled to maintain the behaviours, it provided shared experience of positive behavioural change to build on in later sessions.

Joint therapy continued on a monthly basis, dealing with a wide range of issues in B's family, leisure and social life (which he tends to miscontrue and overreact to) and helping to plan for situations likely to cause difficulty (e.g. family events, holidays, etc.). This was supplemented by the brain injury educational programme, personal issues group and cognitive group (described in chapter 4) plus support from the placement consultant about voluntary work options. The cognitive group was followed by individual guidance in managing memory difficulties at home. (His wife attended the relatives' educational programme and continues to attend bi-annual follow-up workshops – see chapter 18.)

A phased withdrawal of support (monthly > two-monthly > quarterly > follow-up) was planned. However, B remained unable to cope with events outside his daily routine or contain his negative reactions to perceived criticism by others. An edited videotape of B being interviewed about issues that arose repeatedly, interspersed with therapist responses, was produced for B to use in between sessions. However, it was not possible to withdraw support completely without a high risk of relapse. If his wife is unable to break the downward spiral when B reacts negatively to events, then professional input is required to help him to put the event into perspective and regain equilibrium. As B commented, 'I find it very difficult. I do find it very helpful for you to put a rational input from outside, because I can see the common sense of what you say but, in myself, I am so worked up emotionally – primitive emotions, they are too strong for me to be intellectual, to be rational and to be detached about . . . I seem unable to control the deep wall of emotion, it overwhelms me . . . that's why I find other people's input very helpful.'

Outcome

B and his wife continue to be seen on average two-monthly for maintenance therapy – 10 years since he was first seen and 18 years post-injury. The progress in personal and family adjustment has been maintained, with routine daily life stable for much of the time. Discussions over recent years have focused on planning for major events (e.g. preparing for his daughter's wedding, including the father-of-the-bride speech), on containing his reaction to unforeseen negative events and on ongoing concern about a decline in his memory function as he has progressed into his sixties.

B is a prime example of the need for ongoing expert assistance to guide and support people in making and maintaining long-term adjustment to marked cognitive, behavioural and emotional difficulties after TBI. Without ongoing specialist input the strain upon his wife had become intolerable and the marital/home situation unsustainable. As B commented, 'You highlight, you explain, you talk about the characteristics of head injury and I see them reflected in my attitude and behaviour – I can then see that it is not just me, it's the head injury – I find that calming and it cheers me up – it's good to talk to someone who understands head injury and recognises the characteristics of head injury as expressed by me, that makes me feel better . . . I can't talk to other people about it, they don't understand.'

Conclusions

In summary, people with TBI have complex adjustment needs. These can be addressed at different stages in rehabilitation and long-term adjustment through a combination of neurorehabilitation counselling, psychological therapy (for specific disorders) and individual/group neuropsychotherapy. Such interventions offer a structure within which to assist people with TBI in moving forward: in making sense of and accommodating changes in themselves and their lives; in identifying, clarifying and prioritising unresolved personal, family and social issues; in supported problem solving about priority issues; and in exploring a new direction through which to rebuild their lives within the constraints of their TBI. One approach to assessment and intervention with a community context has been outlined, developed from the author's clinical training and neuropsychological rehabilitation experience. The reader is encouraged to explore other approaches to neuropsychotherapy, which may be more suited to a particular service context.

Neuropsychotherapy is highly skilled, requiring integration of neuropsychological, neurorehabilitation and psychotherapeutic expertise. Knowledge of the underlying cognitive, behavioural and emotional difficulties (together with any relevant physical and/or sensory difficulties) allows the experienced practitioner to compensate for these in order to release the person's compromised problem-solving capacity and to guide/support them in tackling high-priority unresolved issues. Neuropsychotherapy is essentially highly personal and usually undertaken on a one-to-one basis. However, it is critical that early interventions are integrated with TBI rehabilitation programmes and later interventions with ongoing community support services, in both cases provided in consultation with the family. Close liaison with TBI rehabilitation and community teams is especially important if psychotherapy input is provided by a therapist who is external to the team and/or does not have specialist TBI expertise. In facilitating adjustment a key consideration is the level of ongoing support that may be required for people with TBI to sustain progress and how this could be provided.

At present, clinical neuropsychologists in the UK are involved primarily in assessment and the early stages of rehabilitation, based within acute, in-patient or community teams. The need for interventions to facilitate long-term psychological adjustment to altered personal, family, vocational and social consequences of brain injury has been identified in the National Services Framework for Long-term Conditions (Department of Health, 2005) and in the National Clinical Guidelines for Rehabilitation following Acquired Brain Injury (RCP/BSRM, 2003). Currently there is a very limited research evidence-base to guide such provision. As such, there is a pressing need both for the development of interventions to facilitate psychological adjustment and for both single case and outcome studies to evaluate their clinical and cost effectiveness.

Recommended Reading

Judd, T. (1999). *Neuropsychotherapy and community re-integration. Brain injury emotions and behaviour.* New York: Kluwer Academic/Plenum Publishers.

Introductory chapter on neuropsychotherapy followed by chapters on theory (neurology and neuropsychology; education and psychotherapy; cognitive rehabilitation) and practice (assessment, interventions, specific problems and social context).

Langer, K.G., Laatsch, C. & Lewis, L. (Eds.) (1999). *Psychotherapeutic interventions for adults with brain injury or stroke: A clinician's treatment resource.* Madison, CT: Psychosocial Press.

Edited book (US authors) with chapters on key aspects of psychotherapy: awareness and denial; depression; transference and counter-transference; cognitive rehabilitation; inattention; group psychotherapy; treating families; and substance abuse.

Ponsford, J. (1995). Dealing with the impact of traumatic brain injury on psychological adjustments and relationships. In J. Ponsford, S. Sloan & P. Snow (Eds.) *Traumatic brain injury: Rehabilitation for everyday adaptive living* (pp.231–264). Hove: Lawrence Erlbaum.

Chapter covering: mild TBI; post-traumatic stress disorder; emotional reactions; self-awareness and self-esteem; emotional and interpersonal problems; depression; anxiety; anger; marital and relationship problems; sexuality; plus two case examples.

Williams, W.H. & Evans, J.J. (Eds.) (2003). Biopsychosocial approaches in neurorehabilitation: Assessment and management of neuropsychiatric, mood and behavioural disorders. *Neuropsychological Rehabilitation*, *13*, Special Issue 1–2.

Articles by leading authors on nature/management of neuropsychiatric, emotional and behavioural difficulties (including depression, anxiety, post-traumatic stress disorder, substance abuse, irritability/aggression; mood change and family/sexual changes).

Useful Resources

There are numerous personal accounts and videotapes providing insights into the experiences of individuals with TBI, available from Headway (the brain injury association in the UK), the Brain Injury Association of America and similar sources.

References

Bach, L.J. & David, A.S. (2006). Self-awareness after acquired and traumatic brain injury. *Neuropsychological Rehabilitation*, *16*, 397–414.

Bannister, D. (1974). Personal construct theory and psychotherapy. In D. Bannister (Ed.) *Issues and approaches in psychotherapy* (pp.115–128). New York: Wiley.

Ben-Yishay, Y. & Lakin, P. (1989). Structured group therapy for brain injury survivors. In D.W. Ellis & A-L. Christensen (Eds.) *Neuropsychological treatment after brain injury* (pp.271–295). Boston: Kluwer Academic.

Brooks, N., Campsie, L., Symington, C., Beattie, A. & McKinlay, W. (1986). The five year outcome of severe blunt head injury: A relative's view. *Journal of Neurology, Neurosurgery and Psychiatry*, *49*, 464–470.

Butler, R.W. & Satz, P. (1988). Individual psychotherapy with head-injured adults: Clinical notes for the practitioner. *Professional Psychology: Research and Practice*, *19*(5), 536–541.

Carberry, H. & Burd, B. (1986). Individual psychotherapy with the brain injured adult. *Cognitive Rehabilitation*, July/August, 22–24.

Carpenter, K. & Tyerman, A. (2006). Working in clinical neuropsychology. In J. Hall & S. Llewelyn (Eds.) *What is clinical psychology?* (4th edn, pp.273–295). Oxford: Oxford University Press.

Cicerone, K.D. (1989). Psychotherapeutic interventions with traumatically brain-injured patient. *Rehabilitation Psychology*, *34*(2), 105–114.

Department of Health (2005). *The National Service Framework for Long-term Conditions*. London: Department of Health. www.dh.gov.uk/longtermnsf.

Ellis, D.W. (1989). Neuropsychotherapy. In D.W. Ellis & A-L. Christensen (Eds.) *Neuropsychological treatment after brain injury* (pp.241–269). Boston: Kluwer Academic Publishers.

Engberg, A.W. & Teasdale, T.W. (2004). Psychosocial outcome following traumatic brain injury in adults: A long-term population-based follow-up. *Brain Injury*, *18*, 533–545.

Fann, J.R., Burington, B., Leonetti, A., Jaffe, K., Katon, W.J. & Thompson, R.S. (2004). Psychiatric illness following traumatic brain injury in an adult health maintenance organisation population. *Archives of General Psychiatry*, *61*, 53–61.

Finset, A., Dyrnes, S., Krogstad, J.M. & Berstad, J. (1995). Self-reported social networks and interpersonal support 2 years after severe traumatic brain injury. *Brain Injury*, *9*, 141–150.

Fleming, J.M. & Ownsworth, T. (2006). A review of awareness interventions in brain injury rehabilitation. *Neuropsychological Rehabilitation*, *16*, 474–500.

Fleminger, S., Oliver, D.L., Williams, W.H. & Evans, J. (2003). The neuropsychiatry of depression after brain injury. *Neuropsychological Rehabilitation*, *13*, 65–87.

Fransella, F., Bell, R. & Bannister, D. (2003). *A manual for repertory grid technique* (2nd edn). Hove: Wiley.

Hoofien, D., Gilboa, A., Vakil, E. & Donovick, P.J. (2001). Traumatic brain injury 10–20 years later: A comprehensive outcome study of psychiatric symptomatology, cognitive abilities and psychosocial functioning. *Brain Injury*, *15*, 189–209.

Johansson, U. & Bernspang, B. (2003). Life satisfaction related to work re-entry after brain injury: A longitudinal study. *Brain Injury*, *17*, 991–1002.

Judd, T. (1999). *Neuropsychotherapy and community re-integration. Brain injury emotions and behaviour*. New York: Kluwer Academic/Plenum Publishers.

Kendall, E. & Terry, D.J. (1996). Psychosocial adjustment following closed head injury: A model for understanding individual differences and predicting outcome. *Neuropsychological Rehabilitation*, 6, 101–132.

Kersel, D.A., March, N.V., Havill, J.H. & Sleigh, J.W. (2001). Psychosocial functioning during the year following severe traumatic brain injury. *Brain Injury*, *15*, 683–696.

Klonoff, P.S., Snow, W.G. & Costa, L.D. (1986). Quality of life in patients 2 to 4 years after closed head injury. *Neurosurgery*, *19*, 735–743.

Laatsch, L. (1999). Application of cognitive rehabilitation techniques in psychotherapy. In K.G. Langer, C. Laatsch & L. Lewis (Eds.) *Psychotherapeutic interventions for adults with brain injury or stroke: A clinician's treatment resource* (pp.131–148). Madison, CT: Psychosocial Press.

Langer, K.G. (1999). Awareness and denial in psychotherapy. In K.G. Langer, C. Laatsch & L. Lewis (Eds.) *Psychotherapeutic interventions for adults with brain injury or stroke: A clinician's treatment resource* (pp.75–96). Madison, CT: Psychosocial Press.

Langer, K.G. & Padrone, F.J. (1992). Psychotherapeutic treatment of awareness in acute rehabilitation of traumatic brain injury. *Neuropsychological Rehabilitation*, 2, 59–70.

Langerbahn, D.M., Sherr, R.L., Simon, D. & Hanig, B. (1999). Group psychotherapy. In K.G. Langer, C. Laatsch & L. Lewis (Eds.) *Psychotherapeutic interventions for adults with brain injury or stroke: A clinician's treatment resource* (pp.167–189). Madison, CT: Psychosocial Press.

Linge, F.R. (1990). Faith, hope and love: Nontraditional therapy in recovery from serious head injury, a personal account. *Canadian Journal of Psychology*, *44*, 116–129.

Mann, D.W.K., Tam, A.S.F. & Li, E.P.Y. (2003). Exploring self-concepts of persons with brain injury. *Brain Injury*, *17*, 775–788.

Miller, L. (1991). Psychotherapy of the brain-injured patient: Principles and practices. *Cognitive Rehabilitation*, March/April, 24–29.

Miller, L. (1993). *Psychotherapy of the brain-injured patient. Reclaiming the shattered self.* New York: W.W. Norton & Company.

Moore, A.D. & Stambrook, M. (1995). Cognitive moderators of outcome following traumatic brain injury: A conceptual model and implications for rehabilitation. *Brain Injury*, 9, 109–130.

Morton, M.V. & Wehman, P. (1995). Psychosocial and emotional sequelae of individuals with traumatic brain injury: A literature review and recommendations. *Brain Injury*, 9, 81–92.

Oddy, M., Coughlan, A., Tyerman, A., & Jenkins, D. (1985). Social adjustment after closed head injury: A further follow-up severe years after injury. *Journal of Neurology, Neurosurgery and Psychiatry*, *48*, 564–568.

Ownsworth, T.L., McFarland, K. & Young, R.M. (2000). Self-awareness and psychosocial functioning following acquired brain injury: An evaluation of a group support programme. *Neuropsychological Rehabilitation*, *10*, 465–484.

Pepping, M. & Prigatano, G.P. (2003). Psychotherapy after brain injury: Costs and benefits. In G.P. Prigatano & N.H. Pliskin (Eds.) *Clinical neuropsychology and cost outcome research* (pp.313–328). New York: Psychology Press.

Ponsford, J. (1995). Dealing with the impact of traumatic brain injury on psychological adjustments and relationships. In J. Ponsford, S. Sloan & P. Snow (Eds.) *Traumatic brain injury: Rehabilitation for everyday adaptive living* (pp.231–264). Hove: Lawrence Erlbaum.

Ponsford, J.L., Olver, J.H. & Curran, C. (1995). A profile of outcome: 2 years after traumatic brain injury. *Brain Injury*, 9, 1–10.

Prigatano, G.P. (1986). Psychotherapy after brain injury. In G.P. Prigatano (Ed.) *Neuropsychological rehabilitation after brain injury* (pp.67–95). Baltimore: John Hopkins University Press.

Prigatano, G.P. (1995). 1994 Sheldon Berrol, MD, Senior Lectureship: The problem of lost normality after brain injury. *Journal of Head Trauma Rehabilitation*, *10*, 87–95.

Prigatano, G.P. (2005). Disturbances of self-awareness and rehabilitation of patients with traumatic brain injury: A 20-year perspective. *Journal of Head Trauma Rehabilitation*, *20*, 19–29.

RCP/BSRM (2003). *Rehabilitation following acquired brain injury: National clinical guidelines* (L. Turner-Stokes, Ed.). London: Royal College of Physicians/British Society of Rehabilitation Medicine.

Sherer, M., Hart, T., Whyte, J., Todd, G.N. & Yablon, S.A. (2005). Neuroanatomic basis of impaired self-awareness after traumatic brain injury: Findings from early computed tomography. *Journal of Head Trauma Rehabilitation*, *20*, 287–300.

Silver, J.M., Kramer, R., Greenwald, S. & Weissman, M. (2001). The association between head injuries and psychiatric disorders: Findings from the New Haven NIMH Epidemiologic Catchment Area Study. *Brain Injury*, *15*(11), 935–945.

Simpson, G. & Tate, R. (2002). Suicidality after traumatic brain injury: Demographic, injury and clinical correlates. *Psychological Medicine*, *32*, 687–697.

Tate, R.L. (2003). Impact of pre-injury factors on outcome after severe traumatic brain injury: Does post-traumatic change represent an exacerbation of pre-morbid traits? *Neuropsychological Rehabilitation*, *13*, 43–64.

Tate, R.L., Lulham, J.M., Broe, G.A., Strettles, B. & Pfaff, A. (1989). Psychosocial outcome for the survivors of severe blunt head injury: The results of a consecutive series of 100 patients. *Journal of Neurology, Neurosurgery and Psychiatry*, *52*, 1128–1134.

Tyerman, A. (1987). Self-concept and psychological change in the rehabilitation of the severely head injured person. Doctoral Thesis, University of London, UK.

Tyerman, A. (1991). Counselling in head injury. In H. Davis & L. Fallowfield (Eds.) *Counselling and communication in health care* (pp.115–128). Chichester: Wiley.

Tyerman, A. & Humphrey, M. (1984). Changes in self-concept following severe head injury. *International Journal of Rehabilitation Research*, *7*, 11–23.

Tyerman, A. & Humphrey, M. (1988). Personal and social rehabilitation after severe head injury. In F.N. Watts (Ed.) *New developments in clinical psychology, Vol. II* (pp.189–207). Leicester: British Psychological Society.

Tyerman, A. & King, N.S. (2004). Interventions for psychological problems after brain injury. In L.H. Goldstein & J. McNeil (Eds.) *Clinical neuropsychology: A practical guide to assessment & management for clinicians* (pp.385–404). Chichester: Wiley.

Tyerman, A., Young, K. & Booth, J. (1994). *Change in family roles after severe traumatic brain injury*. Paper presented at The Fourth Conference of the International association for the Study of Traumatic Brain Injury, St. Louis, September.

Whitehouse, A.M. (1994). Applications of cognitive therapy with survivors of head injury. *Journal of Cognitive Psychotherapy: An International Quarterly*, *8*, 141–160.

Williams, W.H. & Evans, J.J. (Eds.) (2003). Biopsychosocial approaches in neurorehabilitation: Assessment and management of neuropsychiatric, mood and behavioural disorders. *Neuropsychological Rehabilitation*, *13*, Special Issue, 1–2.

Williams, W.H., Evans, J.J. & Fleminger, S. (2003). Neurorehabilitation and cognitive-behaviour therapy of anxiety disorders after brain injury: An overview and a case illustration of obsessive-compulsive disorder. *Neuropsychological Rehabilitation*, *13*, 133–148.

Wilson, B.A., Evans, J., Brentnall, S., Bremner, S., Keohane, C. & Williams, H. (2000). The Oliver Zangwill Center for Neuropsychological Rehabilitation. In A-L. Chistensen & B.P. Uzzell (Eds.) *International handbook of neuropsychological rehabilitation* (pp.231–246). New York: Kluwer Academic/Plenum Publishers.

Yates, P.J. (2003). Psychological adjustment, social enablement and community integration following acquired brain injury. *Neuropsychological Rehabilitation*, *13*, 291–306.

Part IV

Vocational Rehabilitation

14

Return to Previous Employment

Roger Johnson and Sue Stoten

Introduction

A return to work is a high priority for most people following traumatic brain injury. It enables independence in other respects and successful employment is associated with good social integration and improved home and leisure activities (O'Neill *et al.*, 1998). It is often difficult for someone who has sustained a severe brain injury to achieve this because of the level of demand that formal work makes on intellectual functions. Nevertheless, many people do manage to return to work despite persistent and sometimes quite severe neuropsychological disability. This chapter is about the particular vocational rehabilitation opportunities that can be exploited when someone returns to their previous employment.

Traditionally, many patients with head injury are followed up in neurosurgical or other medical clinics and advised to return to their work when they appear to be fit to do so. At this point, follow-up is often discontinued and success or failure to cope with work, and the possibility of persisting neuropsychological disabilities, are therefore not investigated. Formal investigation of the vocational rehabilitation needs of those with brain injury has a history of only about twenty years in the UK. One of the first comments on the possibility of using the workplace as a part of the rehabilitation process was by Fernandez (1967). He drew attention to the benefits of liaison between health service and employers, and to the need to identify alternative forms of employment in assisting those with head injury back into work. He suggested that part-time work, as a first stage in returning to employment, should be more easily available. Glanville (1970) described making use of the previous workplace as a stage in rehabilitation for patients who had sustained head injuries. He was perhaps the first to suggest that the employer should be considered as part of the rehabilitation team.

Studies by Oddy *et al.* (1985) and by Brooks *et al.* (1987) identified the difficulties experienced by those with head injury in returning to work and investigated how success or failure might relate to factors such as age, severity of injury and occupational level. Johnson (1987b) provided evidence to suggest that a return to previous employment, and continued rehabilitation in the workplace, might increase the chances of a successful return to work. In the USA research has focused more on the benefits of job coaching and other methods of support within new working environments (Kreutzer *et al.*, 1991; Wehman *et al.*, 1990, 2003).

Outcome Studies

Figures for return to work after head injury vary widely. This is because there is little uniformity in different study samples. There are wide variations between them in terms of severity of injury, previous employment history and so on (Humphrey & Oddy, 1980; Wehman *et al.*, 1995). The criteria for what constitutes a return to work also vary from one study to another – in one instance 'home making' is included as a successful return to work (Sale *et al.*, 1991).

There is uncertainty about the stability of employment after head injury. Many people change to easier levels of work and there is a tendency for people to change their jobs more frequently too (Wehman *et al.*, 1993; Johnson, 1998). Many outcome studies are based on evaluations within one or two years of injury and there are few studies looking at longer-term outcome. Thomsen (1984) followed up a series of people who had sustained very severe head injuries some 10 to 15 years post-injury and found little change in occupational outcome compared to 2 to 3 years post-injury, apart from some small increase in the number who were in sheltered work at late follow-up. Johnson (1998) reported similar evidence of stability in employment status between about 3 years and about 10 years. This study showed three patterns of outcome. Those who settled back into work within two years of injury tended to remain in stable employment. Those who returned to work and failed at their first attempt usually showed an unstable pattern of work subsequently, with short-lived jobs and frequent changes. A third group, who made little or no attempt to work within two years of injury, remained unemployed. The pattern for any individual was established within the first two years following injury, and follow-up 10 years post-injury showed that few people changed their pattern of work later on. Hoofen *et al.* (2001) followed up people 10 to 20 years after brain injury and noted that many had difficulties in maintaining jobs for any length of time and that this prevented successful vocational rehabilitation.

It has been reported that about 50 per cent of those with moderate to severe head injuries return to work (Groswasser *et al.*, 1999), but an overview of the studies on outcome would suggest that only about 30 per cent of those sustaining a severe head injury make a successful return (Greenwood & McMillan, 1993). Probably few people with mild head injury fail to return to work (Fisher & Williams, 1994; Wrightson & Gronwall, 1981), although other studies have suggested that a significant number may have disabilities sufficient to affect employment (Rimmel *et al.*, 1981). However, it might be concluded that such cases are therefore incorrectly classified as mild injuries (Thornhill *et al.*, 2000), or that it is psychological factors rather then neuropsychological ones that are the basis for the problems they have when they return to work (Wright & Telford, 1996).

Johnson's (1987b, 1998) series of patients sustained very severe injuries – all had post-traumatic amnesia of seven days or more and for the majority (69 per cent) the duration of post-traumatic amnesia was three weeks or more. Of those who returned to their previous employment, 73 per cent settled back into work successfully, and overall the return rate to stable employment for all patients in this study was 42 per cent. This therefore suggests that return to previous employment and continuing rehabilitation into the workplace may lead to a better then average rate of return to work – although it is important to note that further research is needed to substantiate this conclusion.

There is a consensus that if employment (or a return to some structured occupation likely to lead to work, such as voluntary work or a training course) has not been achieved within two years of injury then it is unlikely to be achieved at all (Brooks *et al.*, 1987; Johnson, 1998; Oddy *et al.*, 1985). Failure to return to work once two years have elapsed is not simply a function of the severity or nature of disability. Some people who fail in this way clearly have less disability than others who have made successful returns (Johnson, 1987b). The implication is that there are other consequences of a lengthy period of unemployment which reduce the chances of returning. These may be loss of confidence and the development of emotional difficulties, such as depression, but there are no detailed studies about this for those with brain injury. There is evidence for deterioration in mental health amongst the long-term unemployed in the normal population and it may be that those with head injury are particularly vulnerable to such effects. On the other hand, going back too soon, or without adequate support, will also lead to serious difficulties. The experience of failing at work may be as detrimental to future employment prospects as the direct effects of the head injury itself. Initial failure is almost invariably followed by a pattern of unstable employment (Johnson, 1998). In his series of patients, all of whom had sustained severe head injuries, none who eventually returned to work successfully made an initial return before five or six months post-injury. McMillan and Greenwood (1993) have pointed out the risks to self-confidence and the likelihood of anxiety and depression developing if a return is attempted too early.

Predictors of Employment Outcome

A number of studies have attempted to identify the factors which might predict the likelihood of successful re-employment following traumatic brain injury. Crepeau and Sherzer (1993) reviewed a number of these studies and concluded that there were few reliable predictors of return to work after head injury. The most reliable correlations they found were between unemployment and symptoms of executive dysfunction, emotional disturbance, and a lack of vocational rehabilitation resources. Dikmen *et al.* (1994) found that no single factor can be used as a predictor of work outcome but concluded that the most reliable predictors for a good work outcome were less severe injury, younger age, and a history of stable employment previously.

Age and severity of injury

Both age and severity of injury (as measured by post-traumatic amnesia) are frequently proposed as the best predictors of return to work (Brooks *et al.*, 1987; Oddy, 1984; Ponsford *et al.*, 1995; Wehman *et al.*, 1993, 1995). However, this is not always reliable. There is some consensus that older people may be less likely to work again after severe head injury. For example, Crepeau and Sherzer (1993) said that this applied for those near to retirement and aged over 60 years at the time of injury, while Brooks *et al.* (1987) concluded that once over the age of 45 years a successful return to work became less likely.

Severity of injury may predict outcome at the extremes. Probably few people with an uncomplicated, mild head injury fail to return to work (Fisher & Williams, 1994). However, some mild injuries, and perhaps particularly where there are predisposing factors, may show more significant disabilities (Thornhill *et al.*, 2000). Those with very severe injuries and multiple handicaps are unlikely to attempt to get back to work (Johnson, 1987b).

It is nevertheless evident that where other factors are favourable, including the opportunity for return to the previous workplace, a successful return can be achieved despite severe injury (Johnson, 1987b, 1998). These, and other studies (e.g. Newcombe, 1982; Oddy *et al.*, 1978), show that it is quite possible for those with persistent neuropsychological disabilities to return to formal work. It is therefore very important that factors such as advanced years or a lengthy period of post-traumatic amnesia should not be used to exclude some individuals from support in their attempts to return. Rather, where these factors suggest that the difficulties may be relatively great, they should be seen to indicate the importance of endeavouring to return the person to their previous place of work and their particular need for support and workplace rehabilitation.

Occupational status

The previous level of employment may have some bearing on employment outcome after injury – but this too is controversial. Oddy (1984) suggested that there was no link and those with manual and semi-skilled jobs were as likely to make a successful return as skilled and professional workers were. On the other hand Brooks *et al.* (1987) found more than twice as many people (50 per cent) in managerial and similar-level jobs returned to work after head injury compared to unskilled workers (21 per cent). It may be that those with more years of education and better premorbid ability have better resources to adapt and cope with their disabilities, but it is also likely that there will be more flexibility within the workplace, and support from work colleagues, in skilled and professional jobs. An important conclusion from the study by Johnson (1987b) was that it was equally possible to set up support plans for disabled patients in manual and unskilled jobs as it was in other kinds of workplace. The difference may be that this is less likely to happen spontaneously in the former setting and there is therefore a particular need to approach these employers and give good advice and support about how the person with brain injury might be accommodated when they return to their work. The Disability Discrimination Act 1995 & 2004 (see Thurgood, 1999) now places some onus on all employers to accommodate someone who is returning to work with a disability.

Disabilities

It is the intellectual and behavioural changes that follow head injury, rather than physical disabilities, which are most likely to lead to difficulties with employment (Bond, 1975; Roberts, 1976). There is some evidence that the number and severity of symptoms after brain injury may be a predictor of work outcome (Godfrey *et al.*, 1993; Wehman *et al.*, 1995). Nevertheless, many people with persistent disabilities can make a successful return to work. The relationship between severity of symptoms and vocational outcome appears to be a weak one (Possl *et al.*, 2001). Assisting someone to return to their employment must include providing education to employers and colleagues about the nature of the difficulties the person may have. The poor level of understanding about brain injury in the general population, and guidelines for providing information, have been described by Swift and Wilson (2001). A return to previous work, where the client and the nature of his or her injury are known, may make it relatively easy for a specialist therapist to help them to develop compensatory strategies further by continued '*in vivo*' work with the client.

Some disabilities will inevitably be more easily accommodated in the workplace than others. Physical or sensory handicaps may require practical adaptations but these may be relatively easy to identify and implement. Moreover, the employer's options here under the Disability Discrimination Act are more easily recognised. Intellectual problems are harder to deal with in the workplace because of (a) their 'hidden' nature, (b) the greater difficulties in understanding the nature of these problems, and (c) the more abstract nature of adaptations that might be needed. Probably the commonest cognitive problems at work are poor memory and attention, vulnerability to errors, slow speed and the adverse effects of fatigue. The Disability Discrimination Act does specify that adaptations should be made, where appropriate, in the workload or in the number of hours worked. Provisions of this kind can assist those with neuropsychological impairments. Moreover, the Act proposes that absence from work by those with disability should be allowed where this is for the purposes of receiving therapy.

Groswasser *et al.* (1999) found that overt behaviour disturbance was associated with poor return to work but there was no relationship between cognitive difficulties and work outcome, whereas Brooks *et al.* (1987) reported that cognitive deficits, changes in behaviour and changes in personality were all associated with failure to return to work. Psychiatric symptoms post-head-injury are also associated with poor employment outcome (Hoofen *et al.*, 2001). There is no doubt that behavioural problems are the most difficult symptoms to accommodate at work (Sale *et al.*, 1991; Wehman *et al.*, 1993). Usually, all but the mildest changes in irritability, impulsiveness or motivation will mean that the person is too erratic or unreliable to remain in work for long. Nevertheless, return to previous work, where the person is well known and there is a high level of motivation to help, can mean that there are surprisingly high levels of tolerance. The realities of the work environment may mean that the client becomes better able to accept feedback about behaviour and becomes more motivated to respond to training in self-control strategies (Johnson, 1987a).

Support at Work

The work environment which the brain-injured person encounters may be at least as important to outcome as the impact of neuropsychological or neurophysical impairments. Many of those who fail at work following severe head injury appear to do so because of a lack of appropriate help rather than because they lack the potential to work again.

Interagency working can increase the chances of return to previous work being successful (McLeod *et al.*, 2002). Jobcentre Plus (formerly called The Employment Services) is an executive agency of the Department of Work and Pensions and was launched in April, 2002. It provides help and advice on jobs and training to people with disability. Recently published interagency guidelines on assessment and rehabilitation after brain injury (Tyerman & Meehan, 2004) set out clearly how this can be advantageous. There are a number of government-funded programmes, including 'Access to Work', which is particularly relevant in terms of support in the workplace. This scheme aims to support the disabled person and their employer in order to overcome obstacles that might be preventing return to work. For example, a support worker might be provided to assist with communication or self-care; specialist aids and equipment can be funded to enable the person to function at work, or the scheme can pay for adaptations to the premises. Assistance with the cost of transport to work may also be available.

Return to previous employment may be more successful because help is more likely and more easily set up. Return to a familiar workplace has a number of important advantages:

1 *Support in the workplace*. Jobs can be made easier in a number of ways and while in principle this might be arranged in any work setting, in practice it is much more easily achieved where someone is returning to their old job. In this setting a flexible approach can be adopted whereby skills are tested out and job demands adapted according to change in abilities. Hours can be shortened and only the easier aspects of the job taken on initially. Work demands can be gradually increased as recovery and skills progress. Sometimes, different work within the same company can be identified which is better suited to the person's current abilities. Moreover, support is often available from a previous employer in terms of tolerance over matters such as being late for work, the need for rest periods, or in recognising that work will need to be checked by somebody else for an initial period.
2 *In-vivo training*. Training in compensatory strategies within the context of work is generally much more effective than endeavouring to teach the same techniques on home-based tasks or within therapy sessions. This is because the client is likely to be more motivated, as well as being better able to judge their own performance relative to previous standards. Moreover, they are more likely to accept the judgement and feedback of a manager about shortcomings

than the same information from family or therapist. Training someone to use strategies in the context in which they need to use them is more effective than procedures which depend on transfer of skills from practice tasks to real life situations.

In-vivo strategies may be particularly effective where it is possible to enlist the help of a work colleague. This strategy is illustrated by a client whose work was described as slapdash and inaccurate following a severe injury. Her job involved property valuations for building societies and preparation of reports. Analysis suggested that her ability to monitor her performance and recognise errors was a principal problem. A training plan was devised with her employers whereby a colleague, with whom she had a good relationship, worked alongside her and provided feedback on performance. A fading strategy was used so that initially errors in reports, or the lines where an error occurred, were pointed out and the client endeavoured to make her own corrections. Later, the number of errors in a paragraph, or per page, was given and she had to identify and correct them. Unfortunately, this client eventually lost her job because, despite dramatic improvement in the accuracy of her work, occasional errors persisted in her reports. The potentially serious consequences of these, however infrequent, meant that she could not continue in the job.

3 *Duration of support.* There is evidence that support and training within the workplace needs to continue for a lengthy period of time to be effective. In the study by Johnson (1987b) the average period of support was about 8 months and this is similar to the average duration of support reported by Wehman *et al.* (1990) in their vocational rehabilitation programmes designed to support head-injured patients entering new employment. There is some evidence to suggest that formal schemes through the government Job Centre Plus for return to work after head injury are more likely to help those with head injury if they are of long duration (up to a year) than if they last only a few weeks (Johnson, 1989). Unfortunately, most current schemes to support disabled people in work, such as the Job Introduction Scheme, are of a short duration and aimed at testing out the suitability of a job rather than '*in vivo*' retraining. The supported Placement Scheme is also principally about supporting someone with a disability rather than training, but it can continue indefinitely and may therefore prove useful in circumventing disabilities following head injury that might otherwise prevent a return to previous employment. The need for a lengthy period of training at work after head injury probably reflects the fact that developing the adaptations required to compensate for neuropsychological disability is a slow process, sometimes requiring changes to the habits established over a lengthy working life.

4 *Change in level of work.* Frequently, the outcome of a trial at work is to recognise that some aspects of a job remain possible while others are difficult because of persistent disability. For example, a man who worked for an insurance company was reliable, although slow, at office-based work which depended on his previous knowledge and ability to assess information about claims. On the other hand, he did not do so well in direct work with customers where he had to assimilate information and make judgements more quickly and he could not continue with this part of his job.

> It is common for the level of work to decline following head injury. Many studies have reported this to be the case. This probability may therefore need to be anticipated in advising the client and the employer. It may also highlight a further reason why return to work is more likely to be successful if it involves the previous employer compared to a new job. Clearly in the latter case the opportunity to test out abilities in a way that establishes the level of work which the individual can now manage is unlikely. Usually those applying for new jobs after head injury are too ambitious about achieving their previous level of work and mistakes or other failures are likely to lead to dismissal or a decision to leave. Where a return can be made to the previous place of work there is more scope to gradually work out a level of employment that matches the employee's abilities.

Employment rehabilitation which makes use of the previous workplace may therefore be successful because it accommodates the particular vulnerabilities of people who have sustained a brain injury. It minimises the amount of new learning needed and it can allow the best possible level of support from employer and colleagues. This can continue for the lengthy period of time which appears to be essential to the gradual process of adaptation to neuropsychological disability. Moreover, the client's level of motivation is better in the context of real work and the difficulties which many head-injured people have with insight may also be more effectively circumvented in a real work setting. Old routines, particularly for someone who has worked in the same way for some years, may be quickly re-established even where there is significant brain injury. When return to previous employment is not possible then it is important to try to establish similar conditions in other ways. This might be via the Jobcentre Plus 'Work Preparation' scheme, or by arranging for voluntary work, informal work with a friend or family member, or possibly a period of study at an easy level.

Planning a Return to Previous Employment

This section draws on clinical experience gained by the authors while working as part of a brain injury outreach team which specialised in vocational rehabilitation, although based in an acute NHS Trust. The team comprised a clinical neuropsychologist, occupational therapist, speech and language therapist and physiotherapist. Patients were referred to the team from the in-patient rehabilitation unit, from the neurosurgical outpatient clinics and sometimes directly by general practitioners or other agencies. Patients were seen at home, in their local communities and as out-patients in the hospital setting.

Timescale

Most people who have sustained a brain injury are desperate to return to their previous employment – they feel it is a benchmark for themselves and others that they have made a full recovery. If left to their own devices, many people with brain injury attempt to go back too soon and the chances are that they will fail in their attempt. Returning too soon is fraught with problems:

- Employer or colleagues may recognise continuing brain injury problems and try to accommodate them at the start, but they soon lose confidence if they do not understand the problems well and if they feel unsupported.
- Many of the consequences of head injury which are likely to disrupt work are difficult to detect. For example, the inability to sustain concentration, mild changes in speed or an increased vulnerability to fatigue may only become apparent once the individual is placed under work-like pressures and time constraints. Occasional errors due to poor memory or other mild deficits may seem of little significance in domestic and leisure activities but mistakes of this kind may be costly in a work environment.
- If behavioural changes are present, these may only gradually become apparent in the workplace but will prove difficult for employers and colleagues to tolerate.

Too long a delay before returning to work will also create problems and have an adverse effect on recovery:

- It may be difficult for the client to keep adequately occupied and stimulated.
- They may lose self-confidence and become depressed.
- There may be financial pressures to return after six months when statutory sick pay ends.

Timing of return to work is therefore crucial. On the one hand allowance should be made for a full period of rehabilitation to achieve a good level of recovery first – the majority of the recovery from the brain injury is likely to take place within the first 6 to 12 months. If a return to the previous workplace is possible, and the employer appears tolerant and flexible in his or her approach, then some form of return to work may be beneficial at a fairly early stage as part of the client's rehabilitation programme and to facilitate further recovery and adaptation. On the other hand, for those with severe injuries, or less accommodating employers, then a longer period may be needed to allow time for as full a recovery as possible before formal work is attempted. However, once two years have elapsed since the injury, further significant recovery becomes very unlikely. As a rough guide, following a severe head injury, a return to work should not be attempted earlier than about six months, and not later than 18 months after the injury.

Alternatives to work as stepping-stones

Rehabilitation after brain injury is about a gradual return to home life, to leisure activities and to work. But convincing those who have sustained a brain injury of the importance of this progression can be difficult. Their expectation is often of returning to work shortly after getting home from hospital. Successful community reintegration needs carefully planned goals, finding suitable things to do at each stage, and using these as stepping-stones towards returning to work. Structured leisure and occupational activities play an important part in rehabilitation after head injury and act as excellent training before a return to work is attempted.

Strategies of this sort improve an individual's quality of life. They reduce social isolation and dependency, help to increase confidence and self-esteem, and they motivate the individual. Their value is that they provide the opportunity for assessment in a more normal environment than hospital or rehabilitation settings. They also provide the opportunity to re-establish and learn skills that may have been lost or to develop strategies to compensate for deficits acquired through the brain injury.

The principal occupations that may be used towards the end of a rehabilitation programme and before a return to previous work is attempted are the following.

Voluntary work

Voluntary work is a step forward in a graded rehabilitation programme from structured activity at home. The latter is dependent on internal frameworks, or on carers, to maintain or increase a level of productivity. Voluntary work placements give the opportunity to observe the client's ability to function in the real world. They provide the increased pressure of working in accordance with external demands while at the same time being more flexible than formal employment.

Prior to a voluntary work placement being set up the individual must be thoroughly assessed and their strengths and weaknesses identified. Care should be taken to match the area of work to the individual's interests as it increases their motivation and therefore the chances of success. An interest checklist is a useful tool for this. Sometimes it is possible to make use of work skills the person has within a voluntary setting. To ensure that it is an integral part of rehabilitation, goals should be identified. These can relate to cognitive, behavioural or physical issues that are relevant to the individual's rehabilitation needs. They may be goals relating to work behaviour such as turning up on time, maintaining concentration, being respectful to the supervisor or simply getting along smoothly with fellow volunteers or work colleagues. Once the goals have been identified a meeting can be set up with the manager or supervisor of the voluntary work placement to plan hours of work, the specific tasks to be undertaken and the level of support the client may need.

Informal work within the family

Informal work within the family provides an alternative to a more formal work trial or a voluntary work placement, yet still provides an increase in structure, purpose and satisfaction for the individual. It is particularly useful if it is within a family-owned business so that a meaningful role for the person with a brain injury can be created whilst the family's awareness of the individual's strengths and weaknesses should increase the chances of success. It is important not to assume that the family has a good knowledge of the individual's impairments following the brain injury. Family members can be prone to collusion with the client's view that there is nothing wrong. Despite the work placement being within the family it should none the less be set up carefully so that the expectations of all concerned are fully considered. Just as with other parts of the rehabilitative process, goals must be identified, timescales should be set and evaluation of progress should be made at regular intervals, changing goals where necessary.

Education and training courses

Education courses provide an opportunity to test out many work behaviours and skills such as punctuality, learning new rules, remembering information, and managing time. Finding the right level of course at the right stage in the rehabilitative process is crucial if this strategy is to be a successful stage in returning someone to his or her previous employment. At this early stage, when not yet considered fit to return to work, an easy level of study is needed. Often courses of a more practical nature are the most suitable. Many further education colleges have daytime and evening courses that may be appropriate, and very often they have a special needs coordinator who will help to choose the most suitable course. An interest in the subject will increase a person's motivation to succeed at it and it may be possible to identify a course that is relevant to the skills the person needs to use once they return to their work.

Assessment of work skills

Most clients are concerned to get back to their work as soon as possible and their own insight into the possible difficulties is often impaired. These factors mean that their own account or their strengths and weaknesses may be unreliable. For example, a 52-year-old woman was only referred to the rehabilitation service after she had been suspended from work because she had run into difficulties. She was certain she had recovered well from a severe head injury some months earlier. She had made a full physical recovery and her presentation at interview appeared entirely normal. Her neurosurgical consultant and general practitioner had therefore felt confident in advising her to go back to work. In fact, evidence from her husband indicated she had become more careless and impulsive since her injury and formal assessment of intellectual function revealed signs of poor processing and poor attention. This illustrates the need for a careful evaluation of recovery after head injury rather than deciding on a return to work simply on the basis of the impression a client may make in a clinical interview. Formal assessment is essential. Persistent disabilities need to be recognised and strategies planned to overcome them within the workplace before a return is initiated.

Even so, the ability to apply certain skills competently in a standardised assessment does not mean the individual will be successful in his or her previous work environment. Many deficits which follow severe head injury are difficult to measure outside the work environment. For example, stamina, the ability to sustain concentration, or mild changes in speed are not easily detected by formal tests. The work setting very often needs other skills and behaviours such as working with colleagues, time management and being self-motivated. A combination of neuropsychological assessment and practical assessment is therefore essential to provide a full evaluation of the brain injured person's ability to return to his or her previous employment.

The findings from a thorough assessment can be used to plan retraining directed towards specific areas of deficit. In the rehabilitation programme, tasks and activities can be designed around the impaired skills and behaviours which have been identified. Therapists must take care to grade tasks according to the current level of difficulty, and to make them achievable. Examples include arranging small projects for the client that relate to the previous employment. The client might prepare an account about what his or her job involves and present it to others attending the rehabilitation programme, for example. Graded rehabilitation can help clients to learn and incorporate compensatory strategies into their work performance and to use their strengths to overcome their difficulties. Work psychologists, part of Jobcentre Plus, can provide specific employment assessments which enable clients to identify appropriate and realistic job goals. Their assessment forms the basis for liaison with the disability employment advisor (DEA) and the employer to assist them in retaining their member of staff.

Physical impairments after head injury are relatively unlikely to prevent people returning to their previous employment. They can be more easily assessed using standardised assessments and can usually be overcome by use of adaptations. Cognitive impairments, such as poor memory, slowness and changes in behaviour or attitude are more likely to be the crucial factors that will affect return to work.

It is necessary to investigate the person's previous job demands systematically and to analyse the task requirements in terms of the skills and behaviours that are needed. The expectations of the employer and employee need to be explored in order to understand the demands of a job. It is also important to assess through discussion the willingness of the individual to cooperate with a graded return to their work and how prepared they are to work at a different level or for fewer hours to begin with.

Negotiating with the client

With any rehabilitation goal it is important to involve the client in the negotiation of that goal and work is no exception. It is vitally important that timescales and goals are agreed with the client to maintain his or her cooperation and compliance. The attitude and views of the client will often determine how a return can be managed. This is not simply because they will have their own agenda and views about their return but more particularly because these views are very frequently affected by the brain injury itself. The person is likely to show difficulties in weighing up alternatives and making judgements. Many people lack insight and cannot perceive the nature or implications of the symptoms that they have. This means that a good deal of negotiation is needed and sometimes compromises have to be identified. Thus, for example, an individual may be adamant that he or she is fit to work at a stage when the likelihood is that this will prove premature.

For example, a 28-year-old man was confident that he was fit to return to his work for an insurance company two months after a severe head injury, despite significant cognitive problems, including poor memory. He denied these problems were significant but the rehabilitation team's view was that further recovery was essential before going back to work. The client did recognise that he had problems with fatigue and this was used to persuade him to consider some voluntary clerical tasks for the Citizens Advice Bureau to build up his stamina before approaching his employer. The outcome was that he discovered his memory was unreliable and the work harder than he expected. He therefore postponed his plans to get back to his work. After a further three months a gradual return to his work, supported by his employer, was possible and proved successful.

It may be evident that advice not to return will simply be ignored but a compromise of returning for just a few hours a week may be agreed. This might be arranged as an informal work trial, perhaps without pay, and accompanied by appropriate advice to the employer. An opportunity is thus provided for the client to test out his judgement about his abilities. Strategies of this sort necessarily depend on the employer being amenable to a flexible approach and supportive.

Most clients are highly motivated to return to work. This can be used advantageously in the rehabilitation process to negotiate a plan for a gradual return with them. Dealing with a client who is reluctant or unable to accept advice about return to their work is difficult but seeking the support of a partner or family member can be advantageous. It may also be possible to enlist the help of the employer to delay return to a more appropriate time or to reduce the work responsibilities to suit the current level of impairment. Compromises can nearly always be reached and this is a better solution than risking the breakdown of trust between the client and the rehabilitation team through being too directive.

Negotiating with the employer

Communication with a previous employer must only be with the consent of the client. It is important that the client is fully aware of what is to be said to their employer and anything which is put in writing should be agreed with the client first.

It is difficult for employers to understand the brain-injured person's problems sufficiently well to make adaptations to the job of their own accord. It is therefore crucial to have input from a member of the rehabilitation team to advise and educate them. Establishing a good relationship with the employer will help both with education about the person's difficulties and with determining how they can best be supported in the workplace. It is essential for employers to realise that job reintegration is a lengthy process and is best accomplished by on-the-job training. Special work conditions will need to be maintained over a protracted period and adjusted as progress in the workplace is made. It is important for the brain-injured person to experience success during the return to work process and a graded approach is therefore crucial. The full support of the employer is essential to achieve this.

Identifying an appropriate level of work is a difficult judgement. If work is made too easy, the client may feel discouraged or be reluctant to comply, but it is also very important to avoid failure because things are too difficult. For example, an apprentice electrician returned to work seven months after a severe head injury. Previously he had been experienced enough to work independently but on his return his employers felt it was essential that he started with supervision and only worked on easy tasks where there was no danger to himself or others. This caused him some frustration but the employers' confidence in his ability was quite quickly re-established. He was therfore able to progress to doing easier jobs independently and then more demanding work under supervison. At this level, problems with memory and speed of work became more evident and strategies were needed to accommodate them.

Adjustments in the work conditions or environment will need to be negotiated with the employer. A trial period, perhaps without pay and as a means of assessment, or similar strategies, may help to persuade an employer to allow a brain-injured person's return to the workplace. Other strategies might include extra supervision, more frequent rest periods, working half-days initially or only working daytime shifts. The thorough assessment of the requirements of the job and the client's impairments will enable the rehabilitation team, together with the client and the employer, to decide how best to structure the work environment in each case. The principle strategies are summarised in Table 14.1.

Self-employment

Particular problems arise for people who are self-employed and working on their own. In these cases, an early return to previous work may be of great importance to the client, not least for financial reasons, but the absence of support from others in the workplace means things are particularly likely to break down. Devising a plan for a supported return may nevertheless be possible. For example, a 25-year-old self-employed mechanic was under pressure to get back to his business because he had no income other than benefits and he feared that in his absence his customers would go elsewhere. His head injury resulted in language impairment, poor memory and some sensory loss in his dominant hand. It was uncertain how these symptoms would affect his work performance. He needed to return for a reasonable number of hours or he risked being worse off than if he remained in receipt of benefit.

In lieu of a trial at work a project to restore an old vehicle for a friend was planned. This identified a number of practical problems, including fatigue and difficulties in using his right hand, and he was unsafe with heavy lifting. On this basis a formal contract could be drawn up of those repair tasks he was fit to do but others for which he would need to seek help or to sub-contract, together with a timetable of suitable hours and breaks. In this way a return to his business, working on his own, was possible, together with continued support from the rehabilitation team.

Financial issues

Caution must be exercised to ensure that an informal return to the workplace does not affect company sick pay schemes. This is particularly likely once the six-month period of statutory sick pay has ended and this issue may need to be negotiated through the company personnel officer. Benefits may also be affected but these problems can be circumvented either if work is started on an unpaid basis or if it is defined as part of the client's rehabilitation programme. Under these circumstances, benefits may continue and a small amount can be earned under the 'Permitted Work' scheme. This needs to be agreed with the Department for Work and Pensions.

Health and safety and insurance issues must also be considered. Some company schemes can be invalidated if the insurance company is not informed that an employee is returning to work at a stage when they are not fully recovered from an injury. In the example of the self-employed mechanic described above, a further problem for him was that his liability insurance was not valid unless he was fully

Table 14.1 Strategies in the workplace

Informal return to work	For example, going into the workplace on a social basis to start with, and then progressing to take on small tasks or components of the previous job in an unpaid capacity.
Work trial	This can be extremely useful to determine whether an individual is ready and able to return to their previous employment. The individual might attend work formally, but for a few hours a week only and remain on benefit with minimal pay under the 'Permitted Work' rule. The trial might include testing out their abilities in a range of different jobs or aspects of the work.
Part-time work	In this scenario the client may be able to undertake most or all of the tasks required of them in their previous job but lacks the stamina for full-time work. It may be the case that the brain-injured individual can only perform some of the tasks that made up their previous job and these are best carried out on a part-time basis.
Easier or lower level of work	This might be a job of an easier nature or working on just the easier aspects of previous work. It may be necessary to negotiate this with the employer if the client is not able to carry out their previous duties. This may be a temporary arrangement or one that becomes permanent.
Support from colleagues	A colleague can be detailed to give specific help or perhaps to monitor performance and provide feedback. This depends on a good pre-existing relationship and caution is also needed here to ensure the client is happy with such an arrangement and has given consent for information relevant to that situation to be disclosed.
Skills training programme	Training in skills to counter specific problems arising at work can be carried out by therapists from the rehabilitation service, either within the workplace or through separate therapy sessions.
Job Centre Plus schemes	An interview with the local disability employment advisor (DEA) gains access to schemes to assist disabled people return to their previous employment. For example, the Access to Work scheme can give help to overcome practical problems that may be preventing the head-injured person from returning to their previous place of employment. Special equipment or alterations to suit a particular work need can be funded; a support worker might be provided, or help given towards the cost of getting to work.

fit. In the event, the contract drawn up which defined those jobs he was fit to do proved acceptable to the insurance company and his cover was reinstated.

Specific safety issues may restrict certain aspects of work if there is a disability which could represent a hazard. These are usually medical issues, such as the risk of fits, or about physical and sensory handicaps that might, for example, make working at heights or the use of machinery unsafe. Once the support of an employer has been enlisted, ways to circumvent problems of this sort can usually be devised. In one instance a young man returned to work in an iron foundry where poor balance and uncertainties about his behaviour after a head injury placed him at considerable risk. This was resolved by finding him alternative work in a safer part of the works and he understood that if he ventured outside this area he would be immediately sent home. Particular care may be needed about safety issues where the client is self-employed. In this situation, potential risks can be easily overlooked or the client may be reluctant to consider their importance.

Establishing a formal return to work

Once the rehabilitation team and client have decided that some form of return to work is the appropriate next step, an approach to the employer should be made. This may be done, with the client's consent, by the rehabilitation team, but sometimes it is more appropriate for the client to talk with his or her employer in the first instance. Agreement must be established between the rehabilitation team and the client about exactly what information should be given to the employer about the nature and consequences of the injury. Generally, a detailed account is unnecessary and it is sufficient to identify the predictable areas of disability together with the general principal of the value of a practical assessment to identify other difficulties. Problems can arise where a client lacks insight and would therefore dispute information about disability which might be given to an employer. This can usually be circumvented by advising the employer of the need for a trial of work skills without defining suspected areas of difficulty.

A meeting between therapists, employer and client, in the workplace, is usually then the best means of proceeding. The purpose of the meeting is to determine the conditions under which the client might attend the workplace, and to address issues of pay and, if necessary, safety. It is particularly important that those aspects of work performance that need to be monitored are defined, and the methods and persons responsible for monitoring are identified. For example, this might entail completing a brief checklist of specific goals, on a daily basis, to be completed by the client and his or her immediate manager. Arrangements for further therapy from the rehabilitation team, and perhaps medical review, should also be identified. A timetable needs to be drawn up which defines when formal reviews of progress will be made and how long special conditions will apply before needs are reviewed and changes considered. The plan should be drawn up in writing.

These strategies are not only important to ensure that the return to work is well planned but they will also prove useful in ensuring that the employer feels well supported and that they are not entering into an arrangement that they might find difficult to manage or to end if problems should arise.

Monitoring progress

Performance at work needs to be monitored. This must be on a regular basis and forms an essential part of the feedback needed by the client if they are to develop compensatory strategies and learn to monitor performance for themselves. At the same time it ensures that plans continue to move forward according to progress or in response to problems that arise. Measuring goal attainment, attendance rates, time needed to complete tasks, frequency of specific difficulties – such as errors of memory, and colleague's reactions to the individual, are examples of ways in which progress might be monitored.

Monitoring can be carried out in a variety of ways and the best method will need to be negotiated with the employer and the individual according to the circumstances of the workplace and the individual's particular problems. For example, for manual or office workers it may be appropriate to spend time observing them at work as well as having an informal interview with the employee to review his or her performance and discuss any problems. In addition, it may be appropriate to interview the employer or a supervisor, preferably by meeting with them or alternatively by telephone. Sometimes a written record of performance will prove useful – perhaps maintained independently by both employee and supervisor. This can identify discrepancies in their respective perceptions of the disabilities and how they affect work performance. It may also be appropriate to have a joint meeting with the employer and the brain-injured person but this will depend on how comfortable the employer feels about discussing the brain-injured person's behaviour and performance in their presence.

For how long is support needed?

Support will often prove necessary for much longer than might be expected. The need for support will be clear while the client is re-establishing their skills and during a period of informal employment or a trial at work. Perhaps after six months or more, formal employment may have been reinstated, albeit with a lower level of work, and the brain-injured person may show little sign of difficulties and appears to be coping well. Further help seems unnecessary. This may be because initially tasks are made easier for him or her, or colleagues are concerned to be supportive and expectations are relaxed. Moreover, the person may cope well because previous skills are retained and impairments in their ability to learn new ones, or to apply themselves to work as efficiently as before, only become gradually evident to the employer over a lengthy period of time. Some aspects of cognitive impairment, and mild behavioural changes, may only be expressed under certain circumstances and it may take a considerable period of time before these changes are perceived as problems. Reviews should therefore be continued for some time after a successful return to work appears to have been achieved. A good relationship with client and employer should ensure that as the interval between reviews lengthens they are likely to contact the rehabilitation team if any problems do occur and before the set-up breaks down.

What to do if the work plan fails

Sometimes, after a period back in previous work, an employer may decide that he or she cannot continue to employ the individual or the client may become dissatisfied and decide to leave. In this event there is a need for careful evaluation of the reasons for failure. On this basis, a constructive approach may be possible and the sense of failure may be minimised. The following options should be considered:

1. Any option to remain with the employer, but working on a different basis or in a different capacity, should be explored.
2. Evaluation may indicate that the client needs to consider a different line of work or to retrain.
3. A vocational rehabilitation course or work placement scheme may be an option.
4. It is important that the next step is a successful one. It may be best to seek a very much easier level of work or to revert to voluntary work, or a study course, for example.

The possibility that work may be unrealistic needs to be considered and alternative options, such as sheltered work, should be explored.

Case 14.1

Tom was a highly qualified materials scientist who had been working for 10 months before his injury as a project manager for a world-leading company specialising in the research and development of welding. He was knocked off his bicycle on his way to work and was not found for about eight hours. A CT scan showed diffuse axonal injury with multiple contusions. He had a post-traumatic amnesia of four or five weeks. After a period of in-patient rehabilitation he was discharged to his mother's home, which was some distance away. Six months after the injury he moved back to his own accommodation and was referred to the outreach team. Assessments identified deficits in memory, attention and problem solving and he had significant language and communication difficulties. He was not yet fit for work.

His rehabilitation programme comprised a range of activities both within the hospital and in the community. Several organisations were used to build up a comprehensive programme that was tailored to his needs.

Initial rehabilitation focused on improving his level of activity and on helping him to develop effective compensatory strategies. Problem-solving tasks and projects in the *occupational therapy workshop* demonstrated his difficulties with planning and organising a task and in problem solving when things didn't go according to plan. It was noted that he was poor at initiating conversation with the technician and had difficulty in explaining exactly what he meant. He showed fluctuating low mood in the 6–12 months following his injury and at times this affected his motivation and ability to structure his own time. Nine months post-injury he engaged in a 6-week period of *counselling* organised through his GP surgery. It enabled him to talk about the feelings he had in relation to the accident in a safe and confidential environment.

He had *outreach occupational therapy* sessions at home, which were used for review and assistance in planning good use of his time. He also had out-patient sessions which followed a more structured programme of cognitive rehabilitation aiming to improve the skills in which he had deficits, developing strategies to overcome those that required it and practising these in functional tasks. He took part in an educational programme on brain function to develop awareness of what happens after a brain injury.

He had weekly outpatient *speech therapy* sessions to look at the issues of memory, reading and comprehension, summarising of written material and the pragmatics of speech.

Neuropsychology reviews were held approximately every three months and were used for goal setting. Sometimes they involved the use of formal assessments, the results of which were used to inform and educate him as to the nature of his brain injury. The sessions were designed to be a reflective process aimed at increasing his understanding of his brain injury and moving him forward towards the idea of a planned and managed return to work.

He attended the local *Headway day centre* as part of the plan to structure the use of his time productively. He developed new leisure pursuits and socialised with other young people who had sustained a brain injury.

Prior to his injury he had been extremely fit. Therefore as part of the structured use of his time and to improve his general level of fitness post accident, he started to attend a gym twice a week through a *GP referral scheme to the local gym*. He was also encouraged to get back on his bicycle and join a local group that rode long distances each weekend. He had previously done this sort of activity on his own.

About seven months post-injury he started to go into work on an informal basis for one day each week. The aim was to initiate his *social reintegration in the workplace*. His line manager gave him

Continued

very simple tasks that were useful to the department but not time dependent. This gave him the opportunity to practise in a real environment the strategies he had been taught in occupational therapy and in speech therapy sessions, and it enabled him to socialise and feel part of the team.

Formal *liaison with his previous employers* was initiated eight months post-injury and a dialogue with his employers was started, which was to prove useful in the later stages of his rehabilitation when a work trial was set up.

Ten months post-injury he started some *voluntary work*. With encouragement and initial supervision from the occupational therapist he went along to the local volunteers' bureau for an interview. He decided to volunteer to help two small museums which both required skills related to his previous expertise. He was encouraged to organise the placements for himself but his progress was monitored regularly by the occupational therapist. He then organised himself to help a local environmental group by doing some practical work at weekends.

About one year post-injury, he started to attend a *specialist cognitive rehabilitation* facility funded through his compensation claim. During this 10-week programme the outreach team were involved in discussions with the unit and with his employers in order to devise projects that would be of relevance to his return to work and which would assist in the assessment of his capability to achieve this goal. During this period his employers were involved in the rehabilitation plan and indeed specific goals and targets were identified by his manager and included in his rehabilitation activities at work and at the cognitive rehabilitation facility.

His employers expressed concern about the health and safety issue of the likelihood of Tom having a seizure if he returned to work. His job had previously involved using heavy machinery. A referral back to his *consultant neurosurgeon* was made to obtain the necessary advice.

Informal activities, aimed at facilitating his further recovery, continued at his workplace for about one year. Two years post-injury a formal *work trial* was set up and this lasted for three months. During this time there was close liaison between the outreach team and the employer. The occupational therapist visited the workplace initially each week and then each fortnight to monitor the trial and evaluate it in conjunction with the line manger according to specific goal areas that were identified at the start of the trial. At the end of the three-month period a meeting was held with Tom, the line manager, personnel manager, occupational therapist and psychologist to discuss the progress to date and the way forward. The outcome of this meeting was positive and a recommendation was made to the board of directors that Tom be re-employed in his previous position. This was accepted and he started full-time employment three weeks later. It was agreed that the outreach team would continue to monitor his progress and provide support to Tom's manager as necessary.

At this time Tom continues to do well at work but he has yet to resume all his previous responsibilities. An unanswered question remains over his capability to progress within the company as successfully as had been predicted before his injury.

Summary

There are no reliable predictors for return to work after severe head injury. It can be achieved even where there has been a very severe injury and neuropsychological disability is evident. Clearly many variables affect return to work after brain injury and they are likely to interact in a complex way to determine outcome. Many who fail at work appear to do so because of a lack of appropriate support. Important factors for successful re-employment are a return to previous work, rehabilitation within the workplace aimed particularly at compensatory strategies, and a period of support which lasts a minimum of several months. These factors may lead to a better than average rate of return.

A common beginning to employment problems after head injury is that a return is attempted too soon. At the same time, negotiating a return to previous work relatively early on, as part of a rehabilitation programme, can greatly assist the client's recovery and facilitate the development of compensatory strategies. Careful planning according to the needs of the client and the circumstances of their place of work are essential to success. As a general principle when devising plans for return to previous employment, it is better to err on the side of making the initial return too easy. This is because it is important that the exercise starts successfully for both the client and the employer. It is then easy to gradually increase demands providing things go well. However, if the client starts out at too high a level and fails, then confidence is lost and it can be very difficult to reduce the number of hours or the level of work.

Key points in planning a return to previous employment are as follows:

- The use of alternatives to the workplace, such as voluntary work, for initial training in work-related skills.
- The timing of a first return to work. As a rule of thumb this usually should not be sooner than 6 months after severe head injury but is best initiated within the next 6 to 12 months.
- Assessment of disabilities which may interfere with previous job skills. This should be through both formal testing and practical measures.

- Education and the presentation of information to employee and employer.
- The potentially confidential nature of information which might be usefully given to the employer.
- A formal plan negotiated between the rehabilitation team, the employer and the client which defines goals, a timetable, and how work is to be monitored.
- Changes in working conditions to accommodate neuropsychological disability.
- Continued training and advice to aid the development of compensatory strategies.
- Implications of an informal or partial return for sick pay agreements or benefits.
- Disabilities that might have safety implications in the workplace.
- Support may need to continue for some months.
- After a successful return appears to have been established, reviews are advisable for a further period.
- If return to employment proves unsuccessful then careful evaluation of the reasons, and consideration of easier alternatives, is essential in order to avoid further failure.

The different circumstances of each client will determine exactly how a return to previous employment can be best achieved. Rehabilitation strategy must therefore follow a problem-solving model rather than any more prescriptive set of rules. Finally, it is important to recognise that the time spent in enlisting the support of previous employers and work colleagues to help a brain-injured person return to their previous work is highly cost-effective. Not only does the present evidence suggest it is the most effective method of vocational rehabilitation but it is also likely to be very much less costly than special retraining programmes or formal interventions set up in new places of work.

Further Reading

Brooks, N., McKinley, W., Symington, C., Beattie, A. & Campsie, L. (1987). Return to work within the first seven years of severe head injury. *Brain Injury*, *1*, 5–19.

This paper looks at the relationship between work outcome and the nature of employment, age, and disabilities following head injury.

Crepeau, F. & Sherzer, P. (1993). Predictors and indicators of work status after traumatic brain injury: A meta-analysis. *Neuropsychological Rehabilitation*, *3*, 5–35.

A review of studies with the aim of identifying factors that might predict work outcome. A wide variety of factors are considered including pre-injury variables, the nature of disabilities and post-injury rehabilitation.

Johnson, R.P. (1998). How do people get back to work after severe head injury? A 10 year follow-up study. *Neuropsychological Rehabilitation*, *8*, 61–79.

A follow-up study of patients previously seen about three years post-injury with the aim of evaluating the benefits of return to previous work and identifying management strategies that might facilitate re-employment.

Kreutzer, J.S., Wehman, P., Morton, M.V. & Stonnongton, H.H. (1991). Supported employment and compensatory strategies for enhancing vocational outcome following traumatic brain injury. *International Disability Studies*, *13*, 162–171.
This paper gives an account of methods of employment rehabilitation in the United States, focusing on job coaching within the workplace.

Oddy, M., Coughlan, T., Tyerman, A. & Jenkins, D. (1985). Social adjustment after closed head injury: A further follow up 7 years after injury. *Journal of Neurology, Neurosurgery and Psychiatry*, *48*, 564–568.
A follow-up of patients previously seen two years post-injury with the aim of looking at progress in occupational and social resettlement in the longer term. The paper discusses the needs of people some years after brain injury.

Thomsen, I.V. (1984). Late outcome of very severe blunt head trauma: A 10–15 year second follow up. *Journal of Neurology, Neurosurgery and Psychiatry*, *47*, 260–268.
A description of the long-term changes after very severe head injuries and the problems of establishing a good level of occupation.

References

Bond, M.R. (1975). Assessment of psychosocial outcome after severe head injury. In *Outcome of severe damage to the central nervous system* (pp.141–157). CIBA Foundation Symposium 34 (new series). Amsterdam: Elsevier.

Brooks, N., McKinley, W., Symington, C., Beattie, A. & Campsie, L. (1987). Return to work within the first seven years of severe head injury. *Brain Injury*, *1*, 5–19.

Crepeau, F. & Sherzer, P. (1993). Predictors and indicators of work status after traumatic brain injury: A meta-analysis. *Neuropsychological Rehabilitation*, *3*, 5–35.

Dikmen, S.S., Temkin, N.R., Machamer, J.E., Holubkon, A.L., Fraser, R.T. & Win, R.H. (1994). Employment following traumatic head injuries. *Archives of Neurology*, *51*, 177–186.

Fernandez, R.H.P. (1967). Head injury protection and return to work problems. *British Medical Journal*, *2*, 830–831.

Fisher, J.M. & Williams, A.D. (1994). Neuropsychological investigation of mild head injury: Ensuring diagnostic accuracy in the assessment process. *Seminars in Neurology*, *14*, 53–59.

Glanville, H.J. (1970). Return to work. *Rehabilitation*, *72*, 59–63.

Godfrey, H., Bishara, S.N., Partridge, F.M. & Knight, R.G. (1993). Neuropsychological impairment and return to work following severe closed head injury: Implications for clinical management. *New Zealand Medical Journal*, *106*, 301–303.

Greenwood, R.J. & McMillan, T.M. (1993). Models of rehabilitation programmes for the brain injured adult. I: Current provision, efficacy and good practice. *Clinical Rehabilitation*, *7*, 248–255.

Groswasser, Z., Melamed, S., Agranov, E. & Keren, O. (1999). Return to work as an integrative outcome measure following traumatic brain injury. *Neuropsychological Rehabilitation*, *9*, 493–504.

Hoofen, D., Assaf, G., Eli, V. & Donovik, P.J. (2001). Traumatic brain injury 10–20 years later: A comprehensive outcome study of psychiatric symptomatology, cognitive abilities and psycho-social functioning. *Brain Injury*, *15*, 189–209.

Humphrey, M. & Oddy, M. (1980). Return to work after head injury: A review of post war studies. *Injury*, *12*, 107–114.

Johnson, R.P. (1987a). Modifying the denial of symptoms following severe head injuries. *Clinical Rehabilitation*, *1*, 319–323.

Johnson, R.P. (1987b). Return to work after severe head injury. *International Disability Studies*, *9*, 49–54.

Johnson, R.P. (1989). Employment after severe head injury: Do the Manpower Services Commission schemes help? *Injury*, *20*, 5–9.

Johnson, R.P. (1998). How do people get back to work after severe head injury? A 10 year follow-up study. *Neuropsychological Rehabilitation*, *8*, 61–79.

Kreutzer, J.S., Wehman, P., Morton, M.V. & Stonnongton, H.H. (1991). Supported employment and compensatory strategies for enhancing vocational outcome following traumatic brain injury. *International Disability Studies*, *13*, 162–171.

McLeod, D., Johnson, R. & Jones, S. (2002). In R. Gravell & R. Johnson (Eds.) *Head injury rehabilitation: A community team perspective* (pp.244–269). London: Whurr.

McMillan, T.M. & Greenwood, R.J. (1993). Models of rehabilitation programmes for the brain injured adult. II: Model services and suggestions for change in the U.K. *Clinical Rehabilitation*, *7*, 346–355.

Newcombe, F. (1982). The psychological consequences of closed head injury: Assessment and rehabilitation. *Injury*, *14*, 111–136.

Oddy, M. (1984). Head injury and social adjustment. In N. Brooks (Ed.) *Closed head injury: Psychological, social and family consequences* (pp.108–122). Oxford: Oxford University Press.

Oddy, M., Coughlan, T., Tyerman, A. & Jenkins, D. (1985). Social adjustment after closed head injury: A further follow up 7 years after injury. *Journal of Neurology, Neurosurgery and Psychiatry*, *48*, 564–568.

Oddy, M., Humphrey, M. & Uttley, D. (1978). Subjective impairment and social recovery after closed head injury. *Journal of Neurology, Neurosurgery and Psychiatry*, *41*, 611–616.

O'Neill, J., Hibbard, M.R., Brown, M., Jaffe, M., Sliwinski, M., Vandergoot, D., *et al.* (1998). The effect of employment on quality of life and community integration after traumatic brain injury. *Journal of Head Trauma Rehabilitation*, *13*, 68–79.

Ponsford, J.L., Olver, J.H., Curran, C. & Ng, K. (1995). Prediction of employment status 2 years after traumatic brain injury. *Brain Injury*, *9*, 11–20.

Possl, J., Jurgensmeyer, S., Karlbauer, F., Wenz, C. & Goldenberg, G. (2001). Stability of employment after brain injury: a 7-year follow up. *Brain Injury*, *15*, 15–27.

Rimmel, R.W., Giordani, B., Barth, J.T., Boll, T.J. & Jane, J.A. (1981). Disability caused by minor head injury. *Journal of Neurosurgery*, *9*, 221–228.

Roberts, A.H. (1976). The long term prognosis of severe accidental head injury. *Proceedings of the Royal Society of Medicine*, *69*, 137–140.

Sale, P., West, M., Sherron, P. & Wehman, P.H. (1991). Exploratory analysis of job separation from supported employment of persons with traumatic brain injury. *Journal of Head Trauma Rehabilitation*, *6*, 1–11.

Swift, T.L. & Wilson, S. (2001). Misconceptions about brain injury among the general public and non-expert health professionals: An exploratory study. *Brain Injury*, *15*, 149–165.

Thomsen, I.V. (1984). Late outcome of very severe blunt head trauma: A 10–15 year second follow up. *Journal of Neurology, Neurosurgery & Psychiatry*, *47*, 260–268.

Thornhill, S., Teasdale, G.M., Murray, G.D., McEwan, J., Roy, C.W. & Penny, K.I. (2000). Disability in young people and adults one year after head injury: Prospective cohort study. *British Medical Journal*, *320*, 1631–1635.

Thurgood, J. (1999). The employment implications of the Disability Discrimination Act, 1995 and a suggested format for developing reasonable adjustments. *British Journal of Occupational Therapy*, *62*, 290–294.

Tyerman, A. & Meehan, M. (Eds.). (2004). *Vocational assessment and rehabilitation after acquired brain injury. Inter agency guidelines.* London: Royal College of Physicians.

Wehman, P.H., Kregel, J., Keyser-Marcus, L., Sherron-Targett, P., Campbell, L., West, M., *et al.* (2003). Supported employment for persons with traumatic brain injury: A preliminary investigation of long-term follow up costs and programme efficiency. *Archives of Physical Medicine & Rehabilitation*, *84*, 192–196.

Wehman, P.H., Kregel, J., Sherron, P.D., Nguyen, S., Kreutzer, J.S., Fry, R., *et al.* (1993). Critical factors associated with the successful supported employment placement of patients with severe traumatic brain injury. *Brain Injury*, *7*, 31–44.

Wehman, P.H., Kreutzer, J.S., West, M.D., Sherron, P.D., Zazler, N.D., Groath, C.H., *et al.* (1990). Return to work for persons with traumatic brain injury: A supported approach. *Archives of Physical Medicine and Rehabilitation*, *71*, 1047–1052.

Wehman, P.H., West, M.D., Kregel, J., Sherron, P.D. & Kreutzer, J.S. (1995). Return to work for persons with severe traumatic brain injury: A data based approach to programme development. *Journal of Head Trauma Rehabilitation*, *10*, 27–39.

Wright, J.C. & Telford, R. (1996). Psychological problems following minor head injury: A prospective study. *British Journal of Clinical Psychology*, *35*, 399–412.

Wrightson, P. & Gronwall, D. (1981). Time off work and symptoms after minor head injury. *Injury*, *12*, 445–454.

15

Vocational Rehabilitation Programmes

Andy Tyerman, Ruth Tyerman and Peter Viney

Introduction

Return to work is critical to the restoration of quality of life for people with traumatic brain injury (TBI), yet only a minority return to previous or alternative employment. This has major economic implications as well as far-reaching personal and family consequences. The previous chapter reviewed the literature on vocational outcome and interventions to assist people with TBI in returning to previous employment. This chapter focuses on vocational rehabilitation for those unable to return to their previous occupation. The following chapter focuses specifically on supported employment and job coaching in the workplace.

Common difficulties in return to work were identified by RCP/JCP/BSRM (2004). Without expert advice many return to former duties too quickly, resulting in fatigue, anxiety or depression, which then exacerbates the underlying TBI difficulties. Reduced speed, poor concentration, unreliable memory, headaches and/or fatigue mean that many remain uncompetitive. Emotional vulnerability may reduce the capacity to cope with pressure or responsibility. Irritability or frustration may cause difficulties in work relationships. Disinhibited or aggressive behaviour is rarely tolerated in the workplace. Other specific restrictions (e.g. seizures, physical/sensory deficits, executive or communication difficulties) may compromise return to work depending on the specific requirements of the job. Executive difficulties may limit both clients' awareness of their restrictions and their capacity to monitor and manage them effectively in the workplace. Difficulties may also arise months or years after a seemingly successful initial return. This can result from a wide range of factors, including one or more of the following: build-up of fatigue or anxiety due to prolonged compensatory effort; cognitive overload due to accumulation of new information; introduction of new work duties or practices; departure of familiar colleagues, supervisors or managers; career progression. Others may cope with a return to a previous job but struggle on moving to a new job. Those seeking alternative employment tend to seek jobs consistent with pre-injury qualifications and experience, not taking full account of the restrictions imposed by TBI. Repeated work failure often drains self-confidence and belief, undermining future attempts to return to work.

Vocational needs (i.e. finding working and improving job skills) are reported to be the least likely outstanding needs to be met after TBI (Corrigan *et al.*, 2004). Interventions to address vocational need are a vital component of brain injury rehabilitation. Yet the British Society of Rehabilitation Medicine (2000) notes that the NHS 'has largely lost the culture and skills of facilitating employment as a key element of effective health care'. In a recent survey of vocational rehabilitation for people with brain injury in the UK (Deshpande & Turner-Stokes, 2004), 62 per cent of neurological rehabilitation services report that they address vocational issues, but only 8 per cent provide specialist vocational rehabilitation. Recognising the lack of provision, a specific quality requirement on 'Vocational Rehabilitation' is included in the *National Service Framework for Long-term Conditions* (Department of Health, 2005). This states that 'People with long-term neurological conditions are to have access to appropriate vocational assessment, rehabilitation and ongoing support to enable them to find, regain or remain in work and access other occupational and educational opportunities'. This is accompanied by four 'evidence based markers of good practice':

1 Coordinated multi-agency vocational rehabilitation is provided which takes account of agreed national guidance and best practice.
2 Local rehabilitation services are provided which:
   - address vocational needs during review of a person's integrated care plan and as part of any rehabilitation programme;
   - work with other agencies to provide:
     - vocational assessment;
     - support and guidance on returning to or remaining in work;
     - support and advice on withdrawing from work;
   - refer people with neurological conditions who have more complex occupational needs to specialist vocational services.
3 Specialist vocational services are provided for people with neurological conditions to address more complex problems in remaining in or returning to work or alternative occupation including:
   - specialist vocational assessment and counselling;
   - interventions for job retention, including workplace support;
   - specific vocational rehabilitation or 'work preparation' programmes;
   - alternative occupational and educational opportunities;
   - specialist resources for advice for local services.
4 Specialist vocational rehabilitation services routinely evaluate and monitor long-term vocational outcomes, including the reasons for failure to remain in employment.

Several 'evaluated examples of good practice' are summarised briefly in the accompanying web-based Good Practice Guide (www.dh.gov.uk/long-termnsf). One of these, the Working Out Programme, is outlined below. This chapter reviews approaches to vocational rehabilitation after TBI (including inter-agency working in the UK) and provides both a service example and an individual rehabilitation case example.

Approaches to Vocational Rehabilitation

Vocational outcome for people with very severe TBI from UK rehabilitation centres has in the past been disappointing. For example, of those admitted to the Wolfson Medical Rehabilitation Centre, Wimbledon, only 36 per cent were in full-time employment at two-year follow-up with most working in a reduced capacity rather than in former jobs (Weddell *et al.*, 1980). When seen again at seven years, some had progressed to jobs comparable to pre-injury but none of those unemployed at two years had since found employment (Oddy *et al.*, 1985). A subsequent follow-up of people with very severe TBI (median PTA 10 weeks) from this centre and the former Joint Services Medical Rehabilitation Unit (RAF Chessington) highlighted vocational rehabilitation needs: 5 per cent previous work/study; 11 per cent working in reduced capacity; 4 per cent sheltered work; 5 per cent voluntary work; 11 per cent day centre; 11 per cent readmitted to rehabilitation; 54 per cent at home with no occupation (Tyerman, 1987).

Even when some clients received specific advice and support in return to work, a successful return was accomplished by just 38 per cent of people with very severe TBI (median PTA six weeks) from the rehabilitation unit at Addenbrooke's Hospital, Cambridge, with a further 28 per cent having attempted but failed to return to work (Johnson, 1987). In a 10-year follow-up 34 per cent were employed full-time and 10 per cent part-time with 6 per cent in sheltered work, but 50 per cent remained unemployed (Johnson, 1998). Most of those returning successfully to work did so without pan-disability employment rehabilitation services, which were found to be of limited value, with programmes not geared to the needs of TBI, of too short a duration and offered too late to be effective (Johnson, 1989).

In a large-scale multi-centre rehabilitation study in the USA, employment was less than half the pre-injury level at one-, two- and three-year follow-up, ranging from 17–25 per cent overall and under 40 per cent for those previously employed (Sander *et al.*, 1996). Many of those who do return to work after TBI experience job instability (Kreutzer *et al.*, 2003). Similarly, of those employed prior to injury, at two-year follow-up 33 per cent were employed full-time and 9 per cent part-time, leaving 58 per cent unemployed after very severe TBI in Australia (Ponsford *et al.*, 1995). In a five-year follow-up 32 per cent of those in employment at two years were no longer employed and, of those injured whilst at school, 12 per cent were still in education but only 29 per cent were employed, leaving 59 per cent unemployed (Olver *et al.*, 1996).

Factors associated with the low rate of return to work are reviewed in the previous chapter and also by Ownsworth and McKenna (2004). In a meta-analysis of 41 studies a wide range of predictors and indicators were found to be only weakly or moderately related to post-trauma work status (Crepeau & Scherzer, 1993). However, one of the highest and most reliable correlations was access to vocational rehabilitation services. A number of models of brain injury vocational rehabilitation have been developed over the past 25 years. A few selected models will be outlined.

Brain injury vocational programmes

The New York University Head Trauma Program adds vocational elements to core brain injury rehabilitation in three phases: remedial intervention (intensive individual/group work – 5 hours a day, 4 days a week for 20 weeks, focusing on cognitive remediation, self-awareness and social skills); guided voluntary occupational trials (up to 9 months); and assistance in finding suitable work placements. The occupational trials (generally within the university medical centre complex) involved work under the guidance/supervision/tutoring of a vocational counsellor. In the placement phase participants were: (1) assisted in finding suitable work; (2) familiarised with the new job; and (3), when needed, assisted in making initial adjustments to the new work environment. Of 94 people with very severe injuries 56 per cent were placed in competitive and 23 per cent in sheltered work at six months with outcome holding up well at three years (Ben-Yishay *et al.*, 1987). However, it is noted that the selection criteria excluded those with a prior TBI, significant psychiatric history or drug or alcohol abuse.

A 'coordinated model' of service delivery at the Mayo Medical Center, Minnesota, integrates medical and vocational services through a brain injury nurse coordinator and brain injury vocational coordinator based in the medical centre. The nurse coordinator directs the client through rehabilitation and refers those with vocational issues to the vocational coordinator, who links with community and vocational services. Key elements of the vocational coordinator role include: integrating vocational goals into core rehabilitation; assessing vocational readiness; developing comprehensive return to work plans; providing vocational counselling and evaluation; linking with local work rehabilitation centres; adjustment to disability counselling; on-the-job evaluation; education to employers; and follow-up/support (Buffington & Malec, 1997). Of 138 participants assisted through this approach, 80 per cent were in community-based employment (56 per cent with no support) one year after initial placement (Malec & Moessner, 2006).

An alternative approach is the supported placement model at Virginia Medical College, characterised by one-to-one on-site training, counselling and support by a job coach (Wehman *et al.*, 1988). This model has four phases:

- Job placement: matching job needs to abilities/potential; encouraging employer communication with client; encouraging parent/caretaker communications; establishing travel arrangements/providing travel training; and analysing the job environment to verify all potential obstacles that may arise.
- Job site training and advocacy: behavioural training (e.g. skills acquisition, timekeeping, reducing inappropriate behaviour and communication training); and advocacy on behalf of client (e.g. orientation to workplace, communication with co-workers, parents and care workers and counselling about work behaviours).
- Ongoing assessment: evaluation from both the supervisor and client.

- Job retention and follow along: regular on-site visits; phone calls; reviews of supervisor evaluations; client progress reports and parent/caretaker evaluations.

Of 43 people with severe TBI, over 70 per cent were competitively placed in employment at six months (Wehman *et al.*, 1993). In an analysis of interventions and costs 73 clients required an average of 245 hours of intervention over an average of 18 weeks to achieve job stabilisation plus an average of 2.24 hours per week of support to enhance job retention over the first year, at a total average cost of $10,189 (Wehman *et al.*, 2003).

A cost–benefit analysis of the specialist Work Reentry Program at Sharp Memorial Rehabilitation Center, San Diego, indicates that brain injury vocational programmes are cost-effective. This programme combines elements of work rehabilitation (vocational evaluation, simulated work samples, work hardening, 'work adjustment experience', vocational counselling and job seeking/keeping skills) with supported placements (including provision for an on-site job coach) and an off-site adjustment/support group. Total operational costs over five years were on average $4377 per person. However, taking into account taxes paid and savings in state benefits, the average payback period was just 20 months for individuals who would otherwise most likely face a lifetime of unemployment and dependency on public assistance (Abrams *et al.*, 1993).

Positive outcomes and cost-effectiveness have therefore been demonstrated for specialist brain injury vocational rehabilitation programmes in the USA. The value of specialist vocational evaluation after brain injury is highlighted by Fraser *et al.* (1990). In Australia an evaluation of a 'transition to employment model' highlighted the value of family and social support as well as an on-site key worker (Rees & Storry, 1997). The Clubhouse model, developed to provide peer support for people with psychiatric conditions, is also reported to have potential in assisting people with brain injury in a return to work (Jacobs & De Mello, 1996). Evidence from both Israel and the USA confirms the long-term benefits of specialist brain injury vocational provision (Groswasser *et al.*, 1999; Wehman *et al.*, 2003).

Brain injury vocational rehabilitation in the UK

In the UK specialist brain injury vocational rehabilitation provision is limited, with just 36 programmes identified in a survey by Deshpande and Turner-Stokes (2004). Some of these are specialist brain injury vocational programmes, some brain injury services with an added vocational element and some generic vocational, educational or training providers that accept people with brain injury. Few of these services are able to meet the full range of vocational needs after TBI and in many areas of the country there is currently no access to specialist vocational rehabilitation. Partridge (1996) also highlighted the 'dearth of intervention methods' in vocational rehabilitation in the UK.

Only a very small number of NHS services have developed specialist brain injury vocational rehabilitation programmes (e.g. the Working Out Programme in Aylesbury; the Wolfson Neurorehabilitation Centre, London; the STAR programme at Whitchurch Hospital in Cardiff). However, some brain injury services work in partnership with vocational providers in the independent or voluntary sector (e.g. Northumberland Brain Injury Service and Rehab UK) or educational establishments (e.g. Royal Leamington Spa Rehabilitation Hospital and Warwickshire College). In Northern Ireland the four Health Boards fund eight small brain injury vocational rehabilitation programmes provided by the Cedar Foundation with close links to local Community Brain Injury Teams.

Jobcentre Plus, part of the Department for Work and Pensions, recognised brain injury as an area of specialist provision and developed a National Framework for Contracting for Brain Injury Work Preparation. This specifies the required elements of a specialist brain injury work preparation programme, including job-finding behaviour-development needs, occupational decision-making needs and job-keeping behaviour development needs (see RCP/JCP/BSRM, 2004). In 2003 there were 13 Jobcentre Plus contracted specialist brain injury work preparation providers – 7 in England, 5 in Scotland and 1 in Wales. Whilst two of these programmes are NHS-based, most are in the independent or voluntary sector. Four programmes were provided by Momentum (Aberdeen, Glasgow, Irvine and Kelso) and three by Rehab UK (Birmingham, London and Newcastle). The latter include two elements: a centre-based pre-vocational phase of cognitive rehabilitation; and an in situ vocational trials phase (Murply *et al.*, 2006).

Inter-agency working

The complex needs of people with TBI require close collaboration between brain injury services, Jobcentre Plus disability employment advisors (DEAs)/work psychologists and vocational rehabilitation and support services. For the Working Out Programme (outlined below), early research and development work with Jobcentre Plus continued through a series of specialist brain injury work preparation contracts. This has involved close collaboration with DEAs and/or work psychologists regarding the following: suitability and timing of individual referrals for specialist assessment, work preparation and/or job retention; pooling of assessment results (e.g. neuropsychological assessment and work psychologist's employment assessment); joint goal setting, monitoring and progress review; and joint consideration of ongoing support needs. Whilst ongoing liaison is often by telephone or e-mail, joint meetings with the client and DEA to discuss complex needs and problem situations have proved of particular value. We have also seen the benefit both of joint staff training with Work Psychologists and DEAs and of joint working with the Work Psychologists' Brain Injury Regional Leads Group. The value of joint working lies both in the integration of brain injury and vocational rehabilitation perspectives and in the provision of a coordinated inter-agency approach.

Effective joint working across statutory services and vocational providers is critical in enabling people with TBI to achieve their optimal outcome, yet is currently very patchy. In developing recommendations on vocational rehabilitation for the *National Guidelines on Rehabilitation following Acquired Brain Injury* (RCP/BSRM, 2003), an Inter-Agency Advisory Group on Vocational Rehabilitation after Brain Injury was formed in April 2003. This comprised members of the NHS, Jobcentre Plus, Social Services and independent vocational and educational providers. This group identified a pressing need to develop a joint framework and guidelines for staff of all agencies in working together to facilitate access to appropriate

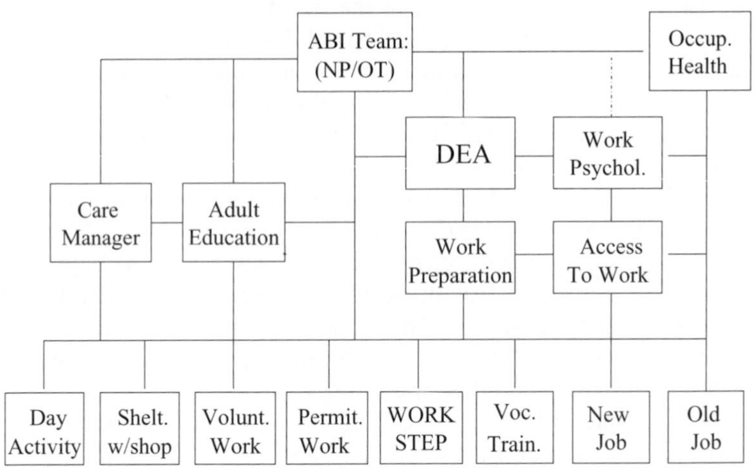

Figure 15.1 Brain injury vocational rehabilitation provision. *Source*: adapted from RCP/JCP/BSRM (2004) with permission from the Royal College of Physicians, London

vocational assessment, rehabilitation and support for people with brain injury (RCP/JCP/BSRM, 2004). These inter-agency guidelines review both specialist vocational rehabilitation and relevant NHS, occupational health, Jobcentre Plus and occupational/educational services. A joint framework for provision of vocational assessment and rehabilitation after brain injury is proposed (outlined below and illustrated in Figure 15.1), along with detailed guidelines for five identified areas of vocational need:

1 *Return to previous employment*. Those able to return to a previous employment position should be assessed and advised by relevant health professionals. Advice and support of Jobcentre Plus services should be sought via the DEA when there is a requirement for ongoing support, significant adjustments to the job or provision through Access to Work.
2 *Employment assessment*. Those unable to return to previous work should be referred for employment assessment by a suitably qualified professional with experience of brain injury and vocational rehabilitation. (Within Jobcentre Plus, after initial assessment by the DEA, such an assessment may be undertaken by the Jobcentre Plus work psychologist, a suitably qualified psychologist in independent practice or a specialist brain injury work preparation provider.)
3 *Vocational rehabilitation*. Those requiring a period of vocational rehabilitation prior to a return to work should be referred to a specialist brain injury vocational rehabilitation programme. This may be accessed via Jobcentre Plus (in the case of a specialist brain injury work preparation provider) or through a direct referral to a specialist vocational programme. (It is recognised that, where there is no specialist provision available, it may be appropriate to refer to a generic work preparation programme, subject to satisfactory brain injury training, support and monitorings.)

4 *WORKSTEP (supported placement programme).* Those requiring a supported placement should be referred via Jobcentre Plus (or directly) to a WORKSTEP provider. WORKSTEP providers accepting clients with brain injury need access to training and support on the nature and effects of brain injury.
5 *Occupational provision.* For those unable to return to employment, responsibility for provision of suitable alternative occupational provision should rest with the NHS and local councils, working with independent and voluntary providers and educational establishments.

In implementing the guidelines it was recommended that local NHS brain injury services, Jobcentre Plus, Local Councils and vocational providers undertake a joint review of services for people with brain injury and develop local protocols, drawing on the framework and guidelines. It was also recommended that key staff from relevant agencies establish ongoing service links (for example, between the brain injury neuropsychologist and/or occupational therapist and the Jobcentre Plus DEA and/or work psychologist) to discuss the complex vocational needs of individuals with brain injury. A joint approach to raising awareness of vocational needs and specialist skills training was also advocated.

In summary, brain injury vocational rehabilitation in the UK is limited, with very little evaluation of existing provision. However, an evaluation of the Working Out Programme in Aylesbury demonstrated that positive vocational outcomes can be achieved for people unable to return to previous occupation after severe TBI in the UK (Tyerman, 1999; Tyerman & Young, 2000). This programme will be outlined.

The Working Out Programme

Working Out is a specialist brain injury vocational rehabilitation programme run by the Community Head Injury Service, Buckinghamshire PCT. Working Out is recognised as an example of good practice by the Department for Work and Pensions (2004) and Department of Health (2005) and was the South-East Regional Winner of the NHS Nye Bevan Modernisation Award 2000. The programme was set up to assist those unable to re-establish themselves in employment after TBI. (Clients able to return to previous occupation are supported by the core rehabilitation team – see chapter 4.) The programme was funded originally as a research and development project by the Department of Health as part of the National Brain Injury Rehabilitation Initiative (1992–1997), with additional funding from the then Employment Service – London & South-East Region (1994–1996). Since 1997 some clients have continued to be funded by Jobcentre Plus through a series of specialist brain injury work preparation contracts.

Programme aims

1 To assess the vocational needs and potential of persons with brain injury.
2 To provide specialist rehabilitation programmes to prepare persons with brain injury for a return to work or alternative occupation.

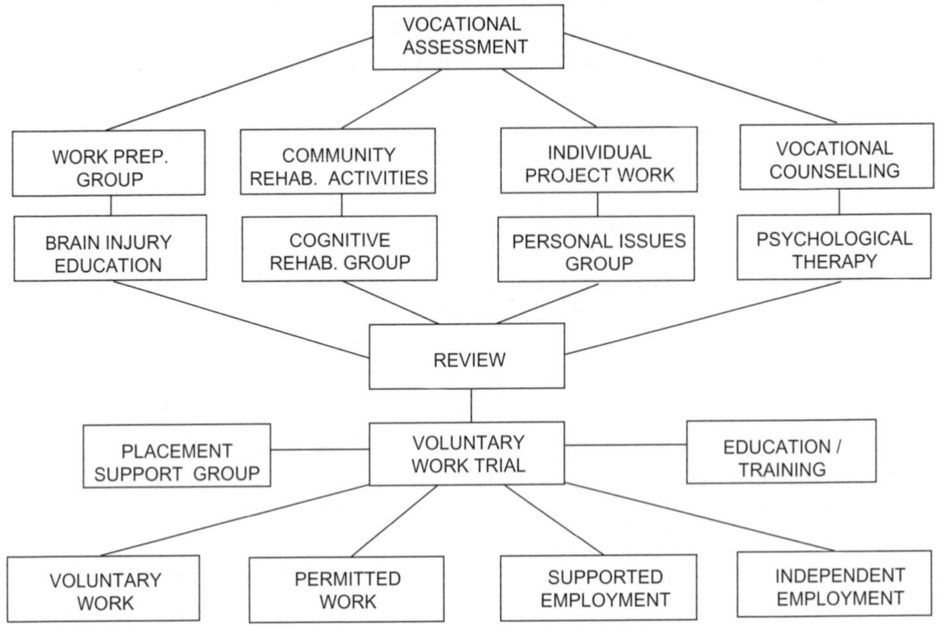

Figure 15.2 CHIS Working Out Programme

3 To find, set up and support voluntary work trials to evaluate alternative occupational options.
4 To find, set up and support suitable long-term work placements for persons with brain injury.

The Working Out programme comprises four interlinked phases: vocational assessment; work preparation; voluntary work trials; and supported placements (see Figure 15.2).

Vocational assessment

All persons referred to the Working Out Programme are seen first for initial suitability assessment. This comprises the following: a Brain Injury Background Interview Schedule (covering personal and clinical history, course of recovery and review of current situation/needs); a Head Injury Problem Schedule (covering physical, sensory, cognitive, behavioural, emotional and social difficulties); a Head Injury Semantic Differential scale (covering changes in self-concept and mood/behaviour); the Hospital Anxiety & Depression Scale (screening of emotional state); and a Family Screening Assessment (when appropriate). (This process is described in detail in chapter 4.) This provides a detailed social, clinical and work history and profile of current problems and work situation, from which individual vocational assessment needs are identified.

The specialist vocational assessment programme combines vocational interviews, formal assessments, group work, and observations/ratings of work attitude, performance and behaviour on practical work activities in the community. Additional assessments (e.g. medical, physiotherapy, speech and language) are completed, as required. The assessment is typically undertaken part-time over one to three weeks, depending on which of the following core components are included:

- neuropsychological assessment;
- Chessington Occupational Therapy Neurological Assessment Battery;
- work preparation group;
- community vocational rehabilitation activities;
- individual project work/assessment;
- vocational ratings;
- vocational guidance interviews.

A neuropsychological assessment is routinely undertaken unless recently completed elsewhere, in which case only selected tests are administered. Assessment has typically included tests of the following: general intellectual ability (i.e. Wechsler Adult Intelligence Scale III); memory and information processing (i.e. Adult Memory and Information Processing Battery) and attention/executive function (i.e. Test of Everyday Attention; Trail Making Test; Six Elements Test or other tests from the Behavioural Assessment of the Dysexecutive Syndrome or Delis–Kaplan Executive Function System), plus other language, perceptual and spatial skills, as appropriate. The assessments employed in the R&D phase of the programme are detailed elsewhere (Tyerman, 1999; Tyerman & Young, 1999).

The Chessington Occupational Therapy Neurological Assessment Battery (COTNAB; R. Tyerman *et al.*, 1986) was designed specifically for assessing return to work after TBI. The battery comprises twelve sub-tests, three in each of four functional areas: Visual Perception (Overlapping Figures, Hidden Figures and Sequencing); Constructional Ability (2D Construction, 3D Construction and Block Printing); Sensory Motor Ability (Stereognosis, Dexterity and Coordination); and Ability to Follow Instructions (Written, Visual and Spoken Instructions). The assessment provides separate Ability and Time grades and combined Overall Performance grades for each sub-test.

The formal assessments clarify the nature of cognitive and sensory-motor difficulties. However, assessment of work attitude, performance and behaviour, as reported and/or observed on practical work activities, is of at least equal importance. As such, clients on assessment typically attend specific components of the work preparation phase of the programme (see below). This may include the work preparation group, one or two community-based vocational rehabilitation activities and/or an individual assessment project set up in the workplace, in the centre, in community settings (e.g. library) or the home. (When the person has recently been in work or on placement, feedback will normally be sought from a relevant supervisor in these settings.) The practical assessments enable the team to observe work attitude, performance and behaviour and complete both a structured 'functional work assessment' and two specialist vocational rating scales – the Functional Assessment Inventory and the Work Personality Profile.

The Functional Assessment Inventory (FAI; Crew & Athelstan, 1981, 1984) has 30 items of vocational strengths/limitations rated on 4-point scale from '0' (no significant impairment) to '3' (severe impairment). The FAI has seven factors: '*adaptive behaviour*' – behaviour, interaction, work habits and social support; '*motor functioning*' – hand and arm function and motor speed; '*cognition*' – learning, reading/writing, memory and perception; '*physical condition*' – mobility, exertion, endurance, sickness and stability of condition; '*communication*' – hearing, speech and language; '*vocational qualifications*' – work history, acceptability, attractiveness, skills, economic disincentives, access to job opportunities and need for special working conditions; '*vision*' – visual impairment. Normative data is reported for 1716 persons consulting vocational rehabilitation counsellors in the USA.

The Work Personality Profile (WPP; Bolton & Roessler, 1986a, 1986b) has 58 items relating to work attitudes, values, habits and behaviours, rated on a 4-point scale from '4' ('a definite strength, an employment asset') to '1' ('a problem area' which 'will definitely limit the chance for employment'). The WPP has five factors: '*Task orientation*' – cognitive skills and good work habits (e.g. learning, initiative, independence, adaptability, responsibility); '*social skills*' – interaction with co-workers in terms of being appropriately sociable, outgoing, friendly and emotionally expressive; '*work motivation*' – willingness to accept work assignments, move readily to new tasks, and work at routine jobs without complaining; '*work conformance*' – appropriate behaviour at work with respect to 'good judgement' in the expression of negative behaviour and the ability to exercise an even temper and 'controlled self-presentation'; and '*personal presentation*' – interaction with supervisory personnel and attention to personal hygiene and appearance. The WPP was standardised on 243 persons receiving vocational rehabilitation in the USA.

The vocational guidance interview undertaken by a placement consultant builds on the initial assessment, providing an in-depth assessment of educational history, vocational qualifications, pre-injury employment (including profiling of past jobs), vocational interests/aspirations and leisure/social interests. However, this has to be balanced by a full understanding of vocational restrictions arising from the TBI, as highlighted by the other assessments. When the person has been on placement or in work post-injury, the placement consultant (or other staff member) will seek feedback from past employers (including, when appropriate, completion of vocational rating scales), visit current and/or recent placements and set up and evaluate on-site work assessment projects.

The results and recommendations of the vocational assessment are discussed with the person and relative at a feedback/planning session, similar to that outlined for the core rehabilitation team (see chapter 4), but focused primarily on vocational needs. Whilst some clients referred are seen for specialist assessment and advice only (typically those at distance with no local specialist service), most require a period of work preparation.

Work preparation programme

The aims of the work preparation programme are as follows:

1 To facilitate further recovery and adjustment.
2 To develop and evaluate coping strategies for work.
3 To assess realistic work potential.

4 To promote more accurate self-appraisal.
5 To foster positive work attitudes and behaviour.

Specific objectives are discussed and agreed with the person and, when appropriate, the DEA or other referring agent. Work preparation programmes are tailored to meet individual needs drawing upon the following core components:

- work preparation group;
- community vocational rehabilitation activities;
- individual project work;
- vocational counselling;
- psychological therapy;
- brain injury educational programme;
- cognitive rehabilitation group;
- personal issues group.

Work preparation group

This weekly group helps people to re-evaluate their strengths and weaknesses, discuss the implications of brain injury for re-employment, explore suitable jobs and manage issues related to brain injury in job applications/interviews etc. The group includes education, workshop elements (role plays, group discussions), peer group sharing/support and 'homework'. The group operates a rolling programme with both individual sessions and short modules planned over a three-month block (see Figure 15.3).

Vocational rehabilitation activities

A variety of community vocational rehabilitation activities have been set up working with voluntary organisations: running an allotment; helping to build an adventure playground; maintenance work at Bucks. Railway Centre; developing a living archive project and a rural life museum; renovating equipment and tools for less economically developed countries at WorkAid; and working on the grounds at Waddesdon Manor, a local National Trust property. At any time two or three half-day activities run each week in which a small group of clients work under the direction of staff of the respective organisations, facilitated by an occupational therapist and technical instructor/assistant psychologist. The assigned tasks need to be completed to the standard required by the organisation. These activities provide an opportunity for clients to progress through a series of graded vocational tasks. Staff observe work attitude, performance and behaviour and help clients to develop greater awareness of their work-related difficulties and strategies to address these in preparation for a return to the workplace.

Individual project work

In parallel with the core rehabilitation activities, an individual project may be set up in the area of work relevant to the particular skills and interests of the client. This has included a wide variety of work projects, for example domestic activities, graded engineering projects, developing questionnaires, assessing and developing computer skills, supporting people with further education courses. This enables staff

PROGRAMME TITLE:	WORK PREPARATION GROUP
AIMS:	To help people re-evaluate their strengths & weaknesses, consider implications for re-employment; To explore issues relating to brain injury and interpersonal skills in the workplace
SUMMARY OF PROGRAMME:	Discussion based, covering a weekly topic, often split into small group work. Programme changes to meet clients' current needs. Areas covered may include: • Brain injury and its effects • Barriers to work • Customer service • Access to work • Job task analysis • Self-evaluation • Strategies • Interpersonal skills • Job application process
LOCATION:	The Camborne Centre
FREQUENCY & LENGTH OF SESSION:	Weekly for 1½ hours
PROGRAMME LENGTH:	Rolling programme
LEAD THERAPIST:	Occupational therapist/Placement consultant
PROGRAMME OPEN TO:	Clients on the Working Out Programme

Figure 15.3 Work Preparation Group, Working Out Programme

to set clients a progressively challenging series of tasks in order to identify potential difficulties in a specific area of work, to develop coping strategies and to evaluate whether this is likely to be a realistic avenue of work to pursue through a voluntary work trial.

Vocational counselling

In parallel with rehabilitation activities clients routinely receive individual vocational counselling. It is essential that this is integrated fully within the vocational rehabilitation process and anchored in an understanding of the personal, family and social context of the individual. For clients with TBI the vocational guidance/counselling process is based in part on past qualifications and experience but balanced by their limitations post-injury, which precludes most clients on the programme from resuming their former career path. Some clients have already tried unsuccessfully to resume former careers, but some others need to experience for themselves (with support) that this is no longer viable. It is often helpful to draw on past experience in the selection of an alternative career (e.g. a frontline policeman becoming a council tax fraud investigator; a tradesman becoming an assistant instructor at a local college). However, for others a complete change of career may be indicated, either due to the skills required or in terms of adjustment – some clients prefer to have a fresh start rather than risk being reminded constantly of what they can no longer do. As such, clients are helped to develop a clear understanding of their vocational aptitudes and resources, the limitations arising from TBI and current opportunities and prospects, which are summarised in a work profile. The client is then assisted in exploring a realistic future vocation through career guidance, job matching and/or through setting up and evaluating 'job tasters'.

Psychological therapy

Many clients on the programme require psychological therapy, addressing issues that are work-related and/or those that reflect the wider effects of brain injury. This may include neuropsychological counselling (i.e. education, advice, promotion of awareness, understanding and coping); specific psychological treatment (e.g. for anxiety, anger, pain, mood and behavioural difficulties); and neuropsychotherapy (i.e. exploring changes in self/lifestyle and help with psychological adjustments – see chapter 13).

Other group programmes

Clients on the programme are routinely invited to attend the brain injury educational programme and may also be invited to join other groups, such as the cognitive rehabilitation group or personal issues group (outlined in chapter 4).

Progress is monitored on an ongoing basis by the programme manager or other assigned key worker (in liaison with the DEA or other referring agent, as appropriate). Formal reviews are held routinely at around three-monthly intervals. Following a work preparation programme the person will usually progress to a voluntary work trial.

Voluntary work trials

When a client is considered to be ready to progress to the workplace the placement consultant works with them to find and set up a suitable part-time voluntary work trial in local services or businesses as close as possible to the person's home. Finding a suitable work trial in the target area of work is often challenging. Avenues worth exploring may arise from existing contacts of the client, family, former work colleagues, staff members or the local DEA, who will be familiar with the local employment market and specific employers. However, it may also involve working with the client to trawl newspapers, Yellow Pages, the internet, employment agencies, Chamber of Commerce and other local employers' groups or trade organisations. Having identified a possible opportunity the placement consultant will make contact initially by telephone and explain the situation with a view to checking out whether this might be a suitable placement in terms of both the work and the employer.

In setting up voluntary work trials care is taken to ensure, as far as possible, that the requirements of the trial match the skills of the client, that the needs of the client are communicated to relevant staff and that appropriate support is provided. It is essential to check that health and safety training and insurance cover are provided by the employer. Trials typically start one or two half-days per week with a graded increase in line with progress and run for about 12 weeks prior to review. Trials usually run in parallel with a reducing work preparation programme, gradually replacing vocational rehabilitation activities and project work. Voluntary work trials serve a number of vital functions e.g.:

- independent assessment of work potential (duties, hours, etc.);
- identification of residual difficulties in the workplace;
- development, evaluation and refining of coping strategies;
- re-establishment of independence, work routines and behaviours;
- supervised and graded rebuilding of self-confidence and self-esteem;
- an independent reference for those applying for jobs.

Placement support group

In parallel with starting a voluntary work trial clients often progress from the work preparation group to a fortnightly placement support group (see Figure 15.4). This promotes understanding and adjustment to the world of work after brain injury. One of the functions of the group is to help clients form a balanced view of any difficulties that arise in the workplace. Whilst those with limited insight may need help to understand how the effects of their brain injury may contribute to difficulties at work, those who have lost confidence in their work skills may assume incorrectly that all work difficulties experienced are attributable to their injury. Ongoing contact with clients helps to alert programme staff to early emergent difficulties, thereby enabling them to provide pro-active advice and support before the difficulties escalate.

Work trials are monitored regularly by the placement consultant. Any major issues highlighted in the trial will be addressed either within the work preparation elements of the programme or in the workplace, as appropriate. On completing the trial a review with the person and supervisor and, as appropriate, with the DEA (or other referring agent) is undertaken to agree further plans. The client usually progresses to one of a wide range of long-term placements depending on their potential.

Long-term supported placements

Long-term supported placements may include full- or part-time employment, vocational training, supported employment, adult education, permitted work and voluntary work. The placement consultant assists the person, as required, in finding and applying for suitable positions, in liaison with the DEA and other agencies, as appropriate. Avenues worth pursuing in seeking long-term placements are similar to those for a voluntary work trial. A key requirement is that the long-term work placement is within comfortable travelling distance of the person's home. Our

PROGRAMME TITLE:	PLACEMENT SUPPORT GROUP
AIMS:	To provide a personnel/welfare function to help clients understand the complexities of the world of work and the necessary adjustment to extract the best from either a voluntary work trial or part-time/full-time employment.
SUMMARY OF PROGRAMME:	Discussion based, covering a weekly topic in small groups (5/6 maximum). Client-centred and geared to meet immediate needs, queries and problems experienced in the workplace. Areas covered may include: • Companies and their different structures; • Stress in the workplace; • Keeping the motivation going; • Dealing with change & the nature of injury; • Getting to know new people when starting work; • Asking and giving help to work colleagues; • The importance of confidentiality; • Looking after yourself at work – avoiding conflict;. • Sharing experience of different strategies that clients use within the workplace.
LOCATION:	The Camborne Centre
FREQUENCY & LENGTH OF SESSION:	Fortnightly for one hour
PROGRAMME LENGTH:	Rolling programme
LEAD THERAPISTS:	Placement consultant/Clinical psychologist/Occupational therapist
PROGRAMME OPEN TO:	Clients on the Working Out Programme plus clients from Rehabilitation Team who have returned to previous jobs

Figure 15.4 Placement Support Group, Working Out Programme

experience is that there is much to be gained from employing placement staff with careers guidance or vocational rehabilitation experience, who adopt a commercial approach in highlighting the positive attributes and potential of the individual. Once a possible opportunity has been identified it is essential to alert employers to relevant restrictions arising from the TBI. The content, timing and process of disclosure of such information require careful planning and agreement with the client. Flexibility is also required as employers vary greatly in terms of the amount of information they seek (or are receptive to), both initially and over time.

Whenever possible the placement consultant is involved in setting up, monitoring and supporting placements. Once established there is usually a phased reduction in support. However, attendance at the placement support group remains open-ended for all clients, some of whom continue regular or intermittent attendance for several years – usually those for whom coping with employment is an ongoing challenge. An open door policy encourages clients to contact staff if they run into difficulties in long-term placements.

Follow-up

Following the establishment of a work placement and the phased withdrawal of ongoing support, the person will be followed up through formal or informal reviews either in person or by telephone, as agreed with the client and the employer. This provides an opportunity to evaluate the long-term viability of the placement and to identify and address any related or unrelated areas of difficulty.

Programme evaluation

The R&D phase of the Working Out Programme was subject to a detailed evaluation of vocational assessment and rehabilitation for the first 45 persons with severe TBI on the programme (Tyerman, 1999; Tyerman & Young, 1999, 2000). Vocational outcomes on completing the programme were as follows: 50 per cent paid employment/vocational training; 12.5 per cent permitted work; 22.5 per cent voluntary work; 5 per cent to pre-vocational education courses; 7.5 per cent referral on for further rehabilitation; 2.5 per cent no regular activity. Outcomes were well maintained, with 50 per cent in paid employment at two-year follow-up.

Ongoing rehabilitation outcomes for people with brain injury on the programme have continued to be encouraging: 67 per cent paid employment or vocational training; 18 per cent permitted work, voluntary work or adult education; 6 per cent referred for further rehabilitation and or other treatment; 8 per cent disengaged during rehabilitation; 1 per cent no occupation. The process of vocational rehabilitation on the Working Out Programme will be illustrated through a case example.

Case 15.1: Example A

Background

A was a junior technician in the RAF and had been recommended for promotion to corporal. He had two years left to serve but was 'loving it' and intended to extend his term. He was in good health with no prior serious illnesses or injuries. He incurred a severe TBI (PTA 3–4 weeks) and injuries to his left radius/ulna, left wrist, right radius, back and neck in a motor cycle accident. On admission he was conscious but very restless, agitated and abusive. He required orthopaedic surgery and was in intensive care for two days. On the ward he was noted initially to be abusive, hallucinating, agitated, confused and very sleepy. He was in hospital for 5–6 weeks and received out-patient physiotherapy for his orthopaedic injuries but no TBI assessment or rehabilitation. A was largely unaware of the effects of his TBI until he returned to work.

A returned to work full-time at six months. He was initially assigned to light duties in the tea bar but was slow with poor concentration and memory (e.g. confusing or losing count of orders and forgetting names) and difficulties in working out money. After his return to his technician role his failure to follow set procedures resulted in a serious health and safety incident. He was then referred for assessment and an electroencephalogram (EEG) showed left frontal damage. He was medically discharged from the RAF at 30 months post-injury. Pending discharge he worked back in the tea bar and also completed a resettlement course on sales and marketing but was not referred for any TBI rehabilitation.

On leaving the RAF, A had six jobs over the next five years, interspersed with periods of unemployment. He reported problems at work with organisation, memory, route-finding and speed, having to complete paperwork in the evenings to keep up. After the first two jobs (surveyor and salesman) he consulted his local disability employment advisor (DEA), completed a Placing Assessment and Counselling Team assessment and was referred for advice and support in seeking employment. After three further short-term jobs (delivering cars and car parts), he returned to see the DEA and was referred to a local employment rehabilitation provider. At 6.5 years post-injury he started a delivery job and received helpful advice and support from the provider in organising loading, routing deliveries, breaking down tasks and implementing daily routines. He continued in this job for a year but was advised to stop by his GP due to problems in lifting due to his back injury. He was also struggling with speed and becoming increasingly despondent, commenting, 'How many times does your head have to be ducked under water before you give up?'

At 7.5 years post-injury A was referred for specialist brain injury vocational assessment/rehabilitation to the Working Out Programme at the recommendation of an independent case manager, whom he had seen for his compensation claim.

Vocational assessment

On initial assessment A presented with physical, cognitive, emotional and behavioural difficulties. His major concerns related to memory,

Continued

poor organisational skills, lack of initiative, frustration, mood swings and lack of emotional/behavioural control. He had a low current self-concept and a mild degree of anxiety and depression. Marked stress on the marital relationship was noted. (He had previously been referred to a psychiatrist due to aggression at home and prescribed antidepressants; he and his wife had also seen a behaviour therapist for a short period.) A vocational assessment on the Working Out programme (including additional speech and language, physiotherapy and marital assessments) was recommended to evaluate the long-term effects of his TBI, identify vocational rehabilitation needs and guide the search for future employment.

Neuropsychological assessment confirmed significant cognitive impairment affecting short-term memory, psychomotor speed, attention, speed of information processing and executive function. Whilst ability scores on the COTNAB were mostly within normal limits, his speed of function was often below average or impaired, notably so on tasks requiring greater planning and application. Physiotherapy assessment confirmed back pain and reduced range of movement of his left arm, likely to cause difficulty with lifting, prolonged driving and tasks involving repetitive movements or rotation of his forearm. On speech and language assessment he was noted to have mild difficulty with the following: processing complex information; auditory memory; providing verbal explanations/descriptions; word retrieval; and planning appropriate verbal output.

On practical rehabilitation activities he demonstrated good knowledge and practical skills in mechanical engineering with great attention to detail. Whilst producing high quality work he was observed to be preoccupied with tasks being completed perfectly, resulting in slow speed of work. Under time pressure he was noted to be anxious, with a further loss of productivity. He was slow in problem solving and in organisational skills. He demonstrated good insight into his cognitive restrictions and was not obviously restricted by his physical difficulties. Confidence and mood were observed to fluctuate with anxiety and the desire to work to a very high standard. On the Functional Assessment Inventory both A and staff rated him as low average in adaptive behaviour, motor functioning, cognition, physical condition (self only) and vocational qualifications. On the Work Personality Profile staff rated him as average except for low average in task orientation – A also rated himself as low average in work motivation (see Figures 15.5 and 15.6).

It was concluded that A had good prospects of sustaining paid employment, provided that this was under supported circumstances

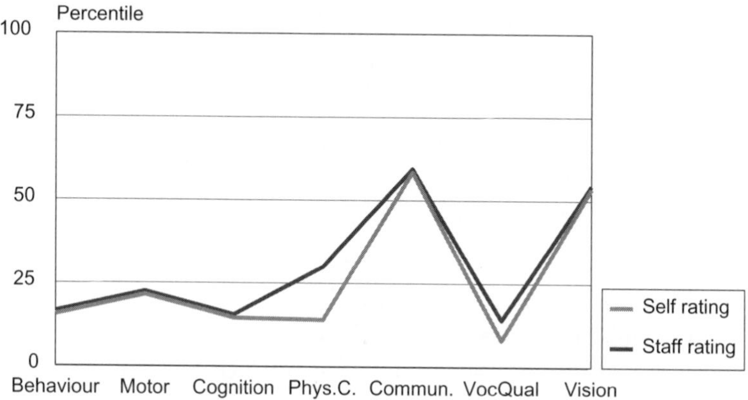

Figure 15.5 Functional Problems (FAI): Example A

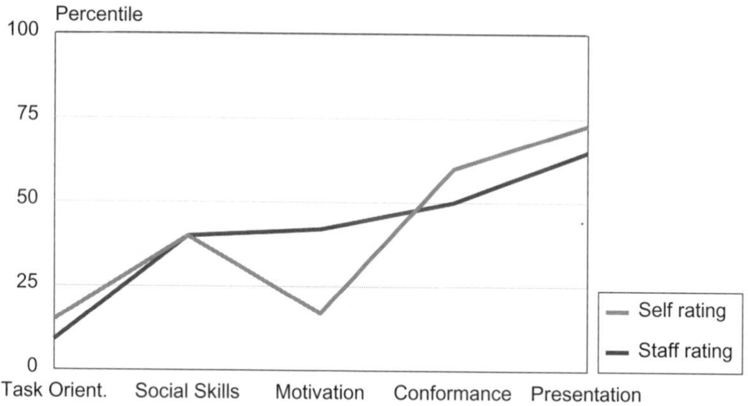

Figure 15.6 Work Personality Profile: Example A

where quality of work was paramount and his slow speed could be accommodated without undue pressure and/or fatigue. A period of specialist vocational rehabilitation was recommended to improve self-management of his cognitive difficulties and to increase confidence and self-belief prior to a return to the workplace.

Reflecting on the value of a specialist vocational assessment A commented: 'Even after $7\frac{1}{2}$ years, a massive relief, a real feeling that everybody understood your situation without you having to sit down and explain it to anyone . . . it was also as much again this labelling process, this underlining "Yes we concur that this problem exists and it affects you in this way" – there is a great deal of comfort

Continued

in that . . . in pinpointing certain other areas where we were not aware, where we knew we had a problem, but for you to say "Well this is why" is again, another major boost.'

Vocational rehabilitation

A attended a work preparation programme comprising the following:

- weekly work preparation group;
- weekly cognitive rehabilitation group;
- weekly community vocational rehabilitation activity;
- individual psychological therapy, focusing on understanding the effects of his TBI, reviewing his self-concept and rebuilding his confidence and self-belief.

Following review after three months we started to look for a suitable voluntary work trial. On starting the trial he ceased attending the community vocational rehabilitation activity. On completion of the cognitive rehabilitation group programme he received individual therapy to assist him in managing his cognitive difficulties on his work trial. On review at six months A was very positive about the benefits of his rehabilitation programme – reduced headaches, improved management of memory and planning/organisational difficulties, 'definite' improvement in behaviour and emotional state with a notable improvement in self-confidence.

A voluntary work trial was set up for two mornings a week in a small company manufacturing fittings for ocean-going yachts where quality (not speed) was paramount. This offered an opportunity for A to use his mechanical engineering skills in sheet metal work drilling, packing and assembly. He lacked confidence initially in his capacity to do the work and required several visits and encouragement. Apart from initial fatigue and a period off work due to pain in his right elbow, the trial progressed well. He was tried on a range of machinery, identifying difficulties and developing strategies to manage them, supported by both the company and the Working Out team. A was positive about the work and was interested in a job with the company should the opportunity arise. Whilst the company were pleased with his progress they were not in a position to offer him paid employment at that time. A was unsure whether to continue on a voluntary basis with the company, in the hope of paid employment becoming available, or to look elsewhere.

Supported placement

After a break before and after the birth of his second daughter A was assisted by the placement consultant in exploring suitable work opportunities. A position was found in a company which made high quality hi-fi speakers for the broadcast and film industry. This was set up initially as a full-time voluntary work trial. On review after a month, the company were very pleased with A's progress, both technically and as a member of the assembly team. The only major reservation related to memory, requiring reminders about what he had been doing the previous day. A was offered a full-time contract with a three-month probationary period. The position was reviewed formally again after two months. The company were generally pleased with A's progress, with his skills noted to lie more with technical assembly. However, problems remained with organisation and memory – A was also concerned about his back and lifting on the job. As such, it was agreed that A would move from building speakers to concentrate on building the circuits for speakers and possibly testing – this was primarily bench-work and a more repetitive job with no significant lifting. A further probationary period was set up in the new role.

A moved to this new position and was also asked from time to time to modify components that did not fit properly, which he particularly enjoyed. He completed successfully a further three-month probationary period and was taken on as a permanent employee without further difficulties. Feedback from the company was that he had become a valued member of the team. Reviewing the value of specialist brain injury vocational rehabilitation A commented: 'I think it very much heightens your awareness of what you should and should not get involved in . . . the Working Out programme makes you aware of the sorts of work that you are going to have problems with so you can flag that up straight away . . . the awareness of what you can and can't do empowers you in a way because . . . when you do take on a job, you are pretty certain that's the one you are going to be successful with . . . It's a dual thing though because, whilst the Working Out programme makes me aware and gives ways of getting around the problems (like diarising things, making notes and such and looking at different ways of doing tasks), it also allows you to talk to the people who are working around you and say, "Look, these are the problems that may crop up, these are the things I may do when I'm working, look out for them". And if you have got the right kind of people around

Continued

with you they start to work with you. So you are not just helping yourself they are helping you as well . . . and, I think, after a while I remember somebody saying "Since you have been here a while, I think you're getting better". You know you're not getting better, it's just the situation is getting better. The thing is they don't realise that they are slotting into you . . . it's like a jigsaw . . . it's their half that fits in with your half as much as the other way round . . . before it was just a game of catch-up where you were just struggling to keep up with things and such but now . . . you can set things up so that they work for you rather than you run around trying to make them work.'

A's experience highlights how, in the absence of brain injury assessment/rehabilitation, significant but not insurmountable difficulties arising from TBI can lead to ongoing and escalating vocational difficulties. Provided with the opportunity of specialist vocational assessment and a combination of core brain injury and vocational rehabilitation, A was assisted in understanding and managing the effects of his TBI and in rebuilding his confidence, thereby enabling a positive and successful return to paid employment.

Conclusions

Currently many people with TBI in the UK do not have the opportunity to return to employment or alternative productive occupation. This reflects a combination of under-developed NHS brain injury services, shortage of specialist brain injury vocational rehabilitation and suitable alternative occupational provision and a lack of joint working both across statutory agencies and with independent providers. There is, however, consistent evidence suggesting that specialist vocational rehabilitation programmes can lead to positive vocational outcomes.

The experience of the Working Out Programme is that a blend of brain injury and vocational rehabilitation expertise, working in partnership with Jobcentre Plus, can assist many people with TBI, who have been unable to return to previous employment, to secure and maintain alternative employment or occupation. The programme has demonstrated the value of assessment of work attitude, performance and behaviour on practical work activities, alongside vocational interviews and formal assessments. It has highlighted the benefits of integrating elements of brain injury rehabilitation with graded vocational rehabilitation activities (i.e. work preparation group, community vocational activities, voluntary work trials and long-term supported placements). The work preparation phase (focusing on understanding and management of work-related difficulties, on rebuilding confidence and on identifying a realistic vocational direction) has provided a valuable interim step between the rehabilitation setting and the demands of the workplace. Evaluated voluntary work trials have proved effective in testing out the viability of alternative career choices. Securing long-term placements has required both an integrated rehabilitation and commercial approach on the part of the placement consultant and the availability of ongoing support, both to guide and support coping strategies and work adjustments and to respond to any emergent difficulties.

In spite of the unmet need and demonstrated value of specialist brain injury vocational rehabilitation, the required service development in the UK has been constrained by lack of funding. The quality requirement on vocational rehabilitation in the National Service Framework for Long-term Conditions (Department of Health, 2005) will hopefully provide a long overdue impetus for brain injury services to prioritise and develop their practice in assessing, preparing and supporting people with TBI in a return to previous or alternative occupation. Addressing the vocational needs of people with TBI who are unable to return to previous occupation is a complex process. We have outlined one UK service example but encourage the reader to explore other models of service provision which may be more suited to a particular service context.

Vocational rehabilitation after TBI in the UK requires joint working across brain injury services, Jobcentre Plus, Social Services and independent/voluntary providers. The inter-agency guidelines (RCP/JCP/BSRM, 2004) provide a framework for joint review of local service provision, both to identify gaps in service provision and to develop protocols to improve joint working. Given the complex needs of people with TBI it is vital that specialist vocational assessment and rehabilitation services are not developed in isolation but rather as one element of a network of services within an integrated, holistic approach. Services will then need to be evaluated to identify the most effective model of brain injury vocational rehabilitation within the UK context.

Recommended Reading

Carew, D. & Collumb, S. (in this volume). Supported employment and job coaching. In A. Tyerman & N.S. King (Eds.) *Psychological approaches to rehabilitation after traumatic brain injury*. Oxford: BPS Blackwell.

Reviews the application of the supported employment model after TBI – job coaching, job profiling/task analysis, neuropsychological interventions, workplace interventions, disengagement and follow-through support, plus an illustrative case example.

Fraser, R.T. & Clemmons, D.C. (Eds.) (2000). *Traumatic brain injury rehabilitation: Practical vocational, neuropsychological and psychotherapy interventions*. Boca Raton, FL: CRC Press.

Chapters covering neuropsychological assessment in vocational planning, counselling, use of assistive technology in vocational rehabilitation and four chapters on supported placements including a chapter on supported employment by Wehman *et al.*

Johnson, R. & Stoten, S. (in this volume). Return to previous employment. In A. Tyerman & N.S. King (Eds.) *Psychological approaches to rehabilitation after traumatic brain injury*. Oxford: BPS Blackwell.

Reviews outcome studies and predictors of return to work after TBI, support at work and practical advice about planning and supporting a return to previous employment after TBI, supported by an illustrative case example.

RCP/JCP/BSRM (2004). *Vocational assessment and rehabilitation after acquired brain injury. Inter-agency guidelines* (A. Tyerman & M.J. Meehan, Eds.). Inter-Agency Advisory Group on Vocational Rehabilitation after Brain Injury. London: Royal College of Physicians, Jobcentre Plus and British Society of Rehabilitation Medicine.

Provides background material (e.g. vocational outcome, approaches to vocational rehabilitation, service provision), proposed joint framework and inter-agency guidelines on provision of services for: return to previous occupation; vocational assessment; vocational rehabilitation; supported placement; and alternative occupation.

Useful Resources

www.jan.wvu.edu

The Job Accommodation Network (USA) website includes papers on brain injury 'Employees with Brain Injuries' (Accommodation and Compliance Series) and a Fact Sheet on 'Job Accommodations for People with Brain Injuries'.

www.jobcentreplus.gov.uk

Jobcentre Plus website includes information on services for people with disability (click on 'Customers' and 'Help for disabled people') – e.g. Access to Work, employment assessment, Work Preparation Programmes, New Deal for Disabled People, Job Introduction Scheme, and WORKSTEP supported employment.

www.vocationalrehabilitationassociation.org.uk

Website for the UK Vocational Rehabilitation Association which 'promotes rehabilitation and return to work for disabled people' – details of membership and Rehab Network magazine.

References

Abrams, D., Barker, L.T., Haffey, W. & Nelson, H. (1993). The economics of return to work for survivors of traumatic brain injury. Vocational services are worth the investment. *Journal of Head Trauma Rehabilitation*, *8*, 59–76.

Ben-Yishay, T., Silver, S.M., Piasetsky, E. & Rattok, J. (1987). Relationship between employability & vocational outcome after intensive holistic cognitive rehabilitation. *Journal of Head Trauma Rehabilitation*, 2, 35–48.

Bolton, B. & Roessler, R. (1986a). *Manual for the Work Personality Profile*. Fayetteville, AR: Arkansas Research & Training Center in Vocational Rehabilitation, University of Arkansas.

Bolton, B. & Roessler, R. (1986b). The Work Personality Profile: Factor scales, reliability, validity & norms. *Vocational Evaluation and Work Adjustment Bulletin*, *19*, 143–149.

British Society of Rehabilitation Medicine (2000). *Vocational rehabilitation: The way forward*. A Working Party Report. London: British Society of Rehabilitation Medicine.

Buffington, A.L.H. & Malec, J.F. (1997). The vocational rehabilitation continuum: Maximising outcomes though bridging the gap from hospital to community based services. *Journal of Head Trauma Rehabilitation*, *12*, 1–13.

Corrigan, J.D., Whiteneck, G. & Mellick, D. (2004). Perceived needs following traumatic brain injury. *Journal of Head Trauma Rehabilitation*, *19*, 205–216.

Crepeau, F. & Scherzer, P. (1993). Predictors and indicators of work status after traumatic brain injury: A meta-analysis. *Neuropsychological Rehabilitation*, *3*, 5–35.

Crewe, N.M. & Athelstan, G.T. (1981). Functional assessment in vocational rehabilitation: A systematic approach to diagnosis and goal-setting. *Archives in Physical Medicine & Rehabilitation*, *62*, 299–305.

Crewe, N.M. & Athelstan, G.T. (1984). *Functional Assessment Inventory: Manual*. Menonomie, Wisconsin, USA: Materials Development Center, Stout Vocational Rehabilitation Institute, University of Wisconsin-Stout.

Department of Health (2005). *The National Service Framework for Long-term Conditions*. London: Department of Health.

Department for Work and Pensions (2004). *Building capacity for work: A UK framework for vocational rehabilitation*. London: Department for Work and Pensions.

Deshpande, P. & Turner Stokes, L. (2004). Survey of vocational rehabilitation services available to people with acquired brain injury in the UK. In RCP/JCP/BSRM (2004).

Fraser, R.T., Clemmons, D.C. & McMahon, B.T. (1990). Vocational rehabilitation counselling. In J.S. Kreutzer & P. Wehman (Eds.), *Community integration following traumatic brain injury* (pp. 169–184). Baltimore: Paul H Brooks Publishing.

Groswasser, Z., Melamed, S., Agranov, E. & Keren, O. (1999). Return to work as an integrative measure following traumatic brain injury. *Neuropsychological Rehabilitation*, *9*, 493–504.

Jacobs, H.E. & De Mello, C. (1996). The Clubhouse model and employment following brain injury. *Journal of Vocational Rehabilitation*, *7*, 169–179.

Johnson, R. (1987). Return to work after severe head injury. *International Disability Studies*, *9*, 49–54.

Johnson, R. (1989). Employment after severe head injury: Do Manpower Services Commission schemes work? *Injury*, *20*, 5–9.

Johnson, R. (1998). How do people get back to work after severe head injury? A 10 year follow-up study. *Neuropsychological Rehabilitation*, *8*, 61–79.

Kreutzer, J.S., Marwitz, J.H., Walker, W., Sander, A., Sherer, M., Bogner, J., *et al.* (2003). Moderating factors in return to work and job stability after traumatic brain injury. *Journal of Head Trauma Rehabilitation*, *18*, *128–138*.

Malec, J.F. & Moessner, A.M. (2006). Replicated positive results for the VCC model of vocational intervention after ABI within the social model of disability. *Brain Injury*, *20*, 227–236.

Murphy, L., Chamberlain, E., Weir, J., Berry, A., Nathaniel-James, D. & Agnew, R. (2006). Effectiveness of vocational rehabilitation following acquired brain injury: Preliminary evaluation of a UK specialist rehabilitation programme. *Brain Injury*, *20*, 1119–1129.

Oddy, M., Coughlan, A., Tyerman, A. & Jenkins, D. (1985). Social adjustment after closed head injury: A further follow-up seven years after injury. *Journal of Neurology. Neurosurgery and Psychiatry*, *48*, 564–568.

Olver, J.H., Ponsford, J.L. & Curran, C.A. (1996). Outcome following traumatic brain injury: A comparison between 2 & 5 years after injury. *Brain Injury*, *10*, 841–48.

Ownsworth, T. & McKenna, K. (2004). Investigation of factors related to employment outcome following traumatic brain injury: A critical review and conceptual model. *Disability and Rehabilitation*, *26*, 765–784.

Partridge, T.M. (1996). An investigation into the vocational rehabilitation practices provided by brain injury services throughout the United Kingdom. *Work*, 7, 63–72.

Ponsford, J.L., Olver, J.H. & Curran, C. (1995). A profile of outcome: 2 years after traumatic brain injury. *Brain Injury*, 9, 1–10.

RCP/BSRM (2003). *Rehabilitation following acquired brain injury: national clinical guidelines* (L. Turner-Stokes, Ed.). London: Royal College of Physicians/British Society of Rehabilitation Medicine.

RCP/JCP/BSRM (2004). *Vocational assessment and rehabilitation after acquired brain injury. Inter-agency guidelines* (A. Tyerman & M.J. Meehan, Eds.). Inter-Agency Advisory Group on Vocational Rehabilitation after Brain Injury. London: Royal College of Physicians, Jobcentre Plus and British Society of Rehabilitation Medicine.

Rees, R.J. & Storry, C.J. (1997). *Plateaus and Summits: Transition to employment for people with acquired brain injury*. South Australia: School of Special Education and Disability Studies, Flinders University.

Sander, A.M., Kreutzer, J.S., Rosenthal, M., Delmonico, R. & Young, M.E. (1996). A multicenter longitudinal investigation of return to work community integration following traumatic brain injury. *Journal of Head Trauma Rehabilitation*, 11, 70–84.

Tyerman, A. (1987). *Self-concept and psychological change in the rehabilitation of the severely head injured person*. Unpublished doctoral thesis, University of London, UK.

Tyerman, A. (1999). *Working Out: A joint DOH / ES traumatic brain injury vocational rehabilitation project*. Project Report available from the author.

Tyerman, A. & Young, K. (1999). Vocational rehabilitation after severe traumatic brain injury: Evaluation of a specialist assessment programme. *Journal of the Application of Occupational Psychology to Employment and Disability*, 2(1), 31–41.

Tyerman, A. & Young, K. (2000). Vocational rehabilitation after severe traumatic brain injury: II Specialist interventions and outcomes. *Journal of the Application of Occupational Psychology to Employment and Disability*, 2(2), 13–20.

Tyerman, R., Tyerman, A., Howard, P. & Hadfield, C. (1986). *The Chessington OT Neurological Assessment Battery*. Nottingham: Nottingham Rehab.

Weddell, R., Oddy, M. & Jenkins, D. (1980). Social adjustment after rehabilitation: A two year follow-up of patients with severe head injury. *Psychological Medicine*, 10, 257–263.

Wehman, P., Kregel, J., Keyser-Marcus, L., Sherron-Targett, P., Campbell, L., West, M., *et al.* (2003). Supported employment for person with traumatic brain injury: A preliminary investigation of long-term follow-up costs and program efficiency. *Archives of Physical Medicine and Rehabilitation*, 84, 192–196.

Wehman, P., Kregel, J., Sherron, P., Nguyen, S., Kreutzer, J., Fry, R., *et al.* (1993). Critical factors associated with the successful employment placement of patients with severe traumatic brain injury. *Brain Injury*, 7, 31–44.

Wehman, P., Kreutzer, J., Wood, W., Morton, M.V. & Sherron, P. (1988). Supported work model for persons with traumatic brain injury: Toward job placement and retention. *Rehabilitation Counselling Bulletin*, 31, 298–312.

16

Supported Employment and Job Coaching

David Carew and Sylvia Collumb

Introduction

This chapter provides an overview of supported employment and the job coaching process for people with traumatic brain injury (TBI). Firstly we provide an overview of the contribution of job coaching to the process of vocational reintegration of people with traumatic brain injury. We then explore in more depth the stages and interventions of job coaching in supported employment. Finally we provide a supported employment case example that is profiled in a step-by-step manner. Each stage is discussed with respect to issues that arose and how these were overcome and their impact minimised.

It is beyond the scope of this review to examine the application of job coaching in other settings such as further education. This overview deals specifically with job coaching in the workplace. However, many of the procedures and issues discussed relate to other environments and can be tailored accordingly to reflect individual circumstances.

Return to work

Work provides many benefits such as income; an opportunity to use skills; develop social relationships; engage in directed activity and many other benefits. It is not surprising that its loss can have catastrophic consequences for the individual. This includes loss of earnings, diminished self-esteem and the disintegration of social and family support structures.

Reports of failure to return to work vary. However, return-to-work rates have typically been poor in the absence of vocational rehabilitation interventions. Neuman *et al.* (1996) found that at six months post-injury 37.5 per cent of previously occupied participants had failed to return to work. Similarly in a 10-year follow-up study Johnson (1998) reported that 34 per cent had failed to return to work or had an irregular work pattern. Interestingly, this study revealed that there was little change in work status after a period of two years since time of injury, suggesting that there is perhaps an optimal time for vocational rehabilitation interventions such as supported employment to be most effective. However, this does not mean that individuals cannot make progress towards work beyond this time span, though it is accepted that prospects diminish over time. Cattelani *et al.* (2002), in a study of 228 TBI survivors, reported lower re-employment rates among individuals as a result of injury severity and post-injury functioning, including cognitive and behavioural competence. In a seven-year follow-up German study of 43 patients of whom 24 had TBI, researchers reported persisting difficulties in maintaining work, highlighting the necessity for attention to be paid to the long-term consequences of reduced capacity for work (Pössl *et al.*, 2001).

The statistics for return to employment post-injury until recently were not particularly encouraging. This was for a number of reasons. Partly long-term studies were few, with little follow-up to track what happened to survivors of traumatic brain injury. It was commonly believed that while a significant number tried to return to work, many were unsuccessful (Brooks *et al.*, 1987). Of the few long-term studies that have been undertaken where poor return to work rates are reported, many highlight the lack of adequate support services to assist individuals in returning to the labour market. For a more detailed discussion of return to work please see chapter 14.

Individuals who survive traumatic brain injury are not immune to unemployment and indeed are further disadvantaged in the labour market as a consequence of their injuries. Therefore they require specialist services to assist them in reintegrating to employment opportunities. In one vocational outcome study researchers noted that unemployment rates increase significantly in individuals with a history of traumatic brain injury. In addition, the authors revealed that 'the rate of unemployment remains high for long periods of time, even if vocational rehabilitation services are provided . . .' (Ben-Yishay *et al.*, 1987).

It is perhaps disturbing that despite individuals receiving vocational rehabilitation services, unemployment rates can remain high among the TBI population. This has demanded that professionals engaged in the delivery of vocational services reconsider how best to reduce the risk of clients with TBI experiencing job loss after vocational services have been discontinued or reduced. The need to provide ongoing support and follow-through assistance to clients and employers has in essence reshaped the provision of vocational resettlement services for people with TBI.

In their paper, Wehman *et al.* (1993) note that vocational resettlement programmes that show most promise provide follow-through support to clients. They cite outcomes from a TBI vocational programme provided to clients in Baltimore in the United States. The programme acknowledges that the needs of clients change over time and there may be an ongoing requirement to provide a vocational service that is reflexive and supportive to both clients and employers alike. This partly reflects structural changes in the employment market in the past number of years where contract work is more the norm. Individuals typically no longer remain with an organisation for long periods of time. In comparison, the careers of individuals are most likely to be punctuated with many changes in roles with a high degree of mobility within the labour market.

Work practices and labour market opportunities

The ever-rapid pace of change in the labour market, coupled with the increasing reorganisation of work practices shaped by technological developments, has provided considerable challenges to vocational rehabilitation providers. Notable among these changes has been the evident shift from a role-dependent culture in organisations to one where people are expected to be flexible and task-focused multi-skilled workers. Improving the employability of people with traumatic brain injury is not easy given the changing trends in employment and the movement towards a knowledge-based workforce.

Yet despite this rather pessimistic picture there continue to be attempts to provide services that are responsive to the work resettlement needs of people who sustain traumatic brain injury. Some studies show encouraging results (West *et al.*, 1990). Usually these are programmes that offer early vocational evaluation and involve a needs-planning approach that is client centred, involving a multidisciplinary team.

Sourcing employment opportunities for people undergoing vocational rehabilitation is a demanding task. Access to current labour market information is important in this process. Some employment sectors are more buoyant and opportunities vary from sector to sector. Sometimes there is an assumption that people with brain injury are only suited to less skilled employment such as that sometimes found in the service sector. Our experience of resettling individuals in employment after traumatic brain injury would suggest that this is not particularly true for every case. In order to accommodate individual needs, there is a need to approach vocational resettlement from the perspective of matching individual ability and interests to the job, thus ensuring a good fit between the individual and the employment opportunity.

Supported Employment Model

Historical perspective

Any discussion about supported employment would be incomplete without alerting readers to the work of Marc Gold. The influence of his work is recognised internationally. Gold contends that it is possible to develop a framework for organising information and strategies for training. Underpinning this framework is a value system. Central to Gold's thesis is the belief that people should be trained to undertake marketable skills to enhance their employability. Other values espoused include the belief that an individual can demonstrate competence if the training meets their needs. Gold further adds that if a person is not learning, the responsibility for failure rests with the trainer for not using appropriate teaching methods. These principles fit well with a supported employment approach for people with TBI.

It would be reasonable to suggest that many of the values proposed are indeed the basis of good rehabilitation interventions. Equally it would be reasonable to hypothesise that Gold was very much from the positivist movement. It is important that these values are seen in both the prevailing political and social context of the time when they first emerged. Gold's ideas were in a sense a very deliberate attempt to depart from the typically traditional approach to vocational reintegration. This largely revolved around the belief that people with disabilities should be trained in large centres or enclaves. In the area of work, Gold proposed ideas that would later become a central cause of the international integration movement. Gold made sure that the value system underpinning supported employment optimised and promoted the abilities of people with disability. His statements about the ever-increasing and overuse of metrics in screening people for work would in a sense limit people in their efforts to achieve.

Perhaps his most regaled statement was that 'labelling is unfair and counterproductive' (Gold, 1980). The legacy left by Gold paved the way for the further development of supported employment. Today it is used widely as a preferred method of vocational integration as it allows for a wider range of job possibilities to be explored in contrast to the rather prescriptive 'train and place model'. The language associated with supported employment has changed in the intervening years and is sometimes termed Systematic Instruction; however, the mission remains the same, i.e. facilitation of full integration in the external world of work on an integrated basis.

Supported employment approach

The supported employment model of vocational integration usually employs the skills of a job coach to facilitate the process of matching the individual's abilities to possible job opportunities. Placement is usually undertaken with an employer in the open labour market. Once a position has been identified, either as an initial placement or actual paid position, the job coach will conduct a comprehensive analysis of the work site. The coach will also request a job specification that describes the duties and responsibilities of the placement or position. Where a job is being created or redesigned to accommodate the needs and abilities of the individual, the job coach will also assist in writing the job description. Subsequently this is agreed with the employer and the client.

As part of the process of evaluating the placement opportunity, the job coach will also conduct a thorough check of the health and safety arrangements in the workplace. It is essential that all parties are aware of who has responsibility for health and safety issues prior to the arrival of the client on the employer's or host company's premises.

To ensure that the benefits of supported placement opportunities are maximised and run smoothly, it is important that the job coach is aware of the expectations of the host company or employer. Underpinning this issue is the need to establish at the outset what role and expectations each party has. This also includes the client. The client should be involved as much as possible in the preparation stage. Doing so will help smooth out any problems that arise initially. More importantly, involvement and clear communication procedures will assist all parties to resolve difficulties that may arise in the course of the placement. Involvement of the client will also assist in helping them develop insight into their skills while helping them to develop effective management strategies to address problems as they arise.

The job coach will provide ongoing responsive, on-site and on-call support as required to the client, workplace colleagues and the organisation or employer. This is an open-ended commitment and one that is increasingly problematic for support organisations due to the difficulty of sustaining resource allocation over a lengthy period of time. Some organisations providing vocational rehabilitation services have entered into partnership arrangements with other providers in order to ensure that support is available in the longer term.

There exists a growing body of research that suggests that the supported employment model holds most promise (Brown *et al.*, 1976; Wehman *et al.*, 1993). Babineau (1998) highlights the benefits of early engagement in supported employment programmes for people with TBI, reporting a success of between 50 and 78 per cent for individuals who find it particularly difficult to get back to work. Others have been critical of traditional approaches to vocational rehabilitation for individuals with TBI, suggesting that approaches based on integrating cognitive rehabilitation with work skills have limited impact (Wall *et al.*, 1998). In contrast, the authors make the case for use of a supported employment model, which combines educational and psychosocial skills training, along with job support. West (1996), in a review of funding for supported employment programmes for people who experience TBI, highlights their positive impact on helping individuals get back to work. In the United Kingdom, encouraging findings from a supported employment programme lend support for this approach to assisting people with TBI return to employment. Tyerman and Young (2000) reported a 50 per cent progression rate to employment with a further 12.5 per cent of programme leavers entering a therapeutic earnings placement, 22.5 to voluntary work and a further 5 per cent to vocational education. This programme is described in chapter 15. At one-year follow-up 51 per cent had sustained employment or training, providing positive evidence for the use of a supported employment approach. Research undertaken in a 10-year follow-up study also highlights the role of in-work training as a part of a supported employment approach and provides further evidence that this model can be effective in helping individuals with TBI to make the transition to work (Johnson, 1998).

Our experience would suggest that a combination approach that includes a period of preparation coupled with a work trial or work placement supported by a job coach and other relevant professionals has the effect of enhancing the success of the outcome for people who sustain traumatic brain injury. Figure 16.1 provides an overview of the key stages and elements involved in the process of operating a supported employment model with people who sustain traumatic brain injury.

Job Coaching and Vocational Reintegration

In the past 15 years, job coaching has attracted significant attention in the traumatic brain injury return-to-work literature. Our own experience of operating a supported employment service for people with traumatic brain injury in Glasgow, Scotland has provided a strong evidence-base for this approach. Outcome rates for service participants using a supported employment model were in the range of 69 per cent with a similar retention rate. Injury severity ranged from mild to severe. The majority of programme participants were in the moderate to severe category of injury

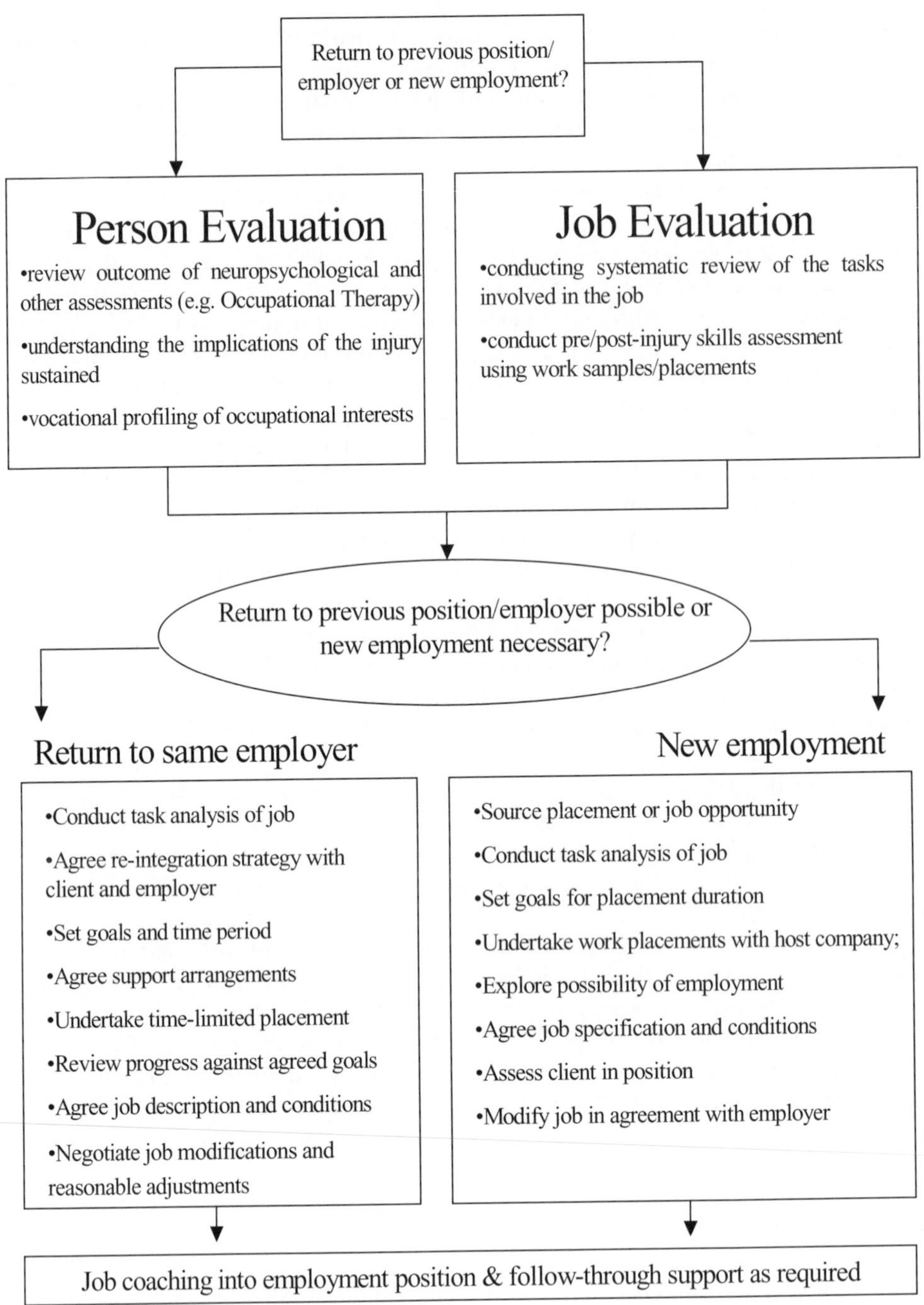

Figure 16.1 Supported employment model for people with TBI – job coaching in the workplace

severity as measured by the Glasgow Coma Scale and duration of post-traumatic amnesia. There was approximately a 50 per cent split between those in employment before injury and unemployed at time of injury. For both groups return-to-work rates were comparative. Significant among the factors associated with achieving positive outcomes was the degree of individual insight and malleability of participants or willingness to engage in vocational rehabilitation.

Additional individual factors which moderated the prospects of a successful return to work or vocational education in the Glasgow programme provided by Momentum Scotland included personal expectations of employment, motivation, attitudes of significant others, level of alcohol intake pre- and post-injury and the existence of premorbid conditions such as mental health difficulties. External factors included employer support policies, supervisor and co-worker understanding. The prevailing labour market conditions did not seem to have any detrimental impact on placement rates, nor did the size of employer. Our experience suggests that employers generally welcomed the support available once they understood what was expected of them and where it could be managed without too much interruption to workflows.

The active involvement of the job coach on site was viewed as a positive way to support employment re-entry for individuals with TBI and we now discuss the specific functions associated with this role within the return-to-work team. Similarly, the rehabilitation team employed an integrated case management approach using a system of individual programme planning to assist the return-to-work process for programme participants. A shared understanding among team members of rehabilitation goals, with high user participation in goal setting coupled with interdisciplinary team working, contributed significantly to placement success.

Function of the job coach

In general terms the function of the job coach is to assist people who are severely disabled achieve competitive employment (Burke, 1996). Stapleton *et al.* (1989) define job coaching as the process of 'teaching traumatically brain injured persons an actual job to be performed in the workplace'. This essentially involves a number of steps or stages:

- reviewing the outcome of neuropsychological and other assessments (e.g. occupational therapy);
- understanding the implications of the injury sustained;
- vocational profiling of occupational interests;
- placement or job opportunity sourcing;
- conducting systematic review of the tasks involved in the job;
- conducting pre/post-injury skills assessment using work samples/placements;
- undertaking work placements with host company;
- job coaching into employment position;
- follow-through support as required.

Before describing in detail the various stages of the application of job coaching skills in the workplace we will review the professional skills necessary for a job coach to be effective in their role.

Job coaching skills

A question that is sometimes asked concerns what skills and qualifications a person needs to work as a job coach. In recent times new qualifications have been developed to assist in the professional training of job coaches. Increasingly, job coaches have to possess a wide repertoire of skills in order to meet the varied demands of resettling people with brain injury in work. As it would be impossible for a job coach to have knowledge of all occupational sectors, it is necessary for job coaches to have a varied range of generic job skills or competencies, some of which are described below:

- ability to adapt to new situations;
- ability to acquire and integrate knowledge quickly and from a variety of sources;
- good communication skills, both verbal and written;
- good analytical and problem-solving skills;
- appreciation of relevant health and safety legislation;
- knowledge of traumatic brain injury; its effects and implications for employment;
- varied occupational experiences in a variety of sectors;
- good marketing and negotiation skills;
- employment market awareness;
- ability to work in a multidisciplinary team;
- ability to drive – possess licence and transport;
- ability to be flexible in working hours and location

As described, job coaches require a number of specific or core competences to be effective practitioners. Broadly speaking, there are four areas of activity that a job coach may be involved in while acting on behalf of the client in assisting their reintegration to the employment market:

- mediator;
- trainer;
- advocate;
- educator.

Most typically, job coaches act as mediators. Here the job coach seeks to gain understanding of the problem that has arisen while the client is on placement or in employment. Resolution will involve the job coach, client and employer in a number of follow-up actions such as developing strategies to enable task completion. In this situation the job coach assumes an advocacy role.

The job coach may also have to advise on the use of particular strategies that the client and/or employer need to adopt for more effective work performance. This may involve the job coach acting as educator, providing information sessions on the effects of brain injury for employees of the organisation. More specifically, the intervention following identification of the problem may involve providing additional or new training to the client as the job may have changed or new tasks been introduced. Here the job coach is acting as trainer.

Specifically, job coaches will carry out such tasks as helping clients prepare job applications and organise mock interviews with employers. Sometimes job coaches will also arrange consultations with welfare officers to provide advice to clients on finance issues. Other tasks include organising induction to the host placement organisation for the client; helping the client to source information on appropriate travel options; analysing tasks associated with a particular job; and training the client at the commencement of placement.

In summary, job coaches require a high degree of flexibility and responsiveness to attend to the various demands placed on their skill base. This can sometimes mean being able to critically appraise a situation and respond quickly with an appropriate approach. Of equal importance, though not shown above, is the need for job coaches to have strong abilities in marketing the skills of people with traumatic brain injury. Essentially this will involve the four aspects of mediation, advocacy, training and raising awareness through education.

Job Profiling and Task Analysis

The process of job profiling and task analysis is central to ensuring a good match between the person and the job or placement. The purpose of conducting job profiling and task analysis is to identify the knowledge, skills and attitudinal components from each of the job duties to promote effectiveness on the job.

Job profiling

Job profiling involves the process of gathering information that describes what the job is about and includes such things as entry requirements or training and qualifications required. It will also provide an overview of occupational sectors where employment opportunities may be available. As such, job profiling may be viewed as part of a broader process that relates to career decision-making or ascertaining occupational interests. It may be appropriate as part of job profiling to gather information on the specific interests of the individual. This may be necessary when return to a previous position is not possible, or where the individual has had little or no work experience.

In younger clients where their most recent experience was school, it is necessary to undertake a period of vocational exploration with the individual to assist them in making informed decisions about employment opportunities. There are many commercially available career interest packages obtainable from a variety of publishers. Some of these are pencil-and-paper based in terms of administration, while others are in computer assisted formats. Costs vary and it is sometimes better to use presentation formats that allow for the particular needs of individuals. For guidance purposes it is suggested that the format presentation needs to be flexible. In our experience, administration can place considerable demands on the client's attention and concentration abilities.

Information gained from this process should be combined with assessment data from other sources. These include feedback from participation in work experience placements; reports on performance from a previous or last employer at the time of injury; neuropsychological findings; performance on work samples; and so on. The importance of considering all available information is central to good vocational rehabilitation programme planning. For an authoritative overview on pre- and post-injury skill analysis, please see Krankowski (1993) and Thomas (1991).

Task analysis

On completion of the information-gathering stage about the individual's occupational interests, it is then necessary to source a suitable placement with a potential host employer. Before this can happen, it is necessary for the job coach to discuss with the client and the vocational rehabilitation team what the aim of the placement will be and decide on the expected outcomes. This can be a difficult stage as expectations may differ. This may be due to limited or diminished insight of the client. It is the task of the rehabilitation team to support the job coach and the client to agree a viable plan that meets the agreed objectives.

Each member of the rehabilitation team has a contribution to make in this process. For example, the neuropsychologist can be instrumental in helping the client and the job coach to decide on appropriate strategies to overcome problems or barriers that might be encountered in the workplace. The contribution of the neuropsychologist is discussed later in this section. Similarly, in some services it might not only be a neuropsychologist who suggests strategies for the workplace. In other services this could be an occupational therapist or occupational psychologist and might on occasion draw usefully on the advice of the physiotherapist for a physical problem or speech and language therapist for a communication difficulty.

The process of task analysis allows the job coach to determine what the skills requirements are for each task as well as gaining insight into the knowledge base required to carry out the task effectively. Each aspect of the job is broken down into its constituent parts, sometimes referred to as task analysis. The purpose of conducting this exercise is to break down each part into 'an achievable or learning component' (Wehman, 1981).

The job coach will also attempt to identify the behavioural competencies required of the client to carry out each task. In the context of retraining people with traumatic brain injury this aspect needs careful consideration. Often it is problems with work-related behavioural skills which impact most on the prospects of successful employment integration and lead to job separation. Ultimately the job coach is attempting to ensure that the best match or fit is found between the client and the prospective job and organisational environment.

Information about the requirements of the job is collected in a variety of ways. Here the relationship with the host placement organisation or employer is important. Gaining access to the worksite can assist the job coach to make an informed decision as to the likely suitability of the work environment. Observation is one of the most common forms of gathering information on the tasks and duties associated with particular jobs. The opportunity to spend time on-site speaking with workers already doing the job can provide valuable information on the complexity of tasks. It can also provide information on the type of training that may be required to help the client to perform the tasks effectively. Similarly, the foundations for supportive working relationships with supervisors and co-workers can be established

Information collection

Other forms of data collection can include desk research. This may involve a review of information gathered, such as job previews or specifications from the employer. TBI individuals should be encouraged to engage in job search activities to encourage independence. While there are no rules as such concerning who the job coach should contact or liaise with in the organisation, there is a need to ensure that all relevant employees that may have contact with the client are aware of the client's role and other issues as necessary. Prior to releasing information to an employer, co-workers or any third party, the job coach should secure the consent of the individual.

In matters of disclosure and information sharing, individuals should be aware of their duties contained in the Data Proctection and Freedom of Information Acts.

In larger organisations it may be appropriate to involve occupational health physicians in the reintegration process. The role of occupational health physicians and nurses can be particularly helpful in facilitating a managed return to work for the employee with brain injury. Co-worker involvement can be helpful to the individual in re-engaging with work activities and settling into the organisation. The human resource department can assist with such matters and can facilitate in a practical sense the dissemination of relevant information through line management prior to the arrival of the client.

It is acknowledged that not all organisations have a human resource department and may operate less formal personnel arrangements. Indeed the majority of organisations in the United Kingdom may be classed as small to medium-sized enterprises. Irrespective of organisation size, it is critical that a named representative of the organisation is appointed to handle the arrangements and liaise with the job coach and unit manager or supervisor as required.

Neuropsychological Interventions

The neuropsychologist may be the first point of contact following referral for vocational rehabilitation. Within the brain injury rehabilitation team the neuropsychologist plays a key role in the identification and management of cognitive, behavioural and emotional constraints. Input from team members can also assist by providing support in the management of such difficulties. It is the strength of the interdisciplinary team to help the individual make progress towards rehabilitation goals, including the resumption of purposeful activities like employment. Occupational therapists and occupational psychologists, physiotherapists and speech and language therapists can all make an important contribution.

As noted earlier, the neuropsychologist may provide advice and guidance to the job coach on such issues as cognitive strategies for overcoming memory deficits; problem identification to identify the relative cognitive and psycho-social demands of tasks; best methods of approach for work-based counselling interventions or helping the client with adjustment issues. The neuropsychologist may also support the job coach in providing awareness and education sessions for the host organisation on issues such as disability management in the workplace.

In addition to providing support in a work-based setting, the neuropsychologist can also provide support to clients external to the work environment. This can provide a valuable opportunity for the client to reflect on their progress and discuss any issues as required. It is sometimes useful to conduct reviews off-site and in conjunction with the job coach. This allows for new strategies to be formulated and involves the client as much as possible in the decision-making process. The neuropsychologist can also provide ongoing assessment information that is valuable in terms of marking progress and planning new approaches as needed. For a comprehensive review of the role of neuropsychology in vocational reintegration please see Kreutzer and Wehman (1990): *Community Integration after Traumatic Brain Injury.*

Work placement and employment contract

The preparation stage of the process is complete once the host company or employer has agreed the expectations, including the terms and conditions. The details of these are normally set out in a contract document. The placement contract contains details of the hours of attendance; payment details if appropriate; duties and responsibilities; contact names in case of difficulty; duration of the placement as well as time points for reviews. The contract will also state the start and finish dates of the placement. The client will sign this with the host company or employer.

Benefits of placements

There are many benefits that can arise from participation in placements with host organisations provided they are well organised and all stakeholders' expectations are clear from the outset. Essentially placements provide a number of opportunities for all parties involved in the agreement. These may be described from three different perspectives as shown in Table 16.1.

While it is acknowledged that there are many benefits for employers from facilitating placements, it is also important to acknowledge issues that can be potential barriers. It is the role of the job coach to address each issue and support the employer in developing awareness through education about traumatic brain injury and its management. Some of these issues include:

- fear that the client may be unreliable;
- feelings that they are not equipped to cope with a person with brain injury;
- concerns about insurance cover and liability;
- fear of client compromising quality if the client makes mistakes;
- concern about not having resource available to provide support;
- concerns about having to do additional paperwork;
- unsure of the benefits for the organisation;
- lack of time to offer support due to organisational demands.

Table 16.1 Benefits of work placements

Client	• Opportunity allows the client to test out new skills and practice in an environment that is supportive. • Provides the client with the opportunity to rebuild self-confidence. • Allows the client to explore the suitability and viability of a particular occupational area, job or employment sector. • Helps the client to gain insight to their abilities and needs through the mechanism of regular reviews with the job coach. • Provides the client with real-life work experience in an integrated setting.
Host organisation	• Provides the host organisation with the opportunity to fill vacancies with trained people through support of the job coach. • Access to support from job coach as needs arise. • Fulfils community responsibility obligations. • Helps organisation meets its legal responsibilities as per the provisions under the Disability Discrimination Act (1995) and the Disability Rights Commission Act (1999). • Helps the organisation to recognise diversity in its workforce. • Assists the organisation in meeting its business objectives by having trained and competent staff.
Rehabilitation team	• Provides team with better insight into the learning potential of the client. • Helps identify individual training needs. • Assists in validating the suitability of the employment environment. • Allows for on-site intervention as required. • Gives a realistic assessment of the client's abilities. • Provides the opportunity to test the client in a variety of situations. • Helps identify possible job opportunities.

Workplace Interventions

The problems that people with traumatic brain injury encounter are well documented in the return-to-work literature. Stapleton and her associates (1989) in Maryland, in a survey of problems identified by job coaches, noted six major problems:

- slow acquisition of job skills;
- verbal memory;
- judgement;
- visual memory;
- inflexibility of thinking;
- anxiety.

Our experience would tend to support Stapleton's findings. We would also add a number of other important factors that may affect work performance. These include:

- inability to work without structure;
- prioritising work duties and tasks;
- distractions and reduced ability to engage in tasks simultaneously;
- diminished communication and assertiveness.

Interventions designed to address these issues must acknowledge the context of the workplace. Involvement of staff or co-workers can help in the design of interventions but more importantly can help to implement them, particularly when the job coach has disengaged from the workplace. Generating solutions to problems identified requires a high degree of creativity on the part of the job coach and the ability to involve others in problem-solving activities. It is very important that the client is involved in this process from the outset. This will help promote the coping skills of the client.

Perhaps one of the more difficult areas of vocational rehabilitation and job coaching concerns addressing psychosocial issues in the workplace. While it is often possible to generate cognitive solutions to solve problems such as route finding, it is arguably more difficult to remediate psychosocial issues. Frustration, distractibility or a clash with supervisors or co-workers because of inappropriate behaviours can lead to conflict in the workplace (Lynch, 1983). It is therefore essential that the job coach have access to additional support. Access to a Work Psychologist can be an effective source of support for in-work issues. Also the wider rehabilitation team can assist in reviewing progress and can suggest methods of approach for emerging problems.

Workplace solutions

It is beyond the scope of this chapter to provide a comprehensive discussion of design of workplace solutions. However, a number of points on good practice are worthy of note. Generating solutions requires a clear definition of the problem. It is also important to ask the client to describe how they see and describe the problem. As a guide, the job coach should adopt a practical approach to resolving the problem. Over-complicated or lengthy procedures are likely to confuse the client as they may have short-term memory problems. It is also useful for the job coach to have insight to the preferred learning style of the client. Information from previous work placements and findings from neuropsychological assessments can be helpful in determining the learning style of the client.

Once the problem and learning style have been defined, it is then necessary to identify the constituent parts of the task in hand. Previous efforts in analysing the tasks of the placement or job can be used here to identify what part of the task the client is experiencing problems with. Whatever solution is ultimately agreed, it is essential that the client fully understands and that it is practical. It may be helpful for the client to translate the solution and record it in their own words.

Table 16.2 Workplace problems and interventions

Problem	Intervention
Inability to work without structure	Timetable/schedule/task list
Route-finding problems in retail outlet	Visual route-map of shop layout
Communication difficulties	Regular reviews/colour-coding system
Punctuality/timekeeping	Self-monitoring form/alarm
Verbal memory	Checklists
Anxiety	Assistance with coping strategies
Slow acquisition of skills	Use task analysis as learning points or components

This will help them recognise it when required. Some possible solutions might involve improving the physical environment for the individual or it may involve designing support materials to enable the individual to carry out a task effectively. Table 16.2 identifies some problems encountered in the workplace and possible interventions.

Job retention

Where a client is returning to a previous position, it may be necessary to undertake a full evaluation of all the tasks and duties contained in the job description. Following this evaluation, it may be necessary for the job coach to recommend a full or part redesign of the individual's job. This may involve negotiating with the employer for a redrawing of the job description to accommodate the change in ability. The revised job description may contain some of the original duties along with some new tasks that may have been reallocated from another position. It is the skill of the job coach to manage this process effectively whereby the employer is able to retain the skills of a valued employee and the client is able to retain employment, albeit altered to reflect the changes in their circumstances.

Returning to a previous position is not always easy and is arguably sometimes more difficult than taking up a new position with another employer. This can be due to anxieties about the perceptions of colleagues, self-perception, client expectations and concerns if it does not work out successfully. In order to reduce the impact of expressed fears, it may be useful for the client to visit the workplace with support on a number of occasions. It is suggested that if such anxieties are significant or persist, it may be prudent to organise a similar placement in another organisation. However, this is not always possible or desirable, particularly if the other organisation is a competitor of the client's employer.

In order to circumvent this problem, it is perhaps worth considering organising a different placement for the client. As such, it does not have to mirror exactly the duties of the client's original employment. In contrast, the alternative placement is used as an opportunity to help the client build up confidence in their abilities and to experience the work environment in a relatively safe way. Following a period of experience, it may then be possible to try a placement with the client's employer.

Workplace health and safety

One of the many challenges facing the job coach is that of creating safe working environments. Health and safety is of the utmost importance in all tasks or duties carried out in the context of the workplace. It is therefore essential that the client is aware of all aspects relating to health and safety.

All risks identified should either be eliminated or reduced so not to cause harm to the client or any other employee. Where a health and safety issue or risk is identified, the job coach should advise the employer or host organisation immediately. It is the responsibility of the organisation to ensure the health and safety of all persons on its premises. Thereafter, the health and safety officer of the organisation should conduct a comprehensive risk analysis assessment. Only when this has been completed and the risk eliminated should the client undertake tasks as per those outlined in the placement agreement or job description with the host organisation or employer. As part of initial preparations for placing clients with host organisations, the job coach should request a copy of the Employer Liability Insurance Certificate. Normally this is displayed prominently in the employer's premises.

Disengagement and Follow-through Support

Supported employment models are based on a number of key principles that guide the process of ensuring a good fit between the individual and the job. This process is underpinned by review structures that involve ongoing assessment. Wehman (1988) notes two aspects to the process, namely, supervisor and client evaluation. The job coach role is to facilitate the review process at particular predefined time points. Checklists that detail different aspects of employability (for example, core skills such as problem solving, trainability, communications) can be helpful in providing an objective view of the client's progress.

As the client gains in confidence and becomes competent performing the duties or tasks, the job coach can begin the process of disengagement. This is sometimes termed 'fading'. Burke (1996) notes that 'the client's work performance throughout the fading process can be viewed as one predictor of their ability to retain the job independently'. Essentially this involves reducing the level of support on a gradual scale from that first needed at induction. The provision of follow-through support is important in enhancing the potential for success of the placement. As part of the disengagement process, the job coach should meet with the employer to agree follow-through arrangements. Both the client and the co-workers should be made aware of whatever arrangements are made. The client should also be encouraged to seek assistance where necessary and make contact with the job coach.

Job coaching outcomes

Why are some job coaching efforts more successful than others? Why do some work and some not? What factors are predictive of success? These are questions that we have often debated, yet each time have come up with different responses. The reason for this, we feel, relates to the fact that not only is everyone who sustains head injury different, but the combination of factors such as personality, previous training and employment experiences, self-expectation and that of others, life events and so on makes each person unique. Stapleton *et al.* (1989) note that 'it is often pre-morbid factors that were exacer-bated by the head injury' that have contributed to placement termination or job loss. There are a number of reasons why job-coaching people with traumatic brain injury may not be successful. These include:

- deterioration in individual's health;
- persistence of alcohol or substance misuse;
- pursuance of compensation claim;
- instability in domestic situation or relationship;
- welfare benefits higher than paid employment;
- starting over – pay less than previous salary;
- significant feeling of loss compared to previous position;
- change in organisational priorities;
- diminished motivation to find paid employment;
- fear of failure and resulting embarrassment
- loss of belief in ability to do the tasks of the job role.

In the final part of this chapter we turn our attention to a supported employment case example to illustrate the process and stages described earlier. Some reasons for the choice of case example are provided, along with a discussion of the key learning points. We conclude with a summary and provide some thoughts on future directions for the use of supported employment approaches in TBI vocational rehabilitation.

Rehabilitation Case Example

The following case example will illustrate the process of coaching a person with TBI in the workplace where return to the original job was not possible following modifications to duties and late on following their injury (about five years). The case provides an overview of the stages involved in assisting the individual find and keep employment, with specific reference to the role of the job coach using a supported employment approach. There are a number of reasons why we chose to profile this case example. First and probably most significantly, it illustrates the point that despite a significant time interval between injury and contact with vocational services, it was still possible to achieve a positive outcome. Second, the individual sustained traumatic brain injuries in the severe range with significant resulting neurological, cognitive and behavioural difficulties. This combination provided many personal challenges, not least for the individual but also for the vocational rehabilitation team. Third, the case demonstrates what can be achieved through interdisciplinary team and interagency working. Above all, the case illustrates the importance of placing the individual at the centre of the vocational rehabilitation process to enable informed choice with the opportunity for self-advocacy and empowerment.

Case 16.1

Background

Jennifer, aged 26, was a trainee secretary working for a recruitment company who sustained a traumatic brain injury as a pedestrian in a road traffic accident. At the time of injury Jennifer was living in the family home with her mother and sister. As a consequence of the accident she sustained severe head and orthopaedic injuries. CT scan on admission revealed the presence of sub-dural haematoma for which neurosurgical intervention for removal was required. Although her Glasgow Coma Scale score was unknown, the length of post-traumatic amnesia was estimated in excess of one month, indicating a very severe injury and one which was likely to result in significant disability.

Subsequently a left hemiparesis was evident, as were post-traumatic seizures. Following the acute surgical management stage, Jennifer was transferred to a specialist national rehabilitation facility to continue functional rehabilitation. She subsequently progressed to a specialist brain injury rehabilitation unit for input where she received speech and language assistance, clinical psychology to aid adjustment and cognitive rehabilitation. Physiotherapy and occupational therapy services were also provided to improve mobility and prepare for independent living. A full neuropsychological evaluation was conducted, which revealed a number of motor, cognitive and behavioural difficulties. These included diminished insight, poor planning ability, problems with short-term memory, reduced attention span and difficulty initiating new activities. These difficulties were compounded by restricted mobility as a consequence of a left sided hemiparesis.

As part of the discharge planning process at the brain injury rehabilitation unit, employment rehabilitation needs were discussed with Jennifer to determine how her return to work could be managed. Following an extensive period of rehabilitation, Jennifer was referred by the clinical psychologist to a specialist brain injury vocational rehabilitation provider for assessment with a view to resuming work activities. Jennifer had not worked since injury and was unsure if she could return to her former position. It was unclear if her previous employer would be amenable in rehiring Jennifer, as it was over four years since she was employed with the company. As a result she required assistance to retrain and find suitable employment.

Rehabilitation programme – work trials

Prior to Jennifer being offered a new employment position, she participated in a total of five work placements. These were organised by the job coach. Jennifer commenced her first work placement after completing a pre-preparation programme for work. This lasted for a period of nine months. This programme comprised group and individual work supported by the job coach, psychologist and work skills facilitator. The purpose of these activities was to help Jennifer develop better self-awareness, relearn core work skills and develop compensatory strategies to overcome and manage the cognitive difficulties she was experiencing. The psychologist and job coach provided vocational rehabilitation counselling sessions to help Jennifer develop coping strategies in preparation for re-entry to the workplace. These support arrangements continued on entry and throughout each work trial.

Jennifer completed a series of short time-limited work trials or placements. These included placement with a bank, a local authority, health board, library and NHS Trust. In each placement, tasks and duties were agreed with input from Jennifer, the employer and job coach. On each occasion the job coach carried out a workplace evaluation supported by the team psychologist. Each placement was viewed as a progression, with new tasks and demands introduced gradually as Jennifer gained confidence. The focus of these placements was to help Jennifer gain insight to what kind of work she was both interested in and could perform competently. These placements also provided the opportunity to try out some of the strategies she gained from the pre-preparation programme and tailor these to new situations.

Progress reviews

Periodic reviews were conducted in each placement to determine progress. the job coach recorded information about the tasks Jennifer could perform effectively and these were then used to build a skills profile to form a curriculum vitae for prospective employers. Throughout the placements the job coach provided a number of worksite interventions to help Jennifer cope with the demands of work. These included:

- introduction of checklists to assist the organisation and priority of work tasks to allow a smooth workflow that would not overwhelm Jennifer;

Continued

- on-site awareness sessions on the effects and management of brain injury for the host employer and co-workers;
- mentoring support for Jennifer to develop procedures for work tasks that could be accessed easily;
- identifying peer support mechanisms in the workplace for times when the job coach was not on-site;
- negotiating a job description and liaising with Jobcentre Plus for funding to access employment;
- providing a communication link to the vocational rehabilitation team and arranging additional support from team members.

Supported employment placement

As part of the ongoing review of Jennifer's vocational rehabilitation plan, she expressed that she liked the work she was doing at the NHS Trust and expressed a desire to find work at the NHS Trust. In consultation with the human resource manager a potential job vacancy was identified. The job coach followed this up with a visit to the worksite to conduct a job analysis. Subsequently it was agreed that Jennifer would be given the opportunity for a time-limited trial period. This was used as a period of extended assessment to ascertain if there was an appropriate job match. Owing to the nature of her difficulties, Jennifer was eligible for sponsorship through the Workstep Programme to help her return to the labour market. Jennifer was also eligible for funding to assist with transport costs as she could not use public transport and required a taxi to and from work. This was provided under the Access to Work programme. With the assistance of the job coach and the office manager, adaptations to the workplace involved a lockable records trolley to enable Jennifer to have a 'mobile office'. This afforded her greater independence in the workplace.

Gradually Jennifer was able to build up her attendance hours. Some tasks she found easier than others. Jennifer particularly enjoyed filing and could do this for extended periods. She also enjoyed writing up notes and her speed and accuracy had improved following the IT skills certificates she had successfully completed while at the vocational rehabilitation centre. Other tasks such as maintaining the business manager's diary required a level of planning, organising and decision making. Jennifer found this difficult. Following discussion, the job description was reviewed and amended to include tasks that she could undertake. Jennifer qualified for Supported Placement Sponsorship, as she was competent in approximately 50 per cent of the tasks. A sponsor was arranged and, with the subsidy, the NHS Trust employed someone to cover the remaining tasks. At the end of the extended assessment period, Jennifer achieved full-time employment status and received all staff benefits. Prior to taking employment, terms and conditions were agreed. These included salary, hours, timekeeping and attendance, holidays, sick pay entitlement, time off for appointments, and pension schemes.

Ongoing support and disengagement

Over the following months the job coach provided ongoing support to Jennifer and her employer. Specifically this included guidance on learning about the workplace culture and expectations. Although Jennifer was slower to learn new skills, her accuracy and high standards often compensated for her lack of speed. She still requires some support with her tasks but her colleagues provide this. Jennifer has settled well in her new position and is keen to develop her range of skills further. She has also made a number of changes in her lifestyle such as quitting smoking and adopting a healthier lifestyle. The job coach agreed a disengagement strategy with Jennifer and her supervisor. This involved reducing the number of site visits, although the job coach could be contacted if a need arose.

Outcome and follow-through support

Following the intervention of the job coach supported by the rehabilitation team, Jennifer has achieved and sustained full-time employment and is still in employment. She continues to gain more skills in the workplace and has recently visited the learning resource centre where she works to avail herself of further training and development opportunities. Achieving this positive outcome has not been without its difficulties. Changes in family circumstances meant that Jennifer had to take some time off due to her mother's illness. Jennifer needed encouragement and support to help her cope over this difficult time. She was able to return to work later. Jennifer is no longer in contact with the vocational rehabilitation team but is aware that she can contact them if she requires assistance.

Reflection on practice

Each individual who sustains a traumatic brain injury is affected in different ways and a complex range of interrelated factors determines their adjustment and recovery. These include degree of insight, malleability, personal expectation and available support in the work context. The case described highlights a number of pertinent points. First, there is no substitute for thorough evaluation to assist the vocational rehabilitation planning process. Second, a deficit model is unhelpful. A good understanding of the medical aspects of TBI is important but should not be overstated. In contrast, emphasis should be placed on maximising residual ability. A third point relates to early engagement with vocational services. In this case there was a significant time interval. However, the outcome illustrates that gains can be made up to five years and in our experience longer periods of time. Fourth, the availability of on-site support provided in a responsive but non-intrusive manner was critical in achieving successful placement. Equally, engaging the employer in problem solving and proposing solutions is important and should be encouraged where possible. Employers know their business well. Involving them will produce good results. Finally, it is important to note that there can and will be setbacks along the way. These are all part of the learning and reintegration process. The issue is not so much that setbacks occur but how the team responds. Creativity and support are key to remaining on track, helping the individual to feel secure and making progression. The ultimate aim is to promote stability in the employment situation and equip the individual to cope with changing situations.

Future directions

The concept of job coaching is relatively new for people with traumatic brain injury in the United Kingdom. Yet despite this, results are encouraging. Some good examples include the Working Out programme in Aylesbury, England and the services provided by organisations like Momentum in Scotland and Rehab UK. International research also provides encouraging support for the use of supported employment within the context of vocational rehabilitation services (Chesnut *et al.*, 1999; Wehman *et al.*, 1989). It may be argued, though, that job coaching is expensive. Intuitively this would be reasonable to assume. However, recent research examining the cost and benefits over a long period provides compelling evidence for the long-term economic value of supported employment programmes (Wehman *et al.*, 2003). Over time the financial benefits for individuals who sustain TBI exceed the costs associated with supported employment services. However, the social and economic costs of a person not being engaged in meaningful activity are considerable by comparison.

While job coaching has shown encouraging results, there are many challenges ahead. As we observed in our introduction, the nature of work has changed and continues to change. This will inevitably place significant demands on people with traumatic brain injury and on employers and supported employment providers. Increasing mobility of the labour force with increased competitiveness, global markets, short-term contract culture and the existence of a more highly skilled workforce may bring additional pressures. Employers and rehabilitation services will have to work in partnership in order to respond effectively to meet the employment needs of people with traumatic brain injury in this changing context.

There is an increasing need to ensure that vocational rehabilitation services are available for people with traumatic brain injury. Recent government employment and welfare legislation has prioritised welfare-to-work programmes and lifelong learning. Vocational rehabilitation providers will need to operate their services in response to changes in employment and welfare legislation. Career development issues for people with traumatic brain injury have not received a lot of attention in the literature. However, this is an area that will need support through the provision of appropriate services in the longer term if people with traumatic brain injury are to retain or avail themselves of new employment opportunities in the changing labour market.

Summary and Conclusion

In our overview we mentioned the influence of Marc Gold and the evolution of supported employment. The vocational reintegration of people with traumatic brain injury is a complex process, though greatly rewarding for teams charged with the responsibility. The supported employment process offers many people with brain injury the chance to re-engage in productive and gainful work activities. The job coach, working within the broader multidisciplinary team, plays a pivotal role in empowering the person with head injury to develop effective self-management skills.

The complexity depends on the inter-relationship of many factors and it requires all the skills of the respective team members to be mobilised in partnership to realise a successful outcome. The availability of natural, technical and professional supports is critical to achieving sustainable outcomes. This not only applies to vocational success but to broader community integration and social inclusion of a person with brain injury. Return to productive activities such as work by many people who are unfortunate to sustain injury is viewed as a benchmark of recovery. For this reason and for many others, efforts to redress such deficits and allow participation in work activities to be optimised are critical to the well-being of the individual.

Future research should focus on evaluating outcomes and integrate new knowledge about methods into rehabilitation interventions. Rehabilitation providers must also ensure that services remain relevant to respond to the changing needs of people in an ever-changing labour market. Managing career development and lifelong learning advice are areas worthy of further exploration and development. This work is necessary to help people with brain injury remain employable throughout their most productive years. This is a worthy undertaking in view of the significant number of people who sustain brain injuries in the United Kingdom each year.

Recommended reading

Burke, W. (1988). Brain injury rehabilitation: Supported employment and TBI. In W.H. Burke, M.D. Wesolowski & W.F. Blackerby (Eds.), *The HDI Professional Series on TBI*, 18. Houston, TX: HDI Publications.

These two publications provide a useful starting point for vocational rehabilitation practitioners assisting people with traumatic brain injury back to work. Both publications provide pragmatic advice and tools such as checklists and other resources that can be used in the workplace. They can be purchased through Amazon.com on the World Wide Web.

Krankowski, T. (1993). Pre and post-injury skill analysis: Determining existing vocational potential for individuals with traumatic brain injury. *Vocational Evaluation and Work Adjustment Bulletin*, *26*(3), 85–88.

A short, though authoritative article that provides a step-by-step approach to pre- and post-injury skill analysis for people who have sustained traumatic brain injury. Include a comprehensive case example that is clearly outlined.

Kreutzer, J.S. & Wehman, P. (1990). *Community integration following traumatic brain injury*. Baltimore: Paul H. Brookes Publishing.

This text is an invaluable resource for rehabilitation professionals involved with all aspects of community integration for people with traumatic brain injury. The sections on work are particularly informative and provide the reader with examples and strategies that could be used in a vocational rehabilitation programme.

Lewis, F. (1999). Brain injury rehabilitation: Developing adaptive work behaviours. In W. H. Burke, M.D. Wesolowski & W.F. Blackerby (Eds.) *The HDI Professional Series on TBI*, 17. Houston, TX: HDI Publications.

Thomas, S.W. (1991). *Vocational evaluation and traumatic brain injury: A procedural manual*. Menomonie, WI: University of Wisconsin–Stout, Material Development Center.

Produced by the Material Development Center, University of Wisconsin-Stout, USA. This manual contains advice on developing viable vocational evaluation services for people with traumatic brain injury. The layout and contents are practical and useful to all vocational rehabilitation practitioners.

Useful resources

www.bounceback.org.uk

A good site for resources, including printable worksheets, to assist in therapy goals when working with clients on their return to work.

www.disability.gov.uk

Information on disability rights and benefits.

www.jobcentreplus.gov.uk/home/customers/HelpForDisabled

This site gives information about disability issues and help available, including Disabled Employment Advisors, Workstep, and the Job Introduction Scheme.

www.newdeal.gov.uk

Gives a good summary of the New Deal for Disabled people.

References

Babineau, J.L. (1998). The value of early placement in a supported programme for individuals with traumatic brain injury. *Work*, *10*(2), 137–146.

Ben-Yishay, Y., Silver, S., Piasetsky, G. *et al.* (1987). Relationship between employability and vocational outcomes after intensive holistic cognitive rehabilitation. *Journal of Head Trauma Rehabilitation*, 2, 35–48.

Brooks, D.N., Campsie, L., Symimgton, C., Beattie, A. & McKinlay, W. (1987). The effects of severe head trauma on patients and relative within seven years of injury. *Journal of Head Trauma Rehabilitation*, 2, 1–13.

Brown, L., Nietupski, J. & Hamre-Neitupski, S. (1976). The criterion of ultimate functioning. In M.A. Thomas (Ed.) *Hey don't forget about me!* (pp.2–15). Reston, VA: Council for Exceptional Children.

Burke, W. (1996). Brain injury rehabilitation: Supported employment and TBI. In W.H. Burke, M.D. Wesolowski & W.F. Blackerby (Eds.) *The HDI Professional Series on TBI*, 18. Houston, TX: HDI Publications.

Cattelani, R., Tanzi, F., Lombardi, F. & Mazzuchi, A. (2002). Competitive re-employment after severe traumatic brain injury: Clinical, cognitive and behavioural predictive variables. *Brain Injury*, *16*(1), 51–64.

Chesnut, R.M., Carney, N., Maynard, H., Patterson, P., Clay-Mann, N. & Helfand, M. (1999). *Rehabilitation for traumatic brain injury. Evidence report No. 2*. Rockville, MD: Oregon Health Sciences University.

Gold, M. (1980). *Did I say that?* Champaign, IL: Research Press.

Johnson, R. (1998). How do people get back to work after severe head injury? A 10 year follow-up study. *Neuropsychological Rehabilitation*, *8*(1), 61–79.

Lynch, R.T. (1983). Traumatic head injury: Implications for rehabilitation counselling. *Journal of Applied Rehabilitation Counselling*, *3*, 32–35.

Neuman, V., Bowen, A., Conner, M. & Chamberlain, M.A. (1996). Lack of occupation after traumatic brain injury: Who is affected? *Brain Injury*, *27*(5), 369.

Pössl, J., Jürgensmeyer, S., Karlbauer, F., Wenz, C. & Goldberg, G. (2001). Stability of employment after brain injury: A 7 year follow-up study. *Brain Injury*, *15*(1), 15–27.

Stapleton, M., Parenté, R. & Bennett, P. (1989). Job coaching traumatically brain injured individuals: Lessons learned. *Cognitive Rehabilitation*, *7*, 18–21.

Tyerman, A. & Young, K. (2000). Vocational rehabilitation after severe traumatic brain injury: II – Specialist interventions and outcomes. *Journal of Occupational Psychology, Employment and Disability*, *2*(2), 13–20.

Wall, J.R., Niemczura, J.G. & Rosenthal, M. (1998). Community-based training and employment: An effective programme for persons with traumatic brain injury. *Neurorehabilitation*, *10*(1), 39–49.

Wehman, P. (1981). *New horizons for severely disabled individuals*. Baltimore: Paul H. Brooks Publishing.

Wehman, P. (1988). *Testimony on national supported employment implementation before House Select Committee on Education*. Washington, DC.

Wehman, P., Kregel, J., Keyser-Marcus, L., Sherron-Targett, P., Campbell, L., West, M., *et al.* (2003). Supported employment for persons with traumatic brain injury: A preliminary investigation of long-term follow-up costs and programme efficacy. *Archives of Physical Medicine and Rehabilitation*, *84*, 192–196.

Wehman, P., Kregel, J., Sherron, P., Nguyen, S., Kreutzer, J., Fry, R., *et al.* (1993). Critical factors associated with the successful supported employment placement of patients with severe traumatic brain injury. *Brain Injury*, *7*(1), 31–44.

Wehman, P., Kreutzer, J., West, M., Sherron, P., Diambra, J., Fry, R., *et al.* (1989). Employment outcomes of persons following traumatic brain injury: Pre-injury, and supported employment. *Brain Injury*, *3*(4), 397–412.

West, M., Fry, R., Pastor, J., Moore, G., Killam, S., Wehman, P., *et al.* (1990). Helping post-acute traumatically brain injured clients return to work: Three case studies. *International Journal of Rehabilitation Research*, *13*, 291–298.

West, M.D. (1996). Assisting individuals with brain injuries to return to work: New paradigms of support. *Journal of Vocational Rehabilitation*, *7*(3), 143–149.

Part V

Family Interventions

17

Brain Injury and the Family: A Review

Michael Oddy and Camilla Herbert

Introduction

Traumatic brain injury is characterised by sudden onset followed by motor, sensory, cognitive and behavioural changes in the individual. It commonly brings with it a recognised pattern of difficulties including not just changes in the victim but also major changes in the family's social and economic position. These factors together make brain injury qualitatively and quantitatively different from other disasters a family may face. There are additional factors that can add to the trauma; for example, family members may have witnessed the accident take place, or may have had some personal involvement in it, such as driving the car. Even where this is not the case the experience of seeing a loved one in a coma or exhibiting disturbing and confused behaviour is an extremely traumatic one. Initially there is uncertainty both about the survival of the individual and about the prognosis for long-term recovery. In the recovery phase that follows it often becomes clear that the very nature of the person is changed and they may exhibit behaviour that is extraordinarily distressing for the family, and there is still uncertainty about the prognosis for recovery. In the long term families frequently find themselves in the position of being the primary caregivers and are subject to the chronic, unremitting stress that caring for someone with a brain injury can entail. In many cases family members struggle to cope with the strain of caring, although it is also recognised that some families do cope well and are very resilient (Perlesz *et al.*, 1992).

Dependency on the family is often increased by the social isolation which develops for people who have suffered a severe brain injury. This is illustrated in a study by Kinsella *et al.* (1989) that found that the primary attachment of 38 head-injured individuals was a member of their family of origin in nearly 50 per cent of cases. This contrasted with only 16 per cent in the control group recruited from friends and acquaintances of the injured participants. In the latter group over 80 per cent of the sources of primary attachment were either spouses or friends.

Whilst no one who has not experienced the position of the family member first hand will ever fully appreciate their predicament, it is important that professionals understand what the family is coping with in order to enable the family to feel supported and understood. It may be important to intervene to try to prevent family members blaming themselves or the person with the brain injury rather than the injury itself. A more detailed understanding of the problems the family faces and of the factors that support or undermine successful coping may enable the professional to help the family alleviate specific problems.

The literature on the distress experienced by family members following an injury to a relative is now extensive. It identifies low mood, raised levels of anxiety and stress and a loss of intimacy as important areas of concern. There are, however, additional and important clinical questions, for example:

1 Can one predict how families will cope with this devastating event?
2 Can a family's response make a difference to the outcome for the person with a brain injury?
3 What input can or should be given to help families cope with this most challenging of tasks?
4 At what stage is it most appropriate to intervene and how should services be organised?
5 To what extent is such support culturally dependent? Do approaches translate across the Atlantic or to different sub-groups of society?

In this review we will first consider the factors that may influence distress for family members, the impact on different family members, and briefly consider the conceptual models that have been used to attempt to understand the impact of brain injury on the family. Second, we will review the range of interventions that have been used to support or address the needs of families. Third, we will consider the difficulties that can arise between professionals and the family in the course of the rehabilitation process and describe ways in which these difficulties can be avoided or overcome. Finally, we will attempt to answer the questions posed above, using the information available in the literature.

Factors Influencing Distress in Families

Time since injury

Distress measured by mood scales has normally been found to be highest in the immediate aftermath of the injury (McKinlay *et al.*, 1981; Oddy *et al.*, 1978). Some studies (Gervasio & Kreutzer, 1997; Gillen *et al.*, 1998) have found no relationship between time since injury and stress levels in family members, but the more consistent finding is of ongoing high levels of distress in the months and years following injury. Many studies have concentrated on the first two years but those studies that have followed families for 7 to 15 years have demonstrated that there are still high levels of distress and chronic strain in the families (Koskinen, 1998; Oddy *et al.*, 1985; Thomsen, 1984).

Severity of injury

Initial severity of injury as indicated by length of post-traumatic amnesia (PTA) or depth of coma has commonly been found not to be predictive of distress in families (Brooks & McKinlay, 1983; Gervasio & Kreutzer, 1997; Gillen *et al.*, 1998; Oddy *et al.*, 1978). A contrary finding is that of Douglas and Spellacy (1996) who found that 58 per cent of variance in family functioning (i.e. communication and conflict) could be explained by severity of injury as measured by PTA in association with residual neuro-behavioural function and adequacy of social support.

Consistent relationships have been found both between the relatives' perception as to the extent of the brain-injured person's deficits and in relation to particular changes in the brain-injured person. Cognitive and personality changes appear to be much more related to family distress than other consequences such as motor and sensory deficits or difficulties in activities of daily living. The description of the individual as 'a stranger' or as 'no longer the same person' is a common experience in clinical practice and studies bear out the significance of such changes for the family (Gosling & Oddy, 1999; Oddy, 1995).

Social isolation

It is not only the individual with the brain injury who experiences social isolation in the months and years following injury. Families also appear to become increasingly socially isolated. This seems to be due to a number of factors. These include the time and energy devoted to caring for the injured person and difficulties in leaving the injured person alone. There can be difficulties involved in inviting people to the home as a consequence of unpredictable or inappropriate behaviour on the part of the brain-injured individual or due to the person's inability to converse in a rewarding way for visitors. A number of studies have indicated the protective effect where families are able to maintain adequate social support (Douglas & Spellacy, 1996; Knight *et al.*, 1998; Leach *et al.*, 1994), although Wallace *et al.* (1998) found no such relationship in a postal study of 61 caregivers one year post-injury.

Male versus female caregivers

There is a generally held view that women find care-giving easier than men. Whilst certain studies have supported this assumption (Gervasio & Kreutzer, 1997), other studies have come to the opposite conclusion (Fitting *et al.*, 1986). In many of these studies the findings may be confounded by the fact that male caregivers have often been looking after females who are injured whereas female caregivers have been caring for males. As Knight *et al.* (1998) point out, it may be the sex of the patient, not the carer, that is important. However, it also seems likely that men and women do go about their care-giving responsibilities in somewhat different ways. Male caregivers often appear to take a more detached, organisational and advocating role rather than being so directly involved in care. They are more likely to continue to go to work and to share direct care-giving with others. Furthermore, it has been argued that men are expected to be helpless at home and are more likely to receive support from friends, family and statutory services. Perlesz *et al.* (1999) found that male relatives of people with a brain injury (the majority of whom were secondary or tertiary carers) reported their distress in terms of anger and fatigue rather than as depression and anxiety. Interestingly, Gervasio and Kreutzer (1997) found that male caregivers of female relatives reported more distress than other combinations.

Parents versus spouses

A common theme in the literature has been to look for differences in the level of distress between spouses and parents of individuals who have suffered a brain injury. The expectation has normally been that spouses will exhibit greater distress and studies by Kreutzer *et al.* (1994b) and Gervasio and Kreutzer (1997) did find more distress in spouses. However, many studies have found no such differences (Gillen *et al.*, 1998; Knight *et al.*, 1998; Livingston *et al.*, 1985; Oddy *et al.*, 1978).

Oddy *et al.* (1985) and Knight *et al.* (1998) did find that parents were more concerned about the future than spouses and in the latter study were more pessimistic about the situation in general. However, as Brooks (1991) has pointed out, it is likely to be more instructive to focus on the qualitative differences between the experience of spouses and parents rather than the quantitative differences.

Impact of Brain Injury on Different Family Members

The experience of brain injury in the family does vary across different family members. If one considers only those living within the same house, this will commonly include parents of adults who have had a brain injury, spouses or partners, children and siblings of the brain-injured individual. As children are being considered in chapter 19, this chapter will focus on parents and partners.

Parents of adults who have had a brain injury

Few studies have looked in detail at the position of parents of individuals who have had a brain injury. As discussed above, there has been an assumption that parents will be less distressed than spouses, and Livingston (1987) suggests that there may be a different time course for distress in mothers than for wives. He found that mothers' distress tended to plateau over the first year whereas wives' distress continued to increase. Clinical experience suggests that this may not be the end of the story and that mothers' distress may increase further later on. Perhaps because of the more intimate relationship, spouses appear to reach an awareness of the situation more quickly than parents.

An early study by Romano (1974), using a bereavement model, found that amongst families of people with brain injuries in New York fantasies about improvement were common. Parents would often deny the existence of behaviour changes making such statements as 'she has always been bad tempered' or 'he has always been a messy eater'. Such denial clearly has its dangers. Unrealistic expectations in the short term can lead to inappropriate pressure on the person with a brain injury and ultimately to feelings of disappointment and hopelessness. However, an alternative perspective on denial arises from a study by Thomsen (1984). This study of people with brain injuries and their families over 15 years found that denial persisted throughout this period. This raises the suggestion that if denial can persist so long, the dangers of disappointment may be over-stated and denial may indeed be a very protective defence against the otherwise overwhelming implications of brain injury. In the experience of the authors, families will often make statements with caveats that suggest they are fully aware of the way in which they are using denial. For example when asked how much a mother felt her son understood she replied, 'I believe he understands everything, I have to. I'm his mother.'

As stated above, parents have been found to be particularly concerned about the long-term future. This concern revolves around the fact that parents realise their life expectancy is less than that of their brain-injured son or daughter and understandably worry greatly about what will become of their son or daughter when they are no longer able to look after them (Knight *et al.*, 1998).

A further consideration is that where there are two parents caring for an individual, not only is the physical work shared but there is another person in exactly the same position with whom the emotional distress can be shared.

Spouses and partners of a brain-injured person

The impact of brain injury on the most intimate of relationships can be immense. Lezak's (1978) description of the spouse 'living in a social limbo, unable to mourn decently, unable to separate or divorce without recrimination and guilt' encapsulates the predicament frequently faced. Even relatively subtle changes in the cognition and behaviour of an individual can make them seem like a stranger to their spouse. These changes are not gradual ones to which a spouse can adapt, but sudden and dramatic. The loss of the original personality makes the bereavement analogy cogent. However, as Lezak points out, the mourning process is complicated by the fact that the old has been replaced by the new. Although occasionally spouses will report welcome changes following brain injury (usually in the form of increased passivity and decreased anxiety and aggression), on the whole the changes are unwelcome ones. Hence the spouse or partner is faced with an unattractive substitute for their loved one demanding intimacy as their right. ('It's like being married to a completely different person; if I'd met him after the accident I wouldn't have married him.') From the perspective of the injured individual, commonly unaware of the full extent of the impact the injury has had on them, the changes in behaviour of the uninjured partner towards them is baffling and disturbing. The significance of the cognitive and behavioural problems is nicely illustrated by an early study by Rosenbaum and Najenson (1976) comparing the wives of brain-injured soldiers with the wives of paraplegics. The former experienced much greater role changes in their marital relationships, disliked physical contact with their husbands more and found their husband's disability more of a social handicap, leading to a greater loss of contact with friends. These wives had significantly more symptoms of low mood.

A study by Gosling and Oddy (1999) used quantitative and qualitative methods to study the nature and extent of the changes in marital relationships, primarily from the perspective of the non-injured partner. The quantitative findings were that partners reported their marital relationship to be significantly worse and their sexual satisfaction in the relationship to be significantly less. More than two-thirds of respondents rated their sexual relationship as worse than before the injury. The participants with brain injuries rated their marital relationship significantly better than did their partners. In common with other studies (Garden *et al.*, 1990; Kosteljanetz *et al.*, 1981; Kreutzer & Zasler, 1989), this study found that around 50 per cent reported that their injured partner's sexual interest had decreased. Fifty per cent reported that their partner's sexual advances felt coercive and this perception of coercion was correlated with lower sexual satisfaction, but more than half indicated that their partner's sexual advances were still welcomed at least some of the time.

The qualitative findings of this study confirmed that severe problems existed in their marital and sexual relationships. 'I was totally unprepared for the changes in our relationship. I knew he'd have memory problems and speech difficulties but I thought we'd still be a couple. The emotional side feels badly damaged, I really miss the intimacy and closeness. Suddenly we had none. There are times when I'd love to be swept off my feet and just loved for me. I don't want to get to 70 and not have felt that warmth and closeness again. I can see the frustrations setting in.'

The change in the nature of the relationship from being a partner to being more like a parent was common. 'Because he's so dependent on me and I'm more like a mother to him, it doesn't feel right that we have sex. I know I'm not the only one who feels like that because in the carers' support group about three other women said they felt the same.'

Another theme was the assumption of an increased range of responsibilities on the part of the non-injured partner: 'all the decisions are mine, especially when it comes to money. I carry all the responsibilities while he just drifts through life with it all being rosy for him.'

A further interesting theme was the ambivalence towards expressions of gratitude by the injured partner. In some cases the injured partner rarely expressed any feelings other than that of gratitude towards their partner. 'I know he is very grateful to me, he puts notes in cards to me at Christmas saying how he couldn't do without me. I wish he wouldn't do this because it reminds me that he is dependent on me and I'm not entirely comfortable with that.'

Not surprisingly perhaps, high rates of marital breakdown have been found in a number of studies. Perhaps the most representative figures come from the National Traumatic Brain Injury Study (Stilwell *et al.*, 1997). They found that 30 per cent of 234 marriages ended in divorce within seven years of severe head injury to one partner, twice the seven-year failure rate in the normal population. Other studies have found figures of 40 per cent (Panting & Merry, 1972; Oddy *et al.*, 1985) or 50 per cent (Tate *et al.*, 1989; Wood & Yurdakul, 1997). In her 15-year follow-up study Thomsen found only two out of nine couples remained together. The critical question is what determines whether couples part or stay together. Wood and Yurdakul (1997) found no relationship between age and relationship status in that male and female partners were equally likely to leave, and nor was there a relationship between the presence of children and the likelihood of separation. The longer the relationship had existed before injury the less likely the couple were to separate, whereas the longer since injury the more likely they were to have separated. Anderson-Parente *et al.* (1990) found that in the third of couples who remained together two years post-injury the injuries tended to be severe and the effects persistent. Those who stayed focused on the positive side of the relationship and viewed their spouse with warmth and respect rather than as a burden were more likely to remain together. Couples who stayed together perceived that the other still cared for them.

In conclusion it would appear that between a third and two-thirds of marriages end in divorce or separation following severe brain injury. The proportion increases with the time since injury, although most of the studies have covered only the first seven years following injury. The numbers in many of the studies are small. However, the separation rate appears to be double or treble that in the general population.

Conceptual Approaches

Over the years a number of approaches have been suggested to explain or explore the impact of brain injury on the family. Following early studies looking at the concept of 'family burden' in psychiatric populations, there were attempts to measure both objective change after brain injury and the relative's perception of the extent of their disabilities. Many authors have been uncomfortable with a concept that implies that the injured person represents a burden on their family, and have introduced concepts such as stress and distress to measure the impact on the rest of the family. Nevertheless, the relationships between 'burden', 'stress' and 'psychological distress' (such as anxiety and depression) are often poorly specified and lack explanatory power. One attempt to explain why members of the same or different families may react in a wide range of ways has been to explore the impact of different styles of coping. However, the literature here is somewhat confusing as some studies have found links between certain coping styles and psychopathology in relatives (Mitchley *et al.*, 1996; Sander *et al.*, 1997), whereas other studies have suggested that the impact of acquired brain injury (ABI) can be so overwhelming for families that coping styles play only a minor role in eventual outcome (Moore *et al.*, 1989, 1991, 1993). More recently, Kreutzer *et al.* (1994a) compared the adaptation of families after traumatic brain injury with more general psychological models of stress and coping, specifically models of coping with chronic illness such as Alzheimer's disease (Vitaliano *et al.*, 1991). This emphasises the 'daily hassle' aspect of stress rather than (or not only) the single traumatic event and may help explain why external circumstances such as improved child care, patient care services and increased social support (Moore *et al.*, 1989, 1991, 1993) can be better predictors of a positive outcome.

A number of authors have looked at the way in which families try to make sense of the brain injury, and according to Willer *et al.* (1991) successful strategies include the ability to develop a realistic but optimistic outlook, maintaining enjoyable activities, the ability to avoid attributing all family problems to the brain injury and keeping the situation in perspective. Other authors have found that families adapt better if they are able to see the impact of the brain injury as both manageable and meaningful (Kosciulek, 1997), and if they can perceive the continuities as well as the discontinuities in the personality of the person with the brain injury (Oddy, 1995).

Another approach has been to look at models of adjustment based around a bereavement process, suggesting that until the emotional task of grieving begins, it is hard for a family to move on from the crisis state brought about as a response to the initial trauma of the injury to cope with the longer-term care needs (Perlesz & McLachlan, 1986; Perlesz *et al.*, 1992). This approach emphasises the importance of recognizing the losses, but acknowledges that with all the uncertainty and variability of the recovery process, the grieving process may be highly disorganised and may be put off indefinitely, which in turn may prevent the family from taking steps to reorganise themselves.

The way in which the impact of the brain injury can reverberate through all members of the family has caused some researchers to draw upon ideas from systemic family therapy. Researchers have used measurement scales developed in family system work (e.g. Gan & Schuller, 2002) to explore adjustment within families, finding changes in family communication, affective involvement and roles (Kreutzer *et al.*, 1994a), and relationships between 'unhealthy' family functioning and improvement on measures such as employment status and Disability Rating Scales (Sander *et al.*, 2002). The hope is that by understanding these complex interactions we may in the longer term be better able to provide appropriate interventions.

Types of intervention

Family education

Rosenthal and Muir (1983) argued that education was particularly useful during the early stages of recovery when there are uncertainties and unanswered questions, and clinical experience does support this in that family members do repeatedly ask for information. Other studies, however, have reported that even when families have had access to an education programme at an early stage, they remain dissatisfied when interviewed later with the amount and type of information they received about the nature and extent of injury (Jacobs, 1991). Although there are few evaluations of the efficacy of particular interventions, it is probable that for many families the process of adjustment affects their ability to take in information. Education programmes at an early stage, therefore, whilst responding to an expressed need, are not sufficient in themselves to address that need. They may, however, serve an important function in establishing communication between the clinicians and the family. Douglas and Spellacy (1996) advocate ongoing practical and emotional assistance for families in order to ensure that community integration of severely brain-injured individuals is achieved. Families are generally ill equipped or reluctant to impose a highly structured environment when the patient arrives home (Sbordone, 1988). As a result of their limited understanding of head injury, and sometimes also as a consequence of their own period of denial, their demands frequently exceed the patient's ability to encode and process information. In turn this results in considerable cognitive and communicative confusion and emotional outbursts that the family may fail to comprehend or find difficult to tolerate.

Kreutzer *et al.* (1994b) suggest (1) education of family members regarding the impact of subtle linguistic and cognitive deficits, (2) consistent and realistic information about behavioural difficulties and their likely impact on the family, (3) ongoing training in behavioural management and (4) counselling and support groups with special attention to grief reactions of spouses.

Support groups

Family support groups may provide education and training or emotional support. They may be 'open' or 'closed' in terms of whether membership is determined at the outset or whether new members can join at later meetings. They may be led by professional staff or they may be self-help groups of family members. Where professionally led, the role of the leader is to prevent one or two members dominating, to avoid criticism or negativity, to prevent the development of erroneous beliefs and minority views, and to draw attention to differences and similarities in the experience of participants. In terms of experience it needs to be recognised that an experienced professional has broader but relatively 'shallow' experience whereas a family member will have or develop 'narrow' but 'deep' experience of brain injury. Toseland *et al.* (1989) found that professional-led groups are more effective than peers in increasing 'well-being', whereas Zarit *et al.* (1987) found that peer-led groups are more effective than professionals in increasing informal support. A study by Whitehouse and Carey (1991) found that parents rather than spouses tend to continue to attend such a support group and that families of the less severely brain injured attended for longer. There was a preference for a semi-structured format to the group, with guest speakers attending 25–50 per cent of the time. An unpublished study by the present authors suggested that it may be those who are in the majority, whether they are spouses or parents, who find such groups of more benefit and hence continue to attend. The finding by Whitehouse and Carey (1991) that families of the less severely brain injured attended for longer may be due to the greater difficulty the relatives of the more severely injured have in leaving their relative unattended. Certainly practical considerations in terms of timing of support groups, venue, frequency of meetings and transport to them need careful consideration if one is to avoid putting even more pressure on the beleaguered relative.

Family therapy

As discussed above, family therapy and theory is readily applicable to families following brain injury. Surprisingly, there are few descriptions of the application of family therapy to such families. Maitz and Sachs (1995) describe the importance of strengthening the parental sub-systems by means such as encouraging the patient to resume parental responsibilities and insisting on the non-injured partner supporting the other even if they disagree with the particular approach being taken. Furthermore, they suggest interpreting aggressive behaviour as resulting from a loss of position and power and addressing the reallocation of roles within the family. A clinical example is that of an 8-year-old son who was struggling to cope with the changes in his father after a stroke that resulted in severe acquired language problems. The son used his inability to comprehend his father's language as a reason not to obey him, his father would become more agitated and his mother was repeatedly required to intervene to defuse conflict. In such cases it is important to give a clear message supporting the shared parental approach and reinforcing the father's role in the family, rather than emphasizing the mother's role. Solomon and Scherzer (1991) have emphasised the more directive nature of family therapy with this patient group. Guidelines for family therapists include the use of logbooks, memory aids, visible reminders, and the role of routine and structure. This includes homework assignments for the family to practise outside the sessions to foster generalisation of behaviour change. Families have been encouraged to look at what is unacceptable behaviour and how they can tackle this. Family therapy has been used explicitly to develop methods for resolving conflicts within the relationship patterns of the family system (Rosenthal & Muir, 1983). For example, members of the family may feel protective towards the injured person and have different ways of dealing with their anxieties. In one case a mother and daughter both had concerns about their husband/father walking to the shops alone along a busy road because of concerns about poor balance and were in conflict as to how to manage this. The mother dealt with it by initially walking with him and then by shadowing him. The daughter refused to let him go to the shops, saying that she hated that road as it was too busy, and insisted that he walked the other way which was less busy. In discussion they were able to see that they had shared concerns, but that their own anxieties affected their approach. Recognising this was important for them in understanding their different roles in relation to their husband/father and the sources of their own conflict. Intervention within the systems model can focus therefore on the notion of role strain as well as the difficulties inherent in the sudden changes that occur following a brain injury to a family member (Laroi, 2003). Roles and 'sub-system' boundaries are emphasised together with related notions such as over involvement, power struggles and specific concepts such as 'the parental child'. Family therapy also uses the concept of circular as opposed to linear causality to explain family dynamics, which has the effect of diffusing the issue of blame within families.

Behavioural family training

For many years support for families has focused on the emotional coping process, particularly in the early stages. More recently there has been greater attention to longer-term support needs and here the literature has described more problem-focused approaches (Jacobs, 1991). Family therapy as it has developed with brain-injured patients has also begun to bridge the gap between family counselling and family training, the primary difference between the two being that the latter has a more focused approach to the behavioural method of problem solving with specific objectives. Behavioural family training has been defined as the establishment of specific operationalised goals and techniques for teaching family members to more effectively manage the problems presented by traumatic brain injury (Muir *et al.*, 1990). They drew a parallel with other areas such as training communication and problem-solving skills to families of people with schizophrenia who relapse (Falloon *et al.*, 1982), and teaching behaviour management skills to families of 'acting out' children (Falloon & Liberman, 1983).

The most thoroughly described model of behavioural family training is that of Jacobs (1991). He focused on the outcome and problem-solving orientation of training programmes in contrast to the process-oriented approach of more traditional therapeutic models. He argued that by emphasising problem-solving techniques and outcomes, rather than processes, the participants take a stronger role in the development of selected interventions and can more concretely measure their accomplishments by the progress they make on specific issues. He had previously argued (Jacobs, 1989) that the nature of treatment following brain injury may facilitate the development of learned helplessness in that patients and families are repeatedly presented with problems rather than solutions, and that they 'learn' that they have no control over major events that affect their lives. They may become dependent, depressed and passive. Jacobs' family training model, with explicit targets and successes, seeks to combat this sense of powerlessness. He argued also that families can learn the critical skills that can be applied to future problems as they develop, rather than placing the responsibility and control of such processes with the therapist.

The overall training model included eight components of education, problem solving, problem identification/problem selection, resource assessment, behavioural assessment, intervention, evaluation, and maintenance/generalisation.

Individual work

There are undoubtedly situations following brain injury where it is necessary to work with one partner rather than the other, sometimes the injured partner, sometimes the other partner. Common themes include accepting that there is a patient and working with disability as part of the system (Doherty *et al.*, 1994), exploring attributions of blame for the accident, exploring resentments both pre- and post-injury and encouraging a problem-solving, experimental approach to problems.

Sexual counselling

Specific interventions may be required where sexual problems are dominant. Several writers have made suggestions for interventions in this area. Price (1985) provides a number of sensible ideas. These include taking a proactive approach to enquiring about such problems but generally intervening at later stages in rehabilitation, discouraging people from taking a dependent role, providing help with broader issues such as self-esteem and social skills and using extinction techniques for sexually inappropriate behaviour. Zencius *et al.* (1990) gives examples of the latter. Griffith and Lemberg (1993) provide a thorough guide, written for families, to sexual issues following brain injury. Elliott and Biever (1996) advocate sex counselling or therapy, as long as the patient has sufficient cognitive abilities to participate actively. They suggest that sex therapy can help evaluate organic impairment and the current level of functioning and then help the couple to adjust to any altered level of function. For the minority with altered sexual function, medical intervention such as prostheses, injections or hormone therapy may be necessary.

Who should provide services for families?

The limited service provision for families means that the question of who should provide support to families is often redundant. Nevertheless, there are some key principles that should guide service provision in this area. The intervention needs to be (a) appropriate to the setting, (b) flexible over time, and (c) based on specialist knowledge. Relatives repeatedly request information but, as has already been described above, there is enormous variation in what, when and how information can be delivered.

In specialist units or units with substantial numbers of clients with ABI it is reasonably straightforward to provide a range of booklets or resources or to employ specialist family workers. In non-specialist services it is important that the needs of families are recognised and that information is provided about where more specialist provision is available. Unfortunately, one common recommendation for counselling via GP services is usually unsatisfactory because it is rare that such counsellors appreciate the specific problems arising from ABI. This often leaves the relative as the 'expert' at a time when they are seeking advice or information. The family member needs to have confidence that they have a shared framework with the person who is working with them.

Why Do Professionals Find Working with Families so Difficult?

It is not uncommon for the relationship between families and rehabilitation staff to become strained, to say the least. In this section we will consider the reasons why this strain arises and how it can be managed.

McLaughlin and Carey (1993) give examples of common comments that families make to clinicians:

> 'If you would give him/her more therapy he would get better.'
> 'If you would keep him/her longer he would get better.'
> 'You are being pessimistic about the outcome, you are giving up on him/her.'
> 'I resent your nurturing role – I feel helpless; I am devastated by my loss, to which you have become a party.'

Few families have any previous experience of brain injury. Instead they have a general familiarity with the medical model that implies a faith in doctors and nurses to actively treat the individual to improve their health. The focus of this model is normally physical well-being and not cognitive and behavioural change. The family's first experience of brain injury is of the life-threatening acute phase. At this stage many may have been told that the person's chance of survival is slim. Where the person with a brain injury does survive, this engenders an optimism amongst the relatives which later leads them to reject or resent notes of caution being sounded by the rehabilitation staff. Gans (1983) described 'hate' as an intrinsic part of the rehabilitation process. The argument here is that powerlessness gives rise to hate and relatives feel powerless during the rehabilitation process. This is for two reasons. One is that they have been forced to relinquish their caring role by the rehabilitation team. One described feeling as though she were giving her husband up to a strange religious cult. Those involved in rehabilitation spoke a whole new and unfamiliar language. Many of their activities were mysterious and carried out behind closed doors. She had to give up her role as a primary carer and her contact with her husband was restricted.

The second reason why families commonly feel powerless is because of their inability to influence the speed of recovery of their relative. This, together with often upsetting behaviour on the part of the individual with the brain injury, leads to frustration and anger. This anger is often directed at staff because the staff are there and they cannot do what the relative wishes or expects them to do, that is, make the person better. Furthermore, a prime role of the relative is to advocate for their currently helpless relative. Therefore they are legitimately involved in ensuring that their relative gets the best possible treatment. In turn it is not surprising that staff can become upset by what they see as constant criticism from the family. Working in brain injury rehabilitation is not easy and is frequently frustrating. Staff are not achieving as much as they would like to achieve. Most staff are highly committed to their work and put a great deal of physical and emotional energy into it. There is a tendency for staff members to start to see themselves as advocates in competition with family members. Sometimes staff may form the view that a relative is not behaving in the best interests of the patient or may be ignoring their advice. These pressures can lead either to rehabilitation staff turning against each other or, as Stern *et al.* (1987) have described, staff mounting a hostile counter attack against the family. Carberry (1990) suggests that the family may become the target of a staff team's frustration if the team's hopes for recovery are not met. Clearly such reactions can be extremely destructive and need to be avoided. The solution is to ensure that all members of the team have an understanding of why family members react as they do and of the possibility and causes of friction between staff and families. All team members need to be able to see the behaviour of family members, particularly critical reactions, as signs of the family's distress and of their means of coping with this. This is not a recipe for complacency but team members need to be taught how to deal with such criticisms calmly, fully and openly. Team members need to be trained to avoid confrontation and encouraged to critically examine their own position. Having done this, if they can reach the conclusion that they are doing all they can then they should be encouraged to have the confidence that they are doing their best, however inadequate this may be in the face of the obstacles imposed by brain injury. Palmer (2005) carried out a qualitative study into the families' perspective of working with professionals and the themes to emerge were that family members valued honesty, professionalism/knowledge, and a willingness to say that they didn't know as the core qualities in professionals.

Conclusions

For over thirty years researchers and clinicians have been studying the effect of brain injury on family members. The high levels of distress are well documented. There is a consistent finding that the physical changes are easier to cope with than the behavioural or emotional changes, and there is broad agreement that there is no simple correlation between the severity of injury and the levels of distress or difficulty in coping as experienced by the extended family. What are less clear-cut in spite of the years of research are the answers to the following clinical questions:

1 *Can one predict how families will cope with this devastating event?* There is some evidence to suggest that the ability of families to cope is related to their pre-injury resources, coping style and way of organising themselves. This is not to say that the outcome is pre-determined, merely that these factors need to form

part of the assessment of a family's ability to cope. However, the very notion of 'coping' is unclear. What do we mean when we say a family is coping or not coping? Attempts are being made to define coping in terms of particular cognitions or cognitive stances. Coping may also be defined in terms of managing at a practical day-to-day level. However, it may also mean that the needs of certain members are effectively valued above those of other family members. Partners or parents may sacrifice their quality of life to salvage some quality for their injured relative. The Holy Grail of trying to identify universal coping strategies may be a fruitless pursuit. Coping may be such an individual process that no generalities are helpful. However, the importance of these questions is so great that attempts to find ways of alleviating distress should not be abandoned. It may be that the achievement of more limited and specific goals will be of greater benefit. For example, ameliorating sexual dysfunction or helping families to reduce challenging behaviour may have more impact than attempts to reduce family distress. For other families the provision of respite care may be more important than any other intervention.

2 *Can a family's response make a difference to the outcome for the person with a brain injury?* Yes. Whilst there is little hard research evidence that the family can influence outcome in terms of impairment, it is clear that if outcome is defined in terms of participation the family's role is considerable. For the majority of those suffering a brain injury, the family will be their main source of support. During the process of rehabilitation the family has a major role in motivating the client and helping them to understand why rehabilitation is necessary. The family also plays a major role in providing information about the person and thus helping the rehabilitation team to gain a better understanding of the influence of premorbid factors in recovery.
3 *What input can or should be given to help families cope with this most challenging of tasks?* The format of the support to be offered remains unclear. The earlier literature focused on the emotional needs of the family, and some of the more recent research has described more problem-focused approaches. The notion of cognitive adaptation seems to combine the two approaches, with an emphasis on finding meaning in the tribulations faced by the family as a whole. Others have argued that it is difficult to find meaning until you have begun the process of grieving. For families it is important that the input is flexible, informed and honest.
4 *At what stage is it most appropriate to intervene and how should services be organised?* The short answer to this is 'when it is needed'. However, service providers do need greater guidance as to when to offer such support and as yet the research has not adequately addressed this issue. The very nature of recovery from brain injury is such that for many families the long-term needs of their relative and their own role in caring for the injured person is not apparent or is denied for a prolonged period. Models which can provide a more flexible but longer-term intervention with the option to 'dip in and out' of provision are generally supported by families. Having to re-engage with services and repeat information to new workers/services is a common complaint from relatives and service users. Continuity of service and ease of access are important, as is knowing that the service has expertise in the field. Unfortunately, structuring a

specialist support service in such a way that the right timing is available to provide intensive input when required is a challenge that health and social services have yet to meet in most cases.

5 *To what extent is such support culturally dependent? Do approaches translate across the Atlantic or to different sub-groups of society?* The structure and values of the family will have a major effect on the way they support their family member through the process of recovery and rehabilitation. Some cultures emphasise family support as the primary if not the sole source of support. Others, notably western cultures, are more likely to turn to 'experts' for help. Some attitudes may have a direct impact on what is acceptable during rehabilitation, for example whether it is acceptable for staff and clients of different genders to work together. Language barriers impose an obvious constraint on rehabilitation and may necessitate having members of the staff team who speak other languages or making arrangements for interpreters.

It is important to recognise that there are many variations within apparently homogeneous cultures. It is impossible to become expert in the ways and beliefs of different cultures but it is imperative to remain open to the range of experiences that families bring and to assess these factors carefully so as to take such considerations into account.

Recommended Reading

Brooks, D.N. (1991). The head-injured family. *Journal of Clinical and Experimental Neuropsychology*, *13*(1), 155–188.
Early but thorough and useful review of the literature.

Jacobs, H. (1991). In J.M. Williams & T. Kay (Eds.) *Family and behavioural issues from head injury: A family matter* (ch. 16). Baltimore: Paul H. Brookes.
Clear and readable description of an approach to family work.

Oddy, M. & Herbert, C. (2003). Intervention with families following brain injury: Evidence-based practice. *Neuropsychological Rehabilitation*, *13*(1/2), 259–273.
Recent review of literature focusing on intervention.

Perlesz, A., Kinsella, G., *et al.* (1999). Impact of traumatic brain injury on the family: A critical review. *Rehabilitation Psychology*, *44*(1), 6–35.
Impressive overview of family issues in brain injury.

Tyerman, A. & Booth, J. (2001). Family interventions after traumatic brain injury: A service example. *Neurorehabilitation*, *16*(1), 59–66.
Helpful, practical account of a comprehensive service for families following brain injury.

References

Anderson-Parente, J.K., DeCesare, A., *et al.* (1990). Spouses who stayed. *Cognitive Rehabilitation*, Jan/Feb, 22–25.

Brooks, D.N. (1991). The head-injured family. *Journal of Clinical and Experimental Neuropsychology*, *13*(1), 155–188.

Brooks, D.N. & McKinlay, W.W. (1983). Personality and behavioural change after severe blunt head injury – a relative's view. *Journal of Neurology, Neurosurgery and Psychiatry*, *46*, 336–344.

Carberry, H. (1990). How to be a really dysfunctional rehabilitation team. *New Jersey Rehabilitation*, *7*, 4–6.

Doherty, W.J., McDaniel, S.H., *et al.* (1994). Medical family therapy. *Journal of Family Therapy*, *16*(1), 31–46.

Douglas, J.M. & Spellacy, F.J. (1996). Indicators of long term family functioning following severe traumatic brain injury in adults. *Brain Injury*, *10*(11), 819–839.

Elliott, M.L. & Biever, L.S. (1996). Head injury and sexual dysfunction. *Brain Injury*, *10*(10), 703–717.

Falloon, I.R.H., Boyd, J.L., McGill, C W., Razani, J., Moss, H.B. & Gilderman, A.M. (1982). Family management in the prevention of exacerbations of schizophrenia: A controlled study. *New England Journal of Medicine*, *306*, 1437–1440.

Falloon, I.R.H. & Liberman, R.P. (1983) Behavioural therapy for families with child management problems. In M.R. Textor (Ed.) *Helping families with special problems* (pp.121–147). New York: Jason Aronson.

Fitting, M., Rabins, P., *et al.* (1986). Caregivers for dementia patients: A comparison of husbands and wives. *The Gerontologist*, *26*(3), 248–252.

Gan, C. & Schuller, R. (2002). Family system outcome following acquired brain injury: Clinical and research perspectives. *Brain Injury*, *16*(4), 311–322.

Gans, J.S. (1983). Hate in the rehabilitation setting. *Archives of Physical Medicine and Rehabilitation*, *64*, 176–179.

Garden, F.H., Bontke, C.F., *et al.* (1990). Sexual functioning and marital adjustment after traumatic brain injury. *Journal of Head Trauma Rehabilitation*, *5*(2), 52–59.

Gervasio, A.H. & Kreutzer, J.S. (1997). Kinship and family members' psychological distress after traumatic brain injury: A large sample study. *Journal of Head Trauma Rehabilitation*, *12*(3), 14–26.

Gillen, R., Tennen, H., *et al.* (1998). Distress, depressive symptoms and depressive disorder among caregivers of patients with brain injury. *Journal of Head Trauma Rehabilitation*, *13*(3), 31–43.

Gosling, J. & Oddy, M. (1999). Rearranged marriages: Marital relationships after head injury. *Brain Injury*, *13*(10), 785–796.

Griffith, E.R. & Lemberg, S. (1993). *Sexuality and the person with a traumatic brain injury: A guide for families*. Philadelphia: F.A. Davis Company.

Jacobs, H. (1989). Long term family intervention. In D.W. Ellis & A-L. Christensen (Eds.) *Neuropsychological treatment after brain injury* (ch. 12). Boston: Kluver.

Jacobs, H. (1991). *Family and behavioural issues.* In J.M. Williams & T. Kay (Eds.), *Head injury: A family matter* (ch. 16). Baltimore: Paul H. Brookes.

Kinsella, G., Ford, B., *et al.* (1989). Survival of social relationships following head injury. *International Disability Studies*, *11*, 9–14.

Knight, R.G., Devereux, R.T., *et al.* (1998). Caring for a family member with a traumatic brain injury. *Brain Injury*, *12*(6), 467–481.

Kosciulek, J.F. (1997). Relationship of family schema to family adaptation to brain injury. *Brain Injury*, *11*(11), 821–830.

Koskinen, S. (1998). Quality of life 10 years after a very severe traumatic brain injury (TBI): The perspective of the injured and the closest relative. *Brain Injury*, *12*(8), 631–648.

Kosteljanetz, M., Jensen, T.S., *et al.* (1981). Sexual and hypothalamic dysfunction in the post-concussional syndrome. *Acta Neurologica Scandinavica*, *63*, 163–180.

Kreutzer, J.S., Gervasio, A.H., *et al.* (1994a). Primary caregiver's psychological status and family functioning after traumatic brain injury. *Brain Injury*, *8*(3), 197–210.

Kreutzer, J.S., Gervasio, A.H., *et al.* (1994b). Patient correlates of caregiver's distress and family functioning after traumatic brain injury. *Brain Injury*, *8*(3), 211–230.

Kreutzer, J.S. & Zasler, N.D. (1989). Psychosexual consequences of traumatic brain injury: Methodology and preliminary findings. *Brain Injury*, *3*(2), 177–186.

Laroi, F. (2003). The family systems approach to treating families of persons with brain injury: A potential collaboration between family therapist and brain injury professional. *Brain Injury*, *17*(2): 175–187.

Leach, L.R., Frank, R.G., Bouman, D.E. & Farmer, J. (1994). Family functioning, social support and depression after traumatic brain injury. *Brain Injury*, *8*(7), 599–606.

Lezak, M.D. (1978). Living with the characterologically altered brain injured patient. *Journal of Clinical Psychiatry*, *39*(7), 592–598.

Livingston, M.G. (1987). Head injury: The relative's response. *Brain Injury*, *1*, 33–39.

Livingston, M.G., Brooks, D.N., *et al.* (1985). Three months after severe head injury: Psychiatric and social impact on relatives. *Journal of Neurology, Neurosurgery, and Psychiatry*, *48*, 870–875.

Maitz, E.A. & Sachs, P.R. (1995). Treating families of individuals with traumatic brain injury from a family systems perspective. *Journal of Head Trauma Rehabilitation*, *10*(2), 1–11.

McKinlay, W.W., Brooks, D.N., *et al.* (1981). The short-term outcome of severe blunt head injury as reported by relatives of the injured persons. *Journal of Neurology, Neurosurgery, and Psychiatry*, *44*, 527–533.

McLaughlin, A.M. & Carey, J.L. (1993). The adversarial alliance: Developing therapeutic relationships between families and the team. *Brain Injury*, 7(1), 45–52.

Mitchley, N., Gray, J.M., *et al.* (1996). Burden and coping among relatives and carers of brain-injured survivors. *Clinical Rehabilitation*, *10*, 3–8.

Moore, A.D., Stambrook, M., *et al.* (1989) Coping strategies and adjustment after closed head injury: A cluster analytical approach. *Brain Injury*, *3*, 171–176.

Moore, A.D., Stambrook, M., *et al.* (1991). Family coping and marital adjustment after traumatic brain injury. *Journal of Head Trauma Rehabilitation*, *6*(1), 83–89.

Moore, A.D., Stambrook, M., *et al.* (1993) Centripetal and centrifugal family life cycle factors in long term outcome following traumatic brain injury. *Brain Injury*, *7*, 247–256.

Muir, C.A., Rosenthal, M., & Diehl, L.N. (1990) Methods of family intervention. In M. Rosenthal, E.R. Griffith & C.R. Bond (Eds.) *Rehabilitation of the adult and child with traumatic brain injury* (2nd edn, pp.407–419). Philadelphia: F.A. Davis.

Oddy, M. (1995). He's no longer the same person: How families adjust to personality change after head injury. In M.A. Chamberlain, V. Neumann & A. Tennant (Eds.) *Traumatic Brain Injury Rehabilitation* (pp.167–179). London: Chapman and Hall.

Oddy, M., Coughlan, T., *et al.* (1985). Social adjustment after closed head injury: A further follow-up seven years after injury. *Journal of Neurology, Neurosurgery and Psychiatry*, *48*, 564–568.

Oddy, M., Humphrey, M., *et al.* (1978). Stresses upon the relatives of head-injured patients. *British Journal of Psychiatry*, *133*, 507–513.

Palmer, S. (2005) *Understanding and coping: An exploration of the family's experience of services and health-care professionals when someone in the family suffers a brain injury.* Unpublished DClin Psych Dissertation, University of Surrey, UK.

Panting, A. & Merry, P.H. (1972). The long term rehabilitation of severe head injuries with particular reference to the need for social and medical support for the patient's family. *Rehabilitation*, *38*, 33–37.

Perlesz, A., Furlong, M., & McLachlan, D. (1992) Family centred rehabilitation: Family therapy for the head injured and their relatives. *Australian and New Zealand Journal of Family Therapy*, *13*, 145–153.

Perlesz, A., Kinsella, G., *et al.* (1999). Impact of traumatic brain injury on the family: A critical review. *Rehabilitation Psychology*, *44*(1), 6–35.

Perlesz, A. & McLachlan, D.I. (1986) *Grieving in abeyance: Head injury and family beliefs.* Paper presented at the Parkville Centre, Melbourne, Victoria, Australia.

Price, J.R. (1985). Promoting sexual wellness in head injured patients. *Rehabilitation Nursing*, *10*, 12–13.

Romano, M.D. (1974). Family response to traumatic head injury. *Scandinavian Journal of Rehabilitation Medicine*, *6*, 1–4.

Rosenbaum, M. & Najenson, T. (1976). Changes in life patterns and symptoms of low mood as reported by wives of severely brain-injured soldiers. *Journal of Consulting and Clinical Psychology*, *44*(6), 881–888.

Rosenthal, M. & Muir, C.A. (1983). Methods of family intervention. In M. Rosenthal, E.R. Griffith, M.R. Bond & J.D. Miller (Eds.) *Rehabilitation of the head-injured adult* (pp.407–419). Philadelphia: F.A. Davis.

Sander, A.M., Caroselli, J.S., *et al.* (2002). Relationship of family functioning to progress in a post-acute rehabilitation programme following traumatic brain injury. *Brain Injury*, *16*(8), 649–657.

Sander, A.M., High, W.M., *et al.* (1997). Predictors of psychological health in caregivers of patients with closed head injury. *Brain Injury*, *11*(4), 235–249.

Sbordone, R.J. (1988) Assessment and treatment of cognitive communicative impairments in the closed head injured patient: A neurobehavioural-systems approach. *Journal of Head Trauma Rehabilitation*, *3*, 55–62.

Solomon, C.R. & Scherzer, B.P. (1991). Some guidelines for family therapists working with the traumatically brain injured and their families. *Brain Injury*, *5*(3), 253–266.

Stern, J.M., Sazbon, L., *et al.* (1987). Severe behavioral disturbance in families of patients with prolonged coma. *Brain Injury*, *2*(3), 259–262.

Stilwell, J., Hawley, C. & Stilwell, P. (1997). *National Traumatic Brain Injury Study.* Warwick: University of Warwick.

Tate, R.L., Lulham, J.M., *et al.* (1989). Psychosocial outcome for the survivors of severe blunt head injury: The results from a consecutive series of 100 patients. *Journal of Neurology, Neurosurgery and Psychiatry*, *52*, 1128–1134.

Thomsen, I.V. (1984). Late outcome of very severe blunt head trauma: A 10–15 year second follow-up. *Journal of Neurology, Neurosurgery and Psychiatry*, *47*, 260–268.

Toseland, R.W., Rossiter, C.M., *et al.* (1989). The effectiveness of peer-led and professionally led groups to support family caregivers. *The Gerontologist*, *29*(4), 465–471.

Vitaliano, P.P., Russo, J., Young, H.M., *et al.* (1991). Predictors of burden in spouse caregivers of individuals with Alzheimer's disease. *Psychology and Aging*, *6*, 392–492.

Wallace, C.A., Bogner, J., *et al.* (1998). Primary caregivers of persons with brain injury: Life change 1 year after injury. *Brain Injury*, *12*(6), 483–493.

Whitehouse, A.M. & Carey, J.L. (1991). Composition and concerns of a support group for families of individuals with brain injury. *Cognitive Rehabilitation*, November/December, 26–29.

Willer, B., Allen, K.M., *et al.* (1991). Problems and coping strategies of individuals with traumatic brain injury and their spouses. *Archives of Physical Medicine & Rehabilitation*, *72*, 460–464.

Wood, R.L. & Yurdakul, L.K. (1997). Change in relationship status following traumatic brain injury. *Brain Injury*, *11*(7), 491–502.

Zarit, S.H., Anthony, C.R., *et al.* (1987). Intervention with caregivers of dementia patients: Comparison of two approaches. *Psychology and Aging*, *2*(3), 225–232.

Zencius, A.H., Wesolowski, M.D., *et al.* (1990). Managing hypersexual disorders in brain-injured clients. *Brain Injury*, *4*, 175–181.

18

Working with Families: A Community Service Example

Andy Tyerman and Sandra Barton

Introduction

Over the past 12 years we have developed and provided specialist services for relatives and close friends of people with traumatic brain injury (TBI). This has reinforced the importance of recognising the needs of the family in their own right and not just as an adjunct to those of the client. However, given the vital role of the family in providing ongoing support, addressing family needs is also a sound investment in meeting the long-term needs of the client. The impact of TBI on the family and approaches to family interventions are reviewed in chapter 17. This chapter outlines a community service example of working with families after TBI. The impact on child relatives and related interventions are reviewed in chapter 19.

In spite of the family impact of TBI, relatives are frequently left to cope with little support, especially if cognitive, behavioural and emotional difficulties are not apparent to extended family and friends. Jacobs (1989) argues that it is unrealistic for families to fulfil all of the survivors' continuing rehabilitation needs by themselves and advocates a 'family training model'. A primary need is development of family education to provide information about physical, cognitive, medical and behavioural status, as well as prognosis, delivered clearly and honestly (Kreutzer *et al.*, 1994b). The importance of information on the psychological effects of TBI is stressed by Whitehouse and Carey (1991) and Junque *et al.* (1997). Holland and Shigaki (1998) advocate a comprehensive three-phase model of family education throughout recovery: acute care; acute in-patient rehabilitation; and out-patient rehabilitation and community re-entry. Smith and Godfrey (1995) reported an example of an evaluated education programme.

As outlined in chapter 17, a wide range of other family interventions are advocated, including family counselling/therapy, marital and sexual counselling, family support groups, family networking, family advocacy and both practical and social support (e.g. Jacobs, 1989; Oddy & Herbert, 2003; Pratt & Baldry, 2002; Rosenthal

& Young, 1988; Smith & Godfrey, 1995; Williams, 1991). Kreutzer *et al.* (2002), for example, describe a brain injury family intervention commonly delivered through family, marital, individual or group therapy in combination with bibliotherapy. The curriculum comprises 16 topics across four areas: recognising and coping with changes; understanding and promoting long-term recovery; effectively managing stress and other problems; working effectively with rehabilitation professionals. Psychological services play a major role in many such family interventions, as detailed by Camplair *et al.* (2003). Sachs (1991) identifies four levels of psychological interventions for families: education; resolving practical problems; ventilation and support; resolving emotional conflict and structural intervention.

The UK *National Clinical Guidelines for Rehabilitation following Acquired Brain Injury* (RCP/BSRM, 2003) stress the need for consultation with the family about treatment and care, assistance with benefits, practical training for carers and advice about the process of compensation. A specific quality requirement on 'Supporting family and carers' is included in the *National Service Framework for Long-term Conditions* (Department of Health, 2005). This states that 'Carers of people with long-term neurological conditions are to have access to appropriate support and services that recognise their needs both in their role as carer and in their own right'. Five 'evidence-based markers of good practice' are identified, as summarised below:

- carers to be offered choice about their caring role, an assessment of their own needs, a written care plan and an allocated contact person;
- training for carers, working in partnership with specialist teams;
- flexible, responsive and appropriate services to support carers (e.g. emergency care, support for children, carer breaks – all culturally appropriate);
- carers who need help to adjust to changes, especially of a cognitive or behavioural kind, to have access to support based (where appropriate) on a whole-family approach and delivered (where necessary) on a condition-specific basis;
- staff working with people with long-term neurological conditions to have carer awareness training.

A number of 'evaluated examples of good practice' in the UK are summarised briefly in the accompanying web-based Good Practice Guide (www.dh.gov.uk/longtermnsf). This chapter outlines the family services developed by one such example, the Community Head Injury Service in Aylesbury.

Service context

The Community Head Injury Service (CHIS) provides specialist assessment and rehabilitation for people with TBI in Buckinghamshire. Referrals vary markedly in severity, time since injury and presenting problems. Some clients require brief interventions, others community rehabilitation over several years, with further input provided late post-injury to promote adjustment and/or prevent deterioration in those at risk of personal, family or vocational breakdown. (See chapter 4 for further details.) A high priority from the outset was to address the needs of relatives.

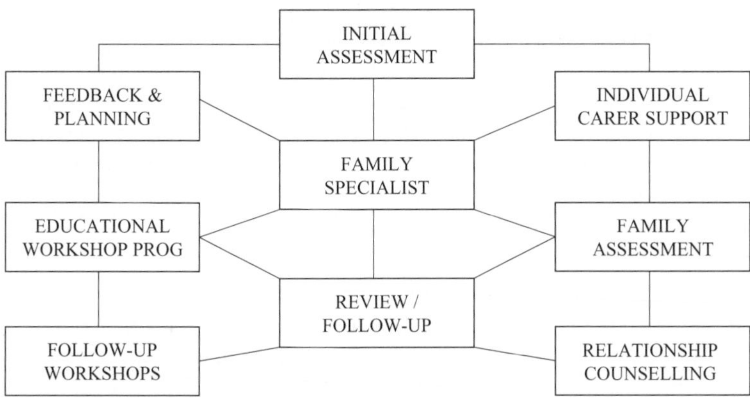

Figure 18.1 CHIS: Working with Families

The development of CHIS family services was informed by a follow-up study of the family impact of severe TBI. This highlighted high levels of stress and distress for primary carers, difficulties in family functioning and changes in family roles, with a marked reduction in the contribution of partners with TBI to practical, social, marital and parental roles (Tyerman *et al.*, 1994). In a further small study a third of marriages were found to have 'very severe problems' (as viewed by partners), with contrasting perceptions of the relationship between partners (Young, 1994). These studies also highlighted the lack of ongoing support in managing complex difficulties after TBI. Relatives stressed the need for those providing support to understand the effects of TBI.

This research helped to shape CHIS family services, which are summarised in Figure 18.1 and outlined below. Provision was made for a family specialist post to coordinate family services, working with a consultant clinical neuropsychologist. This role was combined originally with an existing specialist social worker post and more recently with a brain injury clinical nurse specialist post. The aims of the family services are:

- to increase awareness and understanding of the nature and effects of brain injury;
- to provide information and advice about the management of brain injury;
- to facilitate and promote positive coping and adjustment in family and friends.

Involving the Family

It is essential to involve the family fully in the assessment and rehabilitation process. Within CHIS a relative or close friend is invited routinely to initial assessment, feedback/planning, review and follow-up appointments.

On initial assessment it is important to determine the family context and gain an early impression of the perceptions, priorities and expectations of the family. In establishing the personal, family, social and clinical history (see chapter 4) we address most questions to the person with TBI, but encourage the relative or close friend to assist the person in recalling details (e.g. early in recovery) and in explaining information and also to contribute their own observations. In identifying current difficulties on a Head Injury Problem Schedule, we interview the person and relatives (or close friend) separately. This allows relatives to speak freely about their observations and concerns without risk of upsetting the person or of prompting confrontation over any differences of opinion.

In order to identify the needs of family members, we routinely administer a brief Relatives' Screening Questionnaire with relatives at the end of the separate interview (see Figure 18.2). The original questionnaire was found both to be quick to administer and to provide valuable initial information about the impact of TBI on the family, any support received to date and current family needs (Booth, 2000). Relatives and close friends often take this opportunity to express their concerns and distress about the TBI and its effects, including, on occasions, the trauma of the injury and its early impact, which may not previously have been expressed. As such, the assessment of family needs should only be undertaken by staff with the experience to manage relatives' distress. Services available to the family are outlined on initial assessment, both those provided by the service and by other agencies (e.g. Social Services, carers' organisations and Headway). However, it is important that relatives are not pressed into acknowledging their needs and taking up family support services before they are ready to do so.

Relatives or close friends are invited routinely to feedback sessions to discuss the results of assessment and rehabilitation interventions/goals. This helps to develop a shared understanding of the major issues and priorities. Alongside a debrief of the person's own experience, relatives are invited to contribute observations about how the person coped with the assessments. The involvement of relatives in assessment feedback is critical, to assist both the person with TBI in processing and recalling information and their relatives in understanding the difficulties observed at home. In planning rehabilitation and agreeing goals it is important to consider the family context and the potential impact of interventions on family members.

Ongoing liaison with the family (e.g. by a designated key worker or programme coordinator/manager) is essential, both to facilitate and reinforce interventions and to elicit ongoing feedback about progress at home and any emergent difficulties. Relatives are invited routinely to review and follow-up appointments. Within our community service it is often only when the person with the injury is established in their rehabilitation programme that the relatives voice their own needs and engage in services for families and friends. These services will now be outlined.

Relatives' Educational Programme

We have been providing relatives' educational sessions and discussion groups since 1994. As noted previously (Booth & Tyerman, 2000), originally 10 educational sessions were provided followed by 12 discussion sessions. Whilst the educational sessions were well attended, the discussion groups were less so. Based

Client: ………………………….... dob. …………......… Date of interview: ………......

Relative:………………………..… Relationship: ….…… Interviewer: ………………….

Since your relative's injury, what changes (if any) have there been in

the support provided to the person?

your work/leisure/social life?

work/leisure/social life of family members?

family relationships?

What support (if any) have you received?

Practically:

Emotionally:

How do you feel the family is coping?

How well do you feel you are coping?

Therapists' impressions:

Overall rating: Coping well Coping Struggling Not coping

Information provided/recommendations:

Relatives' Education Prog.

Couple/family counselling

Individual carer counselling for: ……………..

Referral to: SSD/Carers Bucks/GP/other ?

Figure 18.2 CHIS Relatives' Screening Interview II

on our experiences and feedback from relatives we moved to a series of Saturday morning sessions in 1998.

Programme

From 1998 to 2005 an annual relatives' educational workshop programme was provided monthly on Saturday mornings (09.30–12.30) from spring to autumn. The six sessions addressed the following topics: (a) the nature and effects of acquired brain injury; (b) physical and sensory difficulties; (c) cognitive difficulties; (d) emotional and behavioural difficulties; (e) personal impact and adjustment; and (f) family impact and adjustment.

The workshops had a core structure including presentations; illustrative videotape examples; small group discussion; feedback, questions and general discussion:

09.20 Arrival and coffee
09.30 Introduction and aims
09.40 Presentation
10.40 Illustrative videotape example
11.10 Break
11.30 Small group discussions
12.10 Feedback, questions and discussion
12.30 Close and Depart

Whilst the Saturday morning timetabling was endorsed by other relatives, the content could equally well be covered in 10–12 shorter presentations sessions of 90–120 minutes. (Our educational programme for clients, for example, currently comprises 12 sessions of 90 minutes.) Following consultation, the current programme has 11 monthly sessions on a weekday evening from 19.00–21.00 (see Figure 18.3). This provides for sessions throughout the year as well as facilitating the involvement of a wider range of staff, thereby enhancing communication with relatives.

In the revised programme the two-hour sessions are structured as follows:

17.00 Introduction and aims
17.05 Presentation(s)
17.50 Videotape example
18.10 Break
18.20 Group discussion
18.50 Feedback, questions and general discussion
19.00 Close and Depart

Content

At the first workshop the presenter welcomes participants, outlines the programme and invites relatives to introduce themselves briefly in terms of name, relationship to the injured person and the circumstances, nature and time since injury. (The

TIME: 19.00–21.00 Thursdays – monthly (Sept. 2007 – July 2008)

VENUE: The Camborne Centre, Jansel Square, Bedgrove, Aylesbury

CONVENORS: Consultant clinical neuropsychologist/family specialist

PARTICIPANTS: Relatives or close friends of people with acquired brain injury.

AIMS : To increase understanding of the nature & effects of brain injury.
To provide an opportunity for relatives to share experiences & coping strategies and provide peer group support.

FORMAT: Talks, videotape examples, questions and discussion.

Core programme – Presenter

1. Brain function & brain injury – Clinical neuropsychologist
Nature of brain function and how the brain is affected by a brain injury.

2. Physical & sensory difficulties 1 – Consultant in neurorehabilitation
Overview of physical difficulties (e.g. weakness, balance/coordination, fatigue).

3. Physical & sensory difficulties 2 – Consultant in neurorehabilitation
Overview sensory difficulties (e.g. visual difficulties) + headaches, fits & driving.

4. Cognitive difficulties 1. General – Clinical neuropsychologist
Overview cognitive difficulties (e.g. memory, concentration, slow speed etc.).

5. Cognitive difficulties 2. Executive – Clinical neuropsychologist
Overview of executive difficulties (i.e. reasoning, planning, problem solving, insight).

6. Communication and social skills difficulties – Speech & language therapist
Overview of difficulties in speech, language, swallowing and social skills.

7. Behavioural difficulties – Clinical neuropsychologist
Overview of major behavioural changes (e.g. irritability, aggression & disinhibition).

8. Emotional changes – Clinical neuropsychologist
Overview of common emotional changes (e.g. agitation, mood swings, low mood).

9. Vocational difficulties – Occupational therapist
Overview of common difficulties in return to employment, education or training.

10. Personal impact & adjustment – Clinical neuropsychologist
Overview of personal impact and common difficulties in long-term adjustment.

11. Impact on family & friends – Clinical neuropsychologist
Overview of the effects of brain injury on family & friends and family relationships.

Figure 18.3 CHIS Relatives' Brain Injury Educational Programme 2006/7

introductions are repeated at later sessions when new members join.) The first workshop includes a presentation (assisted by videotape material and a model brain) on brain function and brain injury, focusing on TBI. Additional material on other forms of brain injury (e.g. a videotape on stroke) is made available at the time or afterwards, as appropriate.

Presentations in subsequent sessions include a talk (with handout) by a clinical neuropsychologist, medical consultant in neurorehabilitation, occupational therapist or speech and language therapist. The talks cover common areas of difficulties, illustrated liberally with practical examples of how such difficulties affect people in their daily lives. Relatives are encouraged to ask questions during and after the presentations. The talks are illustrated by 15–20-minute videotape examples. In the past these have included the following: a client demonstrating and talking about physical difficulties; a client and his wife talking about cognitive difficulties early post-injury; a client and his parents talking about behavioural and emotional changes; a client and his wife talking about personal impact and adjustment at seven years; and his wife talking about the associated impact on the family. A major advantage of the revised format is the increased scope for videotape examples, which illustrate common difficulties discussed in the presentations and act as a catalyst for the group discussions.

After a break, relatives have been provided with an opportunity for peer group discussion. Depending on numbers, relatives have in the past been divided into separate groups of partners and parents. Other relatives, such as siblings and teenage children of an injured parent, tend to stay with their attending parents. Relatives have been provided with prompt questions as a focus for group discussions, for example:

In your experience . . . :

1 What are the major cognitive difficulties you have observed in your relative?
2 How do these difficulties affect family members?
3 How have you tried to manage these difficulties?

In the past the presenter has not usually joined the group discussions, in order to allow group discussion and peer support, rather than an extended question and answer session. However, the family specialist checks that group discussions are constructive and is available to facilitate and/or provide information, direction and emotional or other support, as required. The groups report back a flavour of their discussions to the large group and any questions for broader discussion. Relatives frequently approach staff at the end of the sessions to raise individual concerns or questions about their injured relative's progress, which are passed on to relevant staff. If discussions raise specific family issues, a time is made to explore these individually.

Participants

The primary carers of people with brain injury seen by the service in the preceding year are invited routinely to attend the sessions, together with any other interested relatives or close friends, including teenage children or siblings. We also re-invite relatives of people referred the previous year as the timing of the last series may have been too early or inconvenient for some relatives. Whilst most relatives attend for just one series, relatives who have attended previously are welcome to attend a second series or specific sessions of particular interest or that may have been missed the first time around.

Feedback and evaluation

Feedback from relatives has been very positive, although those who attend are, of course, likely to be well disposed towards the sessions. The format appears to work well, combining information, videotape examples and the opportunity to ask questions and talk with others in a similar situation. Formal feedback from the first series was very positive, with all elements rated as 'very helpful' or 'helpful' by all except one participant on one occasion, with group discussions most often reported to be the most helpful element. The realisation by relatives that they are not alone in what they experience is observed to be of particular value.

The previous six half-day workshops programme has been implemented by several other brain injury services and formally evaluated by one. In general there was a very positive response, with participants reporting an increase in knowledge and understanding about the effects of TBI, reflected in a change in attitudes and response towards the person with TBI, as well as in developing a greater variety of coping strategies (Hesdon, 2004). Less effect on emotional functioning was reported, but this would in our view be an unexpected bonus from these sessions alone. The sessions have been valued highly by relatives even many years post-injury, as illustrated by videotaped interviews with a wife and daughter who attended the sessions 17 years after their husband/father's TBI:

> *Wife*: 'It was the best thing that ever happened because by explaining it to us . . . the more we got to understand about the brain and how it works and how different impacts will affect personality or the injured person, it just made all the difference to us – it was like a light bulb moment. Just the first time we came . . . that was amazing, we couldn't wait to come back to the next one . . . In order for M to progress he couldn't do that on his own, he needed someone else there to do it with him. If I hadn't been given the understanding I couldn't help him because I would have been against the brick wall again.'
>
> *Daughter*: 'Basically over the course of the months that we've been coming here Mum and I developed a greater understanding as to why Dad does things and we can share . . . it's drawn my Mum and I together so much, it really has – it's brought us so close together. What we find is we sit in these meetings and will go through and we will listen to what everyone has to say and then we will sit in the car journey on the way back and we will start talking about what happened and then we will start re-living scenarios and situations and it will become clear and that is so helpful . . . I don't remember ever sitting down the three of us and having a discussion and it's happening now because we have something similar to talk about. I know that these workshops have been the focus of bringing us all together.'

As well as providing education and facilitating peer group support, the sessions provide feedback on how the relatives view progress in rehabilitation and how they are coping. It enables them to raise concerns, discuss problems, ask questions and pass on information without having to do so in front of their injured family member.

Follow-up Workshops

In response to feedback from relatives, follow-up workshops (usually two a year) have been provided since 1999. The topics, which are usually generated by participants, are less educational and more focused on issues in long-term management and family adjustment (e.g. coping with difficult situations, the stress of ongoing care, independent living, taking risks versus playing safe, effects on siblings, the extended family, sexual relationships, leisure activities, planning for the future, etc.). Whilst some relatives attend the follow-up workshops regularly, others come intermittently to maintain contact and/or when they feel in need of further professional or peer support.

The format of the follow-up workshops is flexible, with staff facilitating the discussions and adding information or comment, as appropriate. After an introduction by a staff member (supported by other videotape examples, as appropriate), relatives typically explore the topic in groups before feeding back themes and issues for further discussion. For example, in discussing 'coping with difficult situations' relatives were first divided into groups and asked to identify common areas of difficulty to work on. These were fed back to the large group and then discussed further in small groups with prompt questions to structure discussions: Could the incidents have been anticipated? Could they (the relatives) have reacted differently? Can they think of ways to reduce the likelihood of such incidents happening again?

Individual Care Support

Individual support is provided for family members by our family specialist. This may be taken up by parents and partners and occasionally by other family members (i.e. adult or teenage siblings and children, grandparents). Support is provided in the family home or the rehabilitation centre as the relative wishes. Common issues for carers include the following: clarification of the challenges resulting from TBI; the need for information and explanation about TBI; coping with stress and loss; adjusting to changes in lifestyle; the sense of obligation and duty to provide care; 'walking on eggshells'; family isolation; clarification of the long-term impact for the carer and family (Tyerman & Booth, 2001).

A recent review of the concerns raised by carers confirms the importance of the psychological effects of TBI, especially behavioural but also cognitive and emotional. For some the latter includes concern over the emotional impact of the person's growing realisation of the extent of their restrictions, but for others the concern is about a reduction in emotional engagement and response. Socially, the person's loss of former work role and friendships are common areas of concern.

Common themes relating to the impact on the carers include: stress; lack of confidence in ability to cope and lack of support; uncertainties and worries about the future; impact on their own work; feelings of guilt and loneliness. Concerns about the impact on the family as a whole have centred on changes in family relationships (including sexual relationships), role change, disruption to family lifestyle and a lack of understanding from the extended family.

The support provided to carers has included the following: empathy and reassurance that the service will also support the family; time to listen and absorb worries, frustrations and distress; information and explanation about the effects of TBI and available services; support in problem solving about current difficulties; the opportunity to reflect upon their situation and express thoughts and feelings that others might not understand (e.g. negative comments about the injured person and their survival); the commitment to provide ongoing support; and the facilitation of adjustment to the long-term effects of TBI (Tyerman & Booth, 2001).

A review of the support currently provided indicates that this is commonly provided across four areas: TBI information and explanation; suggestions to facilitate practical problem solving; exploring, understanding and coping with changes in family relationships; and facilitating carers in expressing their feelings, frustrations and worries, in developing confidence in their coping skills and in accessing support. It is important to develop a relationship of trust within which the family member feels valued in the role of carer and safe to talk openly about their feelings without fear of being judged. Whilst practical suggestions may be offered for some difficulties, this is not always possible. However, the understanding of the family specialist can reassure carers that they are doing all that they reasonably can to manage the situation and support them in continuing to cope.

In this way carers are supported both during active rehabilitation and, not infrequently, after ongoing involvement with the client has ceased. For some families individual carer support is provided in parallel with couple/family counselling.

Couple and Family Counselling

Couple/family counselling is usually provided jointly by a clinical neuropsychologist and the family specialist. Couples or families may be offered such input on assessment, during rehabilitation or later following review or follow-up. Some couples or families may be seen to address difficulties early post-injury, others to facilitate adjustment years post-injury. A number of common issues have been noted in couple and family work: the need to clarify the effects of TBI and their impact on family members, family relationships and family functioning; management advice about cognitive difficulties (especially lack of insight and judgement) and behavioural difficulties (e.g. especially disinhibition, aggression and unpredictability); competing perceptions of TBI and its effects; reduced communication; restricted leisure and social life for family members. For a person with TBI living with parents there may be friction over dependency issues and concerns for the parents about future needs and their capacity to meet them. For partners common issues include: a need to explore changes in the experience and expression of emotion; concerns about role change and dependency; increased responsibility and decision making for partners;

difficulties for people with TBI in relating to their children; reduced sexual relationship; and reduced emotional intimacy.

Family assessment

When a need for relationship counselling has been identified we usually meet with the client and relevant family members separately and together to discuss this possibility. We sometimes complete family assessments to understand more fully the impact of TBI on the family. However, due to the sensitivity of the issues explored, this is only undertaken in the context of established therapeutic relationships with the client and relative(s). If we undertake family assessment the injured person and relatives are typically interviewed separately, with the clinical neuropsychologist interviewing the person and the family specialist the partner or parents. As outlined previously (Tyerman & Booth, 2001), a number of family interviews and rating scales were revised for clinical practice along with family and marital rating scales drawn from the family assessment literature:

1 *Family Impact Interview (FII)*. A structured interview revised from previous family research (Tyerman *et al.*, 1994), including questions and overall ratings about the impact of TBI upon the family as a whole and upon each family member living at home.
2 *Family Head Injury Semantic Differential (FHISD II)*. The FHISD II was developed to explore changes in the family arising from TBI (Tyerman, 1987). Version II comprises 12 adjective pairs rated on a seven-point scale (e.g. from 1 'greatly worried' to 7 'greatly care-free'). Family members are asked to rate the family at 'Present' (last two weeks) and in the 'Past' (6 months prior to injury). On the original scale 25 relatives of people with very severe TBI rated the current family less positively than the 'Past' on 12 of 16 dimensions.
3 *Aylesbury Family Roles Questionnaire II (AFRQ II)*. The AFRQ II (Tyerman *et al.*, 1994) is a 28-item scale in which family members are rated (usually by a primary carer) with respect to the extent to which they undertake practical (9), social (9), marital (4) and parenting (6) roles before and after TBI on a five-point scale from '0' (not at all) to '4' (very frequently). In its original form, marked changes in roles were reported after severe TBI, mainly in the form of reduced contribution to family roles by the person.
4 *Family Assessment Device (FAD)*. The FAD (Epstein *et al.*, 1983) is a self-report scale measuring six dimensions of family functioning: Problem Solving; Communication; Roles; Affective Responsiveness; Affective Involvement; Behaviour Control; as well as General Functioning. The FAD has been reported to be of value after TBI (Kreutzer *et al.*, 1994a; Zarski *et al.*, 1988).
5 *Golombok Rust Inventory of Marital State (GRIMS)*. The GRIMS (Rust *et al.*, 1988) is a screening assessment of marital state, comprising 28 statements rated on a four-point scale ('strongly disagree' to 'strongly agree'). The GRIMS appears sensitive to the effects of TBI (Gosling & Oddy, 1999; Young, 1994).
6 *Personal Assessment of Intimacy in Relationships (PAIR)*. The PAIR (Schaefer & Olson, 1981) comprises 36 statements rated on a five-point scale ('strongly agree' to 'strongly disagree') within five intimacy factors (Emotional, Social,

Sexual, Intellectual and Recreational). Normative data are reported for 192 'non-clinical' couples prior to 'enrichment weekends'. In the context of TBI we find it helpful to obtain ratings for pre- and post-injury. The PAIR can provide valuable information after TBI (Young, 1994).

Clinically, these scales have been used selectively for specific families by experienced practitioners to clarify family difficulties in the context of specialist intervention. Whilst the FII, FHISD II, AFRQ II and FAD are appropriate for both parents and partners, the GRIMS and PAIR are only suitable only for partners. Clinically, the scales have proved valuable in: clarifying the nature and extent of family difficulties; identifying potential avenues for therapy; facilitating engagement; and monitoring change during intervention in individual cases. Their value was supported in a study of assessment results for groups of parents and partners and also in individual case studies (Booth, 2000).

Feedback of family assessment results needs to be handled with great sensitivity and care, so as not to inflame difficult family relationships or fuel disagreement about causal factors. In our experience the foundation for family work is establishing an appropriate understanding of the nature and effects of the TBI. This framework is then used to promote a shared understanding about how family relationships have been affected, with a view to reducing associated conflict and promoting family coping.

Couple counselling

The pattern of couple counselling varies, with some seen only for joint sessions and others also seen individually, with the clinical neuropsychologist seeing the client and the family specialist the partner. If interventions with the family focus primarily on the management of cognitive, behavioural and emotional effects of TBI, then this may be undertaken by a clinical neuropsychologist alone. However, in addressing relationship issues we routinely involve the family specialist – our experience is that the clinical neuropsychologist is often required to facilitate the person with TBI in managing their cognitive, emotional and behavioural difficulties in order to cope with the counselling session. As such, the family specialist is needed to focus in parallel on the needs of the partner, which might otherwise be overlooked. A typical pattern of couple counselling is monthly joint sessions interspersed with monthly individual sessions.

When couples are seen early post-injury, in parallel with the rehabilitation programme, it is often necessary to help them to explore and agree strategies both to manage the effects of TBI (such as irritability and aggression) that are impacting negatively on the family and also to nurture positive interactions with children. It is also vital to facilitate communication between partners, especially when the person with TBI is struggling to express themselves or when competing perceptions of either the nature of TBI or its family impact are undermining communication. It is not uncommon for couples to comment that they only discuss their relationship/family difficulties within the security of the therapy session. Whilst it is rare in our experience for couples to attain an early reconciliation of competing perceptions about TBI and its effects, it is often possible to facilitate movement towards an agreed framework that accommodates their disparate views to enable them to address specific areas of conflict. This may in turn provide an opportunity to guide, encourage and support couples in exploring and starting to rebuild an adjusted relationship that takes into account the effects of the TBI.

In our experience it has often proved possible to reduce some of the friction and stabilise the relationship, with positive change recorded in levels of marital discord and intimacy for some couples. However, couples may have difficulty in maintaining the benefits of intervention once this is phased out, a tendency previously noted after TBI (Perlesz & O'Loughlan, 1998). As such, sources of ongoing support may need to be explored. Two examples of work with families will be illustrated.

Case 18.1: M and J

Background

M and J had been married for six years, had a four-year-old daughter and were expecting their second child. They had a good and settled relationship prior to the injury, sharing many interests and attitudes (Booth, 2000). They had only recently moved to a new area.

M incurred a severe TBI and orthopaedic injuries in a road traffic accident. He was unconscious for a week, in intensive care for 18 days and in hospital for nine weeks with a post-traumatic amnesia of six weeks. His TBI difficulties included: right visual field loss; impaired taste/smell; slurred speech; fatigue; marked cognitive impairment (word-finding difficulties, reduced speed of information processing, impaired verbal memory; lack of awareness/insight); and marked behavioural difficulties (i.e. irritability, frustration, disinhibition, verbal aggression, mood swings). M attended for out-patient rehabilitation before joining a brain injury vocational rehabilitation programme at one year post-injury. After a long period of 'work preparation' he progressed to voluntary work trials. However, at three years post-injury, he accepted that he could not cope with the pressure of paid employment and decided to continue with part-time voluntary work.

Early support for partner

When seen for initial assessment at five weeks post-injury, J reported M's major problems as obsession with returning home, lack of insight, aggression, disinhibition, being overly talkative and being very self-critical. After his return home, J described the family situation as 'horrendous' – M was 'extremely difficult to manage' with no family close by, a four-year-old at home and J pregnant with their second child.

J was seen at home by the family specialist, initially fortnightly, then monthly. (J was invited to relatives' groups but could not easily attend.) She also received considerable support from her parents. As detailed by Booth (2000), early intervention focused on explaining and supporting J in coping with M's cognitive, behavioural and other personality changes and in managing her pregnancy and birth of their second child. Concerns about the family situation in general and M's relationship with his older daughter in particular prompted additional couple counselling.

Couple counselling

At one year post-injury M was not coping well with family life. He appeared preoccupied with his TBI, irritable, frustrated, unable to discuss family matters without becoming irritated, and verbally aggressive if challenged or criticised. He was intolerant of noise and was struggling to cope with a young family – tending to opt out and take refuge on his computer. In his relationship with his older daughter he was not dealing well with discipline or her demands and was not joining in her play. M appeared at this stage to be largely unaware of the impact of his behaviour on the family.

On marital scales M and J both rated the relationship as having 'very severe problems', with low levels of intellectual, emotional and sexual intimacy. Whilst contributing to practical roles within the family (apart from driving), M was contributing less to social roles (i.e. planning, providing advice and support) and less to parental roles (i.e. providing comfort, playing, teaching, discipline and childcare). As a father, J reported that he had 'lost the ability to do anything without being told how to do it'. He was reportedly finding it difficult to get to know his older daughter again and would become 'very irritable, quite quickly'.

Over the next two years couple counselling was provided jointly by a clinical neuropsychologist and family specialist at monthly internals. We sought to guide and support the couple in understanding the family impact of the TBI, in managing his anger, in rebuilding his relationship with his older daughter, in facilitating communication and supporting their relationship. In joint sessions M needed help to compensate for his cognitive difficulties and contain his volatility. (He found it difficult to appreciate others' views – tending to dominate discussions, interrupt frequently and see issues categorically from his own perspective.) Parallel individual support for J from the specialist social worker/family specialist was critical both in helping

Continued

her to raise difficulties (or in alerting us to issues that were difficult for her to raise) and in reflecting on previous discussions.

Guiding M and supporting J in redeveloping his relationship with his daughter proved to be particularly helpful with, as J commented, 'somebody else coming up with positive suggestions away from the house where he perhaps felt I was nagging . . . I think that was quite a positive thing, I think it actually worked – I think it was just simple things like sitting with her reading books or even playing games, very simple games – Snap, things like that – and it made him think "Yes I can do that" and the more success he had with it, (the more) he was prepared to do it, but it never came naturally – it was still "Go on M why don't you go and read her a story".'

With respect to the marital relationship M reported that he no longer experienced feelings of intimacy as a result of his injury and it became clear that there was a risk that focusing on the marital relationship would become increasingly negative for J. At this point M decided that he did not wish to continue with the couple work. Whilst there remained a marked reduction in sharing and intimacy, couple counselling helped M and J to contain areas of confrontation, stabilise the strained marital relationship, open up communication and facilitate some rebuilding of relationships under extremely difficult circumstances.

Ongoing support for partner

When the couple counselling ceased, it was critical that individual support continued for J. Once M settled into part-time voluntary work the family stress and friction eased a little, but substantial difficulties remained. As discussed by Booth (2000), support for J from the family specialist continued on a monthly basis for the next year and then less frequently (from six- to eight-weekly) for the next five years. J was supported in coping with the stress and sense of isolation, in managing the ongoing family situation and in facilitating M's relationships with his daughters and in his role as a father.

The importance of ongoing informed advice and support was vital, particularly because M difficulties and J's need for support were not appreciated by others. As J commented: 'That has been extremely important because I think obviously at the beginning of any experience like this people will understand . . . but I think when people see M now . . . , he doesn't seem to have any problems and therefore people think "What is she talking about" . . . they don't understand any more and, quite rightly 7, 8 years down the road, you can't expect people to realise if they are not living it . . . Seeing (the family specialist) monthly means that there is somebody there who appreciates exactly what's going on and, even if I just moan to her for the hour, it's helpful because she understands.'

On reflecting on the family impact at seven years post-injury, J described the situation as still 'tough', having to facilitate and manage family relationships, especially M's now more volatile relationship with his younger daughter. J would have welcomed further joint sessions to address this relationship but M has not been keen. However, the offer of further couple sessions remains open, as and when he wishes to take this up.

Case 18.2: N's parents

Background

N was aged 14, in good health and progressing very well at school where he was a weekly boarder. He incurred a very severe TBI when knocked off his bicycle. He was transferred from his local hospital to the neurosurgical unit, deeply unconscious. He was in intensive care for 5–6 days then on a high dependency unit where he remained unresponsive for 3–4 weeks. At two months he was transferred to a brain injury rehabilitation unit for three months. At discharge he was walking but weak, with poor coordination, monotonous speech, confused, restless, aggressive and agitated. His progress was monitored by the consultant neurologist at the rehabilitation unit.

N returned to school part-time at six months and as a weekly boarder at one year, but struggled with writing, memory and concentration and was also having absences. He passed a reduced programme of GCSEs at modest grades and started but did not complete A/S courses. On leaving school he completed a two-year GNVQ in Leisure & Tourism and then a two-year HND in Leisure Studies with learning support provision. His parents were then at a loss as to N's future employment. He was therefore referred for brain injury vocational rehabilitation. When seen for initial assessment at eight years post-injury, N presented with some physical restrictions, absences and substantial cognitive (primarily memory) and emotional/behavioural difficulties (i.e. depression, verbal aggression and disinhibition). Whilst N's main concerns were with memory, getting a job, frustration and lost aspirations, his family were also concerned about his absences and limited awareness and acceptance of his disabilities and their implications.

Continued

Family impact

When interviewed separately N's mother and sister reported major difficulties with N's aggression, social isolation, social skills, immaturity and disinhibition. As reported by Booth (2000), N's injury had a major impact on all four family members. In addition to major concerns about the ongoing stress on N's mother and his aggression towards his sister, N's mother also reported concerns about relationships with her husband and her daughter. She felt that the family had been 'devastated', yet had received little help.

The stress on N's mother was not helped by the fact that her husband worked abroad. This required her to split her time between her husband and children, who became full-time boarders when she was abroad. Whilst this ensured continuity in N's schooling, his mother was left for long periods on her own to cope with N's difficulties, including his volatile relationship with his sister, on whom he reportedly took out his aggression. Whilst N's father was now back working in the UK and home at weekends, N had been at home full-time since finishing college and N's mother reported that the situation was 'driving her crazy', commenting, 'I never feel that I have got control over my own life, I always feel that he has invaded my space . . . rarely a week goes by when I don't have most of the week having to think about doing or being somewhere with N and, as my life goes on and I get older, I am finding that more of an imposition on me.'

Family interventions

N's parents were regular attenders at the relatives' educational programme and follow-up workshops. Discussion of issues such as 'independent living' and 'taking risks' in the follow-up workshops were particularly pertinent. N's parents contributed positively to discussions, sharing their own contrasting views on how best to cope with N's needs and also drawing on the experiences of other relatives. The positive experience of the relatives' sessions, coupled with family assessment as part of a research project, facilitated N's parents in taking up the offer of family support.

In the first joint session, accompanied by their daughter, N's parents described the 'total devastation' of N's injury and the ongoing stress, particularly on his mother. His parents subsequently attended for joint sessions, initially monthly, then two- or three-monthly. N's mother and sister were also offered individual sessions. A home visit with N's mother provided an opportunity to focus specifically on her concerns and needs. Whilst some joint sessions with N's parents focused on understanding/managing N's needs and liaison about his vocational programme and future work options, there was a parallel focus on the family, especially the stress on his mother. The joint sessions facilitated discussion between N's parents about issues over which they disagreed, especially about how best to meet N's future needs.

When asked whether family support had helped, N's mother commented as follows: 'The workshops certainly. You realise that you're not the only one that is facing the problems. I feel guilty sometimes about the way I feel about N because he is mine at the end of the day, but you listen to the other people and they've got similar feelings and you think "OK it's not so bad then to feel that way . . . it's not just me", you know, and so that's been a great benefit. I think also listening to the way people cope with things you think that maybe we could have done that and you learn from them . . . and hopefully they learn from you as well. I think probably seeing you made us – certainly made me – able more to speak (to her husband) about the way I feel through you, if you like, rather than sitting down at home and thinking, "Oh God she's going to have another nag at me now", you know. Also other people on the workshops . . . they also have had problems in, if you like, agreeing about what the best way to do things is and you think "well, yes, I can understand that" and certainly it's helped just to talk really about it because I think you're so busy coping with it all at home, you don't tend to just sit down and think about the way forward really, you just muddle on a day at a time.'

Whilst the workshops and support for N's parents were of benefit, the stress of the caring role remained. 'When do we get our lives back, that is what I am waiting for really – I just feel that over the last 11 years my life has been put on hold whilst we have sorted everything out for N.' The team were in the process of a protracted search for a suitable 'live-in' opportunity within the leisure industry when N's father was offered a job in China. N accompanied his parents to China, with his sister remaining in the UK.

Follow-up and ongoing support

N and his parents returned to the UK two years later and requested a review. Whilst the trip had worked out well for N (who had helped in a voluntary capacity in an English-speaking school), his mother had herself incurred a severe TBI and his father had been diagnosed with Parkinson's disease. As such, N's parents were no longer able

Continued

to provide the same degree of support for N and the priority was exploring supported living options. We contacted Social Services on their behalf, highlighting N's needs and those of his parents. N moved into supported accommodation 15 years after his TBI. His parents have since resumed their attendance at the follow-up workshops.

Discussion

In reviewing CHIS family services our experience is that most relatives welcome involvement in assessment and rehabilitation. Understanding the family context (past and present) is essential for brain injury rehabilitation and also the foundation for family interventions. The pattern of family support is variable, with some relatives receiving short-term input in parallel with rehabilitation (e.g. educational programme and carer counselling), others ongoing input (e.g. follow-up workshops and couple counselling). A small number have received individual, couple or family support for several years, as previously noted for couple counselling (Gervasio & Kreutzer, 1997; Perlesz & O'Loughlan, 1998). Some relatives re-engage at five or more years post-injury when the long-term strain becomes difficult to sustain or when new issues arise, for example in response to family life transitions (e.g. adult child seeking to achieve/regain independent living, ill health in carer, new partner, birth of child, etc.). Some relatives have commented that their ability to cope with the long-term effects of TBI is strengthened by the knowledge that support is available to them in the future should the need arise.

The relatives' educational programme has been well received by those attending and appears to be an effective way of providing education, general guidance and support. However, as only a minority of relatives attend it is important to view such programmes alongside other forms of family education and support. It has been suggested that support groups are better suited to parents than spouses (Kreutzer *et al.*, 1994a). Whilst this has been less evident in the educational programme, it is important to be sensitive to the difficulty for partners in attending sessions without the person with the TBI. The fact that clients are invited to similar sessions probably helps to reduce their concerns.

We view our family services as facilitating and supporting relatives in understanding, coping with and adjusting to the effects of TBI. In working with families it is vital that we are realistic in our expectations and do not risk adding to their stress and distress by seeking a level of adjustment that is not realistically attainable, the pursuit of which could de-stabilise further a precariously balanced situation. Relatives often value family support very highly even when the effects of TBI (e.g. marked behavioural difficulties) are such that there is no easy or early resolution of the difficulties that they face. In couple work particularly, we need to be careful not to set out to keep couples together when a managed/supported separation may be best for one or both partners and/or any children.

We have found it helpful to have a designated team member with responsibility for addressing the needs of family members, working with clinical neuropsychologists.

Such a joint approach, combining specialist family and neuropsychological and/or brain injury expertise, is also advocated by Solomon and Scherzer (1991) and Laroi (2003). Our experience is that a family specialist role ensures that the impact on the family is taken into consideration in rehabilitation planning. This reduces the risk that we may exacerbate inadvertently the stress on primary carers or foster changes in family roles and relationships that may be difficult to reverse (e.g. inappropriate use of family members in a therapy role). The family specialist role facilitates take-up of family services and ensures that the views and needs of the family are expressed and addressed in couple and family counselling. Within CHIS the role has been fulfilled in the past by an experienced social worker and currently by a nurse with community mental health experience. However, staff providing our family services have not had specialist post-qualification training in family therapy and it has been critical for us to remain within the bounds of our expertise. As such, our family services have focused primarily on education, management of the effects of TBI within the family context and facilitation of family adjustments rather than on applying a model of family therapy. For a discussion of family therapy after TBI see Solomon and Scherzer (1991), Zarskii and Depompei (1991), Miller (1993), Maintz and Sachs (1995) and/or Laroi (2003).

We have developed our family services through family specialist sessions. Whilst liaison with families could be provided through a key worker or primary nurse, the educational programme requires TBI and teaching expertise and family interventions require TBI expertise combined with experience of working with families. Whilst our family specialist sessions have been filled by existing staff members, an alternative would be to employ a family therapist or counsellor and provide training on the effects of TBI. In providing information, advice and support, links with local Headway groups (some of which have family support workers), benefits advice services and carers' organisations should be explored. Joint work with Relate in couple counselling may also be worth considering.

In our experience it is critical that those working therapeutically with families have experience of and/or undertake training in brain injury rehabilitation, counselling skills, family work and interdisciplinary team working. Staff providing family services need specialist supervision by a practitioner experienced in working with families, which may need to be accessed externally. Close liaison both with key workers and other members of the rehabilitation team (including attending team meetings if possible) and with other agencies involved is vital. However, this raises complex boundary and disclosure issues which will need to be considered carefully within supervision.

In meeting family needs it is vital, in our experience, not to view relatives as patients requiring treatment. Whilst a small proportion of relatives warrant referral to their GP or mental health services (e.g. for post-traumatic stress disorder, anxiety or depression), an overly clinical approach may be rejected by relatives who ascribe family difficulties solely or primarily to TBI, with a risk that they will not then engage in family services. In our experience, within a community service, a light touch and a flexible open-door approach is productive, allowing relatives to recognise and adjust to the effects of TBI as far as possible at their own pace and to opt in and out of family services as they wish. However, when there are concerns about risk to family members, especially children (see chapter 19) or vulnerable adults, active intervention may be required. Within in-patient rehabilitation settings, a

Table 18.1 Auditing family liaison and support services

a. On assessment – do you or your team:
   Establish the family context of your clients?
   Include the family in assessment process?
   Elicit family perceptions of client difficulties?
   Check how family are managing these difficulties?
   Check how family members are coping?
   Identify family priorities (as well as client's)?
   Debrief family member (as well as client) after assessment?
   Include family in feedback of assessment results?
b. In rehabilitation – do you or your team:
   Involve family in programme planning/goal setting?
   Provide training for family members in managing difficulties?
   Consider/monitor impact of rehabilitation on the family?
   Facilitate family member involvement?
   Include family in ongoing review & follow-up:
   - Elicit feedback on progress from family?
   - Provide feedback on progress to family?
   Consider the needs of family in future planning?
c. How does your team address family needs?
   Provide education about brain injury (incl. siblings & children)?
   Consider (and assess) the needs of the family?
   Provide information about support services?
   Provide or facilitate referral for:
   - Individual support (incl. children & siblings)?
   - Relationship/family counselling?
   - Sexual counselling?
   Facilitate peer support for family members?

proactive approach to family liaison, education, training, discharge planning and any pressing family issues is advocated (Kreutzer *et al.*, 1997; McLaughlin & Carey, 1993; Ponsford, 1995; Webster *et al.*, 1999). In acute rehabilitation Sachs (1991) recommends that family therapy should be available on a weekly basis.

In reviewing how well brain injury rehabilitation services work with families it might be helpful to consider the questions about family involvement and addressing family needs, set out in Table 18.1.

Conclusions

The *National Service Framework for Long-term Conditions* (Department of Health, 2005) requires services to support families and carers, in terms of education, liaison and practical support but also in assisting families in adjusting to cognitive and/or behavioural changes. Brain injury services will therefore need to review their practice against the 'evidence-based markers of good practice' of Quality Requirement 10. It is also recommended that services are audited against the relevant guidelines (G30–32; G168; G170) in the *National Clinical Guidelines on Rehabilitation following Acquired Brain Injury* (RCP/BSRM, 2003). It might also be helpful to review services against the questions about liaison with the family and about family needs in Table 18.1.

Our experience within a community head injury service is that routine inclusion of relatives in assessment and rehabilitation combined with specialist family services can make a valuable contribution to meeting some of the short- and longer-term needs of the family after TBI. Family services (educational programme, follow-up workshops and carer, couple and family counselling) have all been favourably received by relatives. There are now a few studies evaluating such family services (e.g. Albert *et al.*, 2002; Brown *et al.*, 1999; Carnevale *et al.*, 2002; Hibbard *et al.*, 2002; Mann, 1999; Perlesz & O'Loughlan, 1998; Smith & Godfrey, 1995). The cost-effectiveness of family services is also beginning to be considered (Camplair *et al.*, 2003). However, there remains a pressing need both for the development of services for families of people with TBI in the UK and for further controlled studies of the benefits of family interventions. In developing and evaluating such services we need to be wary of underestimating their value by relying inappropriately on methodologies and measures designed for evaluating the efficacy of clinical treatments.

Recommended Reading

Daisley, A. & Webster, G. (in this volume). Familial brain injury: Impact on and interventions with children. In A. Tyerman & N.S. King (Eds.) *Psychological approaches to rehabilitation after traumatic brain injury.* Oxford: BPS Blackwell.
Reviews theory and research on the impact of TBI on child relatives and provides practical advice on assessment and interventions, including two illustrative examples.

Kreutzer, J.S., Kolakowsky-Hayner, S.A., Demm, S.R. & Meade, M.A. (2002). A structured approach to family intervention after brain injury. *Journal of Head Trauma Rehabilitation, 17*, 349–367.
Summary of family intervention service and curriculum – 16 topics in four areas: recognising and coping with changes; understanding and promoting long-term recovery; effectively managing stress and other problems; working effectively with professionals.

Oddy, M. & Herbert, C. (in this volume). Brain injury and the family: A review. In A. Tyerman & N.S. King (Eds.) *Psychological approaches to rehabilitation after traumatic brain injury*. Oxford: BPS Blackwell.
Reviews theory and research on both the impact of TBI on the family and issues in and approaches to family interventions.

Sachs, P. (1991). *Treating families of brain injury survivors.* New York: Springer.
Detailed account of family assessment and intervention – includes reviews of family impact, assessment, psychological therapy, specific treatment issues for specific family members and issues (e.g. behavioural control, sexuality, denial) plus personal accounts.

Smith, L.M. & Godfrey, H.P.D. (1995). *Family support programs and rehabilitation. A cognitive-behavioural approach to traumatic brain injury.* New York: Plenum Press.
A cognitive–behavioural approach to TBI rehabilitation within a family context in New Zealand – illustrates how families are involved in the rehabilitation process, with a specific chapter on 'Fostering family adaptation' including information provision.

Useful Resources

www.carers/gov.uk > www.direct.gov.uk/CaringForSomeone
Provides information about assessment for carers, support services, carers' rights, money matters, links to carers' organisation and support.

www.headway.org.uk
Headway, the brain injury association (UK), website provides information on TBI, access to local Headway groups and branches which provide support to carers.

References

Albert, S.M., Im, A., Brenner, L., Smith, M. & Waxman, R. (2002). Effects of a social work liaison program on family caregivers to people with brain injury. *Journal of Head Trauma Rehabilitation*, *17*, 175–189.

Booth, J. (2000). Evaluation of family needs and interventions following severe traumatic brain injury in the context of a community head injury service. M.Sc. by Research, University of Hertfordshire, Hatfield, UK.

Booth, J. & Tyerman, A. (2000). Relatives workshops following severe TBI: Experience in a community service. In J. Booth (2000) *Evaluation of family needs and interventions following severe traumatic brain injury in the context of a community head injury service* (pp.111–121). M.Sc. by Research, University of Hertfordshire, Hatfield.

Brown, R., Pain, K., Berwald, C., Hirschi, P., Delehanty, R. & Miller, H. (1999). Distance education and caregiver support groups: Comparison of traditional and telephone groups. *Journal of Head Trauma Rehabilitation*, *14*, 257–268.

Camplair, P.S., Butler, R.W. & Lezak, M.D. (2003). Providing psychological services to families of brain injured adults and children in the present health-care environment. In G.P. Prigatano & N.H. Pliskin (Eds.) *Clinical neuropsychology and cost outcome research: A beginning* (pp.83–107). New York: Psychology Press.

Carnevale, G.J., Anselmi, V., Busichio, K. & Millis, S.R. (2002). Changes in ratings of caregiver burden following a community-based behavior management programme for persons with traumatic brain injury. *Journal of Head Trauma Rehabilitation*, *17*, 83–95.

Department of Health (2005). *The National Service Framework for Long-term Conditions*. London: Department of Health. www.dh.gov.uk/longtermnsf.

Epstein, N.B., Baldwin, L.M. & Bishop, D.S. (1983). The McMaster Family Assessment Device. *Journal of Marital and Family Therapy*, *9*, 171–180.

Gervasio, A.H. & Kreutzer, J.S. (1997) Kinship and family members' psychological distress after traumatic brain injury: A large sample study. *Journal of Head Trauma Rehabilitation*, *12*, 14–26.

Gosling, J. & Oddy, M. (1999). Rearranged marriages: Marital relationships after head injury. *Brain Injury*, *13*, 785–796.

Hesdon, B. (2004). Evaluating the effectiveness of a family education/support group. Unpublished manuscript available from the author.

Hibbard, M.R., Cantor, J., Charatz, H., Rosenthal, R., Ashman, T., Gundersen, N., *et al.* (2002). Peer support in the community: Initial findings of a mentoring program for individuals with traumatic brain injury and their families. *Journal of Head Trauma Rehabilitation*, *17*, 112–131.

Holland, D. & Shigaki, C. (1998). Educating families and caretakers of traumatically brain injured patients in the new heath care environment: A three phase model and bibliography. *Brain Injury*, *12*, 993–1009.

Jacobs, H.E. (1989). Long-term family intervention. In D.W. Ellis & A.L. Christensen (Eds.) *Neuropsychological treatment after brain injury* (pp.297–316). Boston: Kluwer Academic.

Junque, C., Bruna, O. & Mataro, M. (1997). Information needs of the traumatic brain injury patient's family members regarding the consequences of the injury and associated perception of physical, emotional and quality of life changes. *Brain Injury*, *11*, 251–258.

Kreutzer, J.S., Gervasio, A.H. & Camplair, P.S. (1994a). Primary caregivers' psychological status and family functioning after traumatic brain injury. *Brain Injury*, *8*, 197–210.

Kreutzer, J.S., Kolakowsky-Hayner, S.A., Demm, S.R. & Meade, M.A. (2002). A structured approach to family intervention after brain injury. *Journal of Head Trauma Rehabilitation*, *17*, 349–367.

Kreutzer, J.S., Sander, A.M. & Fernandez, C.C. (1997). Misperceptions, mishaps, and pitfalls in working with families after brain injury. *Journal of Head Trauma Rehabilitation*, *12*, 63–73.

Kreutzer, J.S., Serio, C.D. & Bergquist, S. (1994b). Family needs after brain injury: A quantitative analysis. *Journal of Head Trauma Rehabilitation*, *9*, 104–115.

Laroi, F. (2003). The family systems approach to treating families of persons with brain injury: A potential collaboration between family therapist and brain injury professional. *Brain Injury*, *17*, 175–187.

Maintz, E.A. & Sachs, P.R. (1995). Treating families of individuals with traumatic brain injury from a family systems perspective. *Journal of Head Trauma Rehabilitation*, *10*, 1–11.

Mann, D. (1999). Community-based empowerment programme for families with a brain injured survivor: an outcome study. *Brain Injury*, 13, 433–445.

McLaughlin, A.M. & Carey, J.L. (1993). The adversarial alliance: Developing therapeutic relationship between families and the team in brain injury rehabilitation. *Brain Injury*, *7*, 45–51.

Miller, L. (1993). Family therapy of brain injury: Syndromes, strategies, and solutions. *The American Journal of Family Therapy*, *21*, 111–121.

Oddy, M. & Herbert, C. (2003). Intervention with families following brain injury: Evidence-based practice. *Neuropsychological Rehabilitation*, *13*, 259–273.

Perlesz, A. & O'Loughlan, M. (1998). Changes in stress and burden in families seeking therapy following traumatic brain injury: A follow-up study. *International Journal of Rehabilitation Research*, *21*, 339–354.

Ponsford, J. (1995). Working with families of traumatically brain–injured individuals. In J. Ponsford, S. Sloan & P. Snow (Eds.), *Traumatic brain injury: Rehabilitation for everyday adaptive living* (pp. 265–294). Hove: Lawrence Erlbaum Associates.

Pratt, C. & Baldry, K. (2002). Families and carers. In R. Gravell & R. Johnson (Eds.) *Head injury rehabilitation: A community team perspective* (pp.291–309). London: Whurr Publishers.

RCP/BSRM (2003). *National clinical guidelines on rehabilitation following acquired brain injury*. (L. Turner-Stokes, Ed.). London: Royal College of Physicians and British Society of Rehabilitation Medicine.

Rosenthal, M. & Young, T. (1988). Effective family intervention after traumatic brain injury: Theory and practice. *Journal of Head Trauma Rehabilitation*, 3, 42–50.

Rust, J., Bennun, I., Crowe, M. & Golombok, A. (1988). *The Golombok Rust Inventory of Marital State.* Windsor: NFER.

Sachs, P.R. (1991). *Treating families of brain-injury survivors.* New York: Springer Publishing Company.

Schaefer, M.T. & Olson, D.H. (1981). Assessing intimacy. The PAIR inventory. *Journal of Marital and Family Therapy*, *7*, 47–60.

Smith, L.M. & Godfrey, H.P.D. (1995). *Family support programs and rehabilitation. A cognitive–behavioural approach to traumatic brain injury.* New York: Plenum.

Solomon, C.R. & Scherzer, B.P. (1991). Some guidelines for family therapists working with the traumatically brain injured and their families. *Brain Injury*, *5*, 253–66.

Tyerman, A. & Booth, J. (2001). Family impact and interventions after traumatic brain injury. A service example. *NeuroRehabilitation*, *16*, 59–66.

Tyerman, A., Young, K. & Booth, J. (1994). *Change in family roles after severe traumatic brain injury.* Paper presented at The Fourth Conference of the International Association for the Study of Traumatic Brain Injury, St. Louis, September.

Tyerman, A.D. (1987). *Self-concept and psychological change in the rehabilitation of the severely head injured person.* Unpublished doctoral thesis. University of London.

Webster, G., Daisley, A. & King, N.S. (1999). Relationship and family breakdown following acquired brain injury: The role of the rehabilitation team. *Brain Injury*, *13*, 593–603.

Whitehouse, A.M. & Carey, J.L. (1991). Composition and concern of a support group for families of individual with brain injury. *Cognitive Rehabilitation*, Nov/Dec, 26–29.

Williams, J.M. (1991). Family support. In J.M. Williams & T. Kay (Eds.) *Head injury: A family matter* (pp.299–312). Baltimore: Paul H. Brooks Publishing.

Young, K. (1994). Marriage after head injury: Investigating both partners' views. Unpublished dissertation, Leicester: British Psychological Society, UK.

Zarskii, J.J. & Depompei, R. (1991). Family therapy as applied to head injury. In J.M. Williams & T. Kay (Eds.) *Head injury: A family matter* (pp.299–312). Baltimore: Paul H. Brooks Publishing.

Zarski, J.J., DePompei, R. & Zook, A. (1988). Traumatic head injury: Dimensions of family responsivity. *Journal of Head Trauma Rehabilitation*, *3*, 31–41.

19

Familial Brain Injury: Impact on and Interventions with Children

Audrey Daisley and Guinevere Webster

Introduction: Why Focus on Children?

As recognition of the psycho-social impact of traumatic brain injury (TBI) on the families of the injured has increased, the provision of support to adult relatives has become a component of many rehabilitation programmes (Tyerman & Booth, 2001). However, rather less attention has been given to the child relatives of people with TBI; little is known about their experiences or about the extent to which their needs are recognised and addressed in this context (Urbach & Culbert, 1991). Nevertheless, a small but growing body of research and the publication of key government guidelines indicate that children with brain-injured relatives are at increased risk for the development of psychological problems and require (like their adult counterparts) the provision of specialist services to support them (Butera-Prinzi & Perlesz, 2004; Daisley, 2002; Department of Health, 2005); this finding is consistent with a large body of evidence from research on children exposed to other types of familial illnesses (e.g. parental cancer; Compas *et al.*, 1994).

Research also indicates that children's problems, if not addressed, might have a significant impact on the rest of the family system too (Maitz & Sachs, 1995). This has some empirical support; Harris *et al.* (2001) found that psychological adjustment problems in children in the family were a significant source of stress for the adult relatives of TBI patients, which in turn can affect the rehabilitation outcome of the injured person (Sander *et al.*, 2002).

Additionally, government recommendations (Department of Health, 2005) now require services to address the needs of the child relatives of people with chronic, disabling conditions. In the case of TBI this has significant implications as a large proportion of TBI occurs in people under the age of 35 (i.e. people in their peak child-rearing years), resulting in potentially large numbers of children having parents who might be affected (Urbach & Culbert, 1991). Definitive figures are difficult to obtain; the National TBI Report (Stilwell *et al.*, 1997) indicated that 32 per cent of

507 patients surveyed had dependants under the age of 18. If the term 'parent' were broadly construed to include step-parents and co-habiting partners, these numbers would increase further. There are also potentially large numbers of children affected by TBI in other close family members, such as siblings or grandparents, although there are no easy ways to obtain national data on this.

Despite compelling arguments for working with child relatives of the brain-injured, they remain an under-served population. There is limited understanding of the issues faced by children exposed to familial TBI, a lack of child-specific practice guidelines and no published reports of well-controlled evaluations of child-focused interventions in this context. This neglect of children's issues is reflected in the dearth of child-focused approaches within neurorehabilitation services (House of Commons Select Committee on Health, 2001; Webster & Daisley, 2005b).

This chapter aims to address this gap. Current knowledge on the impact of familial TBI on child relatives is discussed (child relatives will be simply referred to as 'children' throughout, and refers to those under the age of 18 who are close relatives of a brain-injured person, e.g. offspring, stepchildren, siblings, grandchildren). The challenges that familial TBI presents to children are described, the existing empirical research on child outcomes and interventions is summarised and the chapter concludes with consideration of process and practice issues. The discussion is focused around some key questions: What are the experiences and needs of child relatives? How do children understand, respond to and cope with familial TBI? What determines that response? And are there effective interventions to enhance outcomes for children in this context?

We draw upon relevant research findings and our experience of developing and providing clinical psychology services to support children affected by familial acquired brain and spinal cord injury in post-acute rehabilitation settings to illustrate the points raised. Insights are also gained from the wider neurorehabilitation (adult-focused) family literature and the research on children affected by other types of familial illness, although neither of these vast literatures is reviewed extensively here. While the focus of interest in this chapter is TBI, we also consider that much of the work outlined may be applicable to working with children who have experienced other types of acquired brain injury (ABI) in a relative (such as stroke and tumour). Children who have relatives with progressive brain diseases face additional and different challenges (readers are referred to Segal & Simkins, 1993).

It is hoped that the information provided in this chapter will raise awareness of the issues facing child relatives and will highlight how services might begin to address these. However, since many TBI rehabilitation professionals may have limited or no child-focused training or experience, the information is written for the non-specialist reader.

The Impact of Familial Brain Injury on Children

Child relatives – the forgotten victims of TBI?

Children with brain-injured relatives have been referred to as the 'neglected victims' of TBI (Florian & Katz, 1991). But why have children's issues been overlooked? Webster and Daisley (2005b) conducted a national survey of TBI rehabilitation professionals' work with child relatives. Of the 263 staff who responded, only 50 (19 per cent) reported undertaking planned, focused work with the children of their patients. A number of reasons for this emerged. First, staff reported that they had little or no access to training, resources or support structures for undertaking such work; this is compounded by the limited evidence-base. As a result, some staff were unaware of both the potential impact of familial TBI on children (and did not, therefore, consider them to be an 'at risk' population who require input) and of ways in which to work with them. This is not unique to TBI settings. Titler *et al.* (1991) found that staff in a critical care unit had limited understanding of the effects of parental illness and hospitalisation on children; similarly, there has been slow recognition at a service level of the needs of children affected by parental mental health problems (Thompson *et al.*, 2000). This may be exacerbated by the fact that most services are typically organised around meeting the needs of individual patients rather than family units, so staff may not routinely enquire about the needs of family members other than a spouse or partner. They, or their managers, might consider family work to be outside their professional role.

This failure of services to recognise children's issues may be further compounded by adult family members' tendency not to request help for their children in the context of familial illness (McCue & Bonn, 2003). This may in part be due to them failing to notice children's issues because they are themselves preoccupied with the needs of their sick relative or with their own distress or from a misguided effort to protect children, thereby limiting opportunities for staff to identify and respond to their needs (Titler *et al.*, 1991).

Familial TBI – the challenges to children

Illness or injury in a family member can be a hugely complex adaptational experience for a child. Overall, a large body of research suggests that familial illness exerts a negative influence on children's adjustment – for example, reports of children experiencing a wide range of emotional and behavioural problems are common (Armistead *et al.*, 1995, Downey & Coyne, 1990; Fisman *et al.*, 1996). However, more recent research also points to positive child outcomes such as increased maturity and responsibility (McCue & Bonn, 2003). In the late 1980s a number of key papers were published that suggested that TBI in the family might present children with a similar set of adaptational challenges and outcomes (Lezak, 1988; Urbach, 1989).

First, there is the direct impact of post-injury symptoms in the changed relative that children must try to comprehend and cope with (alongside the accompanying range of difficult and sometimes conflicting feelings about this). Urbach (1989) suggested that this might be especially difficult for children faced with the relative who survives TBI but sustains emotional, behavioural and personality changes, or for those who experience the death of the relative or have a family member in a permanent vegetative state. Children must also face the task of trying to make sense of the events surrounding the onset of the injury, including understanding its cause, any separation from the relative due to hospitalisation, the role of the hospital, the staff and therapies.

Second, children, like their adult counterparts, may also be faced with the challenge of having to renegotiate and redefine their relationship with their injured relative and other family members. Considerable research has pointed to the dramatic role and relationship changes that can occur following TBI and the accompanying alterations in family routines, responsibilities and to the dynamics of family power and control (Thomsen, 1984; Moore *et al.*, 1993). As such it is not uncommon for children to experience role reversals; they may become 'parentified' and treat the injured parent as though they were a child; or they may become the injured relative's carer or take more responsibility for the care of younger children in the family, often alongside managing the demands of school. When parenting ability is compromised by the TBI, children may be at risk for not being properly cared for themselves. In the case of sibling injury, the non-injured child may feel unimportant and forgotten about and may feel as if their own needs are secondary to those of the injured sibling. They may be asked to perform additional family duties and assume different roles within the family. The long-term nature of TBI suggests that these will not be temporary adjustments for most children.

Third, stressful circumstances arising from the TBI may also affect children. TBI typically imposes social consequences on families (Brooks, 1991) to which children must also adapt. Financial hardships, unemployment and increased likelihood of house moves are not uncommon TBI outcomes and these can lead to insecurity and embarrassment for children as well as restriction of normal childhood experiences. Family restructuring (e.g. divorce, separation) is also common after TBI and can further hinder children's efforts to adjust (Webster *et al.*, 1999).

Fourth, TBI can also challenge children via its impact on other family members, perhaps most notably the non-injured parent. The stresses associated with a spouse's injury can deplete the resources that the 'well' parent has available to meet their children's needs or to maintain important routines (Pessar *et al.*, 1993). Uysal *et al.* (1998) reported that spouses of TBI patients reported fewer feelings of love and acceptance towards their children compared to controls. Additionally, they found that parents with TBI reported significantly less involvement in parenting. In this context, children could be said to experience a degree of loss of both parents.

The next section summarises the small empirical research literature on how children respond to and are affected by the challenges just described.

Familial brain injury – how are children affected?

Much of what is known about how children are affected by familial TBI is based on clinical observation rather than rigorous empirical research (Butera-Prinzi & Perlesz, 2004); as such the factors involved in determining children's reactions are not well understood. However, research on children's adaptation to other types of familial illness points to the important role of children's cognitive and emotional development in this process (Lobato, 1990) and we propose this as a useful framework for considering children's adjustment to familial TBI. As some of the readers may not be familiar with child development theory, a brief overview is provided (readers are referred to Sylva & Lunt 1982 for further information).

Developmental considerations in understanding children's reactions to familial TBI

Children's social and psychological development (the basis for their understanding of the world) is a continuous process. However, a series of different, predictable stages that are said to be influenced by age, biological predispositions, life experience and interactions with others have been identified. Children's understanding of, and beliefs about, the world and events that they experience are said to be influenced, in part, by their stage of cognitive development. In simple terms, as children get older their understanding of the world is said to become more sophisticated. This is thought also to apply to how children's understanding of illness develops (Bibace & Walsh, 1980), including TBI (Sachs, 1991), although the latter has not been empirically tested.

Awareness of these different stages of development is important for any rehabilitation professional (especially those without child experience) who might be considering work with child relatives. A summary of some of the key issues that might arise at each stage of development is next (based partly on Sachs, 1991, and Tonin *et al.*, 1996).

Infants (0–2 years) learn through exploration of their environment using their senses and motor skills. The concept of injury is said to be limited or largely incomprehensible at this stage, beyond simple notions such as 'sick' or 'hurts', and as such, there is often an erroneous belief that infants are not 'affected' by something they do not understand. However, even very young children are sensitive to, and can be affected by, changes in family life and routines (particularly if it involves the prolonged absence of a family member who is in hospital). Infants' primary needs are for intense physical care and consistent, predictable relationships and routines; they are vulnerable to fears about separation or abandonment and are often afraid of strangers. Disruption to routines and relationships can lead to general distress as well as more specific problems such as with feeding and sleeping.

While the *pre-school (2–4 years)* stage is characterised by the development of language and an increased understanding of the world, these children remain typically concrete and egocentric (i.e. believing that everything revolves around them) in their thinking. This can result in them being vulnerable to believing that they might have caused the relative's injury through their own misbehaviour or wrongdoing; they may perceive the TBI as them being punished and they may feel guilty (it is important to note, however, that children do not typically offer this information without prompts). Understanding of TBI remains at a rudimentary level and only the clearly observable and non-abstract aspects are easily understood, e.g. they can understand that because of the TBI 'mum cannot walk', but may be unable to comprehend its less visible consequences such as cognitive problems. Pre-schoolers' view of recovery is based on their own personal experience (e.g. take medicine to recover from illness) and therefore they usually expect the relative to make a full recovery. Children at this stage lack the inner resources to cope with stressful life events on their own and are dependent on others for explanation and reassurance. They have a tendency to ask many questions and require simple explanations. They are vulnerable to developing a range of fears (e.g. of the dark, monsters and of harm coming to themselves or other family members) and as a result can become clingy and anxious, have tantrums and show regressive behaviours such as bedwetting. However, some children can appear to be doing 'too well' with few or no observable problems; this requires careful monitoring.

Younger school-aged children (5–12 years) develop basic logic and can begin to consider the multidimensional aspects of a situation or event, e.g. they may be able to recognise that their relative has both cognitive and behavioural problems; however, they will struggle to understand that these problems are related. They have a broader view of treatment but may still believe in a full recovery. Children's key needs at this stage are for information about events and reassurance about their own health. They worry about being different (and fear the reactions/teasing of others), losing friends and falling behind at school. They often show resentment about lack of attention from adults (when the attention is focused on the injured person), anger towards the injured person, and physical complaints (e.g. stomach aches); they, too, may blame themselves for the relative's injuries and may try to compensate for this by trying to help the relative recover – either through trying not to misbehave or by becoming overly helpful at home. They may also be sad or withdrawn and may fall behind their peers in academic work.

Adolescents' and young adults' (13–18 years) thinking and reasoning becomes more sophisticated, resulting in an increased understanding of the multidimensional nature of illness, and they will have better understanding of the severity, seriousness, degrees of recovery and permanence of it. Children at this stage need complete information about events, privacy and respect and to be able to maintain close peer relationships; they are typically concerned about their own independence, their physical appearance, social issues and how they compare to their peers. TBI can place demands on them to take on other household duties or care responsibilities for their ill relative, and consequently, they can be vulnerable to becoming tired, isolated, missing school or falling behind academically. They may react to this with anger (towards the 'world' and the injured relative), 'anti-social' behaviour, hostility and mood swings; some may engage in new drug or alcohol use. They may be pre-occupied with justice and the wish to avenge the relative's injury. They may also feel distant from the relative and be embarrassed about the changes seen in them. Typically, teenagers will find these issues difficult to talk about.

What types of child outcomes are reported in the literature?

The literature tends to focus on the negative impact of familial TBI on children. The types of child adjustment problems reported are generally similar across studies, but there are too few studies to allow indication of any specific constellation of symptoms that can be considered 'typical'. Emotional and behavioural problems are focused on more frequently, with other areas of functioning, such as physical, social and educational functioning, quality of life and family or peer relationships, receiving much less attention.

Qualitative investigations (involving interviews with children or their non-injured parent) reveal a range of emotional responses to TBI that include crying, sadness, despair, worry, anger, resentment and jealousy of the attention given to the injured relative (Butera-Prinzi & Perlesz, 2004; McLaughlin, 1992). Urbach and Culbert (1991) reported (in a study of three school-aged children with head-injured fathers) children experiencing embarrassment, feelings of rejection, altered self-image, fear of being abandoned, ignored or bullied by the injured parent, as well as difficulties adapting to the changed parent and family roles. Children fearing the changed relative has also been reported; LaMata *et al.* (1960), Rosenbaum and Najenson (1976) and Thomsen (1984) documented that children were afraid of the changed father and avoided him, resulting in clinginess and increased dependency on their mothers.

Other such regressive behaviours and actual loss of developmental milestones (such as the re-emergence of bedwetting in older children) have also been documented in the child literature (McLaughlin, 1992).

There are also reports of children experiencing specific injury and safety-related fears concerning themselves or the non-injured parent (McLaughlin, 1992). Fisher (2002) suggested that children might be vulnerable to developing symptoms indicative of post-traumatic stress disorder (PTSD) since TBI occurs unexpectedly, can have an enormous effect on children's lives which they are generally powerless to change, and can result in the loss of the relative as they were. She suggested that problems such as nightmares, sleep disturbance, lack of emotional responsiveness and irritability might be symptomatic of the disorder. This is pertinent to the findings of Conder *et al.* (1988) who reported a possible cluster of post-injury child reactions that included sleep and behavioural disturbance, social withdrawal, decreased stress tolerance and heightened sensitivity and preoccupation with family and personal safety. The detailed findings of this study have not been published. Oppenheim-Gluckman *et al.* (2003) reported that 4 of the 19 children (with relatives with TBI) studied had 'pathological' anxiety. Similarly, Pessar *et al.* (1993) found that children in 4 of the 25 families they investigated (where one parent had a TBI) had significant emotional difficulties, while Orsillo *et al.* (1993) studied 13 siblings of TBI patients and found that they reported obsessive-compulsive thinking and paranoid ideation.

Uysal *et al.* (1998) found higher (but not clinically significant) levels of self-reported depression in children compared to normal controls. These symptoms were said to reflect feelings of ineffectiveness, negative mood and poor self-esteem. To the authors' knowledge there have been no reports of suicidal ideation or acts in the TBI child relatives' literature.

There are also reports of children presenting with a range of behavioural problems following familial TBI, such as impulsivity, disobedience, aggressiveness and anti-social behaviour. Pessar *et al.* (1993) found that 21 per cent of families in their study specifically reported children's 'acting out' (temper outbursts, absenteeism from school, disobedience) as a significant problem. Similarly, Ducharme and Rushford (2001) describe a case study in which a son's non-compliance at home was the major presenting problem following TBI in his father. Daisley (2002) and Smiton (2005), the only two known UK studies, found that children with brain-injured parents had significantly more emotional and behavioural problems than children in the general population.

Family relationship problems have also been observed; Pessar *et al.* (1993) noted that just under half (42 per cent) of the families studied reported a substantial increase in relationship problems between the injured parents and their children. A 15-year follow-up study of head-injured fathers indicated that the 'relationship between the patients and their children had developed badly in all cases' (Thomsen, 1984, p.264).

Child relatives have also been reported to show impaired social and educational functioning (e.g. Hansell, 1990; Pessar *et al.*, 1993; Smiton, 2005) but this has not been consistently investigated. This is a significant gap in the research, as such problems have been found to be prevalent in children who are faced with other types of parental illness and loss (Dowdney, 2000).

Is it all bad?

The small body of research just summarised suggests that child relatives are at risk for psychological adjustment problems. However, the numbers of children reported to show clinically significant levels of maladjustment vary across studies, depending partly on the measures used and who is asked (Daisley 2002; Orsillo *et al.*, 1993; Pessar *et al.*, 1993; Smiton, 2005). This suggests that 'clinical caseness' or maladjustment is not necessarily the only or most common outcome for children; it also suggests that not every child exposed to TBI will experience difficulties. For example, Hansell (1990, cited in Pessar *et al.*, 1993) found that self-reported psychological functioning of children whose fathers had sustained TBI did not differ significantly from that of a normative sample, and similarly, McMahon *et al.* (2001) assessed depressive symptoms, self-concept and behaviour in siblings of head-injured children and failed to find any statistically significant differences between them and a control group.

Research has also suggested that children might exhibit positive personal growth as a result of the injury experience. Uysal *et al.* (1998) reported that non-injured parents described their children as being 'stronger' as a result of the injury experience. Similarly, Butera-Prinzi and Perlesz (2004) reported that children identified positive outcomes such as greater availability of the injured parent, an increased sense of personal strength and spiritual development. Smiton (2005) found that all the children in her study ($n = 40$) could identify positive areas of personal growth including a sense of increased maturity, independence, compassion, perceptiveness of the needs of others and the acquisition of coping skills since their parent's TBI. Taken together these studies offer the preliminary, but important, suggestion that the experience of familial TBI need not be uniformly bleak.

In summary, although existing research into children who have brain-injured relatives is limited, some tentative conclusions can be drawn. First, familial TBI is likely to be associated with at least moderate levels of psychological distress in some children. Second, familial TBI does not guarantee negative outcomes for children and there is likely to be considerable variation in children's adjustment (even within the same family). The factors that might determine children's responses and the modification of these in interventions are discussed next.

Sink or swim – what determines children's responses to familial TBI?

The factors involved in influencing children's response to familial TBI are not yet well understood. Consistent with the research on adult relatives' adjustment, attention has been given to the role of both socio-demographic factors (such as children's/relative's gender, ages and social class) and injury variables (such as injury severity). While few firm conclusions can be drawn from this small, largely atheoretical body of research, it has been suggested that factors such as the presence of behavioural problems in the injured relative (Daisley, 2002) and depression in both the injured and non-injured relatives (Hansell, 1990; Pessar *et al.*, 1993; Uysal *et al.*, 1998), may be associated with poorer outcomes for children. There has also been interest in (but little empirical investigation of) some other potentially important predictors of adjustment such as psychosocial factors. For example, Daisley (2002) found that children's use of the coping strategy 'self-blame' (for the parent's injury and problems) was associated with poorer child adjustment. It was also found that children who used positive strategies such as 'cognitive restructuring' (e.g. trying to see the good side of things) reported fewer adjustment difficulties.

Research into children's responses to parental or sibling illnesses other than TBI provides useful pointers to other potentially important psychosocial factors that might influence children's responses to TBI. These include the provision of both good quality, age-appropriate information for children about the relative's illness (Craft, 1993) and supportive counselling (Faux, 1993), children's participation in the relative's treatment (Flickinger & Amato, 1994), the maintenance of children's relationships with the injured relative (Lewis *et al.*, 1993) and effective family communication (McKeever, 1983). A consistent finding that has emerged is that these psychosocial variables are often the most powerful mediators of child adjustment (Lobato, 1990; Sloper & While, 1996) and, on an encouraging note, these are also the factors most likely to be amenable to intervention.

The next section discusses how many of the factors above are already being incorporated into interventions with child relatives.

Interventions for Children Affected by Familial Brain Injury

The wider literature on children's adjustment to familial illness and disability contains many examples of interventions to inform and support children. This work includes individual and group interventions (e.g. Craft, 1993; Lobato & Kao, 2002) as well as indirect work via parents (e.g. Beardslee *et al.*, 2003). It focuses on educating and informing children about the condition, providing opportunities to ask questions and discuss concerns, and supporting them in developing helpful coping strategies. The literature suggests a number of key principles in providing services to this group of children, which are summarised below. Despite the dearth of research on the efficacy of such approaches, encouraging results have been reported with intervention packages in the literature on parental depression (Beardslee *et al.*, 2003) which has received greater research attention.

The literature on interventions for children following familial TBI is not well developed. In fact there is currently little evidence for the most effective ways to intervene with adult relatives of brain-injured people (Oddy & Herbert, 2003), although there are various reports and practical examples of interventions. For example, Rosenthal and Young (1988) stress the importance of viewing brain-injured people systemically in the context of their families, and give an overview of the types of intervention that should be available to families. These include education, advocacy, family therapy, marital and sexual counselling, support groups and 'family networking' (facilitating problem solving jointly with local communities and other families who have experienced ABI).

This section will focus on considerations in the assessment of children's needs following familial brain injury, and approaches to intervention with this group. We look at both direct approaches to working with the child and indirect interventions via parents and other professionals. Ways in which the whole interdisciplinary team can be involved in supporting children are suggested, followed by two clinical case examples.

Engaging children and assessing their responses to familial TBI

Children may come to the attention of rehabilitation staff in a variety of ways. Some services might routinely make contact with all family members, including children, to 'screen' for any concerns, or help may be requested for children in a crisis situation (for example, where there are concerns about their safety). There may be considerable expertise within the rehabilitation team such that children's difficulties, if identified, can be addressed 'in-house'. However (and more likely), there may be teams with little experience of, or specialist skill in, working with children and in these situations careful consideration should be given to who is the most appropriate person to carry out an initial assessment of children's issues. There are no specific published measures available to assess children's reactions to, or understanding of, familial brain injury. The following points act as a guide to some of the key issues that we have found it useful to address in trying to understand a child's situation in this context.

It is useful to gain a picture of the child's understanding of causes of the TBI. Allow children to 'tell the story' of the accident or injury from their perspective, and note in particular whether the child witnessed or was involved in it. Explore children's (and adults') understanding and appraisal of the TBI and subsequent disabilities. Particular emphasis should be placed on children's ideas about injury causation and likelihood of recovery (Springer *et al.*, 1997; Tonin *et al.*, 1996). Ask about children's recent behaviour and emotional status – it is especially important to ask about changes in these areas since the TBI because it may be that the child's problems pre-date the injury. Take a broad perspective, asking about children's health, relationships with family and friends, school performance and social competence. It is important to be aware of symptoms suggestive of post-traumatic stress in children who were present at the time of the injury. Urbach *et al.* (1994) offer a useful list of probes for assessing children's symptoms, but a review of published clinical measures of child adjustment goes beyond the scope of this chapter.

It is helpful to explore the coping strategies that children (and adults) have been using to deal with the situation. It is useful to include a focus on positive aspects such as the child's resilience, any positive outcomes of the situation (e.g. more contact with an injured parent who is no longer employed), and the child's strengths, competencies, sources of support and other resources which can be drawn on to facilitate adjustment. Seek multiple sources of information; include interviews with children, parents and staff. Because of emotional stress non-injured relatives can have difficulty making an accurate assessment of the impact of events on children, so it may be helpful to seek permission to contact a schoolteacher or significant other outside of the family who can offer an alternative picture. It can be informative to observe children interacting with the injured relative. It is not unusual for both parents and children to deny or minimise problems; children are often reluctant to report difficulties, for fear of upsetting their parents further. Parents fear being judged as 'not coping' so try to maintain a 'brave face'. In such cases it can be helpful to normalise and describe possible child and adult post-injury reactions with generalisations such as 'It is common for children to feel . . .'.

It is important to place any involvement with children within a family systemic approach, to consider the child's needs within the context of the whole family (Aldridge & Becker, 1999; Maitz, 1991). Therefore, try to obtain information about the family's adjustment, both currently and before the TBI. Obtain information on the current family social context: e.g. financial worries and availability of social support, to obtain a picture of family stressors and resources. Obtain information on the injured relative's main impairments and prognosis. This provides a context for understanding children's reactions and for planning psycho-education.

Be aware of risk issues. Indications that children may be experiencing severe adjustment difficulties, such as severe mood disturbance or thoughts of self-harm, severe conduct problems or exclusion from school, will require further specialist assessment as a matter of urgency. Any concerns regarding children's vulnerability to abuse or neglect will also need to be referred on to the appropriate Social Services departments. Local child protection policies should be followed.

Considerations for planning interventions

Systemic approaches can be helpful in formulating cases and planning action, as is illustrated in the case examples below. Use of a developmental framework in planning interventions that will be meaningful and helpful to children according to their age and developmental stage is vital; approaches used with adults cannot always be adapted. This also means that the needs of different-aged children within the same family should be considered separately. Faux (1993) recommends that when planning child-focused interventions, clinicians should take account of children's level of existing knowledge and experience of the relative's condition (ascertained in assessment), use age-appropriate vocabulary and explanations and address the commonly seen reactions and concerns (discussed in the first section). Particularly with informational/educational and group interventions, the activities need to be fun – play approaches and games are helpful (Gosling & Herbert, 1996; Lobato, 1990). Peer support is a useful ingredient of many group interventions, for all children but especially adolescents (Heiney *et al.*, 1990; Pinyerd, 1983). Finally, it is helpful to normalise the need for support; providing interventions that all can benefit from, with additional specialist help for those with greater needs, reduces the stigma for children and their families in seeking support following a relative's TBI (Tyerman & Booth, 2001).

Sachs (1991) offers treatment recommendations specific to children with brain-injured relatives, with respect to the developmental level of the child. These are outlined below and are useful to bear in mind when planning interventions for children:

- *Infants (0–2 years)*: intervention is directed towards the primary carer to minimise changes in the child's routines. Allow infants to visit their relative and to explore the rehabilitation unit.
- *Pre-schoolers (2–5 years)*: visits to the relative, creative play therapies, use of stories or other concrete activities to aid understanding. Allow the child to express feelings in words or actions, e.g. drawing.

- *Younger school-age children (6–12 years)*: include diverse modalities, e.g. involve children in rehabilitation tasks, model ways of interacting with their relative, use verbal and non-verbal expressive therapies.
- *Adolescents (12–16 years)*: verbal and non-verbal psychotherapy, peer group therapy or activities. It could be preferable to seek help outside the rehabilitation unit to ensure confidentiality.

Interventions provided directly to children

Although little research has been conducted into the differential effectiveness of particular approaches to work on children with brain-injured relatives, published studies all place emphasis on the need to address gaps in children's knowledge about familial TBI in order to help them understand, adapt and cope with change. Educational interventions, orientation programmes and the provision of support are commonly the 'first-line' approaches employed and are described in the following section. If difficulties persist, more specialist therapies can be offered and these are also outlined. All the approaches described rely heavily on joint working within the rehabilitation team. The case examples highlight some of the issues encountered in clinical practice.

Psycho-educational approaches

Psycho-education is recommended as a basis for interventions with adult relatives, with the rationale that informed families cope better, have lower stress levels and more realistic expectations (Frye, 1982; Lezak, 1988). Interventions involving psycho-education have been used successfully with children with other types of familial chronic illness (e.g. Carpenter *et al.*, 1990; Heiney *et al.*, 1990; Lobato & Kao, 2002; Williams *et al.*, 2003) and have been shown to be effective in increasing children's understanding of illness-related concepts (Williams & Binnie, 2002).

Studies recommending psycho-education propose that the provision of ongoing age-appropriate information to children might achieve the following goals: correct children's injury-related misconceptions or misattributions (especially about causation); increase knowledge of possible post-injury reactions; increase perceived control; address unrealistic fears and hopes; provide ongoing feedback about important decisions and plans for the relative, and significant changes to the family situation; and indirectly address adults' misunderstandings. In the context of familial TBI, Butera-Prinzi and Perlesz (2004) found that children expressed a desire to be informed from the outset about their parent's TBI, despite their fears about what they might be told.

McLaughlin (1992) reported an educational 'activity group' intervention for children of brain-injured parents aged 6 to 13, which provided them with the opportunity to learn about and participate in aspects of the rehabilitation process (e.g. undertake physiotherapy exercises, try out wheelchairs). Urbach and Culbert (1991) reported the use of individual psycho-educational interventions to help children understand the nature of brain injury, particularly its behavioural consequences. Neither of these studies reported the use of outcome measures.

Information can be conveyed using a variety of media such as video clips, drawings and photographs; booklets and information leaflets are useful as they allow repeated presentation of materials and are non-threatening. However, there is a dearth of published child educational materials on TBI. Webster and Daisley (2005a) have compiled a resource pack listing materials currently available.

In order to meet the needs of children with complicated adjustment problems, it may be preferable to develop personalised information materials collaboratively with them (Daisley & Webster, 1999). The latter provide general information about familial TBI, which is then closely linked to the child's own concerns and experiences of the injury. But providing information in this way requires time, creativity and a good working knowledge of how to make age-specific modification to content.

Child involvement in the rehabilitation programme

There is a consensus in the TBI rehabilitation literature about the importance of involving adult relatives in patients' rehabilitation (Oddy & Herbert, 2003). This has clear benefits to both the adult family members in terms of facilitating their psychosocial adjustment and also the injured person by improving rehabilitation outcome (Sander *et al.*, 2002; Serio *et al.*, 1997). From a systemic perspective, it is helpful to include children in this, because children's adjustment problems also affect rehabilitation outcome for the injured person through their influence on the whole family's functioning (Harris *et al.*, 2001).

It has been proposed that efforts should be made to create a child-friendly environment in hospitals, to familiarise children with professional staff and ways of working and to involve them actively in the relative's treatment – particularly important for younger children who learn most effectively through 'seeing and doing' (Craft, 1993; McKeever, 1983). Such an approach is said to demystify treatment, increase children's knowledge, foster relationship maintenance by increasing the relative's accessibility, and help children understand and cope with necessary separation from the relative.

The success of this, however, relies heavily on the cooperation and enthusiasm of rehabilitation staff. In the first author's centre, children routinely visit therapy departments to meet and question staff working with the relative. They frequently participate in therapy activities with the relative (e.g. computer work in occupational therapy, or word games in speech and language therapy), and in doing so, can develop understanding and tolerance for the relative's difficulties and learn appropriate ways to assist them. This also provides the opportunity to watch the relative progress and to be aware of their relative's strengths. Such approaches have been reported to foster a sense of mastery and competence in children (Faux, 1993).

Children's safety and privacy on the unit are maximised by the provision of a designated family room, equipped with toys and games. Staff are committed to maintaining relative–child communication; e.g. therapy sessions are often used to assist injured persons in writing or audio-taping letters to child relatives. This work is staff intensive, time consuming and requires careful planning, since the presence of children in therapy areas can be disruptive to other patients.

It may be necessary or appropriate to provide child relatives with training on participation in aspects of their family member's rehabilitation (McLaughlin, 1992). This would be likely to occur particularly in situations when children's participation is needed in order for them to be able to maintain a relationship with the brain-injured relative. For example, if the relative has severe communication problems, children will benefit from advice on interacting with the person and using communication aids, in the same way as adult family members.

At times it may be appropriate to train older children in aspects of care, if they become involved in care tasks either when visiting the relative during rehabilitation or following the relative's return home. This might include tasks such as how to manoeuvre the relative's wheelchair, apply the brakes, fold it up to put in a car and so on; the correct way to feed a relative who has swallowing problems and what sorts of food can be eaten safely; or how to orientate an amnesic relative.

The following points are important to bear in mind when teaching children these skills: check that children are keen to be involved, and make it clear to them that it is not obligatory; tailor the teaching methods and the specific skills that are taught to the child's age, ability to understand, and ability to cope with the task emotionally; collaborate with non-injured parents, e.g. include children in a teaching session for the whole family; try to avoid children becoming 'parentified' in taking on caring roles, for instance by supporting the brain-injured person in directing helpful tasks to be carried out, rather than children taking responsibility for doing them.

Wherever possible it is preferable for children not to be carrying out significant levels of care-giving because of the negative impact of this on their psychological adjustment (Pakenham *et al.*, 2006). It is therefore essential to ensure that children are not acquiring these skills as an alternative to professional carers or adult relatives providing care. The reason for involving children should be primarily to benefit the children themselves, e.g. in being able to maintain their relationship with the brain-injured person and carry out helpful tasks as part of their natural wish to show support and care (Aldridge & Becker, 1999). Monitor the amount of caring tasks children are carrying out, review this with the whole family if necessary, and facilitate other ways of providing this care if it is burdening children. In situations where this is unavoidable, children may gain useful support from organisations for young carers.

Child-focused support

There are many consequences of TBI that cannot be altered and therefore it is necessary to support children in adapting to these. Supportive interventions for adult relatives have been reported in the literature (e.g. Lauer-Listhaus, 1991), but to date there are few reports of their application to children with brain-injured relatives.

While primarily an educational intervention, McLaughlin's (1992) 'activity group' also provided a forum for children to receive mutual support, peer validation and to learn vicariously about ways in which other children cope with familial brain injury. In a related area, parental multiple sclerosis, Blackford (1992) proposed the teaching of peer-counselling skills to children, to enable them to support each other, to feel accepted, less isolated and to have a more positive identity from being a member of the group.

Various studies of group interventions for children who have siblings with chronic illness have been conducted. Lobato and Kao (2002) carried out a group programme for parents and siblings of children with chronic illness or developmental disability, which was effective in increasing children's knowledge, reducing behavioural problems and enhancing their relationships with their siblings. Studies of interventions for siblings in paediatric cancer have found that group interventions are effective in increasing children's knowledge of their sibling's condition as well as reducing specific fears, facilitating peer support and allowing expression of negative feelings (Carpenter *et al.*, 1990; Heiney *et al.*, 1990). Williams *et al.* (2003) carried out a randomised controlled trial of an intensive residential 'camp' group intervention for siblings of children with chronic illness. The intervention aimed to improve children's knowledge, behaviour problems, self-esteem, attitude, mood and social support. The study found the intervention to be effective in all these areas, and of significant benefit compared to the control conditions.

Individual supportive counselling sessions for children have also been reported (Romano, 1976). These help to allow the expression and normalisation of difficult emotions, such as anger, resentment or guilt. Issues that commonly arise include ambivalence about reincorporating the relative into the family after discharge, especially if the separation has been lengthy, or the need to ventilate anger about the injustice of the family situation. Individual sessions also facilitate discussion and development of coping strategies to manage problematic situations, e.g. preparing for other people's reactions towards the relative.

It is important to establish links with the local child and family mental health service regarding referral routes and criteria, so that any children requiring specialist help can be referred on quickly and appropriately. It may also help to provide these services with information about TBI, because they may lack a detailed understanding of the issues affecting children in this situation.

Specialist advice and psychological therapies

In practice, for most children, information and support are adequate to help them cope with familial brain injury. Some, however, require more intensive intervention or specialist advice (Urbach *et al.*, 1994). On the basis of the TBI literature and clinical experience, children who might be at risk for this include those who have pre-existing adjustment difficulties (although it is not always easy to gain information about this), who have experienced multiple losses (e.g. both parents were injured), whose injured parent is the sole carer, or who themselves are providing significant amounts of care to their injured relative. Children who were involved in the accident with the relative may need to be assessed for post-traumatic reactions or to address issues such as survivor guilt. Children whose non-injured parent is depressed (or experiencing other adjustment difficulties) are likely to be vulnerable. Children who present with ideas of suicide, self-harm or have severe and persisting conduct problems may also need urgent referral. In such cases, local child mental health services should be consulted.

If there are concerns about children's safety, for instance when a child reports incidents suggestive of abuse or neglect, or a parent or staff member raises concerns, it is essential to contact the local Social Services child protection team for advice and guidance. In the first instance this can be sought without identifying the family, to establish whether the concerns warrant further action. NHS Trusts are required to have detailed policies and procedures for child protection; staff should be familiar with these in order to be able to respond promptly and appropriately if concerns are raised.

Psychological therapies for children with brain-injured relatives can take various forms depending on the age of the child and the presenting problems. Unless there is specific child expertise within the rehabilitation centre, this work is normally undertaken by outside services (ideally where the child lives).

Romano (1976) reported the use of play therapy (dolls, puppets and special stories) to help young children prepare for disability in the parent. Urbach and Culbert (1991) reported applying a range of cognitive and behavioural techniques such as relaxation training, self-monitoring and cognitive restructuring with school-aged children following parental brain injury, to manage severe and long-lasting reactive symptomatology. Child-focused interventions were conducted alongside couples' sessions for the parents, family therapy and educational interventions. Significant improvements were reported in children's functioning and resolution of emotional difficulties following treatment.

Cognitive approaches may also be useful to help children process the traumatic discontinuity of experience caused by familial brain injury. Anthony (1970) noted that this discontinuity can cause a state of pathological mourning, just as severe as that seen after parental death.

As with all child-focused interventions, individual work should be undertaken with an awareness of the systemic context and ideally encompass working with parents or other significant family members. The cases reported below exemplify this.

Family interventions and therapy are reviewed in chapter 17. Family therapy approaches may be indicated when family relationships appear problematic. Such interventions ensure that no one person is focused on as the source of the family's problems, and may be useful for addressing power struggles or role reversals (e.g. the 'parental child'). Family therapy can foster group problem solving and provide opportunities for the family to hear each other's stories. It can also be used to strengthen the parental subsystem, helping parents resume roles and responsibilities in the family that might have shifted to the children (Maitz & Sachs, 1995). Pertinent issues where children are involved include ensuring that cognitively impaired parents are not overwhelmed or undermined by children who may be cognitively or linguistically superior to them since TBI. Children need to be protected from possible post-injury effects in the relative, such as inappropriate language, disinhibition or decreased emotional control, which may become more evident in a stressful family session (Zarski & DePompei, 1991).

Special treatment issues for different groups

Parents with TBI

A primary problem for children with a brain-injured parent is likely to be disruption to their relationship. This may be due to separation from the parent during prolonged hospitalisation and rehabilitation, but may also continue after community re-entry if the parent has marked personality, cognitive or behavioural sequelae (Urbach, 1989). A focus on encouraging and supporting children and the injured parent in maintaining their relationship is helpful, alongside ensuring that the child's needs for consistent and supportive care-giving are being met in the parent's absence.

Open and honest family communication is important whichever relative is injured, but may be particularly problematic in parental injury because of parents' worry about whether their children can cope with honest information about parental vulnerability (Altschuler & Dale, 1999).

When an immediate family member is brain-injured, children are vulnerable to disruption of their usual routines, and the financial difficulties and social isolation that often accompany brain injury (Brooks, 1991). Help for the family as a whole in maintaining familiar routines as far as possible is beneficial. Advice on financial matters such as benefits, and contact with other families affected by TBI, may also help.

Finally, the non-injured parent's psychosocial adjustment is of immense importance (Compas *et al.*, 2002). Interventions to support the non-injured parent both for themselves and with guidance in supporting their children will benefit children's adjustment (Pessar *et al.*, 1993; Siegel *et al.*, 1990).

Siblings with TBI

When a sibling is brain-injured, children have similar needs to those coping with parental brain injury, including open communication within the family (Adams-Greenly *et al.*, 1987), information about the injury and treatment (Craft & Wyatt, 1986), opportunities to maintain a relationship with the injured family member and age-appropriate involvement in rehabilitation (Craft & Wyatt, 1986; Menke, 1987). With an injury in the immediate family, the issues of financial problems, social isolation and disruption to family routines and living circumstances (e.g. house moves) also apply. Parents of brain-injured children are at risk for stress-related psychological disorders such as depression (Hawley *et al.*, 2003), and this clearly places other children in the family at risk from the effects of parental adjustment problems, so provision of support to parents is essential in the same way as for families coping with parental brain injury (Fisman *et al.*, 2000).

Additional issues specific to children who have brain-injured siblings include: rivalry, jealousy and resentment of parental attention directed towards the injured sibling (Faux, 1993; Peretti & Abderholden, 1995); children compensating for the sibling's disability by taking on responsibility for meeting parental expectations of achievement or good behaviour (Nodell, 1990); effects of birth order, for instance a young child close in age to the injured sibling may be most negatively affected by lack of parental time and attention, while older siblings may be more affected by needing to shoulder additional responsibilities (McKeever, 1983); survivor guilt and feelings of responsibility (Adams-Greenly *et al.*, 1987; Nodell, 1990), especially when children are unclear about the cause of the injury.

Here it is important to support parents in helping children to manage these issues, and to balance the needs of the injured sibling with those of the other children (Fleitas, 2000). For instance, it can be helpful if parents make time for activities with the child while someone else cares for the injured sibling (Kahn, 1997; Menke, 1987). To minimise jealousy and resentment it can help if parents focus on each child's personal strengths and specialness (Kahn, 1997; Sears & Sears, 2002), while acknowledging and praising children's helpful behaviours. This could help to promote positive outcomes in children (Craft & Wyatt, 1986).

Professionals and parents need to help children to balance their feelings of love, support and concern for the injured sibling with negative feelings such as jealousy and resentment (Fleitas, 2000); address children's fears of contagion and parents' over-protectiveness (Kahn, 1997); assist children in coping with social embarrassment and teasing (Adams-Greenly *et al.*, 1987; Tozer, 1996), and with helping their friends accept the disabled sibling (Kahn, 1997). It is important to normalise the child's desire to have fun without feeling guilty (Adams-Greenly *et al.*, 1987; Edwards & Davis, 1997).

Other relatives with TBI

Children may also be significantly affected by injury to relatives outside the immediate family (e.g. grandparents, aunts, uncles, cousins etc.). The impact on children is likely to depend on closeness, frequency of contact and the function of the relationship (e.g. providing care). Thus it is important to check this out with the child and family rather than assuming that a child will be unaffected by injury to a more distant relative. In the absence of disruption to care-giving relationships (e.g. if the relative resides with the family) or family routines, the most pertinent issues may be to address the child's fears of contagion or of similar events occurring in the immediate family.

Indirect intervention: working with parents and others

It is possible to target, indirectly, the adjustment and well-being of children by supporting parents in the management of their own stress and in their parental role (Siegel *et al.*, 1990).

Parent guidance and support has the following aims: to increase parental knowledge about children's understanding of familial TBI, the nature of its impact and the possible range of adjustment reactions; to enhance parental competence in providing children with appropriate information and support; to help parents recognise and manage personal stress; to help them continue their parental role, maintain routines and balance the needs of individual family members. Parent guidance and support can be delivered in various forms: information booklets, parent discussion groups, or individual sessions.

The impact of TBI on parenting abilities and parent–child relationships has received scant attention (Uysal *et al.*, 1998). How to support people with TBI in their parental role has been largely unexplored, with the notable exception of studies carried out by Ducharme and Rushford (2001); these have demonstrated that interventions aimed at enhancing brain-injured parents' parenting skills can have benefits for both parents and children. Rehabilitation teams should routinely ask parents with TBI about their concerns regarding parenting and relationships with children and rehabilitation plans should incorporate goals aimed towards addressing these issues.

Indirect work can often usefully involve liaison with teachers and other professionals who may be involved with children (e.g. health visitors). Such professionals represent a resource to children in assisting their coping with the situation. However, professionals working outside TBI or the health service are unlikely to have a detailed understanding of the issues children are facing following familial TBI and may require information and guidance on this before they can adequately support children. Altschuler *et al.* (1999) note how children's school performance and behaviour may be affected by familial chronic illness or disability. For instance, worrying about their relative may affect children's concentration, or they may be tired or unable to complete homework tasks if they are carrying out care at home. Families may require support from the rehabilitation team in helping teachers and other professionals to be aware of the impact of familial TBI on children.

Interdisciplinary team working

A truly systemic approach to supporting families after TBI is possible only through close and effective teamwork. Supporting children with brain-injured relatives in the context of family involvement is no exception. Staff from all disciplines may be involved in interventions to support children coping with familial brain injury; it may help to have one person in the team who coordinates the service to child relatives. As well as working directly with children, team members can facilitate children's adjustment in many ways, such as by targeting and prioritising rehabilitation for problems in the injured relative that children find particularly distressing. They can also provide a supportive and welcoming environment for the involvement of children in the rehabilitation process. In direct work with children, different professionals may contribute in a variety of ways and may blur professional boundaries in order to work closely together.

The following are some examples of input from different team members:

- Medical staff may provide information about TBI (e.g. by explaining to a child relative why damage to the brain means the injured person can no longer walk).
- Nursing staff may help children and injured relatives maintain their relationship (e.g. by facilitating regular play sessions on the ward).
- Physiotherapists may involve children in therapy sessions to explain treatments used and demonstrate the progress injured relatives have made (e.g. by playing a ball game together).
- Occupational therapists may also include children in treatment sessions and activities (e.g. by taking the child on a community trip with the injured relative).
- Social workers may involve children in discharge planning (e.g. by explaining the options, gaining their views, updating them on progress).
- Speech and language therapists may teach children specific skills (e.g. by teaching a child how to use a communication book to interact with a dysphasic relative).
- Clinical psychologists may focus on enhancement of children's coping skills (e.g. by explaining why disinhibited behaviour occurs and suggesting ways children can cope with this).

Rehabilitation teams require good support and supervision for all involved in interventions with children, because children's issues can be particularly upsetting and challenging for staff.

Rehabilitation Clinical Case Examples

Case 19.1: The Smith family

Tom Smith, an in-patient nearing the end of his rehabilitation, asked the clinical psychologist to see his daughter, Angela (aged 15), as he was concerned that their relationship had become increasingly strained over his past three weekends at home. He described her as rude, unhelpful and distant, while his younger child, Marie (aged 12), was said to be kind and willing to help him. He and his wife had been arguing about Angela's attitude.

Background

Tom, aged 50, a research scientist, had sustained a severe head injury (via a fall) eight months previously (GCS not known, PTA two weeks, CT scan showed multiple contusions and facial fractures, craniotomy to evacuate a left frontal intracerebral haematoma). He had been admitted five months previously for rehabilitation to focus on high-level cognitive problems; during this time he had decided to 'retire' early somewhere else in the country. His two daughters lived at home and his wife was a part-time secretary. They had a history of marital problems, including a trial separation before Tom's accident, but were now reunited.

Key assessment findings

Angela and Marie described their feelings about their father's injury. Marie said that she had coped well with her father's accident, had read about TBI, and felt that she understood his problems. She had hoped for a full recovery but knew this was unlikely. Angela reported resentment and anger towards her father. He was described as controlling, obsessed with rules and as running the home in a military fashion. His behaviour embarrassed her and she no longer wished to bring friends home. Previously, her father's work had often taken him away from home, so that he had played little part in setting limits for the girls. He was now seen as interfering and they dreaded his permanent return home. Angela expressed guilt about these feelings, had trouble sleeping and was tearful and depressed. She reluctantly admitted that she had twice recently cut her arm superficially when she was upset. It had immediately made her feel better but now disgusted her. She thought there was a high chance that she might repeat this. She had told Marie about it, who had been trying to look after her since. The girls were pleased that their parents no longer had plans to separate, but did not want to move house. The team social worker met with Mr and Mrs Smith to gain their views on the current situation. A family meeting was agreed to plan intervention.

Intervention plan

A formulation was developed collaboratively to account for Angela's and other family difficulties. It was acknowledged that at a time when the girls would have preferred to develop their independence, their father's TBI had pulled them closer into the family. It was suggested that his over-controlled (and controlling) presentation was both his attempt to reorder his life and a cognitive consequence of the TBI; this was difficult for the girls to tolerate. They had clearly developed different ways of coping with this; Marie took on the role of caring for everyone, while Angela expressed her distress through self-harm. Although reasonably informed about TBI, neither girl had been told that resentment and anger were normal responses for adolescents. Thus they were feeling guilty about their reactions. By contrast, their mother appeared to have taken a 'back seat' on issues and admitted to being preoccupied with thoughts of what the future would hold for the marriage. See Figure 19.1 for a diagrammatic representation of the formulation.

The family was interested in and accepted this formulation as a useful way of understanding the current issues facing the family. Intervention involved the following components:

- A family education session about family responses to TBI was organised, focusing particularly on normalising Angela's reaction. This was attended by the family and was accepted.
- Angela was offered individual therapy to focus on the development of alternative coping strategies for managing distress. Following this, her GP agreed to monitor episodes of self-harm.
- The clinical psychologist worked jointly with the speech and language therapist and the family. A meeting was held to review appropriate techniques for helping Tom manage cognitive and language problems. In addition, fortnightly planning meetings were scheduled, involving the whole family, where activities and priorities for the weekends ahead were agreed jointly. Initially Tom found this difficult but reported that it was a worthwhile undertaking.

Continued

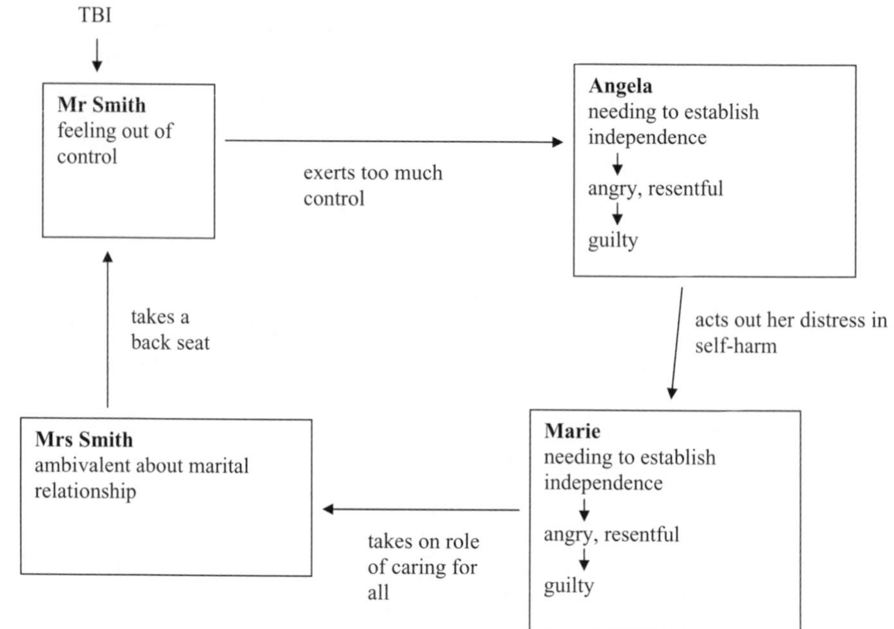

Figure 19.1 The Smith family – diagrammatic formulation

- The parents agreed to attend marital counselling to talk about the relationship difficulties that they had not previously addressed. They also reflected on the strain and changes the TBI had placed on their parenting roles.

Outcome and comment

Tom's initial return home (two months later) was troublesome, as he found the joint scheduling of activities challenging without the support of therapists. There were reports of many arguments among the family members; during this time Angela engaged in one episode of superficial self-harm, which her GP supported her through. The activity scheduling was re-implemented. Tom and his wife decided to stay together but not to move house. One year on, the family was doing well. Angela had taken a year out and was living with family in Australia.

Case 19.2: The Brown family

Mrs Brown had recently been admitted for a period of in-patient rehabilitation. Her husband asked the clinical psychologist to see their four children (aged 3, 5, 8 and 10 years) because they were reluctant to visit their mother at the rehabilitation centre and had been highly distressed on seeing her for the first time since the injury two weeks ago; in particular John (aged 5) had started bedwetting and waking up in the night after this visit. Mr Brown was also concerned about how to talk to the children about their mother's injury when her prognosis was unclear.

Family and clinical background

Mrs Brown, a 38-year-old teacher, had sustained a severe head injury as a passenger in a car accident two months previously (GCS 3, PTA five weeks, CT scan showed right-sided frontal contusion and left fronto-parietal contusions and sub-arachnoid bleeding). After a two-week period of coma she had made a good physical recovery but presented as disorientated, distressed, verbally disinhibited and physically aggressive towards staff.

Prior to the injury Mrs Brown had divided her time between part-time work and looking after the children. Mr Brown was employed as a senior manager for a large company.

Key assessment findings

Play techniques, drawing and stories were used to elicit the children's perceptions and understanding of the current situation. This revealed that they had limited understanding of their mother's injuries (Peter, aged 8, said 'Her brain's all gone now') and unrealistic expectations of full recovery (except Lisa, aged 10, who was afraid that her mother would not recover and that their life would always be 'horrible'). The children were confused about the time lapse (John reported that his mother had been in hospital for two years) and the course of events since the accident. They had little understanding of the reasons for her transfer to the rehabilitation centre. They reported that they had not been allowed to visit her in the other hospital but did not know why. Lisa said that she had eavesdropped on her father's conversation with a friend and had heard her mother

Continued

had been 'totally smashed up'. They reported that they had seen her again a few weeks ago and she had shouted at them for making a noise. She had also called them by the wrong names and this had made them laugh at her. They said that they did not want to see her again until she was better. The children also expressed concern for their father whom they described as sad. They reported that the maternal aunt, both grandmothers and several family friends had been looking after them.

The clinical psychologist also interviewed Mr and Mrs Brown, the children's maternal grandmother, and nursing staff. Mr Brown reported feeling overwhelmed since his wife's accident and was struggling to cope with the children. He feared that they were suffering, but could not bring himself to talk to them in case he 'broke down'. He felt that the children wanted to (and should) see their mother but that her behaviour frightened them. He did not know how to tackle this, and so far he had been forcing them to visit. He thought his wife did not notice the effect on the children and this was a shock to him. John's bedwetting and frequent night waking was causing extra disruption. Aside from concerns about the children, he had many questions about the nature of his wife's impairments and her prognosis.

It was difficult to gain Mrs Brown's views because she was agitated and found it hard to concentrate. She reported that the children had possibly gone away on holiday, or that they had forgotten about her. She could correctly identify them from photographs in her room and did not report any concerns about them. The grandmother reported that the whole family was in shock. She felt that the children were very confused and needed to see their mother every day to help her remember them. She had a limited understanding of her daughter's post-injury problems.

Nursing staff reported that the children were brought to the ward every evening to see their mother. Visits were noisy, unstructured and chaotic, with the children running up and down the corridors, crying; Mrs Brown shouted at them frequently and Mr Brown always asked for nurses' help to calm her down. Other patients had complained about the disruption. Mrs Brown talked about the children frequently to staff but was often confused about their names and ages. Staff were concerned that Mr Brown was becoming depressed.

Observation of two of the children's visits with their mother confirmed the description provided by nursing staff. Mrs Brown appeared over-stimulated by the children's loud voices and their running around and there was little or no structure to their time together. Visits were frequent and lengthy.

Intervention plan

Formulation highlighted that the children had experienced an abrupt separation from their mother; they did not understand why or what had happened and had unrealistic ideas about the future. After lengthy separation they were 'reunited' with her in an unfamiliar environment, without preparation for how she had changed. This had been so distressing for them that they were now trying to avoid further contact. Further, their father was frequently absent, resulting in them having several different carers. In addition, Mr Brown himself was overwhelmed by the many demands placed on him and the new roles that he had had to adopt, and did not know how to help his children. Intervention therefore focused on the following components:

- It was essential to help the children understand their mother's impairments and treatment, teach them strategies to cope with upsetting events, and keep them informed about what was happening to her. To achieve this, a personalised scrapbook was developed collaboratively with the children. This included information on TBI generally, their mother's problems specifically and about the therapy team working with her. Written information was supplemented by drawings and photographs (many of which the children took of their mother in therapy sessions), to aid the understanding of the younger children. The children were encouraged to talk about their feelings as they carried out this activity. Coping strategies (such as trying to avoid everyone talking to mum at the same time) were discussed, role played then recorded in the scrapbook. Information was compiled over twelve 60-minute sessions in all, with responsibility for keeping the book updated passed over to the family. 'Homework' tasks were given (e.g. make a calendar for mother) to both maintain the children's experience of the therapy process between sessions and encourage discussion between Mr Brown and the children about their mother. The children entered into this process enthusiastically and were very proud of the book; one was reported to have taken it to school to show their teacher. Despite the differences in age they were all able to play some part in its development.

Continued

- In order to provide the children with enjoyable time with their mother, a graded approach to reintroducing them to her was recommended. This started with the children drawing up a rota of who would visit on their own with dad, and being supported in communicating in other ways with her outside of these times (e.g. letters, cards). Children were also involved (individually and eventually together) in Mrs Brown's therapy sessions. This provided a safe and structured means of interacting with her, with a focus on her abilities rather than difficulties. This approach was complemented by the provision of written guidelines for Mr Brown on structuring children's visits, to minimise distress for all parties. He applied these to good effect. Nursing staff observed less distress during visiting times.
- Mr Brown was offered supportive counselling sessions with the unit's social worker to discuss his own issues, and a fortnightly meeting with the psychologist to discuss children's issues. In addition, a referral to the family health visitor was made to provide support in managing John's bedwetting and night waking.

Outcome and comment

The intervention described proved successful in addressing the information and support needs of both the children and Mr Brown, and facilitated the re-establishment of Mrs Brown's relationship with her children. Four months into their mother's rehabilitation programme the children were able to visit her all together, with no visible evidence of distress. By this time the children had developed a large information book, and were making another, with their father's help, which addressed future issues. At six months, Mrs Brown began having successful overnight and weekend stays at home. At follow-up one year post-injury, Mrs Brown was living back with her family, and, along with a nanny, was responsible for the children's care. She had not returned to work, and had no plans to do so, but her husband had resumed his full-time job. The children were reported to be happy and doing well at home and at school. The health visitor agreed to maintain a watching brief to monitor the situation.

Process and Practice Issues

Working with children and other family members in the context of TBI can be a challenging and complex undertaking. There are a number of key process and practice issues to bear in mind when carrying out this work.

Working in partnership with the family and rehabilitation team is the basis for all intervention. The success of the interventions described relies heavily on the cooperation, commitment and enthusiasm of the rehabilitation team and family members. Incorporating a child-focus into adult settings is challenging, time consuming, staff intensive and complex. However, team working offers children the skills of several professionals and guards against the stress associated with being an individual worker in complex situations. The provision of different interventions from each discipline within the team, working closely together (as described above in the section on interventions and illustrated in the case examples), delivers a more comprehensive service to children, but requires better awareness of roles to avoid role confusion within the team when there may inevitably be some role blurring. When deciding to work as a team, clarification of roles and responsibilities with respect to different family members, regular case review and peer supervision go towards more effective working (Webster *et al.*, 1999).

Confidentiality is often a difficult issue when working with children, and can be further complicated when working with more than one family member, or when more than one agency is involved. Staff should, therefore, be aware of their own particular professional codes of confidentiality. This is especially pertinent to situations where difficulties arise, such as child protection.

It is essential that brain injury services providing support to children with brain-injured relatives recognise the limits of their professional competence in working with children. Many brain injury rehabilitation staff may work mainly with adults and may have had little training or experience with children's issues. It is therefore helpful to seek guidance from specialist child and family services, both for individual families (e.g. in the case of severe adjustment difficulties or child protection concerns, as discussed above in the sections on assessment and intervention), and for general staff training purposes. Child and family services could provide training on local agencies and service structures, referral routes and criteria, and how to identify and respond to problems requiring urgent specialist help. NHS Trusts often require staff who are regularly working with children to undergo an enhanced police check and receive yearly training on child protection awareness. Depending on local Trust policy, this may apply to staff who aim to carry out work with children with brain-injured relatives.

Child work is typically characterised by considerable consultation and liaison with outside agencies; it is important to build up good links with local child mental health services, Social Services, education and the voluntary sector.

Child disturbance may reflect undetected psychological distress in the non-injured parent, which again underlines the importance of taking a family systemic perspective. The fact that not all children with brain-injured relatives present to services highlights the complex nature of the association between familial illness and child adjustment.

The needs of children following familial TBI and other chronic conditions have been gaining prominence at a policy level in recent years, suggesting that the time is right to explore ways of providing more systematic support to this group (Department of Health, 2005; House of Commons Select Committee on Health, 2001; International Working Party Report on PVS, 1996). It will be important to identify and address the barriers to service development that currently exist (Webster & Daisley, 2005b). A first step would be to raise awareness among rehabilitation teams of the need for such services and provide training. Secondly, provision of a child-friendly environment such as a designated family room or play area is helpful in creating a physical context for the service. Within this framework, multi-level interventions for children provided by the whole interdisciplinary team can be developed as discussed above.

Summary and Conclusions

Despite the prevalence of TBI in child-rearing adults, there is little research on its impact on children. As a result, child-focused interventions have received scant attention; those that are reported in the literature are often methodologically weak and are generally based on clinical intuition. Despite the dearth of research, there is evidence that children with brain-injured relatives, like their adult counterparts, are additional victims of TBI. For each child the experience of living with a brain-injured relative is unique, but there are some common experiences and challenges. Children must adjust to a condition that is often invisible, unpredictable and complex. The difficulty of this task can be compounded by limitations in their understanding, by psychological distress and a lack of appropriate information and support. An interdisciplinary approach, combining the expertise of both adult and child-focused services – working together – is essential to pool resources in providing appropriate support to families.

Finally, it is not suggested that services with a predominantly adult focus should merely be complemented by an 'added-on' child-focused service. Rather, this chapter aims to enhance clinicians' awareness of issues relating to children with brain-injured relatives, and to provide a starting point for considering interventions. The challenge will be to apply this to a truly systemic approach in which the needs of children are acknowledged as an integral part of the family system and rehabilitation provision.

Recommended Reading

Butera-Prinzi, F. & Perlesz, A. (2004). Through children's eyes: Children's experience of living with a parent with an acquired brain injury. *Brain Injury*, *18*(1), 83–101.

Gives a summary of the published empirical research on child with brain-injured parents literature.

Lobato, D.J. (1990). *Brothers, sisters, and special needs: Information and activities for helping younger siblings of children with chronic illnesses and developmental disabilities.* Baltimore: Paul H. Brooks Publishing

Segal, J. & Simkins, J. (1993). *My mum needs me: Helping children with ill or disabled parents*. Harmondsworth: Penguin.
These references give more general (non-head-injury specific) information about working with children facing familial illness.

McLaughlin, A.M. (1992). Addressing the psychological needs of children of brain-injured relatives: An activity group model. *Journal of Cognitive Rehabilitation*, March/April, 12–18.
Sachs, P.R. (1991). *Treating families of brain injury survivors*. New York: Springer.
Webster, G. & Daisley, A. (2005a). A family resource pack for working with children affected by familial acquired brain injury. *Clinical Psychology*, *46*, 26–29.
These references provide useful ideas for assessment of and intervention with children.

Urbach, J.R. (1989). The impact of parental head trauma on families with children. *Psychiatric Medicine*, *7*(1), 17–36.
Urbach, J.R. & Culbert, J.P. (1991). Head injured parents and their children. *Psychosomatics*, *32*, 24–33.
These references provide a useful discussion of the issues facing child relatives.

References

Adams-Greenly, M., Shiminski-Maher, T., McGowan, N. & Mayers, P.A. (1987). A group program for helping siblings of children with cancer. *Journal of Psychosocial Oncology*, *4*(4), 55–67.
Aldridge, J. & Becker, S. (1999). Children as carers: The impact of parental illness and disability on children's caring roles. *Journal of Family Therapy*, *21*, 303–320.
Altschuler, J. & Dale, B. (1999). On being an ill parent. *Clinical Child Psychology and Psychiatry*, *4*(1), 23–37.
Altschuler, J., Dale, B. & Sass-Booth, A. (1999). Supporting a child when a parent is physically ill: Implications for educational psychologists and schools. *Educational Psychology in Practice*, *15*(1), 25–32.
Anthony, E.J. (1970). The impact of mental and physical illness on family life. *American Journal of Psychiatry*, *127*, 138–146.
Armistead, L., Klein, K., & Forehand, R. (1995). Parental physical illness and child functioning. *Clinical Psychology Review*, *15*(5), 409–422.
Beardslee, W.R., Gladstone, T.R.G., Wright, E.J. & Cooper, A.B. (2003). A family-based approach to the prevention of depressive symptoms in children at risk: Evidence of parental and child change. *Pediatrics*, *112*(2), 119–131.
Bibace, R. & Walsh, M.E. (1980). Development of children's concepts of illness. *Paediatrics*, *66*, 912–917.
Blackford, K.A. (1992). Strategies for intervention and research with children or adolescents who have a parent with multiple sclerosis. *Axon*, December, 50–54.
Brooks, D.N. (1991). The head-injured family. *Journal of Clinical and Experimental Neuropsychology*, *13*(1), 155–188.
Butera-Prinzi, F. & Perlesz, A. (2004). Through children's eyes: Children's experience of living with a parent with an acquired brain injury. *Brain Injury*, *18*(1), 83–101.
Carpenter, P.J., Sahler, O.J. & Davis, M.S. (1990). Use of a camp setting to provide medical information to siblings of pediatric cancer patients. *Journal of Cancer Education*, *5*, 21–26.

Compas, B.E., Langrock, A.M., Keller, G., Merchant, M.J. & Copeland, M.E. (2002). Children coping with parental depression: Processes of adaptation to family stress. In I.H. Gotlib & S.H. Goodman (Eds.) *Children of depressed parents: Mechanisms of risk and implications for treatment* (pp.227–252). Washington, DC: American Psychological Association.

Compas, B.E., Worsham, M.L., Epping-Jordan, J.E., Grant, K.E., Mireault, G., Howell, D. C., *et al.* (1994). When mom or dad has cancer: Markers of psychological distress in cancer patients, spouses and children. *Health Psychology*, *13*(6), 507–515.

Conder, A.A., Conder, R., Levy, L. & Faulkner, P. (1988). Psychological reactions of intact children to their parent's traumatic head injury: Measurement and treatment. *Abstracts of the Proceedings of the 12th Annual Conference of the Postgraduate Course on Rehabilitation of the Brain-Injured Adult and Child* (pp.54–55). Williamsburg: Virginia Commonwealth University.

Craft, M.J. (1993). Siblings of hospitalized children: Assessment and intervention. *Journal of Pediatric Nursing*, *8*(5), 289–297.

Craft, M.J. & Wyatt, N. (1986). Effect of visitation upon siblings of hospitalized children. *Maternal–Child Nursing Journal*, *15*(1), 47–59.

Daisley, A. (2002). *Psychological adjustment of children to parental brain injury*. Unpublished doctoral dissertation, University of Newcastle, UK.

Daisley, A. & Webster, G. (1999). Involving families in brain injury rehabilitation: Children's information books. *Proceedings of the British Psychological Society*, *7*(1), 71.

Department of Health (2005). *The national service framework for long term conditions*. Crown Copyright.

Dowdney, L. (2000). Annotation: Childhood bereavement following parental death. *Journal of Child Psychology and Psychiatry*, *7*, 819–830.

Downey, G. & Coyne, J.C. (1990). Children of depressed parents: An integrative review. *Psychological Bulletin*, *108*, 50–76.

Ducharme, J.M. & Rushford, N. (2001). Proximal and distal effects of play on child compliance with brain-injured parent. *Journal of Applied Behaviour Analysis*, *34*, 221–224.

Edwards, M. & Davis, H. (1997). *Counselling children with chronic medical conditions*. Leicester: BPS Books.

Faux, S.A. (1993). Siblings of children with chronic physical and cognitive disabilities. *Journal of Pediatric Nursing*, *8*(5), 305–317.

Fisher, B.C. (2002). Children who are forgotten: The child of the brain-injured parent. http://www.brainevaluation.com.

Fisman, S., Wolf, L., Ellison, D. & Freeman, T. (2000). A longitudinal study of siblings of children with chronic disabilities. *The Canadian Journal of Psychiatry*, *45*, 369–375.

Fisman, S., Wolf, L., Ellison, D., Gillis, B., Freeman, T. & Szatmari, P. (1996). Risk and protective factors affecting the adjustment of siblings of children with chronic disabilities. *Journal of the American Academy of Child and Adolescent Psychiatry*, *35*(11), 1532–1541.

Fleitas, J. (2000). When Jack fell down . . . Jill came tumbling after: Siblings in the web of illness and disability. *American Journal of Maternal Child Nursing*, *25*(5), 267–273.

Flickinger, E.E. & Amato, S.C. (1994). School-age children's responses to parents with disabilities. *Rehabilitation Nursing*, *19*(4), 203–306.

Florian, V. & Katz, S. (1991). The other victims of traumatic brain injury: Consequences for family members. *Neuropsychology*, *5*, 267–279.

Frye, B.A. (1982). Brain injury and family education needs. *Rehabilitation Nursing*, *7*, 27–29.

Gosling, S. & Herbert, A. (1996). What about me? Groups for the siblings of disabled children. *Clinical Psychology Forum*, February, 6–9.

Hansell, A.G. (1990). *The effects on children of a father's severe closed head injury*. Unpublished doctoral thesis. University of Michigan, Ann Arbor, USA.

Harris, J.K.J., Godfrey, H.P.D., Partridge, F.M., & Knight, R.G. (2001). Caregiver depression following traumatic brain injury (TBI): A consequence of adverse effects on family members. *Brain Injury*, *15*(3), 211–223

Hawley, C.A., Ward, A.B., Magnay, A.R. & Long, J. (2003). Parental stress and burden following traumatic brain injury amongst children and adolescents. *Brain Injury*, *17*(1), 1–23.

Heiney, S.P., Goon-Johnson, K., Ettinger, R.S. & Ettinger, S. (1990). The effects of group therapy on siblings of pediatric oncology patients. *Journal of Pediatric Oncology Nursing*, *7*(3), 95–100.

House of Commons Select Committee on Health (2001). Third Report – Head Injury: Rehabilitation. Retrieved May 15, 2001, from http://www.parliament.the-stationery-office.co.uk.

International Working Party Report on the Persistent Vegetative State (1996). London: Royal Hospital for Neurodisability.

Kahn, P. (1997). Siblings of children with brain injuries. *Rehab Update*, Winter, 1–4.

LaMata, R., Gingras, G. & Wittkower, E. (1960). Impact of sudden, severe disablement of the father upon the family. *Canadian Medical Association Journal*, *82*, 1015–1020.

Lauer-Listhaus, B. (1991). Group therapy for families of head-injured adults. *Counselling Psychology Quarterly*, *4*, 351–354.

Lewis, F.M., Hammond, M.A. & Woods, N.F. (1993). The family's functioning with newly diagnosed breast cancer in the mother: The development of an explanatory model. *Journal of Behavioural Medicine*, *16*, 351–370.

Lezak, M.D. (1988). Brain damage is a family affair. *Journal of Clinical and Experimental Neuropsychology*, *10*(1), 241–249.

Lobato, D.J. (1990). *Brothers, sisters, and special needs: Information and activities for helping younger siblings of children with chronic illnesses and developmental disabilities*. Baltimore: Paul H. Brooks Publishing Co.

Lobato, D.J. & Kao, B.T. (2002). Integrated sibling–parent group intervention to improve sibling knowledge and adjustment to chronic illness and disability. *Journal of Pediatric Psychology*, *27*, 711–716.

Maitz, E.A. (1991). Family systems theory applied to head injury. In J.M. Williams & T. Kay (Eds.) *Head injury: A family matter* (pp.65–79). Baltimore: Paul H. Brookes.

Maitz, E.A. & Sachs, P.R. (1995). Treating families of individuals with traumatic brain injury from a family systems perspective. *Journal of Head Trauma Rehabilitation*, *10*, 1–12.

McCue, K. & Bonn, R. (2003). Helping children through an adult's serious illness. *Paediatric Nursing*, *29*(1) 47–51.

McKeever, P. (1983). Siblings of chronically ill children: A literature review with implications for research and practice. *American Journal of Orthopsychiatry*, *53*, 209–218.

McLaughlin, A.M. (1992). Addressing the psychological needs of children of brain-injured relatives: An activity group model. *Journal of Cognitive Rehabilitation*, March/April, 12–18.

McMahon, M., Noll, R.B., Michaud, L.J. & Johnson, J.C. (2001). Sibling adjustment to pediatric brain injury: A controlled case pilot study. *Journal of Head Trauma Rehabilitation*, *16*(6), 587–594.

Menke, E.M. (1987). The impact of a child's chronic illness on school-aged siblings. *Children's Health Care*, *15*(3), 132–140.

Moore, A., Stambrook, M. & Peters, L. (1993). Centripetal and centrifugal family life cycle factors in long-term outcome following traumatic brain injury. *Brain Injury*, *7*(3), 247–255.

Nodell, S. (1990). The forgotten feelings, fears and family: Sibling issues from a parent's perspective. *Cognitive Rehabilitation*, *8*, 6–7.

Oddy, M. & Herbert, C. (2003). Intervention with families following brain injury: Evidence-based practice. *Neuropsychological Rehabilitation*, *13*(1/2), 259–273.

Oppenheim-Gluckman, H., Marioni, G., Virole, B., Aeschbacher, M.T. & Canny-Verrier, F. (2003). Personal experience of children with a brain injured parent: Preliminary study. *Annales de Readaptation et de Medecine Physique*, *46*, 525–538.

Orsillo, S.M., McCaffrey, R.J. & Fisher, J.M. (1993). Siblings of head injured individuals: A population at risk. *Journal of Head Trauma Rehabilitation*, *8*, 102–115.

Pakenham, K.I., Bursnall, S., Chiu, J., Cannon, T., & Okochi, M (2006). The psychosocial impact of care giving on young people who have a parent with an illness or disability: Comparisons between young care givers and non-caregivers. *Rehabilitation Psychology*, *51*, 113–126.

Peretti, P.O. & Abderholden, P. (1995). Effect of imputed or implied loss of parental affection due to the brain-damaged child in the family on sibling rivalry. *Indian Journal of Clinical Psychology*, *22*(2), 23–26.

Pessar, L.F., Coad, M.L., Linn, R.T., & Willer, B.S. (1993). The effects of parental traumatic brain injury on the behaviour of parents and children. *Brain Injury*, *7*(3), 231–240.

Pinyerd, B.J. (1983). Siblings of children with myelomeningocele: Examining their perceptions. *Maternal/Child Nursing Journal*, *12*(1), 61–70.

Romano, M.D. (1976). Preparing children for parental disability. *Social Work in Health Care*, *1*(3), 309–315.

Rosenbaum, N. & Najenson, T. (1976). Changes in life patterns and symptoms of low mood as reported by wives of severely brain-injured soldiers. *Journal of Consulting and Clinical Psychology*, *44*, 881–888.

Rosenthal, M. & Young, T. (1988). Effective family intervention after traumatic brain injury: Theory and practice. *Journal of Head Trauma Rehabilitation*, *3*(4), 42–50.

Sachs, P.R. (1991). *Treating families of brain injury survivors*. New York: Springer.

Sander, A.M., Caroselli, J.S., High, W.M., Becker, C., Neese, L. & Scheibel, R. (2002). Relationship of family functioning to progress in a post-acute rehabilitation programme following traumatic brain injury. *Brain Injury*, *16*(8), 649–657.

Sears, W. & Sears, M. (2002). *The successful child*. New York: Little, Brown & Co.

Segal, J. & Simkins, J. (1993). *My mum needs me: Helping children with ill or disabled parents*. Harmondsworth: Penguin.

Serio, C.D., Kreutzer, J.S. & Witol, A.D. (1997). Family needs after traumatic brain injury: A factor analytic study of the Family Needs Questionnaire. *Brain Injury*, *11*(1), 1–9.

Siegel, K., Mesagno, F.P. & Christ, G. (1990). A prevention programme for bereaved children. *American Journal of Orthopsychiatry*, *60*, 168–175.

Sloper, P. & While, D. (1996). Risk factors in the adjustment of siblings with cancer. *Journal of Child Psychology and Psychiatry*, *37*(5), 597–607.

Smiton, A. (2005). *Children's coping with parental brain injury*. Unpublished doctoral dissertation, University of Oxford, UK.

Springer, J.A., Farmer, J.E. & Bouman, D.E. (1997). Common misconceptions about traumatic brain injury among family members of rehabilitation patients. *Journal of Head Trauma Rehabilitation*, *12*(3), 41–50.

Stilwell, J., Hawley, C., Stilwell, P. & Davies, C. (1997). *National Traumatic Brain Injury Study: Report*. Coventry: Centre for Health Services Studies, University of Warwick.

Sylva, K. & Lunt, I. (1982). *Child development: A first course*. Oxford: Blackwell.

Thompson, A., Whitney, L. & Whyte, J. (2000). Developing links between child and family psychiatry and an adult mental health service. *Clinical Psychology Forum*, *140*, 21–23.

Thomsen, I.V. (1984). Late outcome of very severe blunt head trauma: A 10–15 year follow-up. *Journal of Neurology Neurosurgery and Psychiatry*, *47*, 260–268.

Titler, M.G., Cohen, M.Z. & Craft, M.J. (1991). Impact of adult critical care hospitalization: Perceptions of patients, spouses, children and nurses. *Heart and Lung*, *20*(2), 174–182.

Tonin, J., Daisley, A., & Wheatley, J. (1996). Children's understanding of parental brain injury. *European Journal of Neurology (abstracts)*, *3*(Supplement 2), 66–67.

Tozer, R. (1996). My brother's keeper? Sustaining sibling support. *Health & Social Care in the Community*, *43*(3), 177–181.

Tyerman, A. & Booth, J. (2001). Family interventions after traumatic brain injury: A service example. *NeuroRehabilitation*, *16*, 59–66.

Urbach, J.R. (1989). The impact of parental head trauma on families with children. *Psychiatric Medicine*, *7*(1), 17–36.

Urbach, J.R. & Culbert, J.P. (1991). Head injured parents and their children. *Psychosomatics*, *32*, 24–33.

Urbach, J.R., Sonenklar, N.A. & Culbert, J.P. (1994). Risk factors and assessment in children of brain-injured parents. *Journal of Neuropsychiatry*, *6*, 289–295.

Uysal, S., Hibbard, M.R., Robillad, D., Pappadopolus, E. & Jaffe, M. (1998). The effects of parental traumatic brain injury on parenting and child behaviour. *Journal of Head Trauma Rehabilitation*, *13*(6), 57–71.

Webster, G. & Daisley, A. (2005a). A family resource pack for working with children affected by familial acquired brain injury. *Clinical Psychology*, *46*, 26–29.

Webster, G. & Daisley, A. (2005b). *Including children in family focused acquired brain injury rehabilitation: A national survey of practice*. Manuscript submitted for publication.

Webster, G., Daisley, A. & King, N. (1999). Relationship and family breakdown following acquired brain injury: The role of the rehabilitation team. *Brain Injury*, *13*(8), 593–603.

Williams, J.M. & Binnie, L.M. (2002). Children's concepts of illness: An intervention to improve knowledge. *British Journal of Health Psychology*, *7*, 129–147.

Williams, P.D., Williams, A.R., Graff, J.C., Hanson, S., Stanton, A., Hafeman, C., *et al.* (2003). A community based intervention for siblings and parents of children with chronic illness or disability: The ISEE study. *The Journal of Pediatrics*, *143*, 386–393.

Zarski, J.J. & DePompei, R. (1991). Family therapy as applied to head injury. In J.M. Williams & T. Kay (Eds.) Head injury: A family matter (pp.283–297). Baltimore: Paul H. Brookes.

Index